Video Atlas *of* Ophthalmic Ultrasound

Video Atlas *of* Ophthalmic Ultrasound

Bernadete **Ayres**, MD
Assistant Professor
Department of Ophthalmology and Visual Sciences
W. K. Kellogg Eye Center
University of Michigan
Ann Arbor, Michigan

Norma **Allemann**, MD
Adjunct Professor and Head of Discipline
Department of Ophthalmology and Visual Sciences
Federal University of São Paulo—UNIFESP
São Paulo, Brazil;
Department of Ophthalmology and Visual Sciences
University of Illinois at Chicago
Chicago, Illinois

Hakan **Demirci**, MD
Associate Professor and Director of Ocular Oncology
Department of Ophthalmology and Visual Sciences
University of Michigan
Ann Arbor, Michigan

ELSEVIER

Elsevier
1600 John F. Kennedy Blvd.
Ste 1800
Philadelphia, PA 19103-2899

VIDEO ATLAS OF OPHTHALMIC ULTRASOUND ISBN: 978-0-443-10712-2

Executive Content Strategist: Kayla Wolfe
Senior Content Development Manager: Somodatta Roy Choudhury
Publishing Services Manager: Deepthi Unni
Senior Project Manager: Nayagi Anandan
Design Direction: Amy Buxton

Printed in India
Last digit is the print number: 9 8 7 6 5 4 3 2 1

To my mother, Lourdes, with deepest gratitude and love.
To my beloved husband, Manuel, who has walked every step of this journey with me.

Bernadete Ayres

To my partner and exemplary professional, Wallace; my daughter, Laura; and my parents, Renato and Thereza, for their continuous support over the years.
To my colleagues and students at UNIFESP, who share my love for the art of ultrasound.

Norma Allemann

To my dear family for their continuous support in my endeavors over the years.

Hakan Demirci

Contributors

Carla Moreira Albhy, MD
Assistant Physician
Ultrasound Service
Department of Ophthalmology and Visual Sciences
Federal University of São Paulo – UNIFESP
São Paulo, Brazil

Norma Allemann, MD
Adjunct Professor and Head of Discipline
Department of Ophthalmology and Visual Sciences
Federal University of São Paulo—UNIFESP
São Paulo, Brazil;
Department of Ophthalmology and Visual Sciences
University of Illinois at Chicago
Chicago, Illinois

Bernadete Ayres, MD
Assistant Professor
Department of Ophthalmology and Visual Sciences
W. K. Kellogg Eye Center
University of Michigan
Ann Arbor, MI

Ana Marisa Pires Castello Branco, MD
Assistant Physician
Ultrasound Service
Department of Ophthalmology and Visual Sciences
Federal University of São Paulo – UNIFESP
São Paulo, Brazil

Zelia M. Correa, MD, PhD
Professor
Director of Ocular Oncology
Bascom Palmer Eye Institute
University of Miami
Miami, FL

Suzanne Daly, BSN
Department of Ophthalmology
Columbia University Irving Medical Center
New York, NY

Hakan Demirci, MD
Professor
Department of Ophthalmology and Visual Sciences
W. K. Kellogg Eye Center
University of Michigan
Ann Arbor, MI

Victor Elner, MD, PhD
Professor
Department of Ophthalmology and Visual Sciences
W. K. Kellogg Eye Center
University of Michigan
Ann Arbor, MI

Renato Landre Fileti, MD
Assistant Physician
Ultrasound Service
Department of Ophthalmology and Visual Sciences
Federal University of São Paulo – UNIFESP
São Paulo, Brazil

Thiran Jayasundera, MD, MS, FACS
Associate Professor
Department of Ophthalmology and Visual Sciences
W. K. Kellogg Eye Center
University of Michigan
Ann Arbor, MI

Mark W. Johnson, MD
Professor
Department of Ophthalmology and Visual Sciences
W. K. Kellogg Eye Center
University of Michigan
Ann Arbor, MI

Liliane Andrade Almeida Kanecadan
Assistant Physician
Ultrasound Service
Department of Ophthalmology and Visual Sciences
Federal University of São Paulo – UNIFESP
São Paulo, Brazil

Olivia Killeen, MD
Assistant Professor
Department of Ophthalmology and Visual Sciences
W. K. Kellogg Eye Center
University of Michigan
Ann Arbor, MI

Melina Correia Morales, MD, PhD
Assistant Physician
Ultrasound Service
Department of Ophthalmology and Visual Sciences
Federal University of São Paulo – UNIFESP
São Paulo, Brazil

Sayoko Moroi, MD, PhD
Professor and Chair
Department of Ophthalmology and Visual Sciences
Wexner Medical Center
Ohio State University
Columbus, OH

Christine C. Nelson, MD, FACS
Professor
Department of Ophthalmology and Visual Sciences
W. K. Kellogg Eye Center
University of Michigan
Ann Arbor, MI

Gabriela Assumpção Brito Pereira Pellegrini, MD, PhD
Attending Physician
Department of Ophthalmology and Visual Sciences
Federal University of São Paulo – UNIFESP
São Paulo, Brazil

Rosana Cristina Sciencia da Silva Pizarro, MD
Ophthalmologist
Ocular Ultrasound
Department of Ophthalmology and Visual Sciences
Federal University of São Paulo – UNIFESP
São Paulo, Brazil

Maria Helena Mandello Ramos, MD
Assistant Physician
Diagnostic Center in Ophthalmology
Fleury Medicina e Saúde
São Paulo, Brazil

Therese Sassalos, MD
Assistant Professor
Department of Ophthalmology and Visual Sciences
W. K. Kellogg Eye Center
University of Michigan
Ann Arbor, MI

Ronald H. Silverman
Department of Ophthalmology
Columbia University Irving Medical Center
New York, NY

Camile Freitas Tonin, MD
Assistant Physician
Ultrasound Service
Department of Ophthalmology
Universidade Federal de São Paulo
São Paulo, São Paulo, Brazil

Raksha Urs, PhD
Department of Ophthalmology
Columbia University Irving Medical Center
New York, NY

Foreword

In the realm of ophthalmic and medical imaging, ophthalmic ultrasound plays a unique role in the clinical care of patients to increase the precision of clinical diagnoses. As a technology, it is available for use and interpretation by ophthalmologists and optometrists in all specialties, in settings from the office to the operating room, and for first-year learners to decades-long experienced physicians. This technology has transformed how we view and understand the intricate structures of the eye, its illnesses, and the mechanisms of many diseases, providing unparalleled insights beyond the reach of traditional exam visibility.

As you delve into the chapters of this book, you will embark on a practical journey, based on decades of experience by our esteemed colleagues, Dr. Bernadete Ayres, Dr. Norma Allemann, and Dr. Hakan Demirci, through the fascinating world of ophthalmic ultrasound. This compendium features high-definition images and video clips to understand the dynamic nature of important eye and orbit disorders. Moreover, the video atlas is rich in ultrasound evidence to support learning and enhance the accuracy of our clinical diagnoses.

Ultrasonography is still an operator-dependent technique, and practitioners need to have the appropriate skills and knowledge to perform and interpret ultrasound examinations. The book comprises sixteen chapters written by ophthalmologists with comprehensive experience in the major areas of ophthalmology, particularly ophthalmic ultrasound, who have accessed hundreds of real-patient cases. This is an invaluable resource for teaching and learning for all levels of practitioners.

The book presents best practices and guidance for image acquisition and helps develop interpretation skills of various conditions. The editors have carefully chosen contributing authors, each being an enthusiastic academic and expert in their field of eye care. The video atlas will be the most recent reference of outstanding value to ophthalmologists, residents, and ophthalmic clinical personnel.

The field of ophthalmology has always been at the forefront of medical progress, and ultrasound imaging is a shining example of this tradition. By harnessing the power of sound waves, ophthalmic ultrasound allows us to peer into the essence of ocular anatomy, enabling early detection, precise diagnosis, and effective treatment of ophthalmic conditions.

This video atlas is more than a collection of technical details; it is an exploration of the symbiotic relationship between technology and ophthalmology. It highlights the tireless efforts of researchers, clinicians, engineers, and innovators who have dedicated their careers to pushing the boundaries of what is possible.

As you read through the pages, you may be inspired by the ingenuity and dedication that have shaped the field of ophthalmic ultrasound. Whether you are a seasoned professional, a student, or simply a curious reader, this video atlas will provide a comprehensive understanding of this remarkable technology and its profound impact on eye care.

So, with curiosity and enthusiasm, let us embark on this enlightening journey together. May the knowledge within these pages illuminate your path and deepen your appreciation for the marvels of ophthalmic ultrasound and what we can do together in service of our patients today and tomorrow.

Paul P. Lee, MD, JD
Executive Director, University of Michigan Medical Group
Senior Associate Dean, Clinical Affairs
Professor, Ophthalmology and Visual Sciences
Former Director, W.K. Kellogg Eye Center

Foreword

It is with great pleasure and honor that I contribute the Foreword to the *Video Atlas of Ophthalmic Ultrasound.* While ophthalmic ultrasound is often regarded as a "mature" discipline, the field continues to evolve with the advent of innovative instrumentation, refined techniques, and novel clinical applications. And unlike OCT, conducting the ultrasound exam is as much an art as a science.

The editors—Drs. Bernadete Ayres, Norma Allemann, and Hakan Demirci—have done a masterful job curating a comprehensive volume that brings together leading experts in every facet of ophthalmic ultrasonography. The chapters cover a broad range of topics, including imaging physics and technology, examination techniques, acoustic anatomy of the eye and orbit, axial length measurement, intraocular tumors, trauma, and pediatric applications. Particularly noteworthy are the contributions on imaging superficial structures such as the anterior segment, conjunctiva, eyelids, and lacrimal system. Of special interest is the discussion of Doppler imaging, a technique that has only recently become a mainstream tool in ophthalmology.

As someone who has witnessed—and contributed to—the extraordinary progress of ultrasound in ophthalmology over the past half-century, I view this *Video Atlas* as a significant and timely resource. It will be of immense value to all who practice ophthalmic ultrasound, whether ophthalmologists or sonographers. I envision it becoming the go-to reference for both learning and addressing clinical questions.

Sincerely,
D. Jackson Coleman, MD
Professor Emeritus of Ophthalmology
Columbia University Irving Medical Center

Preface

Ultrasound remains one of the most frequently used and valuable modalities for imaging, diagnosing, and guiding interventional treatments in ophthalmology. Over the years, ultrasound technology has evolved, and new instruments and examination techniques have emerged that are more accurate and offer improved image resolution.

This book intends to be a useful and practical reference source for those using ophthalmic ultrasound in their clinical practice and serves as a go-to guide for producing diagnostic sonograms for ophthalmic physicians, radiologists, residents, fellows, and allied personnel.

The concept of this book arose from the need for quick, easy, objective, and precise technical and clinical information on ultrasound scanning techniques and presenting the features of common ocular and orbital conditions.

The book is organized as an atlas, structured in 16 chapters. Each chapter is concise yet provides a comprehensive overview of cases based on high-quality images and digital streaming videos uploaded from a website. The quality of images and video clips combined with an objective and practical explanation of image features in the examples provided are valuable tools in this book. The introductory chapters cover the aspects of physics, instrumentation, and exam techniques. In the ocular diagnosis chapters, the features are described and criteria for the identification of the most common diseases are presented. In the orbital chapters, ultrasound imaging is complemented with computed tomography scans and magnetic resonance imaging, providing critical information and a better understanding of orbital lesions.

One of the major accomplishments of this video atlas is addressing major questions when performing ophthalmic ultrasound exams in a practical and objective format that facilitates understanding and using scanning techniques to capture key images and understand differential criteria of diagnosis using multimodal techniques of ultrasound: A-scan, B-scan, ultrasound biomicroscopy, and color Doppler.

This atlas is not intended to replace the comprehensive textbooks available. Rather, it was designed to supplement those sources with dynamic and updated higher-resolution images.

The editors of this book are extremely grateful to the many contributors in their ophthalmic specialties.

We thank Tanya McClendon, CDOS, ROUB; Ericca Nickles, COA, ROUB; Erin Manno, COT, OSA; and the Photography Division of Kellogg Eye Center for their help in patient examination and the collection of illustrations and videos.

We would like to thank the Department of Ophthalmology and Visual Sciences at UNIFESP—Federal University of São Paulo, Brazil, and its faculty for the continued opportunity to develop and improve the art of ophthalmic ultrasound examination.

It is our hope that this atlas will help clinicians and technicians perform, understand, and interpret ultrasound images of the eye and orbit by applying effective exam techniques and using this reference as a guide in their daily practice.

Bernadete Ayres, MD
Norma Allemann, MD
Hakan Demirci, MD

Contents

Video Contents

5 Intraocular Inflammation

6 Glaucoma

7 Anterior Segment Tumors

8 Tumors of the Posterior Segment

8.1 B-scan exam of a choroidal nevus.
8.2 B-scan exam of an atypical choroidal nevus with subretinal fluid at the margins.
8.3 Choroidal melanoma with positive internal vascularity and associated retinal detachment.
8.4 Dynamic view of a mushroom-shaped choroidal melanoma with positive intrinsic vascularity and retinal detachment at margins.
8.5 Dynamic ultrasound localization of radioactive episcleral plaque.
8.6 Dynamic ultrasound of choroidal metastasis of right eye on transverse and longitudinal views.
8.7 Circumscribed choroidal hemangioma with typical high internal reflectivity and shallow shoulders.
8.8 Dynamic ultrasound of diffuse choroidal hemangioma with total closed funnel retinal detachment.
8.9 Bilateral choroidal osteomas. Axial B-scan of choroidal osteoma in the right eye (OD). In the sequence, the video shows a choroidal osteoma in the left eye (OS).
8.10 Bilateral Retinoblastoma. B-scan ultrasound of non-calcified retinoblastoma in the right eye (OD). In the sequence, the video shows a retinoblastoma with intrinsic calcification in the left eye (OS).
8.11 Dynamic B-scan ultrasound sequence videos of multiple retinoblastomas in a patient with a positive family history.
8.12 Dynamic B-scan ultrasound of a retinal hemangioblastoma. Note the lesion does not involve the choroidal layer.
8.13 Dynamic B-scan ultrasound of a juxtapapillary retinal hemangioblastoma.
8.14 Dynamic ultrasound of an astrocytic hamartoma characterized by high reflectivity and acoustic shadowing.
8.15 Multifocal, plaque-like hyperreflective with marked acoustic shadowing in sclerochoroidal calcification.

9 Orbit Tumors and Tumor-Like Lesions

9.1 Dynamic B-scan ultrasound of a superficial dermoid cyst.
9.2 Dynamic B-scan ultrasound of a respiratory epithelial orbital cyst.
9.3 Dynamic B-scan ultrasound of an orbital mucocele.
9.4 Dynamic B-scan ultrasound using a modified immersion technique of superficial infantile hemangioma.
9.5 Dynamic ultrasound B-scan of an infantile hemangioma extending deep in orbit.
9.6 Dynamic transverse and longitudinal B-scan ultrasound of cavernous venous malformation.
9.7 Dynamic transocular and paraocular B-scan of an orbital venous-lymphatic malformation with intrinsic hemorrhage.
9.8 Dynamic B-scan ultrasound with provocative Valsalva maneuver shows a dilated orbital varix and increased blood flow.
9.9 Dynamic B-scan ultrasound using a modified immersion technique for lacrimal gland assessment.
9.10 Dynamic transverse and longitudinal B-scan ultrasound of adenoid cystic carcinoma of the lacrimal gland.
9.11 Dynamic transverse B-scan ultrasound of an orbital lymphoma.
9.12 Dynamic transverse B-scan of an orbital leukemic tumor.
9.13 Dynamic ophthalmic ultrasound of an orbital rhabdomyosarcoma.
9.14 Dynamic axial B-scan of an optic nerve glioma.
9.15 Dynamic B-scan ultrasound of an orbital metastasis attached to extraocular muscle.
9.16 Dynamic longitudinal B-scan ultrasound of an orbital alveolar soft-part sarcoma.

10 Orbital Inflammatory Diseases

10.1 IgG4-related dacryoadenitis. Transverse B-scan ultrasound shows a medium reflective enlargement of the lacrimal gland.
10.2 Orbital sarcoidosis. Transverse B-scan ultrasound shows a large, low reflective sarcoid orbital mass.
10.3 Thyroid eye disease. Longitudinal B-scan ultrasound shows a low reflective enlarged extraocular muscle with normal tendon.

12 Pediatric Ophthalmic Ultrasound

12.1 B-scan ultrasonography of a 9-months-old male infant presenting with leukocoria in the right eye. Cynetic exam allows observation of low-reflectivity vitreous membranes with no adherence to the retina and a rectilinear membrane (hyaloidal stalk) extending from the optic disc to the posterior lens capsule, through the center of the vitreous cavity – in this example, persistent fetal vasculature stalk is thin.

13 Axial Eye Length Measurement

13.1 Immersion A-scan technique.
13.2 Immersion A-scan of a phakic eye.
13.3 Alignment of the sound beam to the visual axis.
13.4 Axial eye length measurement using contact A-scan technique.
13.5 Horizontal axial B-scan.
13.6 Horizontal axial B-scan demonstrates a posterior staphyloma.

14 Ocular Trauma

14.1 Axial B-scan with pseudoimmersion. Suggestive of posterior lens capsule rupture and lens material in the anterior vitreous, observed as linear membranes with medium reflectivity adherent to the posterior capsule.
14.2 Transversal B-scan showing a highly reflective lens positioned anteriorly to the detached posterior hyaloid and surrounded by a dense cluster of echoes.
14.3 Longitudinal B-scan showing the highly reflective lens with internal opacity positioned anterior to the detached posterior hyaloid and surrounded by a dense cluster of echoes.
14.4 After four months, new longitudinal B-scan exam showed a small lens positioned anteriorly to the detached posterior hyaloid.
14.5 Longitudinal B-scan of the ocular wall rupture.
14.6 Transverse B-scan of the ocular wall rupture.
14.7 Longitudinal B-scan of the ocular wall rupture one month after trauma.
14.8 Transverse B-scan of the ocular wall rupture, one month after trauma.
14.9 Longitudinal peripheral B-scan showing the proximity of the IOFB with the lens. No eye movement during the video.
14.10 Longitudinal peripheral B-scan during eye movement, showing that the position of the IOFB does not change and remains fixed to the lens.
14.11 Transverse peripheral B-scan showing the hyper-reflective IOFB fixed to the hyper-reflective lens.
14.12 Metallic foreign body removal from the anterior chamber. (Video from CP Araujo and cols.)

15 Color Doppler in Ophthalmology

15.1 Color Doppler showing blood flow of normal retrobulbar vessels. Linear 3–12 MHz probe. B-scan image shows the shadow of the optic nerve (ON). In the center of the ON, two parallel vessels observed: central retinal artery and central retinal vein. At each side of the ON, the vessels observed are the posterior ciliary arteries. And placed posteriorly into the orbit, a larger vessel is detected, the ophthalmic artery.
15.2 Linear 3–12 MHz probe of the ophthalmic artery blood flow. Color Doppler shows a spectral profile similar to the internal carotid, with a maximum systolic peak, a dicrotic notch, and a smooth slope of the diastolic flow.
15.3 Orbital Varix. Color Doppler showed a regular caliper of the superior ophthalmic vein with continuous anterograde flow prior to the Valsalva maneuver. During the maneuver, a brief period of retrograde flow was noted at maximal distension of the vein. Immediately after the Valsalva maneuver, a rush of anterograde flow was seen within the enlarged vessel, followed by a rapid return to the regular size of the vessel.
15.4 Carotid-cavernous fistula. Color Doppler demonstrates an enlarged superior ophthalmic vein with arterial flow, color-coded in red. In spectral analysis, the flow appears positive and arterialized.
15.5 Color Doppler of a choroidal hemangioma as a dome-shaped lesion with high internal reflectivity and diffuse internal vascularization.
15.6 Color Doppler of a choroidal melanoma. Solid, with medium-to-low internal reflectivity, dome-shaped lesion presenting internal vascularization.

1

Ultrasound Physics and Instrumentation

RONALD H. SILVERMAN, RAKSHA URS, AND SUZANNE DALY

What Is Ultrasonography?

Ultrasonography is one of the primary modalities used for diagnostic imaging of the eye. Unlike optical and CT imaging, which utilize electromagnetic radiation, ultrasound is a form of *mechanical* radiation.

As with any sound wave, ultrasound is a pressure wave comprised of regions of compression and rarefaction propagating through a medium. While sound waves perceptible to the human ear have a frequency in the range of 20–25,000 cycles per second (Hz), diagnostic ultrasound systems operate in millions of cycles per second (MHz).

As with other wave phenomena, wavelength and frequency are defined by the relation $c = \nu\lambda$, where c is the speed of sound, λ is wavelength, and ν is frequency as shown in Fig. 1.1. The speed at which the pulse travels through a medium is related to the medium's composition and temperature. The speed of sound is high in dense tissues such as bones, slower in water, and slower still in oils. In water, $c \approx$ 1500 m/sec at room temperature. Speed of sound is largely independent of frequency.

Physical Principles

The basic principle of ultrasound imaging is that when a propagating acoustic wave encounters an interface that differs in acoustic impedance (density × speed of sound) from the surrounding medium, some acoustic energy is reflected. If the speed of sound in the medium is known and the time (t) from transmission of the ultrasound wave until reception of an echo is measured, then the range to the interface is simply $ct/2$ (the factor of 2 is needed to account for sound traveling to and from the reflector). This is illustrated in the biometric A-scan shown in Fig. 1.2.

Transducers and Probes

Transducers convert an electrical voltage spike into an ultrasound pulse. When echoes interact with the transducer, these generate minute voltages that are then amplified and processed for imaging and biometry. The process whereby an acoustic pulse is launched and reflection converted to voltage is illustrated in Fig. 1.3.

The transducer (Fig. 1.4) is comprised of a *piezoelectric* element that emits and receives ultrasound, a backing layer for damping, a focusing element, and a coaxial cable to excite the piezoelectric element with a voltage spike and send voltages produced from echo data to an amplifier. When excited, the rapid expansion and contraction of the piezoelectric element is communicated to the fluid or tissue with which it is in contact. Conversely, when echoes compress and decompress the transducer element, it generates proportional voltages.

The piezoelectric element is most often a ceramic material, such as lead zirconate (PZT), although lead-free piezoelectric materials are being developed.[1] A backing layer is used to dampen vibrations of the piezoelectric element to shorten pulse duration and improve axial resolution. Polyvinylidene fluoride (PVDF), a polymer, is often used as the piezoelectric element in very high-frequency (e.g., 50 MHz) ultrasound biomicroscopy (UBM) transducers. Ultrasound probes can use either a single piezoelectric element or an array of elements.

Whether ceramic or polymer, single-element transducers have a fixed focal length. While A-scan interrogates one line of sight, B-scan and UBM probes are mechanically scanned (Fig. 1.5). B-scan probes typically are designed to have a focal length of 20–24 mm so that the focal point falls in the posterior vitreous near the retina in a normal adult eye. UBM probes typically focus at around 12 mm, which is suitable for imaging the anterior segment. Note that while 10–20 MHz B-scan probes are sealed, UBM probes generally are not, leaving the transducer exposed. UBM exams thus require the use of a water bath, scleral shell, or a disposable water-filled ClearScan membrane (ESI, Inc., Plymouth, MN) to contact with the eye in order to avoid the attenuation that would otherwise be caused by the cap of a sealed probe. Similarly, UBM exams are performed with open lids to avoid attenuation by the eyelids.

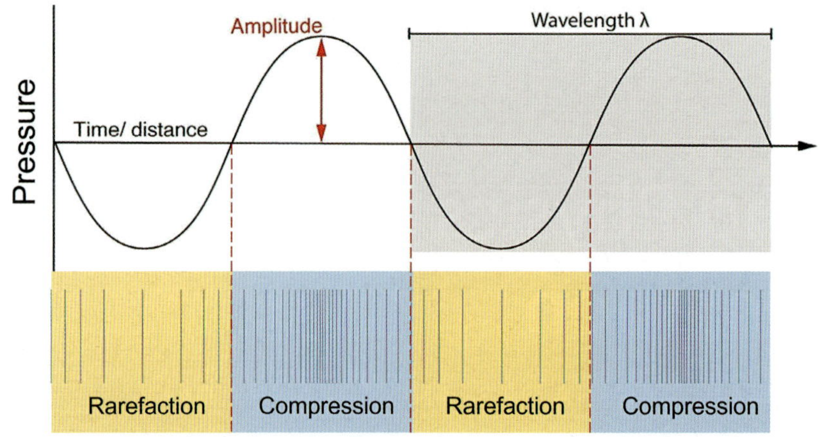

• **Fig. 1.1** The transducer emits an acoustic pulse characterized by pressure amplitude and wavelength that propagates at a speed characteristic of the medium.

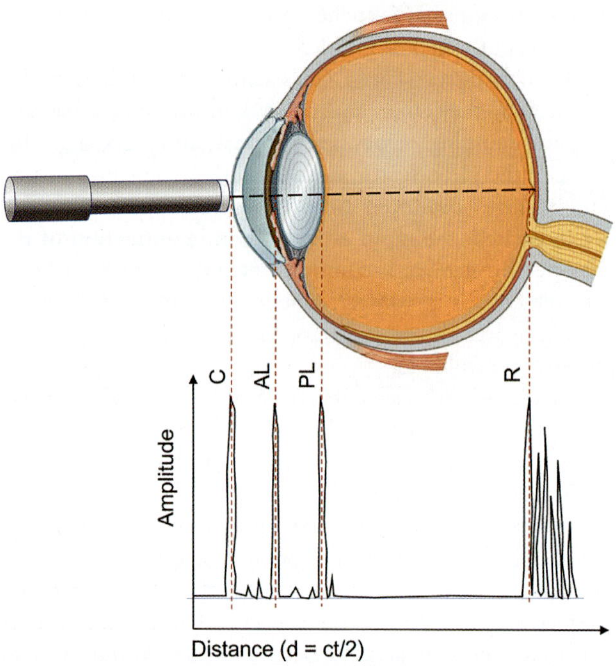

• **Fig. 1.2** For a medium of known speed of sound, the range to an acoustic reflector is readily determined from the time of flight. This is the principle of a biometric A-scan used to determine axial length.

A recent technological development in ophthalmic ultrasound is the annular array, which in form is similar to a single-element probe but comprised of several (e.g., 5 or 6) concentric piezoelectric rings, each of which can independently transmit and receive ultrasound.[2] The advantage of an annular array is that by precise timing of excitation of the individual elements, the transmitted wavefronts can be made to converge at different ranges from the probe. Thus, annular arrays overcome the fixed focus limitation of conventional single-element probes and are advantageous for smaller eyes in pediatric exams, and long staphylomatous or myopic eyes. Furthermore, by rapidly transmitting a series of waves at increasing focal depths and combining echo data, an image can be formed with an extended depth of focus, improving the evaluation of axially extended structures such as the vitreous.

In clinical specialties outside ophthalmology, linear array probes predominate. Linear arrays typically consist of on the order of 100 independent piezoelectric elements, spaced a wavelength apart and allow B-mode imaging without any moving parts. This is accomplished by having successive small sub-apertures of the array transmit a focused wavefront, receiving echoes, and then iterate this process from one end of the array to the other. This produces a rectilinear rather than a sector-shaped image.

While mechanical B-scan systems typically provide 10–20 images per second, linear array-based systems can provide several hundred images per second. Although ophthalmology has historically been neglected by the manufacturers of linear array systems, some manufacturers are now providing instruments with an ophthalmic setting compliant with regulatory standards for the eye, which are more stringent than in any other organ.[3] Linear array-based systems require substantially greater technologic complexity than mechanically scanned systems in that they must be able to control on the order of 100 transducer elements versus just one element in a typical B-scan or a handful of elements in an annular array system.

While A- and B-mode systems specifically designed for imaging the eye are by design compliant with FDA guidelines for ophthalmic safety, this is not the case for linear array-based systems that are designed for general purpose imaging unless the manufacturer has included a specific ophthalmic mode. General purpose systems, however, display acoustic output, typically the mechanical index (MI), which under FDA guidelines should be under 0.23 for ocular imaging versus 1.9 for other clinical specialties.[3]

Fig. 1.6 illustrates the variable focal lengths that can be emitted by annular and linear arrays, and how single-element and annular array probes must be physically moved to obtain a B-scan while the beam itself can be scanned in a linear array.

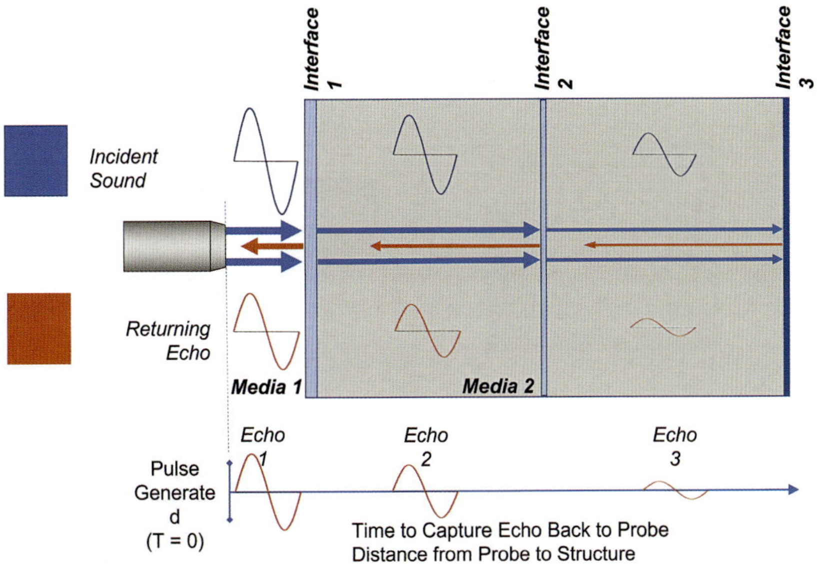

• **Fig. 1.3** Partial reflection occurs whenever a propagating ultrasound pulse encounters an interface between media of different acoustic impedance.

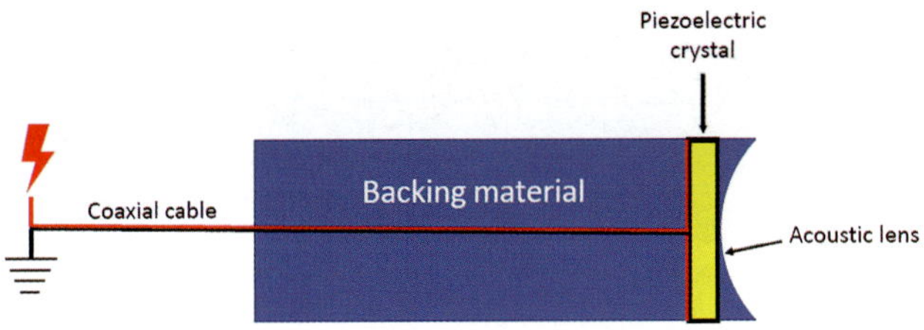

• **Fig. 1.4** The transducer converts a voltage spike into ultrasound. Reflections interacting with the piezoelectric element then produce voltages, which are processed for imaging and biometry.

Imaging Modes

A-scan ultrasonography: In A-scan ultrasonography (see Fig. 1.2), reflections from the cornea, lens, and retina are used to measure axial length. A-scan probes, typically around 10 MHz in center frequency, incorporate a fixation light enabling alignment of the ultrasound beam axis with the visual axis. Ultrasound systems using A-scan for determination of axial length incorporate software that utilizes

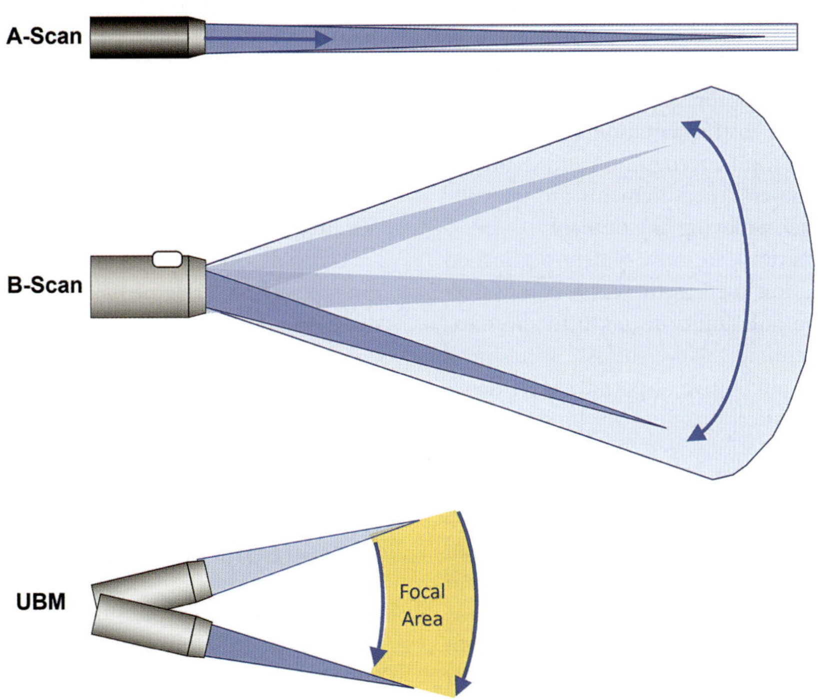

• **Fig. 1.5** An A-scan probe incorporates a fixation light to facilitate biometry along one line of sight corresponding to the optic axis. B-scan probes incorporate a transducer that is pivoted within the probe housing to sweep out a sector image. In UBM, the transducer has a short focal length and is mechanically pivoted or linearly translated to produce a B-scan centered on the focal region.

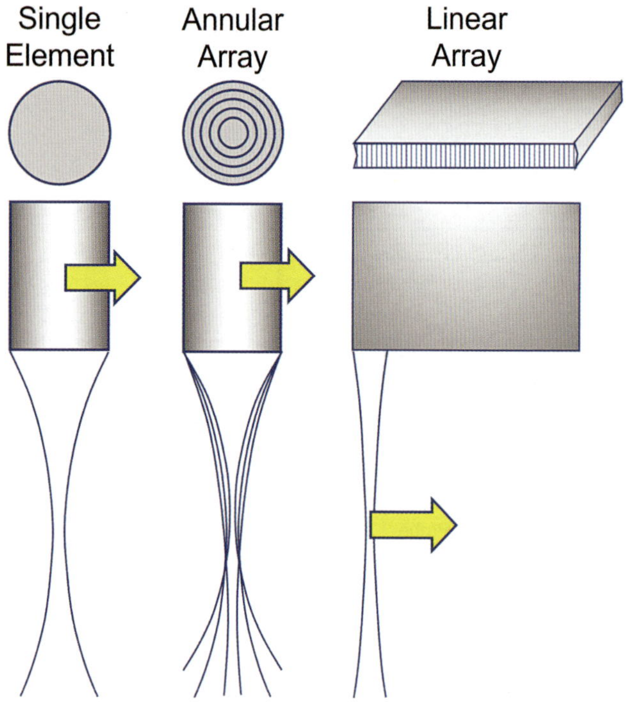

• **Fig. 1.6** Single-element probes produce a fixed focus, while annular arrays can vary the focal range or combine data from several focal ranges to extend the depth of field. Linear arrays can do the same but can produce B-scans electronically without any physical motion.

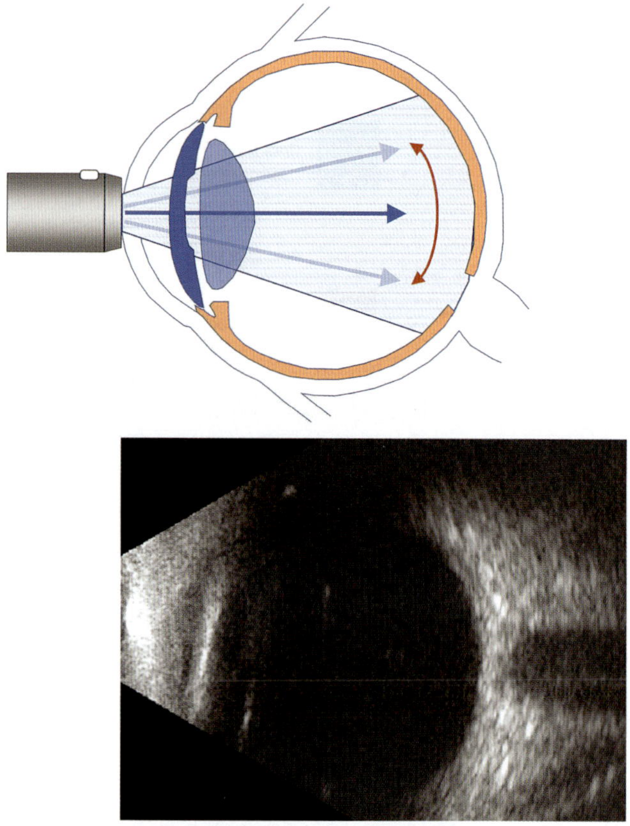

• **Fig. 1.7** B-scans represent acoustic reflection amplitude as pixel brightness.

appropriate values of the speed of sound for the aqueous and vitreous for normal, dense cataractous lenses, pseudophakic, and aphakic eyes. A-scans can be performed in contact mode, where the probe touches (without compressing) the corneal surface, or in immersion mode using a scleral shell. While the contact method can produce with care comparable results to immersion,[4] the latter is generally considered preferred as it obviates potential corneal compression and underestimation of axial length.[5] A-scan instrumentation also generally includes the capability of real-time recognition and recording of well-aligned A-scans. Several measurements are typically recorded and averaged after removing any outliers.

Axial length determinations are now widely performed with optical instrumentation such as the Zeiss IOLMaster because of their precision and ability to perform the measurement without eye contact. Nevertheless, ultrasound remains an indispensable alternative, especially with dense cataracts or where other optical opacities are present along the visual axis.

Ultrasound pachymetry is a contact A-scan technique for the measurement of corneal thickness. Pachymetry probes operate at 20–50 MHz. They do not include a fixation light as they may be used to measure thickness at multiple positions of the cornea.

B-scan ultrasonography: B-scan ultrasonography provides two-dimensional cross-sectional images of ocular anatomy. Systems using a focused single-element probe (the most common setup in ophthalmic B-scan systems) produce B-scan images by moving the probe mechanically. Newer instruments are equipped with annular array transducers. In 10–20 MHz systems, the transducer and motor are within a permanently sealed housing, and the transducer is pivoted during scanning to sweep out a sector-shaped scan plane, as shown in Fig. 1.7. Images are then formed by taking account of the orientation of the probe and the range to each reflector and setting pixel brightness at the appropriate position proportional to the reflection amplitude. B-scan instruments allow adjustment in brightness (gain) and contrast and may include a depth-dependent brightness option to compensate for attenuation (time-gain control).

UBM is essentially a B-mode system operating at frequencies of 35 MHz or higher. UBM transducers were first developed and applied to ophthalmic imaging by Sherar, Foster, and Pavlin in the early 1990s.[6–8] In UBM systems, the probe may be scanned in a sector or linearly.

In linear array-based systems, B-mode images are formed electronically without any moving parts. Linear arrays can produce hundreds of images per second.

Resolution

Axial resolution describes how close together two reflectors can be along the propagation axis of the ultrasound beam and still be distinguished from each other. While transducers are characterized by their center frequency, they actually emit a pulse comprised of a range or "band" of frequencies about the nominal center frequency. *Bandwidth* refers to this range. Broadband probes are well-damped

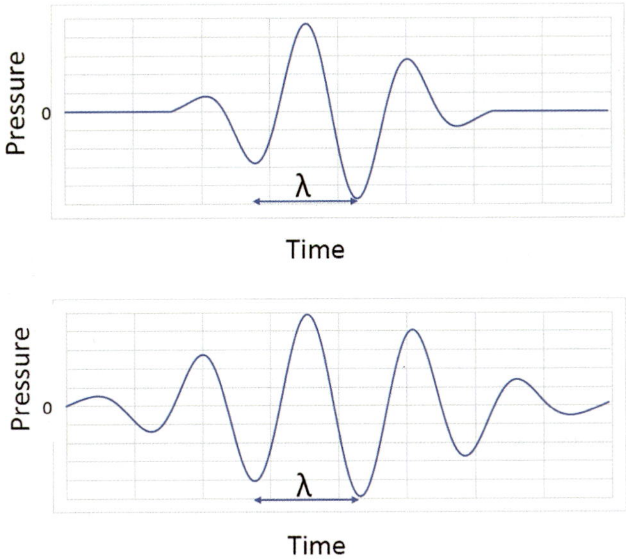

• **Fig. 1.8** Although axial resolution generally improves with frequency, two probes of the same frequency may differ in bandwidth (*corresponding to pulse-length*). A poorly damped (*narrow bandwidth*) probe will give poor resolution.

and provide good axial resolution. Narrowband probes of the same frequency offer relatively poor resolution. Thus, we cannot assume that resolution will always improve as frequency increases without knowing the transducer bandwidth. Fig. 1.8 illustrates two waveforms of the same frequency but with one highly damped and the other poorly damped.

The speed of sound, c, in the vitreous, is 1532 m/sec. For a typical ophthalmic ultrasound system operating at a frequency of 10 MHz, $\lambda = c/\nu = 153$ µm. This would correspond to axial resolution in a fully damped probe.

Lateral resolution describes how close together two reflectors adjacent to each other with respect to the propagation axis of the ultrasound beam can be and still be distinguished from each other. This is affected by both the frequency and aperture of the transducer. As the transducer aperture increases, lateral resolution will improve, but at the cost of decreasing the depth range over which good lateral resolution is achieved.

Reflection

Acoustic reflection is related to the impedance mismatch of an interface with respect to its surrounding media. As a consequence, both an air bubble and a metallic foreign body will produce bright reflections in ultrasound.

When imaging a surface, reflection amplitude will be greatest when the angle of incidence of the ultrasound beam is normal to the interface. This has practical consequences when performing an exam, as the sonographer must orient the probe as normal as possible to the structure of interest (Fig. 1.9). Specular (mirror-like) surfaces such as the cornea or an intraocular lens (IOL) optic tend to be particularly difficult to visualize when imaged even slightly obliquely because the reflection may entirely diverge from the probe. Surfaces that are less specular, such as the posterior of the eye or the iris, tend to scatter ultrasound and are thus more forgiving when the angle of incidence is somewhat oblique.

Because of the specularity of the cornea and the limited depth of field of UBM transducers, scans produced by conventional UBM systems are unsuited for mapping the layered biometry (epithelial and stromal thickness) over the full corneal width. To address this limitation, Silverman and colleagues developed a UBM probe system that scans in an arc such that the beam axis maintains normality with respect to the corneal surface and maintains the cornea within the focal zone over its full lateral extent.[9] By scanning over a series of clock hours, depictions of the thickness of the cornea, epithelium, and stroma could be produced that proved of great value in the detection of keratoconus and in planning of corneal refractive surgery.[10–13]

Refraction

Ultrasound is refracted when propagating across an interface between media differing in speed of sound and, like light, is subject to Snell's law. This is of particular importance

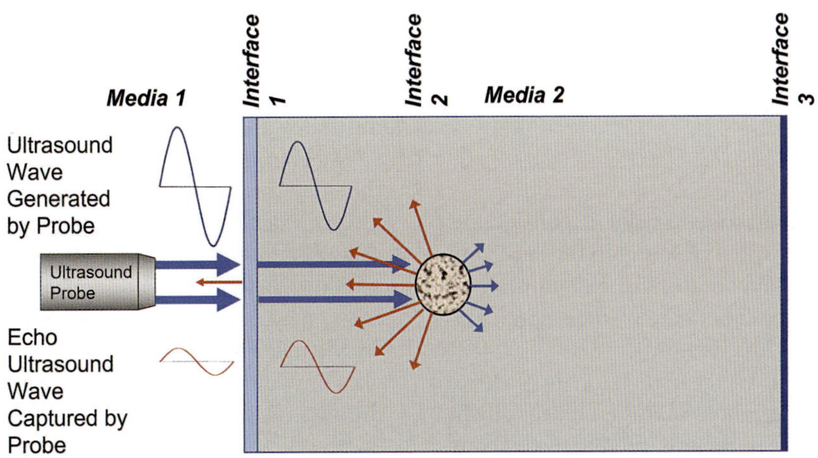

• **Fig. 1.9** Ultrasound echo dispersion due to surface irregularity of structure.

when the ultrasound path encounters the crystalline lens; whereas light is brought to a focus by the lens, ultrasound is defocused because the speed of sound in the lens is faster than that of aqueous and vitreous, whereas the opposite is the case for light. While an A-scan aligned normal to the lens suffers only small distortion on its way to the retina, a B-scan will be noticeably distorted when crossing the lens. Thus, a B-scan imaging plane should avoid the lens when evaluating the posterior pole. Note, however, that refraction of ultrasound in ocular tissues is far less than that of light; in the cornea the optical refractive index (ratio of speed of light in vacuum versus tissue) of light is 1.34 compared to the refractive index of ultrasound (ratio of speed of sound in normal saline versus tissue) which is approximately 1.05.

Attenuation

Attenuation of ultrasound occurs as it propagates through tissue as a consequence of reflection, scattering, and absorption. Attenuation is expressed in logarithmic form in decibel (dB) units, defined as 20 log (A/A_0), where A/A_0 is the ratio of acoustic pressure amplitudes across a tissue depth. Acoustic amplitude decreases exponentially with depth. While tissues differ significantly in their attenuation coefficients, a "rule of thumb" for soft tissues is an attenuation of approximately 0.5 dB/cm-MHz. As transducer frequency increases, attenuation increases exponentially. It is for this reason that UBM probes operating at 50 MHz cannot be used to image the posterior area of the eye; at this frequency, even the vitreous significantly attenuates the ultrasound wave.

Speckle

If acoustic impedance inhomogeneities that are too small to be resolved are present in a tissue, they will cause acoustic backscatter. If sufficient numbers of such scatterers are present, reflections from the many scatterers will undergo random constructive and destructive interference; this results in an artifactual granular textured appearance of the tissue that degrades image quality. Because resolution is related to frequency and bandwidth, speckle is more pronounced with low frequency or narrowband transducers. Speckle is often present in images of tissues such as tumors, hemorrhage, orbital fat, and the sclera in UBM. Fig. 1.10 provides an example of a speckle of orbital tissue.

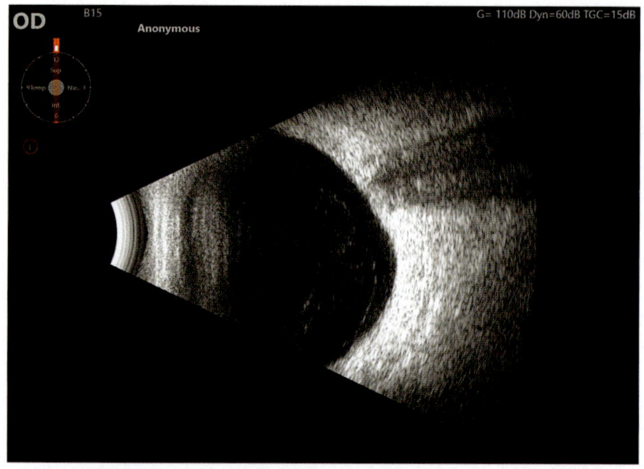

• **Fig. 1.10** Constructive and destructive interference from unresolvable reflectors in the orbital fat produces a mottled appearance (*speckle*).

Artifacts

When B-mode imaging is performed axially in a phakic eye, refraction due to the higher speed of sound in the lens compared to vitreous can result in an artificial elevation of the posterior wall of the eye on either side of the image. This artifact is referred to as "Baum's bumps."

In an immersion B-scan, the structures of the anterior segment can produce strong echoes that then reflect off the transducer surface and back to the eye, producing a second "ghost" image in the vitreous. This "reduplication" artifact can be recognized by varying the range of the probe from the eye during the exam—the artifactual ghost image will move twice the distance as the primary reflection. Fig. 1.11 illustrates these artifacts in an immersion B-scan.

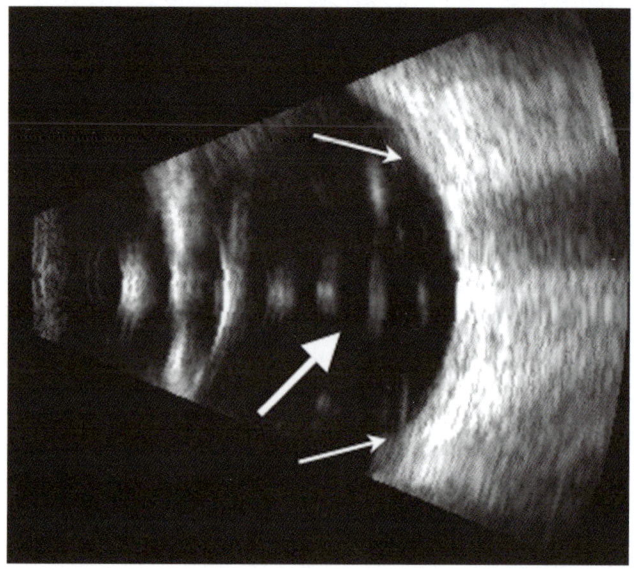

• **Fig. 1.11** In this immersion B-scan, refraction of ultrasound by the lens (*high speed of sound*) produces artifactual "Baum's bumps" (*small arrows*). Bright reflections from the anterior segment structure produce a ghost image of the anterior segment (*bold arrow*) in the mid-vitreous (*reduplication artifact*).

When a structure reflects or absorbs ultrasound strongly, this may cast an acoustic shadow on the deeper structures. This can occur with a densely cataractous lens, calcified tissues, or a foreign body such as a rock fragment.

A reverberation artifact, appearing as a comet-tail of reflections, may occur when imaging a foreign body (Fig. 1.12) with parallel reflective surfaces such as a sliver of metal or glass or with spherical objects such as gas bodies or silicone oil droplets. Reverberation occurs when ultrasound is reflected back and forth between the two regular surfaces, with partial reflection towards the transducer with each pass.

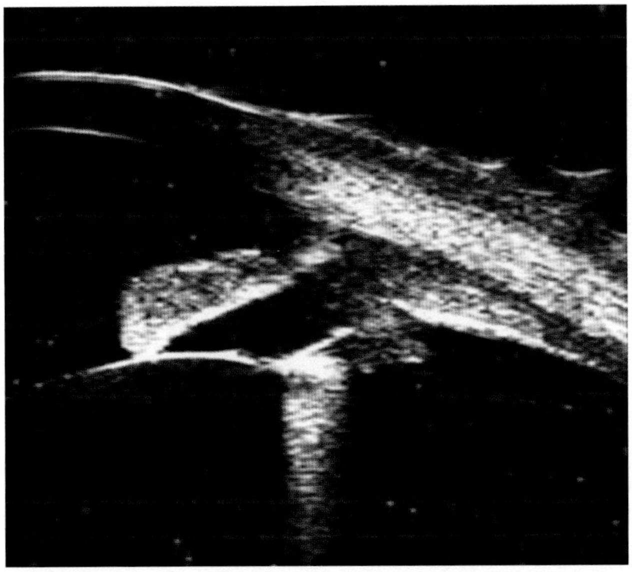

• **Fig. 1.12** Comet-tail artifact resulting from metallic foreign body in UBM image.

Doppler

When a reflector (e.g., flowing blood cells) is moving towards or away from the transducer, a *Doppler* shift in the frequency of the acoustic reflection occurs; if blood flow is moving towards the transducer, the waveform is compressed, resulting in an increased frequency with respect to the waveform emitted by the transducer. The opposite occurs when blood moving away from the transducer.

Continuous-wave Doppler entails measurement of a Doppler frequency shift along a line of sight interrogated by a continuous ultrasound wave, with one transducer transmitting and another receiving within a single probe. This narrowband waveform is very sensitive for detection of Doppler frequency shifts but provides only the direction and not the range to a blood vessel.

Pulsed Doppler entails measurement of the frequency shift in short acoustic pulses, which enables detection of flow together with direction and range. In the context of B-mode imaging, pulsed Doppler requires rapid iterative transmit/receive along each line of sight in order to detect frequency shifts. Because of their low scan rate, pulsed Doppler is not implemented on systems utilizing mechanically scanned probes but is found on linear array-based systems that offer much higher scan rates and pulse repetition frequencies (PRFs). In duplex imaging, regions of blood flow are depicted by superimposing color over the grayscale structural image. Flow towards the transducer, considered arterial flow, is depicted in red, and flow away, considered venous flow, in blue. Power Doppler imaging depicts the magnitude of the Doppler shift without directional or velocity information but is more sensitive to flow than standard color Doppler.

Aliasing is an apparent change in the direction of blood flow in high-velocity areas resulting from undersampling, that is, an inadequate PRF. Obtaining accurate flow velocities requires acquisition of data at a rate such that aliasing is avoided. For pulsed Doppler, the required PRF is $2f_t(v/c)$. Note that in order to measure flow over the cardiac cycle (i.e., peak systolic and end-diastolic velocities), the dwell time over a vessel must be at least one cardiac cycle or about one second. In addition to flow velocity, Doppler systems provide resistance indices, which are related to the ratio of end-diastolic to peak systolic velocities.

Virtually all commercial linear array-based systems offer duplex color flow imaging and measurement of flow velocity. Only some systems, however, offer an ophthalmic setting compliant with regulatory standards. At present, such systems offer color flow imaging (Fig. 1.13), but pulsed Doppler measurement of flow velocity is not presently offered at acoustic intensities within FDA ophthalmic guidelines.

Emerging Technologies

Ultrafast Plane Wave Imaging

Conventional linear arrays generate images by transmitting a converging wavefront from a small subarray, waiting to receive echo data, and then iterating this from one end of the array to the other. If we consider 50 µsec to be the two-way transit time from the probe to the orbit, then the minimum time to produce a B-scan from a 100-element array would be approximately 5 msec for a scan rate of 200 images/sec.

Plane wave imaging is an alternative strategy in which all of the array elements transmit together to produce one unfocused wavefront. Beamforming is then performed on the received data to bring the image into focus.[14] This strategy allows formation of B-mode images at the system PRF. In the example above, this could generate 20,000 images/sec. This ultrafast imaging is ideal for characterizing transient tissue motions such as blood flow or shear waves.

Compounding images from transmits at multiple angles improves resolution and image quality.[15] This, however, reduces the acquisition rate to PRF/n, where n is the number of angled transmits used to form each compound image. So, if, for example, 10 angled transmits were made and combined, 2000 compound images per second could be acquired.

A particularly important aspect of plane wave imaging is that acoustic intensity is significantly reduced compared to that of conventionally scanned arrays because the transmitted wavefronts are unfocused.[16] Because of this, it is possible to produce color-flow Doppler images and measure flow velocity over the cardiac cycle while in compliance with ophthalmic ultrasound safety guidelines, as illustrated in Fig. 1.13.[17,18] We have utilized this methodology in clinical and preclinical studies of retinopathy of prematurity,[19] preeclampsia,[20] and glaucoma.[21]

3D Imaging

3D and even 4D (3D + time) ultrasound imaging has a long history, and is widely used in clinical specialties outside of ophthalmology.[22] It is possible to acquire 3D ultrasound

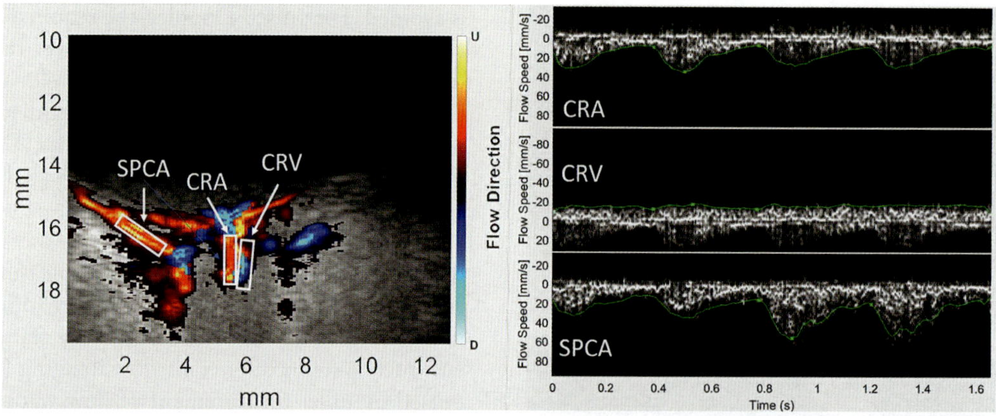

• **Fig. 1.13** Left: Color-flow Doppler image depicting blood flow derived from 18 MHz plane wave scan of a preterm neonatal eye. Right: Spectrograms depict flow in the central retinal artery (CRA), central retinal vein (CRV), and a short posterior ciliary artery (SPCA). Eye was scanned from six angles over a ±9° range and the angled data combined to form 3000 compound images per second.

data by attaching a B-scan probe to a linear translation stage or by rotating it.[23–25] It is also possible to attach an accelerometer to the probe and construct 3D images from probe positional data in a handheld scan.[26] The ideal system for 3D acquisition, however, is the 2D array transducer.[27] This is similar to a linear array but with transducer elements arranged in a 2D grid in a configuration such as a square. Although this is now available at low frequencies for imaging internal organs such as the heart, only research prototypes with higher frequencies suitable for ophthalmic imaging have been demonstrated.[28] This is because, as in a linear array, transducer elements should be no more than a wavelength apart to avoid imaging artifacts. For a square 10 × 10 mm, 15 MHz matrix probe, we would need 10,000 elements 0.1 mm apart. This is difficult and expensive to fabricate, connect, process, and control.

Several approaches towards reducing the complexity and cost of matrix-based probes for 3D and 4D imaging have been explored, including sparse arrays[29] and row-column (RC) arrays.[30–32] RC arrays consist of rows of elongated transducer elements and columns of elements orthogonal to the rows. RC arrays would consist of only 2n elements rather than the n^2 elements of a fully populated matrix. Thus, for the example given above, we would require just 200 instead of 10,000 elements. RC array architecture is inherently suitable for transmission of plane waves, and by transmitting on rows and receiving on columns and then transmitting on columns and receiving on rows, ultrafast volumetric imaging can be achieved.

Elastography

Ultrasound has also been investigated as a tool for characterizing tissue viscoelastic properties. It is possible to "palpate" tissues with acoustic radiation force (stress) and use the same probe to measure acoustic radiation force-induced tissue displacement (strain).[33,34] Ocular tissue elastic properties have also been investigated by measuring the speed of propagation of shear waves induced by an exogenous vibrator.[35] Corneal elasticity has been measured using endogenous variations in intraocular pressure as a source of stress while measuring strain with high-frequency ultrasound.[36]

Conclusions

Ophthalmic ultrasound has been utilized clinically for over 50 years. While it may be considered a mature technology, it is also dynamic, with innovations in transducer design, imaging, signal processing, and technology under continuous and intense development. Technologies now limited to the laboratory will rapidly make their way from bench to bedside.

References

1. Chen R, Jiang L, Zhang T, et al. Eco-friendly highly sensitive transducers based on a new KNN-NTK-FM Lead-free piezoelectric ceramic for high-frequency biomedical ultrasonic imaging applications. *IEEE Trans Biomed Eng*. 2019;66(6):1580–1587. https://doi.org/10.1109/tbme.2018.2876063.
2. Silverman RH, Ketterling JA, Mamou J, Coleman DJ. Improved high-resolution ultrasonic imaging of the eye. *Arch Ophthalmol*. 2008;126(1):94–97. https://doi.org/10.1001/archopht.126.1.94.
3. Abramowicz JS, Adhikari S, Dickman E, et al. Ocular ultrasound: review of bioeffects and safety, including fetal and point of care perspective: review of bioeffects and safety, including fetal and point-of-care perspective. *J Ultrasound Med*. 2022;41(7):1609–1622. https://doi.org/10.1002/jum.15864.
4. Hennessy MP, Franzco, Chan DG. Contact versus immersion biometry of axial length before cataract surgery. *J Cataract Refract Surg*. 2003;29(11):2195–2198. https://doi.org/10.1016/s0886-3350(03)00224-4.
5. Olsen T, Nielsen PJ. Immersion versus contact technique in the measurement of axial length by ultrasound. *Acta Ophthalmol (Copenh)*. 1989;67(1):101–102. https://doi.org/10.1111/j.1755-3768.1989.tb00732.x.

6. Sherar MD, Foster FS. The design and fabrication of high frequency poly(vinylidene fluoride) transducers. *Ultrason Imaging.* 1989;11(2):75–94. https://doi.org/10.1177/016173468901100201.
7. Sherar MD, Starkoski BG, Taylor WB, Foster FS. A 100 MHz B-scan ultrasound backscatter microscope. *Ultrason Imaging.* 1989;11(2):95–105. https://doi.org/10.1177/016173468901100202.
8. Pavlin CJ, Harasiewicz K, Sherar MD, Foster FS. Clinical use of ultrasound biomicroscopy. *Ophthalmology.* 1991;98(3):287–295. https://doi.org/10.1016/s0161-6420(91)32298-x.
9. Silverman RH, Reinstein DZ, Raevsky T, Coleman DJ. Improved system for sonographic imaging and biometry of the cornea. *J Ultrasound Med.* 1997;16(2):117–124. https://doi.org/10.7863/jum.1997.16.2.117.
10. Reinstein DZ, Silverman RH, Raevsky T, et al. Arc-scanning very high-frequency digital ultrasound for 3D pachymetric mapping of the corneal epithelium and stroma in laser in situ keratomileusis. *J Refract Surg.* 2000;16(4):414–430. https://doi.org/10.3928/1081-597x-20000701-04.
11. Reinstein DZ, Archer TJ, Gobbe M, Silverman RH, Coleman DJ. Epithelial thickness in the normal cornea: three-dimensional display with Artemis very high-frequency digital ultrasound. *J Refract Surg.* 2008;24(6):571–581. https://doi.org/10.3928/1081597x-20080601-05.
12. Reinstein DZ, Archer TJ, Gobbe M, Silverman RH, Coleman DJ. Stromal thickness in the normal cornea: three-dimensional display with artemis very high-frequency digital ultrasound. *J Refract Surg.* 2009;25(9):776–786. https://doi.org/10.3928/1081597x-20090813-04.
13. Silverman RH, Urs R, Roychoudhury A, Archer TJ, Gobbe M, Reinstein DZ. Epithelial remodeling as basis for machine-based identification of keratoconus. *Invest Ophthalmol Vis Sci.* 2014;55(3):1580–1587. https://doi.org/10.1167/iovs.13-12578.
14. Tanter M, Fink M. Ultrafast imaging in biomedical ultrasound. *IEEE Trans Ultrason Ferroelectr Freq Control.* 2014;61(1):102–119. https://doi.org/10.1109/tuffc.2014.6689779.
15. Montaldo G, Tanter M, Bercoff J, Benech N, Fink M. Coherent plane-wave compounding for very high frame rate ultrasonography and transient elastography. *IEEE Trans Ultrason Ferroelectr Freq Control.* 2009;56(3):489–506. https://doi.org/10.1109/tuffc.2009.1067.
16. Urs R, Ketterling JA, Silverman RH. Ultrafast ultrasound imaging of ocular anatomy and blood flow. *Invest Ophthalmol Vis Sci.* 2016;57(8):3810–3816. https://doi.org/10.1167/iovs.16-19538.
17. Bercoff J, Montaldo G, Loupas T, et al. Ultrafast compound Doppler imaging: providing full blood flow characterization. *IEEE Trans Ultrason Ferroelectr Freq Control.* 2011;58(1):134–147. https://doi.org/10.1109/tuffc.2011.1780.
18. Demené C, Deffieux T, Pernot M, et al. Spatiotemporal clutter filtering of ultrafast ultrasound data highly increases doppler and fUltrasound sensitivity. *IEEE Trans Med Imaging.* 2015;34(11):2271–2285. https://doi.org/10.1109/tmi.2015.2428634.
19. Silverman RH, Urs R, Jokl DH, et al. Ocular Blood Flow in Preterm Neonates: A Preliminary Report. *Transl Vis Sci Technol.* 2021;10(2):22. https://doi.org/10.1167/tvst.10.2.22.
20. Silverman RH, Urs R, Wapner RJ, Bearelly S. Plane-wave ultrasound doppler of the eye in preeclampsia. *Transl Vis Sci Technol.* 2020;9(10):14. https://doi.org/10.1167/tvst.9.10.14.
21. Silverman RH, Urs R, Tezel G, Yang X, Nelson I, Ketterling JA. Retrobulbar blood flow in rat eyes during acute elevation of intraocular pressure. *Exp Eye Res.* 2021;207:108606. https://doi.org/10.1016/j.exer.2021.108606.
22. Smith SW, Pavy HR, von Ramm OT. High-speed ultrasound volumetric imaging system. I. Transducer design and beam steering. *IEEE Trans Ultrason Ferroelectr Freq Control.* 1991;38(2):100–108. https://doi.org/10.1109/58.68466.
23. Helms RW, Minhaz AT, Wilson DL, Örge FH. Clinical 3D imaging of the anterior segment with ultrasound biomicroscopy. *Transl Vis Sci Technol.* 2021;10(3):11. https://doi.org/10.1167/tvst.10.3.11.
24. Downey DB, Nicolle DA, Levin MF, Fenster A. Three-dimensional ultrasound imaging of the eye. *Eye (Lond).* 1996;10(Pt 1):75–81. https://doi.org/10.1038/eye.1996.11.
25. Cusumano A, Coleman DJ, Silverman RH, et al. Three-dimensional ultrasound imaging. Clinical applications. *Ophthalmology.* 1998;105(2):300–306. https://doi.org/10.1016/s0161-6420(98)93211-0.
26. Kim T, Kang DH, Shim S, et al. Versatile low-cost volumetric 3D ultrasound imaging using gimbal-assisted distance sensors and an inertial measurement unit. Sensors (Basel). 2020;20(22): 6613. https://doi.org/10.3390/s20226613.
27. Smith SW, Trahey GE, von Ramm OT. Two-dimensional arrays for medical ultrasound. *Ultrason Imaging.* 1992;14(3):213–233. https://doi.org/10.1177/016173469201400301.
28. Correia M, Provost J, Tanter M, Pernot M. 4D ultrafast ultrasound flow imaging: in vivo quantification of arterial volumetric flow rate in a single heartbeat. *Phys Med Biol.* 2016;61(23):L48–L61. https://doi.org/10.1088/0031-9155/61/23/l48.
29. Yen JT, Steinberg JP, Smith SW. Sparse 2-D array design for real time rectilinear volumetric imaging. *IEEE Trans Ultrason Ferroelectr Freq Control.* 2000;47(1):93–110. https://doi.org/10.1109/58.818752.
30. Jensen JA, Schou M, Jorgensen LT, et al. Anatomic and functional imaging using row-column arrays. *IEEE Trans Ultrason Ferroelectr Freq Control.* 2022;69(10):2722–2738. https://doi.org/10.1109/tuffc.2022.3191391.
31. Demore, Christine, Lockwood GR. Theoretical assessment of a crossed electrode 2-D array for 3-D imaging. *Proceedings of the IEEE Ultrasonics Symposium.* 2003;1:968–971. https://doi.org/10.1109/ULTSYM.2003.1293560.
32. Sauvage J, Poree J, Rabut C, et al. 4D Functional imaging of the rat brain using a large aperture row-column array. *IEEE Trans Med Imaging.* 2020;39(6):1884–1893. https://doi.org/10.1109/tmi.2019.2959833.
33. Urs R, Lloyd HO, Silverman RH. Acoustic radiation force for non-invasive evaluation of corneal biomechanical changes induced by cross-linking therapy. *J Ultrasound Med.* Aug 2014;33(8):1417–1426. https://doi.org/10.7863/ultra.33.8.1417.
34. Silverman RH, Urs R, Lloyd HO. Effect of ultrasound radiation force on the choroid. *Invest Ophthalmol Vis Sci.* 2013;54(1):103–109. https://doi.org/10.1167/iovs.12-10773.
35. Qian X, Li R, Lu G, et al. Ultrasonic elastography to assess biomechanical properties of the optic nerve head and peripapillary sclera of the eye. *Ultrasonics.* 2021;110:106263. https://doi.org/10.1016/j.ultras.2020.106263.
36. Clayson K, Pavlatos E, Pan X, Sandwisch T, Ma Y, Liu J. Ocular pulse elastography: imaging corneal biomechanical responses to simulated ocular pulse using ultrasound. *Transl Vis Sci Technol.* 2020;9(1):5. https://doi.org/10.1167/tvst.9.1.5.

2

Patient Care and Exam Techniques

BERNADETE AYRES, NORMA ALLEMANN, AND OLIVIA KILLEEN

Exam Technique

Ophthalmic ultrasound is a noninvasive technique that allows a reliable and reproducible detection, differentiation, and measurement of intraocular and orbital lesions. A systematic method to assess the eye and orbit employs "standardized echography," which refers to the combined use of standardized A-scan, B-scan, and Doppler ultrasound.[1]

The anterior segment is better evaluated using a higher-frequency (50–100 MHz) transducer providing greater resolution of more superficial structures.[2,3]

Patient Care

The first step of the ultrasound exam is a brief review of the patient's medical history, ophthalmic exam, and the indication or reason for the sonographic examination. This information will guide the investigation more objectively and effectively.

Effective communication between the sonographer, patient, and physician is essential for accurate diagnoses and optimal patient care. Explaining the procedure and answering questions will build a trustful and cooperative sonographer/patient relationship, leading to succesful outcome in the exam.

Patient, Instrument, and Sonographer Positions

The patient is comfortably accommodated in a reclining examination chair and can be examined supine, inclined, or upright. The examination should be performed preferentially with the patient supine.

Position the ultrasound machine on the patient's right side with the screen facing the examiner (Fig. 2.1). With this disposition, the examiner can face both the patient and the ultrasound screen, scanning with the right hand and manipulating buttons on the machine with the left hand; therefore, the probe, the eye, and the image can be tracked simultaneously. Position the monitor of the ultrasound equipment such that its display is at eye level and perpendicular to your line of sight.

Musculoskeletal disorders have been identified in sonographers and are increasing in incidence. An ergonomic workstation plays a significant role in mitigating these injuries. Sonographers must take the time to optimize the ergonomic features of the workstation equipment and working postures.

The ambient room light must be dimmed. This allows enough light intensity for the operator to adequately see the patient and the ultrasound device. In addition, it provides comfort for dilated pupil patients.

Scanning of the Posterior Segment and Orbit

Once the patient is appropriately positioned, topical anesthetic drops are administrated to the indicated eye(s). A methylcellulose fluid or a lubricant eye gel is applied to the probe face. The probe is placed opposite the area being examined. The exam can be performed either with an open eye or through closed lid. The open-eye method is advantageous because it produces less sound attenuation by the eyelids and allows the sonographer to observe the proper probe position and the patient's eye direction.

The ultrasound beam is aligned with reflective surfaces in the B-mode probe, producing a sector scan of the eye and orbit. The B-scan is a two-dimensional cross-section image generated by mechanically sweeping the transducer over an angle of 50–60° with the probe oriented on a specific axis.[4]

The B-scan probe has a white mark on its tip (Fig. 2.2) that indicates the plane of the scanning motion. This mark corresponds to the top of the sonogram, despite where the probe is positioned.

TEACHING POINT

Probe marker. It is always useful to confirm which side of the probe corresponds to the top side of the screen to identify the correct orientation of the image.

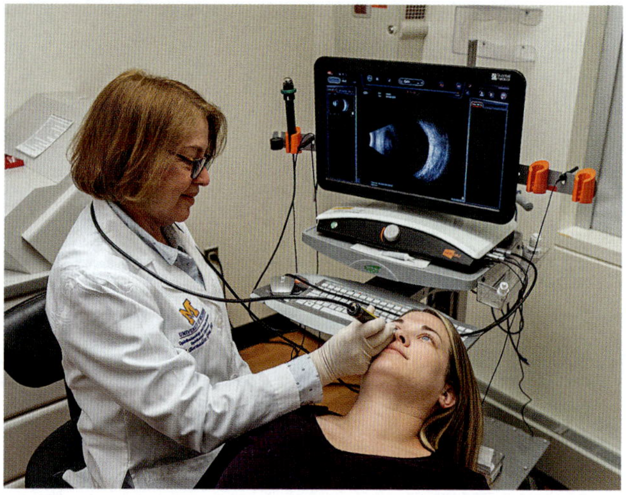

• **Fig. 2.1** Workstation for an ultrasound exam. The patient is comfortably accommodated in a supine position on the right side of the sonographer. The sonographer should be able to see both the patient and the instrument.

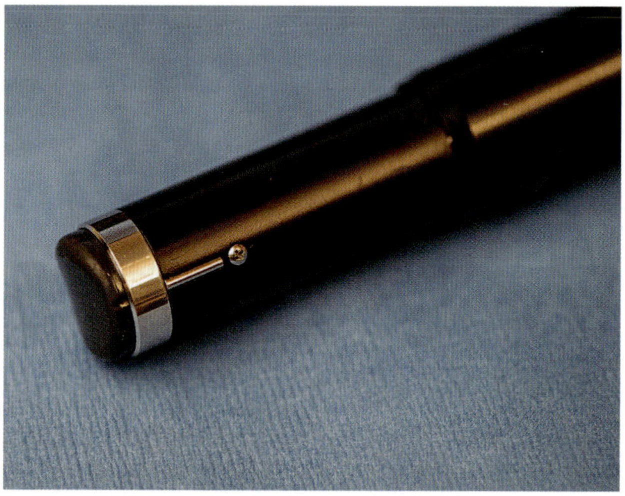

• **Fig. 2.2** Probe Marker. The B-scan probe has a mark that designates the plane of the transducer scanning plane and indicates the upper zone of the sonogram.

Exam Assessment

The eye and orbit can be assessed using two basic ultrasound exam techniques: transocular and paraocular approaches.

Transocular Approach

In the transocular approach, the sound travels through the globe, assessing the intraocular and extraocular spaces (Fig. 2.3).

Paraocular Approach

In the paraocular approach, the sound beam is aimed to surround the eye, assessing the anterior orbit and eyelids (Fig. 2.4).

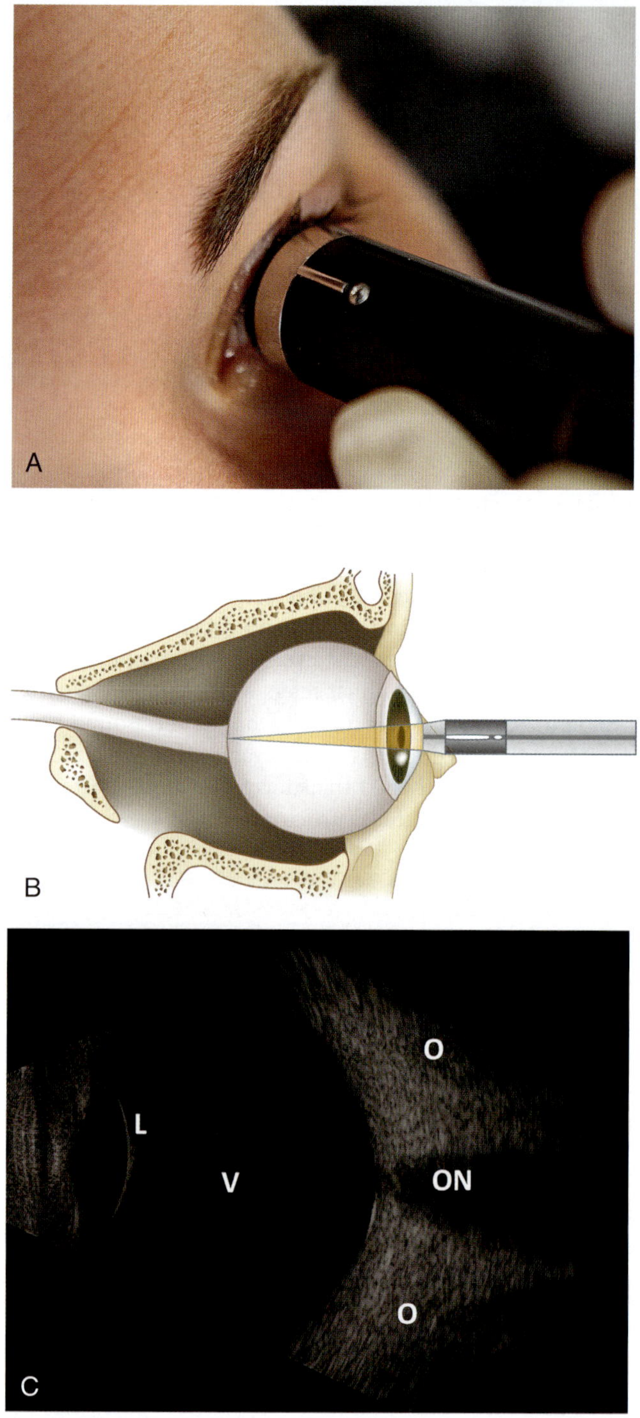

• **Fig. 2.3** Transocular Approach. **(A)** The probe is placed over the eye **(B, C)**, assessing the intraocular and extraocular spaces. *L*, Posterior lens capsule; *O*, Orbital tissue; *ON*, optic nerve; *V*, vitreous.

Furthermore, the scanning planes of the B-mode ultrasound are transverse, longitudinal, and axial. In transverse and longitudinal scans, the probe is placed on the corneoscleral limbus, and the patient is oriented to look in the direction of the meridian to be scanned. In an axial scan, the probe is placed on the center of the cornea having the patient fixating in the primary gaze (Fig. 2.5). Since the

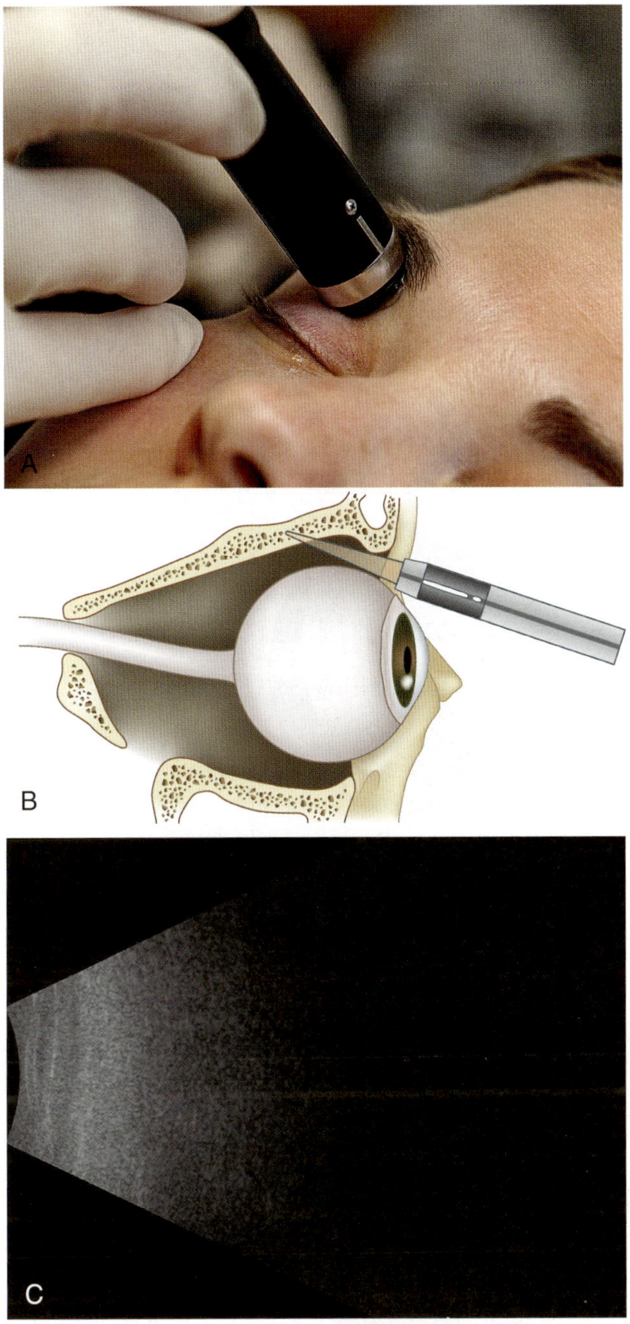

• **Fig. 2.4** Paraocular Approach. **(A)** The probe is placed on the upper or lower eyelid with the sound beam surrounding the eye **(B, C)**, assessing the anterior orbit region and lids.

sound beam bypasses the lens in transverse and longitudinal scans, deeper tissue penetration is obtained.

Transverse Scan

The probe is placed on the limbus on transverse scanning, with the transducer oscillating parallel to the limbus, producing a circumferential slice through the opposite quadrant, extending for six meridians. The probe mark can be oriented:

- Upright for a transverse vertical scan of the nasal or temporal fundus (Fig. 2.6 and Videos 2.1 and 2.2).
- Nasally for transverse horizontal scan of the superior or inferior fundus (Fig. 2.7).
- Upright for transverse oblique scans of the superonasal, inferonasal, inferotemporal, and superotemporal fundus images (Fig. 2.8).

Initially, the posterior pole is screened, with the sound beam directed toward the optic disc and juxtapapillary area. Soon after, the probe is slowly shifted to the fornix; therefore, the quadrant is screened sequentially from the posterior pole to the periphery. It is important to keep the angle of the ultrasound beam perpendicular to the object area.

TEACHING POINT

Perpendicularity. Position the probe perpendicular to the target; therefore, more ultrasound waves will be reflected to the transducer, and fewer will be scattered away, resulting in a better resolution image.

Longitudinal Scan

On the longitudinal scan, the probe is placed on the limbus, with the transducer oscillating perpendicular to the limbus, generating an anteroposterior slice of the opposite meridian. The probe's mark is always oriented towards the cornea (Fig. 2.9 and Videos 2.3 and 2.4). The acquired image shows the optic nerve on the lowest area of the screen, while the globe periphery is displayed at the highest portion of the screen. Shifting the probe over the periphery of the cornea reaches a more posterior view, whereas moving the probe to the fornix assesses more the fundus periphery at the level of the ciliary body.

The longitudinal scan is useful for displaying the lesion location and its relationship with the optic nerve, midperiphery, or periphery. For example, defining an insertion of a membrane at the edge or into the optic disc.

The longitudinal scan aimed temporally is the best approach to locating the macula, which is centered about 4.0 mm from the optic disc (Fig. 2.10 and Video 2.5).

TEACHING POINT

Macula position. Longitudinal scans aimed at the 9-o'clock meridian in the right eye or the 3-o'clock meridian in the left eye are valuable approaches for macula evaluation.

Axial Scan

On the axial scan, the probe is placed on the center of the cornea with the patient in primary gaze fixation. The image generated shows the posterior lens capsule, central vitreous cavity, and two opposite meridians crossed by the optic disc. One disadvantage of this scan is the sound attenuation caused by the lens or intraocular lens implant, decreasing the resolution of the posterior regions. The axial scan is practical to evaluate the macula, the optic nerve, or the correlation of these structures to a posterior pole or retrobulbar pathology.

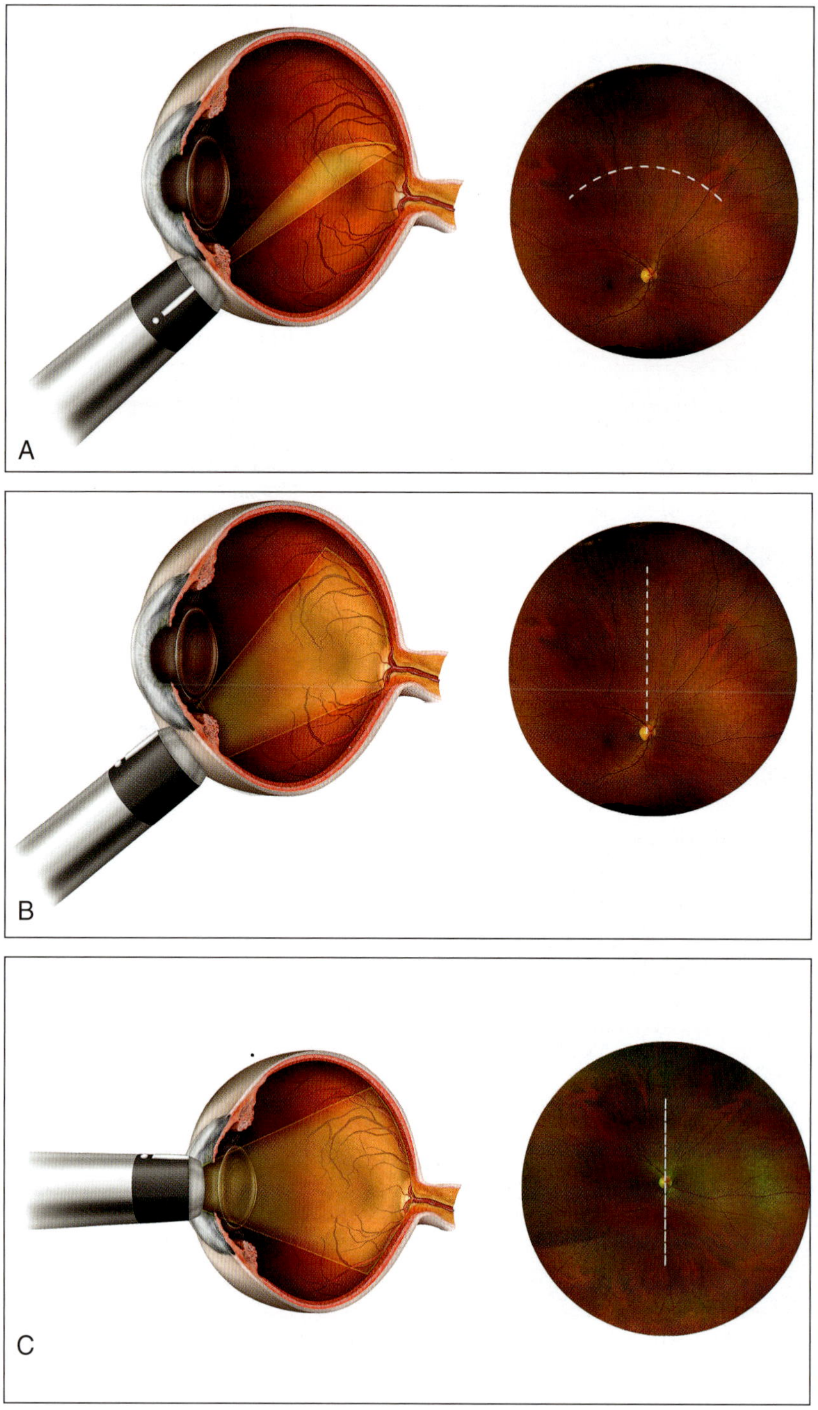

• **Fig. 2.5** Scanning Planes. **(A)** Transverse, **(B)** longitudinal, and **(C)** axial scans and corresponding fundus area.

The probe mark can be oriented:

- Upright for vertical axial scan, imaging the superior area of the posterior pole on the top of the screen, the optic disc at the center, and the inferior area at the bottom (Fig. 2.11).
- Nasally for horizontal axial scan, imaging the nasal side at the top of the screen, the optic disc at the center, and the temporal side at the bottom (Fig. 2.12). The macula is situated just below the optic disc.
- Toward 10:30 or 1:30 meridians for oblique axial scans, imaging the 10:30–4:30 and 1:30–7:30 meridians.

A systematic screening of the globe and orbit must use the transverse scan to sweep all quadrants in the following order: first, the superior quadrant, then the nasal, then the inferior, and last the temporal quadrant. If any abnormality is detected, a longitudinal and axial view must be performed for complementary scanning.

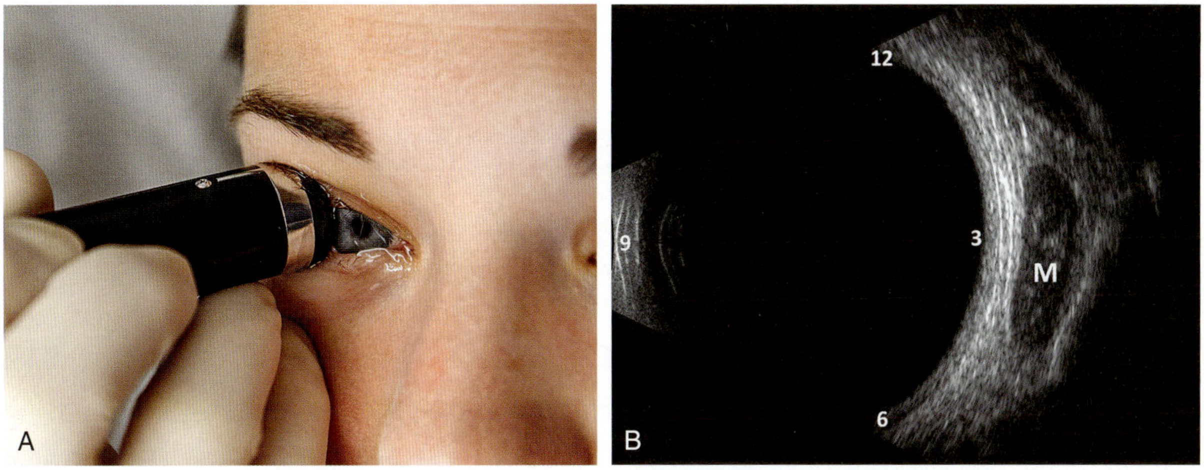

• **Fig. 2.6** Transverse Scan Nasally, Right Eye. **(A)** The patient is left gaze, and the probe is placed on the temporal limbus with the marker oriented upright with the sound sweeping across the nasal fundus from 12- to 6-o'clock, centered at the 3-o'clock meridian. **(B)** The corresponding sonogram in transverse view. *M*, Medial rectus muscle in cross-section.

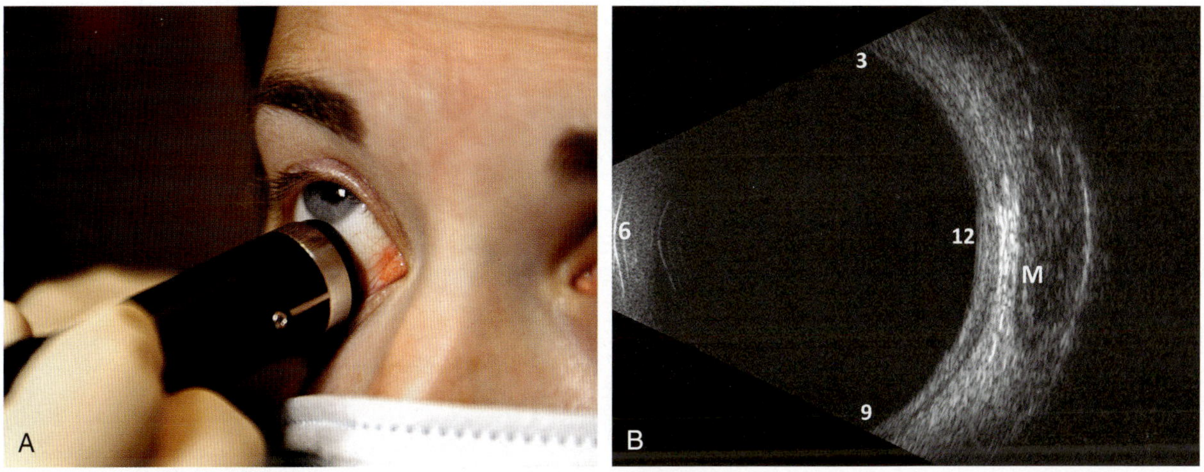

• **Fig. 2.7** Transverse Scan Superiorly, Right Eye. **(A)** The patient fixates on an upward gaze. The probe is placed on the inferior limbus with the marker oriented nasally with the sound sweeping across the superior fundus from 9- to 3-o'clock, centered at the 12-o'clock meridian. **(B)** The corresponding sonogram in transverse view shows the superior rectus muscle in cross-section (M).

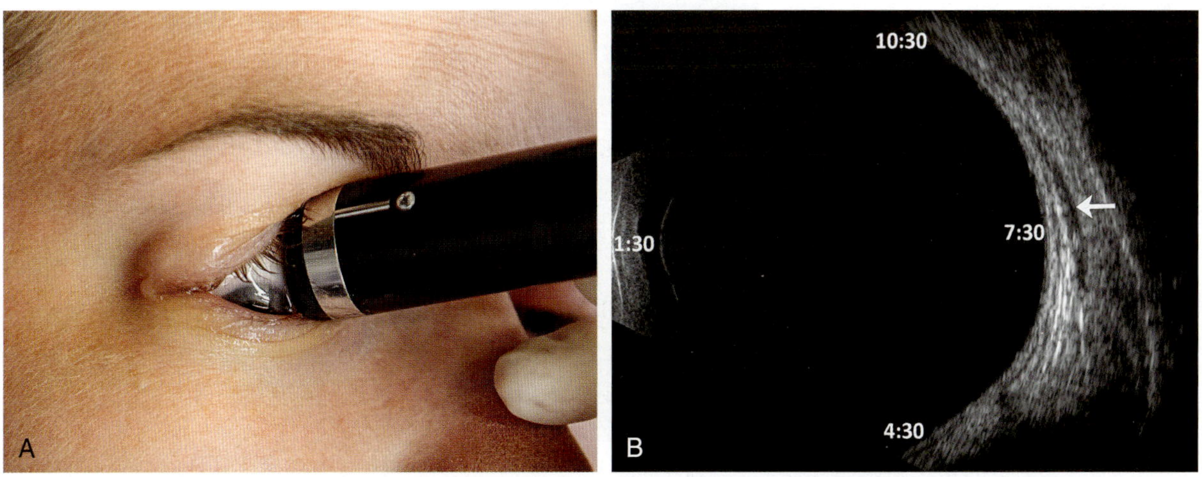

• **Fig. 2.8** Oblique Transverse Scan Inferotemporally, Right Eye. **(A)** The patient fixates on the right and downgaze. The probe is placed on the superonasal limbus with the marker oriented upright with the sound sweeping inferotemporally from 4:30- to 10:30-o'clock, centered at 7:30-o'clock meridian. **(B)** Corresponding sonogram of oblique transverse inferotemporally imaging the inferior oblique (*arrow*).

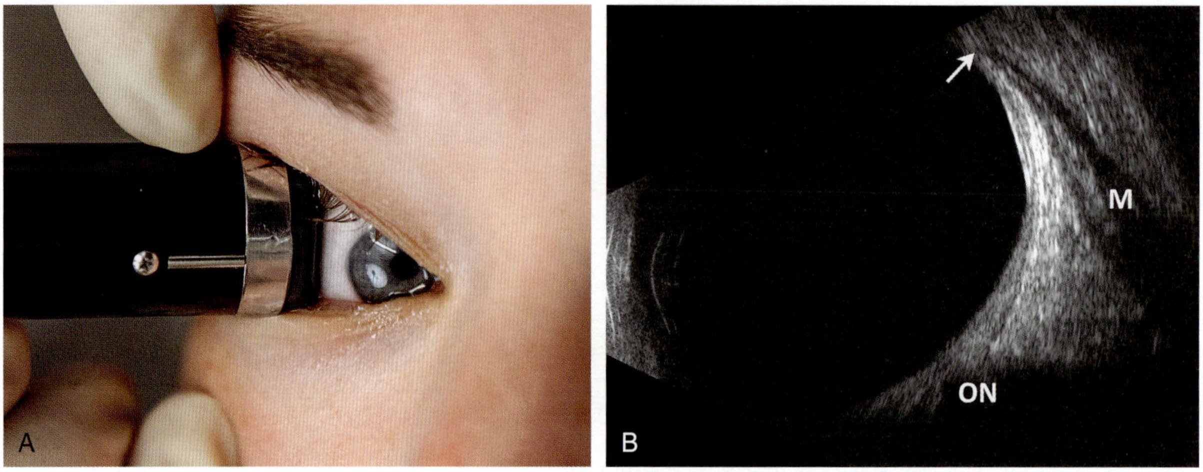

• **Fig. 2.9** Longitudinal Scan Nasally. **(A)** The patient is left gaze, and the probe is placed on the temporal limbus with the marker oriented towards the cornea with the sound sweeping along a specific meridian of the nasal fundus. **(B)** The corresponding sonogram in longitudinal view, where the optic nerve and posterior pole are imaged on the lower portion of the echogram, while the fundus periphery is imaged on the upper portion of the echogram. The medial rectus muscle insertion (*arrow*), located anterior to the equator, is an echographic landmark for the topographic ultrasound. *M*, Muscle; *ON*, optic nerve.

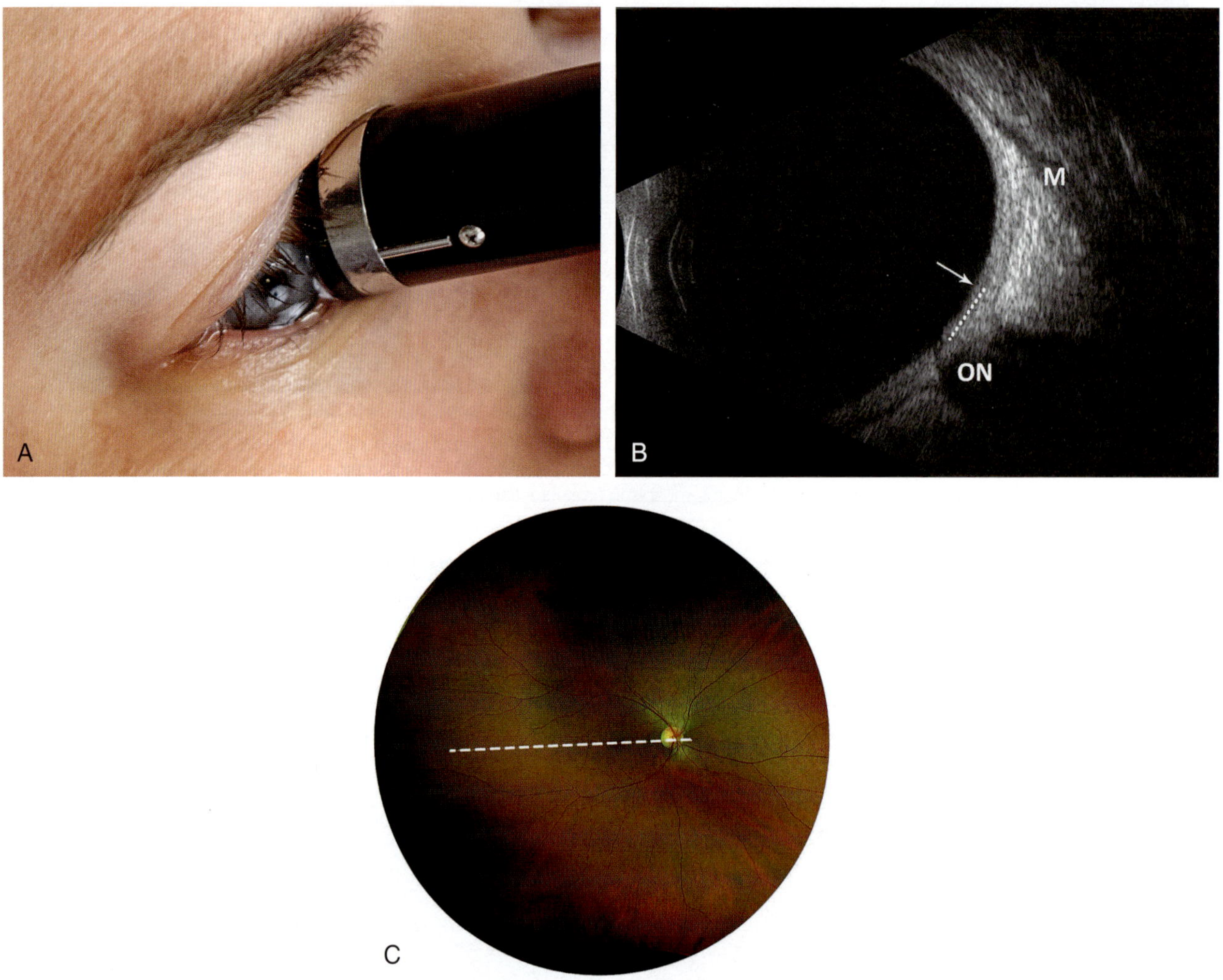

• **Fig. 2.10** **(A)** Longitudinal scan of the macula, right eye. The patient fixates on the right gaze and slightly down towards the 8:30 meridian **(B)**. The corresponding sonogram of the longitudinal macula. The center of the macula (*arrow*) is estimated to be approximately 4 mm from the edge of the optic disc. **(C)** Fundus photography indicates the macula location. *M*, Lateral rectus muscle; *ON*, optic nerve.

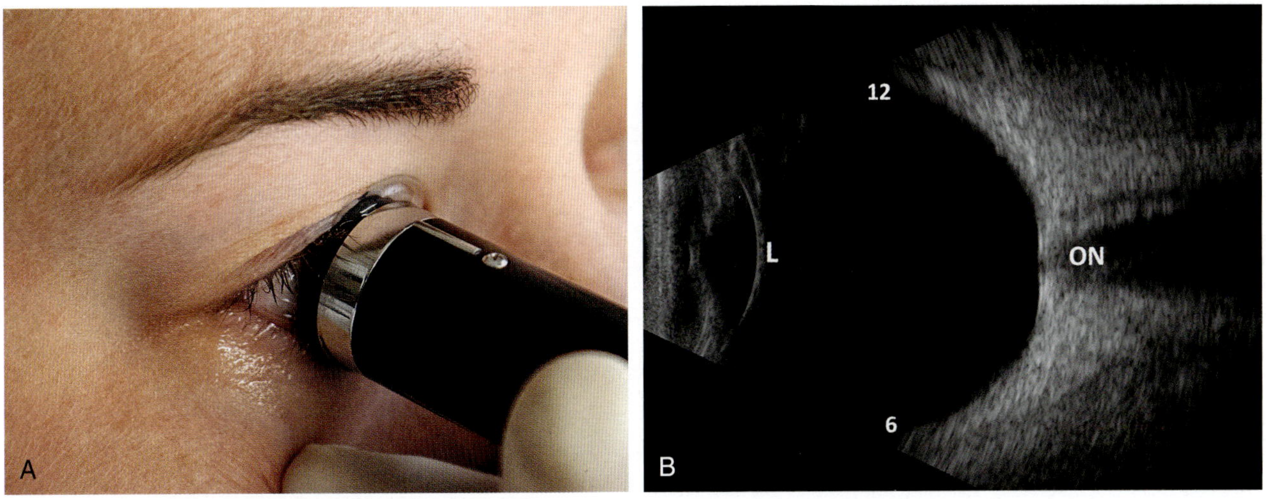

• **Fig. 2.11** Vertical Axial Scan. **(A)** Having the patient in primary gaze, the probe is placed on the center of the cornea with the marker oriented upright with the sound sweeping from 12:00- to 6:00-o'clock. **(B)** The corresponding sonogram displays the superior fundus hemisphere above the optic disc and the inferior fundus hemisphere below the optic disc. *L*, Posterior lens capsule; *ON*, optic nerve.

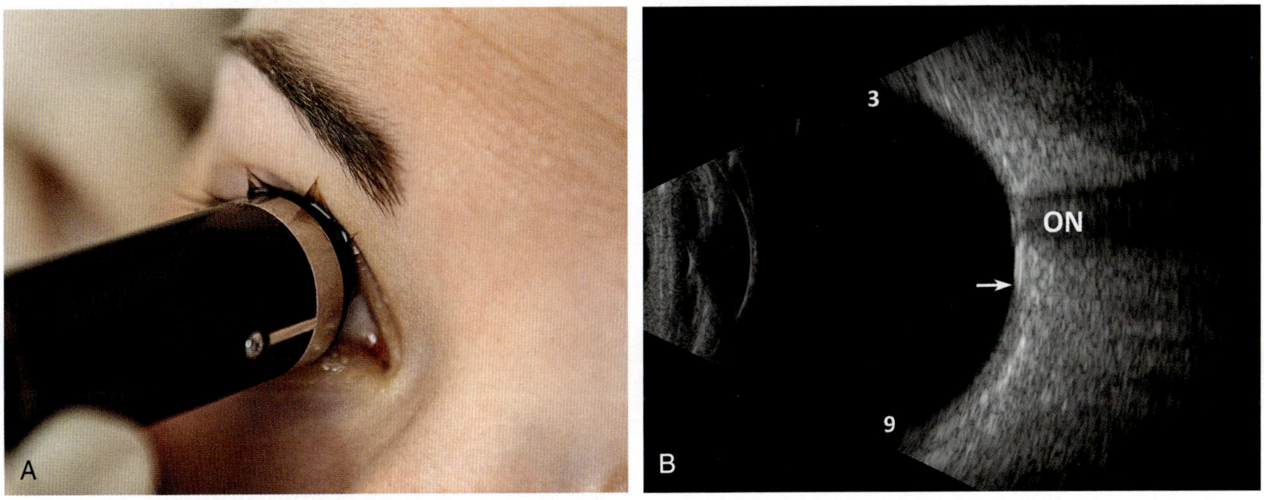

• **Fig. 2.12** Horizontal Axial Scan, Right Eye. **(A)** Having the patient in primary gaze, the probe is placed on the center of the cornea with the marker pointing nasally. **(B)** The corresponding sonogram displays the nasal fundus above the optic disc and the temporal fundus (macula included) below the optic disc. *ON*, Optic nerve; *arrow*, macula center.

TEACHING POINT

Whole globe screening. Use transverse scans to screen all quadrants shifting the probe from limbus to fornix avoiding missed area and misinterpretation.

The exam should first be performed using a higher gain level, and soon the gain is adjusted as necessary to optimize the brightness for better image resolution.

A successful interpretation of a B-scan ultrasound relies upon the capacity of the examiner to think in three dimensions while scanning in two dimensions. The users mentally integrate many two-dimensional images to form an impression of the anatomy and pathology in three dimensions.

Diagnostic Parameters

Once a lesion or an abnormality is detected by the sonographic screening, the topographic, quantitative, and kinetic parameters are analyzed.

Topographic Parameters

A combination of transverse, longitudinal, and axial scans assesses a lesion's location, extension, shape, contours, size, and relationship with adjacent structures.

The lesion is initially evaluated with a transverse scan to define its location and lateral extension. Shifting the probe from the limbus to the fornix can determine the approximate location of the lesion. Then, a longitudinal scan is employed

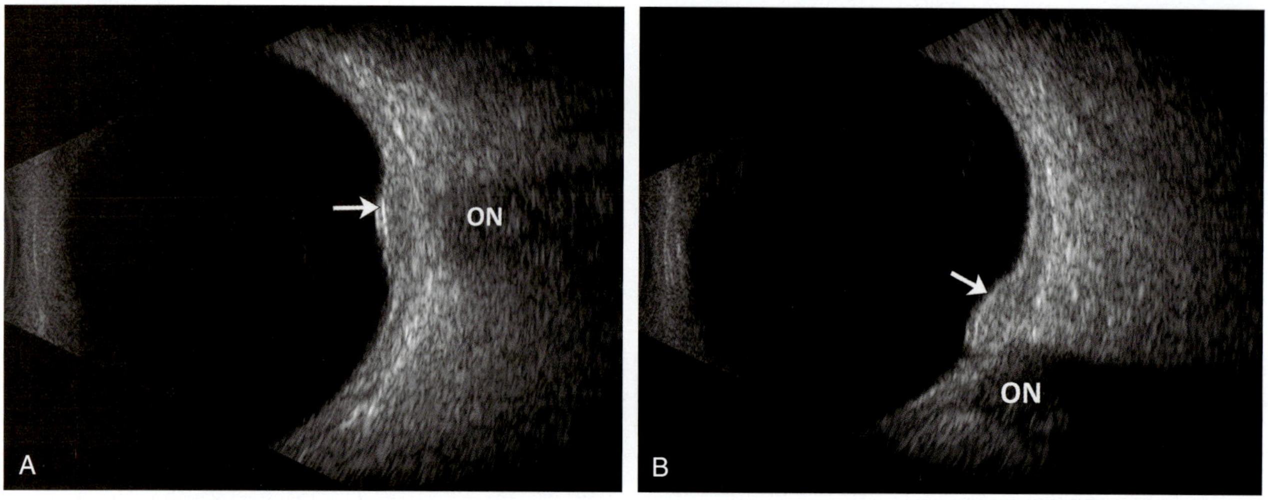

• **Fig. 2.13** Lesion Location. **(A)** A transverse scan displays a focal, solid, mass-like fundus lesion (*arrow*) extending for approximately two meridians laterally. (B) Longitudinal B-scan displays the lesion (*arrow*) at the posterior pole, touching the optic disc. *ON*, Optic nerve.

to assess its radial extension and relationship with the optic disc, macula, and peripheral zone (Figs. 2.13 and 2.14).

The shape of the lesion or finding on ultrasound can be described as punctiform, membranous, mass-like, or irregularly shaped (Fig. 2.15).

The lesion or any finding on ultrasound must be carefully scanned in transverse and longitudinal positions for measurements, sweeping the sound beam from margin to margin to estimate the maximal elevation and basal diameters (Fig. 2.16 and Video 2.6).

TEACHING POINT

Echographic landmarks. The optic nerve is an important anatomic landmark to identifying the scanning plane at the posterior pole. The insertions of the recti muscles are the sonographic reference for the region anterior to the equator.

Quantitative Parameters

After a lesion has been detected and localized, the internal structure, reflectivity, and sound attenuation are analyzed. Ophthalmic ultrasonography devices with better image resolution currently offer a reasonable evaluation of these properties with a B-scan mode. A standardized A-scan, at tissue sensitivity, through the area of greatest interest can complement the B-scan exam to define the quantitative parameters further.

Reflectivity

For greater accuracy, the reflectivity of the lesions should be evaluated with a standardized A-scan at tissue sensitivity and having the probe facing a lesion in maximal perpendicularity (Fig. 2.17). Reflectivity is the amplitude of the lesion spikes, expressed as a percentage of the total echogram height. According to the height of spikes, the A-scan reflectivity measured at tissue sensitivity can

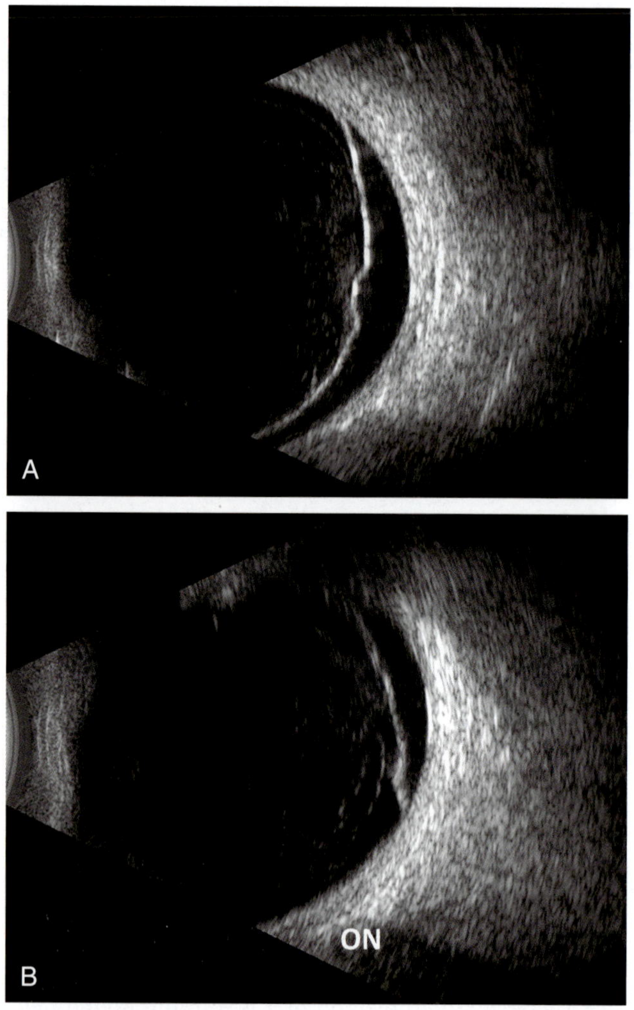

• **Fig. 2.14** Topographic Information. Abnormal Finding Location. **(A)** Transverse B-scan showing a retinal detachment extending for approximately five meridians laterally. **(B)** Longitudinal B-scan showing the anteroposterior extension of a retinal detachment from the midperiphery to the ora serrata region. *ON*, Optic nerve.

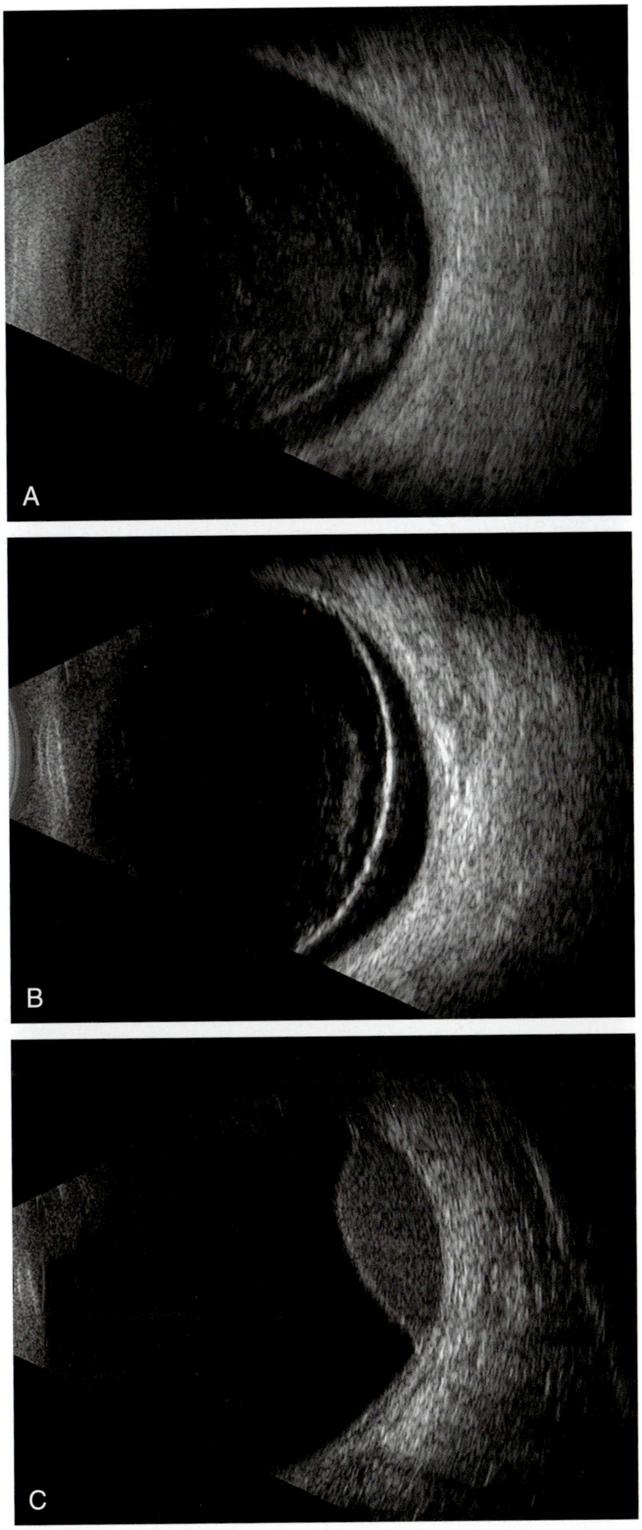

• **Fig. 2.15** Shape of Ultrasonographic Findings. Distinct shapes, **(A)** punctiform, **(B)** membranous, and **(C)** mass-like.

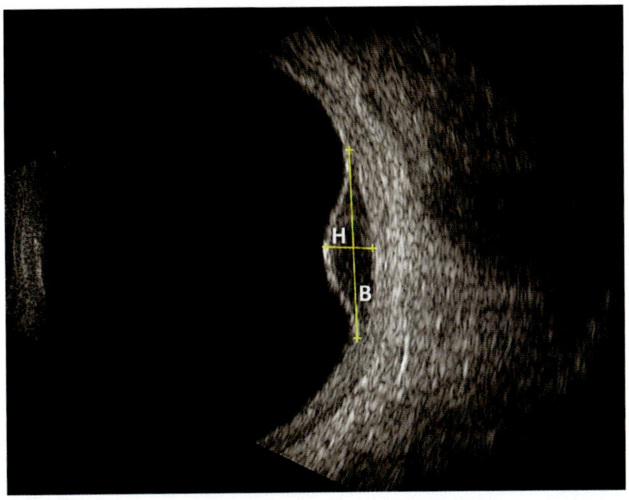

• **Fig. 2.16** Lesion Measurement. Electronic calipers measure the maximal height (H) and largest basal diameter (B) of a tumor.

TABLE 2.1 Levels of Reflectivity Using A-Scan at Tissue Sensitivity Setting

Level	Spike Height (%)
Markedly low	0–5
Low	5–40
Medium	40–60
Medium-high	60–80
High	80–100

be classified as markedly low (0–5%), low (5–40%), medium (40–60%), medium-high (60–80%), and high (80–100%) (Table 2.1).[5] A detached retina is a classic example of highly reflective tissue (Fig. 2.18). Vitreous hemorrhage can produce spikes of low to high reflectivity, depending on the organization of the blood over time (Fig. 2.19).

The reflectivity of the tissues can be grossly estimated on B-scan mode observing the intensity of signal brightness compared to the hyporreflective normal vitreous or the hyperreflective scleral tissue. This technique does not offer as high accuracy as the A-scan because the intensity of the echoes changes with the gain setting.

Internal Structure

The internal structure of a mass lesion or a subretinal or suprachoroidal space can be evaluated with a B-scan or A-scan, shifting the probe to different lesion areas. The internal lesion structure is directly correlated to its histological architecture. For a more homogenous, compact histological arrangement in the entire lesion, the echotexture is more regular; conversely, if the histological arrangement is heterogeneous in different areas of the lesion, the echotexture is irregular (Fig. 2.20).

Sound Attenuation

Sound energy can be progressively attenuated through scattering and absorption by a medium. Sound attenuation is manifested by the progressive decrease in the strength of the echoes on the B- or A-scan. The "angle kappa" is the angle formed by

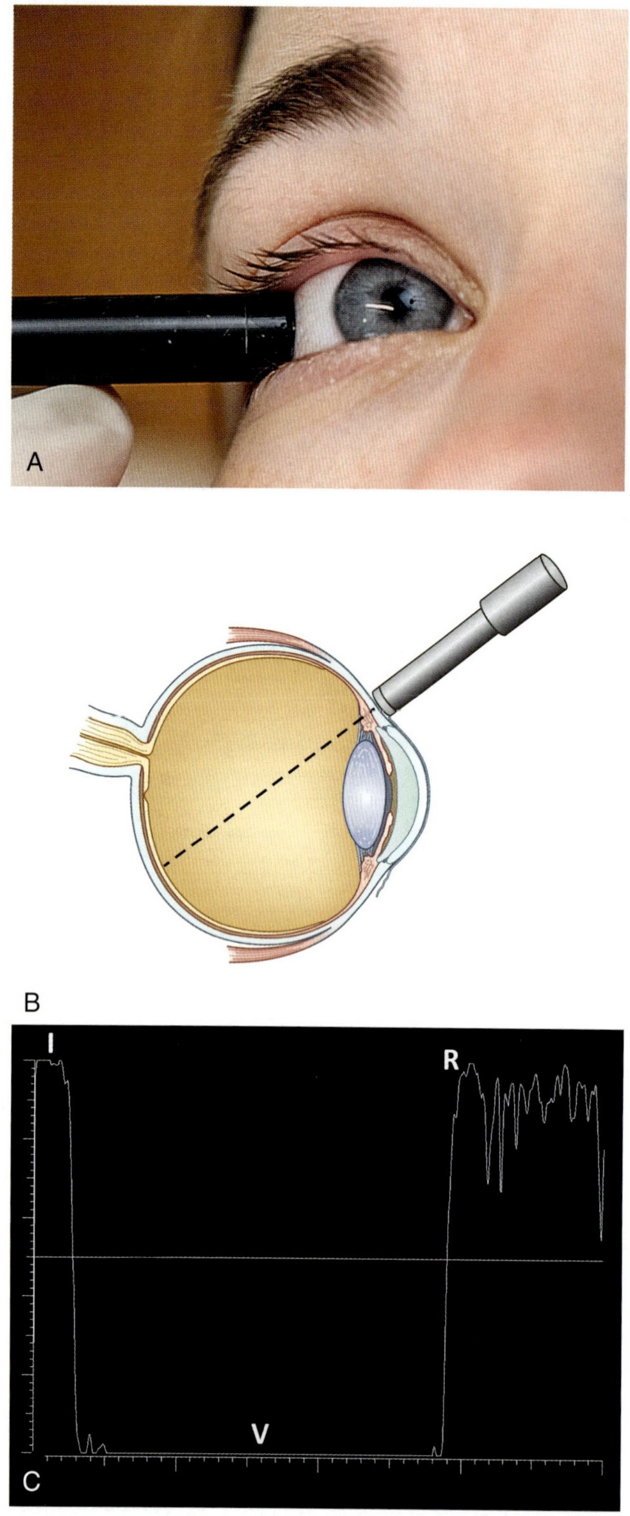

• **Fig. 2.17** **(A)** Standardized A-scan at tissue sensitivity exam for tissue reflectivity and structure evaluation. **(B)** The probe is placed opposite the area to be examined while the patient looks in the direction of the meridian to be examined. **(C)** A-scan of a normal eye. *I*, initial spike pairing the probe tip and ocular wall. *R*, Retina; *V*, vitreous cavity.

drawing a line through the peaks of the internal lesion spikes and intersecting the horizontal baseline of the A-scan echogram. The steeper the angle, the greater the sound attenuation.

Some tumors attenuate sound waves substantially, whereas others attenuate sound very little (Fig. 2.21). Marked sound attenuation causes an acoustic shadow following the lesion on B-scan. Strong sound attenuation is characteristic of specific lesions such as intraocular foreign bodies or those containing calcium or bone, for example, choroidal osteoma, retinoblastoma, drusen, phthisis bulbi, etc. (Fig. 2.22).

Kinetic Parameters

Ultrasound makes it unique among other imaging techniques in that it permits active evaluation and, therefore, significant functional information. Kinetic echography assesses the vascularity, aftermovement, convection motion, and consistency (compressibility).[6]

Vascularity

Having the patient's eye steady and holding the probe fixed on the globe allows the examiner to assess the internal vascularity of a tumor. Spontaneous motion with fast, low-amplitude flickering within the lesion indicative of vascular flow can be detected with B-scan (Fig. 2.23 and Video 2.7). On a standardized A-scan, vascularity is indicated by the very fast vertical movement of the spikes. Moreover, vascularity may be observed along portions of the retina and choroid.

Aftermovement

Following cessation of eye movement, typical mobility of vitreous gel, membranes, or fluid level can be evaluated with B-scan. The probe is held steady on the globe, and the patient is directed to move in the same direction of the sound beam, that is, up and down for vertical transverse and left to right for horizontal transverse (Fig. 2.24 and Video 2.8).

Convection Motion

This type of slow, spontaneous movement is caused by the circulation of fine particles (blood, lipids, or silicone oil droplets) within a cavity or anatomic space, for example, the motion of fine particles of a diffuse hemorrhage in the vitreous cavity in a vitrectomized eye or lipids in the subretinal space in long-standing retinal detachment (Fig. 2.25 and Video 2.9).

Consistency

The compression test is helpful in evaluating the firmness of orbital masses. Hard or soft tissues respond differently to a mild probe pressure over the eye (Fig. 2.26 and Video 2.10).

Orbit

In orbital disorders, multimodal imaging has helped improve the ability to diagnose and guide the therapy of many pathologies. Ultrasound is a cost-effective, dynamic real-time imaging modality adjunct to computed tomography and magnetic resonance imaging in orbital diseases.

The methods employed to assess the orbit are transocular and paraocular approaches.

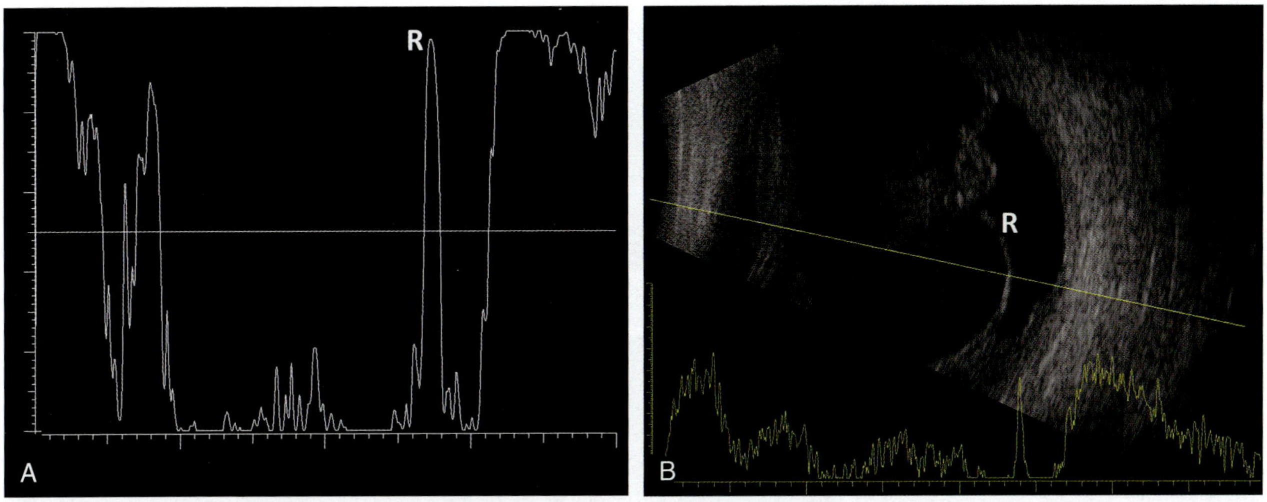

• **Fig. 2.18** Reflectivity on Standardized A-scan. **(A)** Highly reflective spike produced by a detached retina (R). **(B)** The corresponding B-scan showing a retinal detachment (R). *R*, Retina.

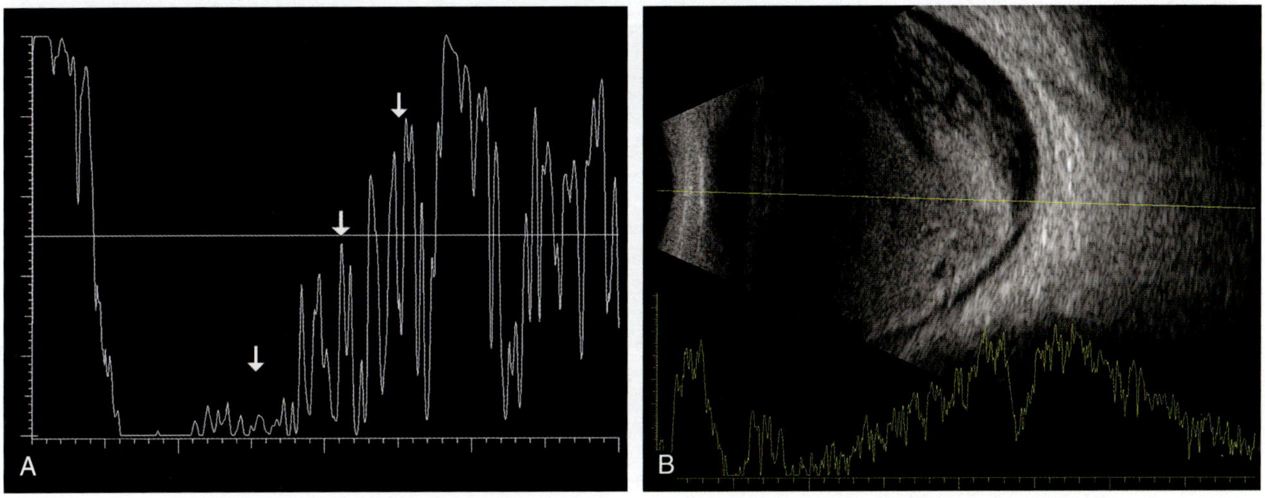

• **Fig. 2.19** Reflectivity on Standardized A-scan. **(A)** Low to medium-high reflective spikes produced by vitreous hemorrhage (*arrows*) near the fundus. **(B)** The corresponding B-scan shows a dense vitreous hemorrhage. *R*, Retina.

The transocular approach evaluates lesions located in the mid- and posterior orbit (see Fig. 2.3), with the transducer scanning in axial, transverse, and longitudinal positions.

The paraocular approach is used to assess the lids and anterior orbit (see Fig. 2.4). The probe is placed over the lids, and the orientations employed are transverse and longitudinal. This technique shows the interaction of an orbital lesion with the globe and orbital wall. A paraocular modified immersion technique, using a scleral shell or a finger of a glove filled with water, displays images of superficial lesions located within the eyelid or the anterior margin of an anterior orbital lesion (Fig. 2.27 and Video 2.11).

The B-scan orbital examination is generally conducted with a medium gain setting. It is a good practice to examine the orbit bilaterally, mainly in subtle changes, comparing the same area of both sides using the same scan orientation.

B-scan mode is used to evaluate the topographic features of an orbital disorder (location, size, shape, borders, extension, and integrity of orbital bone). A-scan is employed to assess the quantitative features (internal structure, reflectivity, and sound attenuation).

It is important to note the limitation of the ophthalmic ultrasound to image the orbital apex because the penetration into the orbit is expected to be less than achieved with a lower frequency probe.[7]

TEACHING POINT

Gain setting in the orbital exam. Since orbital soft tissues are hyperreflective, adjusting the gain to a medium level improves the ability to distinguish irregularities of orbital structures.

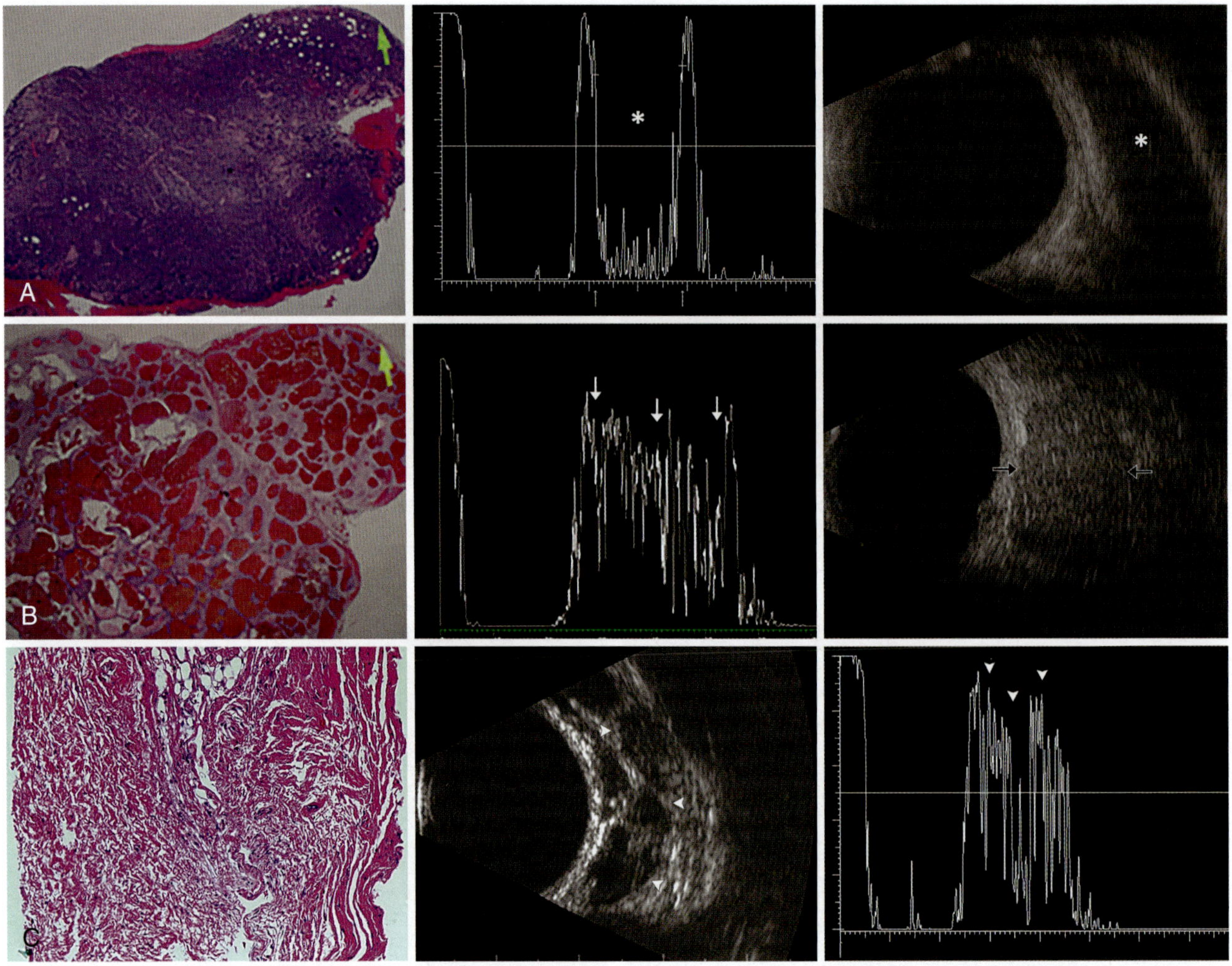

• **Fig. 2.20** Histopathological and Sonographic Correlation in Orbital Lesions. **(A)** Histology of a single type of small cells compactly arranged in lymphoma, and corresponding sonograms presenting as low reflective with homogeneous texture (*asterisk*). **(B)** Pathology of large vascular spaces with homogeneous distribution in cavernous hemangioma matching highly reflective spikes with the regular internal structure on ultrasound (*arrows*). **(C)** Histological appearance of a lymphangioma showing lymph-filled spaces of varying sizes and corresponding ultrasound with heterogeneous echoes (*arrowheads*).

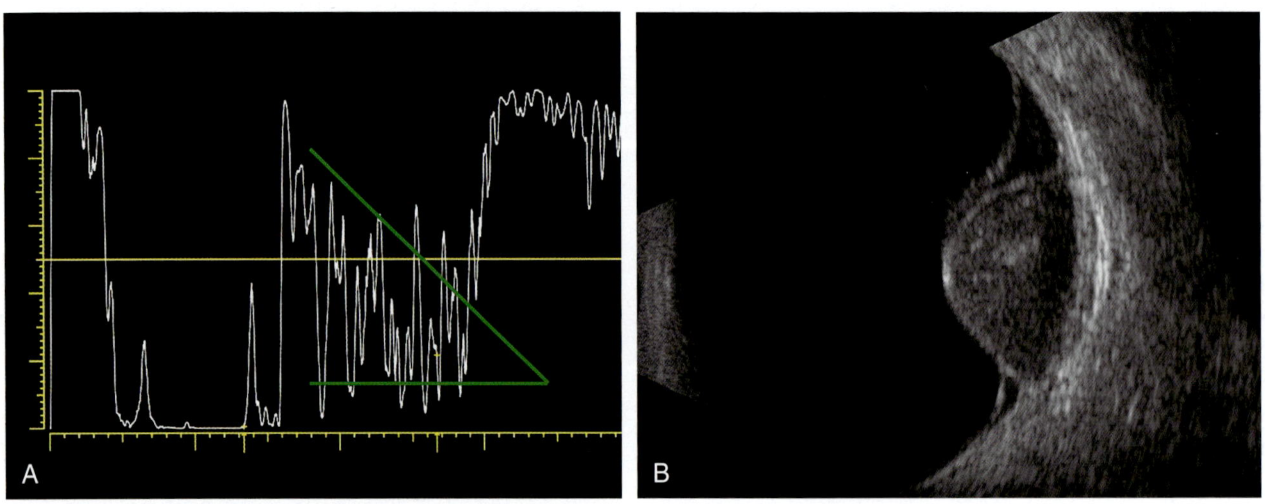

• **Fig. 2.21** Sound Attenuation. **(A)** A-scan of an intraocular mass showing decreasing spikes heights defining an angle kappa (in green). **(B)** Corresponding B-scan of the intraocular tumor showing echolucent area at the tumor's base.

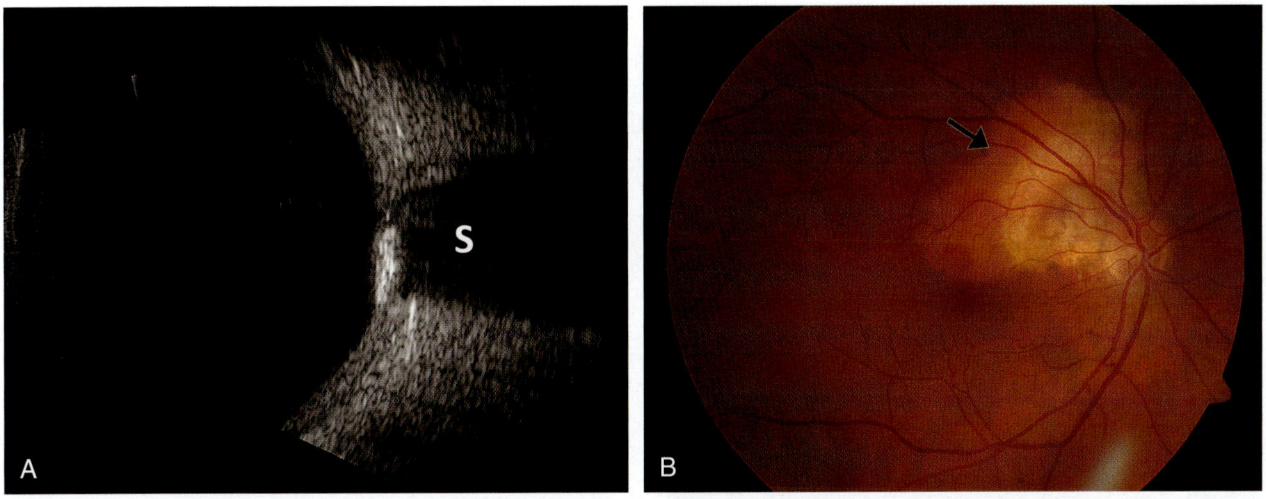

• **Fig. 2.22** Sound Attenuation. **(A)** Longitudinal B-scan displaying a marked calcified plaque-like fundus lesion causing a distinct acoustic shadow (S) in the posterior tissues. **(B)** Fundus photography of the calcified lesion (*arrow*) superotemporal to the optic disc.

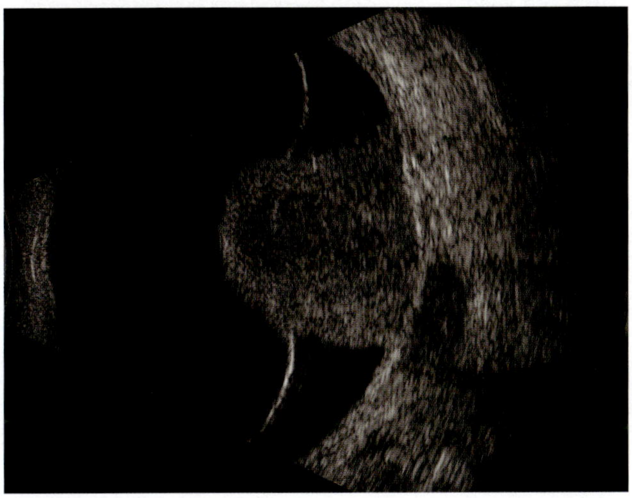

• **Fig. 2.23** Captured still image from the video of intrinsic vascularity of a tumor.

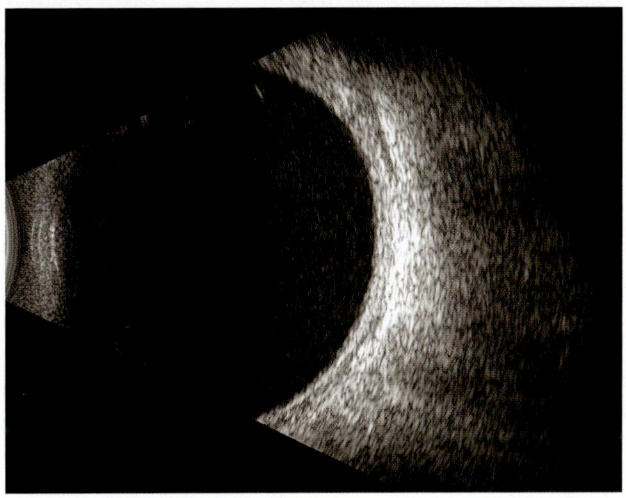

• **Fig. 2.25** Captured still image from the video of a convection motion of blood in the vitreous cavity.

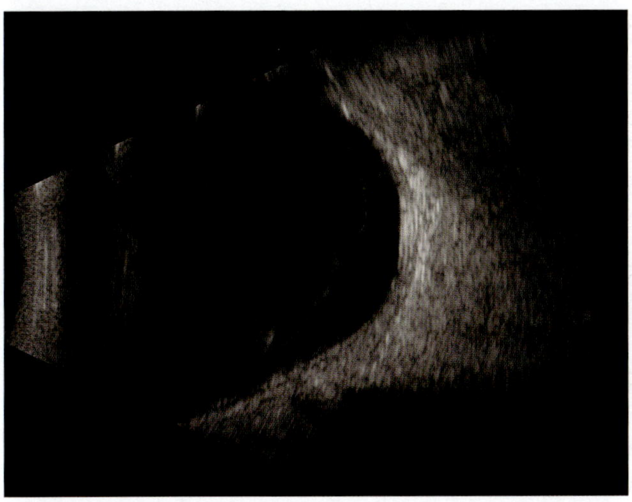

• **Fig. 2.24** Captured still image from the video of aftermovement of a membrane.

Scanning the Anterior Segment

High-frequency ultrasound biomicroscopy (UBM) provides high-resolution imaging of the anterior segment. The technology is based on a 50- to 100-MHz transducer incorporated into a B-mode clinical scanner. The tissue penetration is approximately 5 mm.[2]

The direction of the movement of the transducer is oriented by a mark, usually a white line located on one side of the probe. The marker may direct an image both from the left or from the right edge of the screen; such information should be provided in the manufacturer's user manual.

The UBM examination technique is analogous to B-mode ultrasound for the posterior segment. The patient is examined in a supine position facing the ceiling in a dim lightroom. After topical anesthesia, a single-use distilled water-filled bag or a reusable immersion conical scleral shell filled with saline

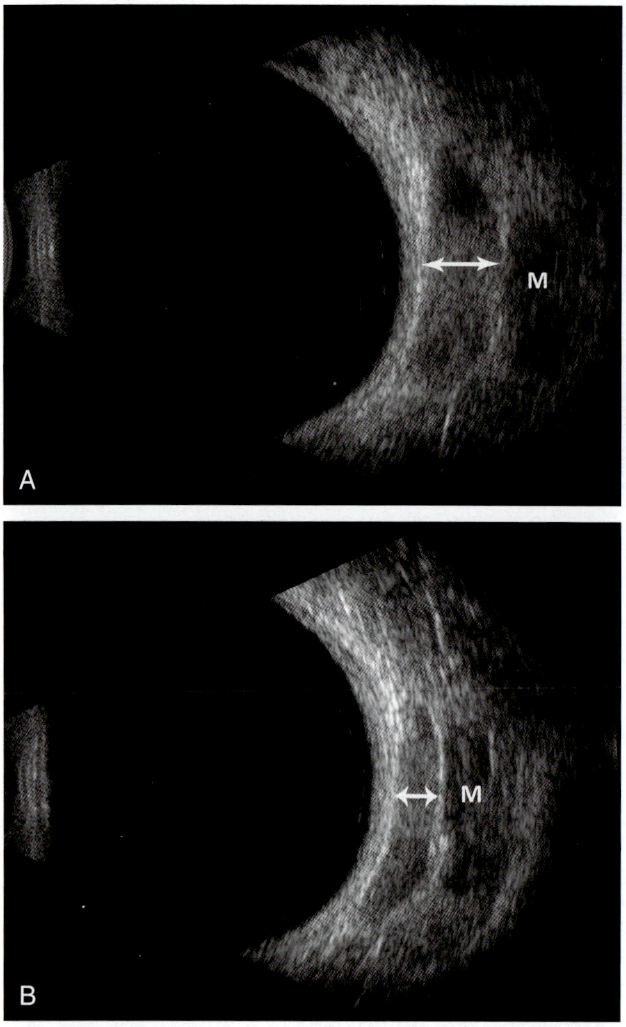

• **Fig. 2.26** Compression Test. **(A)** Orbital lesion (*connected arrows*) prior to probe pressure over the eye. **(B)** Decreased diameter of the lesion under probe pressure. *M*, Extraocular muscle.

solution is used to separate the eyelids and produce a coupling medium between the transducer and the eye. A distilled water-filled bag device (Fig. 2.28A) has the advantage of comfort for the patient, and the exam can be performed in an upright sitting position. The reusable immersion conical scleral shells (Fig. 2.28B) are available in 18–22 mm diameters.

It is critical to adjust the internal bag pressure in the water bag method, especially in patients with low intraocular pressure.

TEACHING POINT

Air bubbles. Air forms a barrier to sound and casts a shadowing artifact. Care should be taken to remove air bubbles from the water-filled bag or a reusable immersion conical scleral shell for the UBM exam.

UBM assessment of the anterior segment can be performed using axial, longitudinal, and transverse scans.

TEACHING POINT

UBM scanning. In contrast to the posterior segment B-scan, in which the probe is placed opposite to the area to be examined, in UBM, the probe is placed directly over the site to be examined.

On the axial scan, the probe is placed on the center of the cornea with the patient in primary gaze fixation. The scan can be oriented in the horizontal, vertical, or oblique planes. The image generated shows the cornea, anterior chamber, anterior lens capsule, iris, camerular angle, and anterior portion of the ciliary body (Fig. 2.29 and Video 2.12). This view is the first choice for evaluating the centralization of intraocular lens implants.

For longitudinal and transverse scans, the patient looks slightly opposite the examined area, creating more space for probe contact.

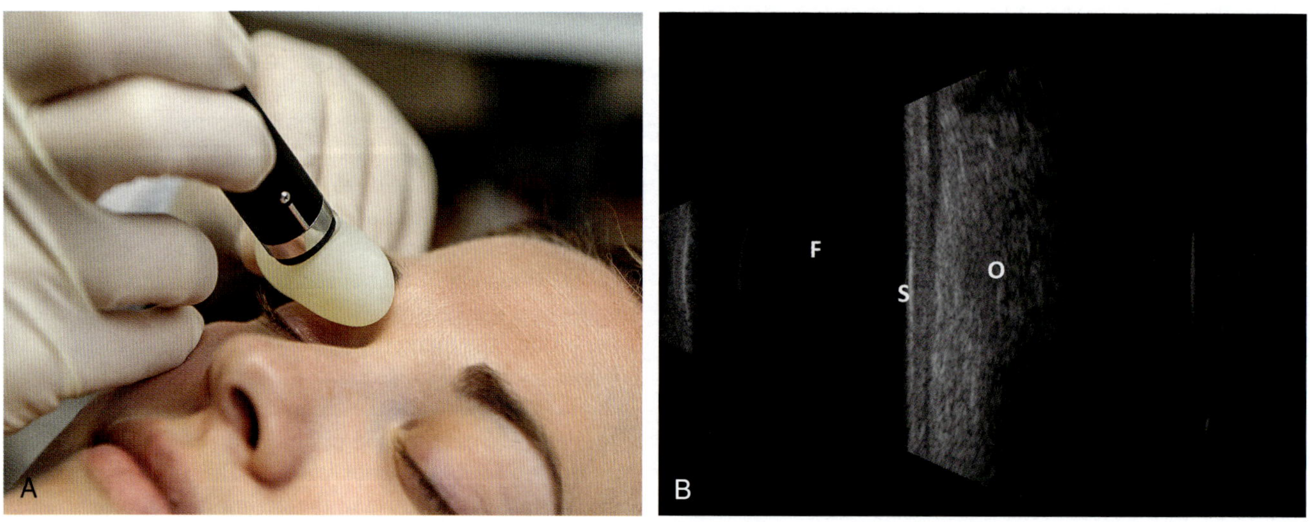

• **Fig. 2.27** **(A)** Paraocular modified immersion using a finger of a glove filled with water. **(B)** Resulting echogram. *F*, Fluid; *S*, skin; *O*, soft orbital tissue.

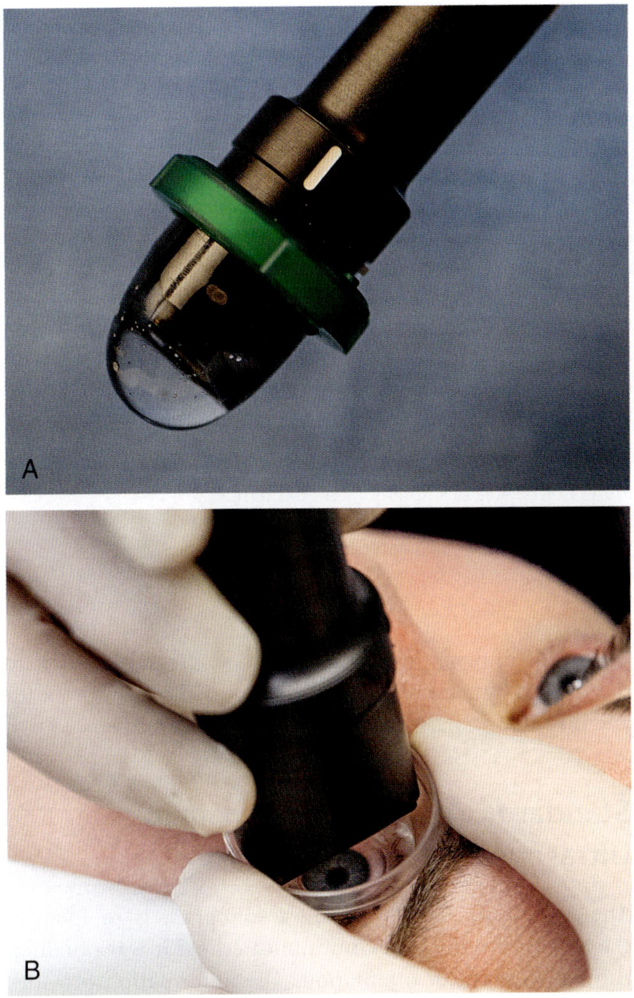

• **Fig. 2.28** **(A)** 50 MHz UBM probe covered with a distilled water-filled bag. **(B)** UBM exam using a fluid-filled scleral shell.

On the longitudinal scan, the probe is placed over the limbus, radially, with the sound beam oriented perpendicular to the limbus (Fig. 2.30 and Videos 2.13 and 2.14). This orientation is the choice to evaluate the anterior chamber angle and identify the scleral spur, allowing qualitative and quantitative angle assessment (Fig. 2.31). Moreover, the anteroposterior extension of the iris and ciliary body lesion is defined using this orientation.

On the transverse scan, the probe is placed parallel to the limbus, on the paracentral zone of the cornea. The probe is then shifted toward the pars plana; thus, the ciliary body and ora serrata can be imaged. This orientation is appropriate for showing the lateral (i.e., circumferential) extent of a lesion (Fig. 2.32 and Videos 2.15 and 2.16).

A recommended screening sequence uses axial horizontal and vertical first, followed by longitudinal and transverse scans in the cardinal clock hours, shifting the probe from the cornea to ora serrata.

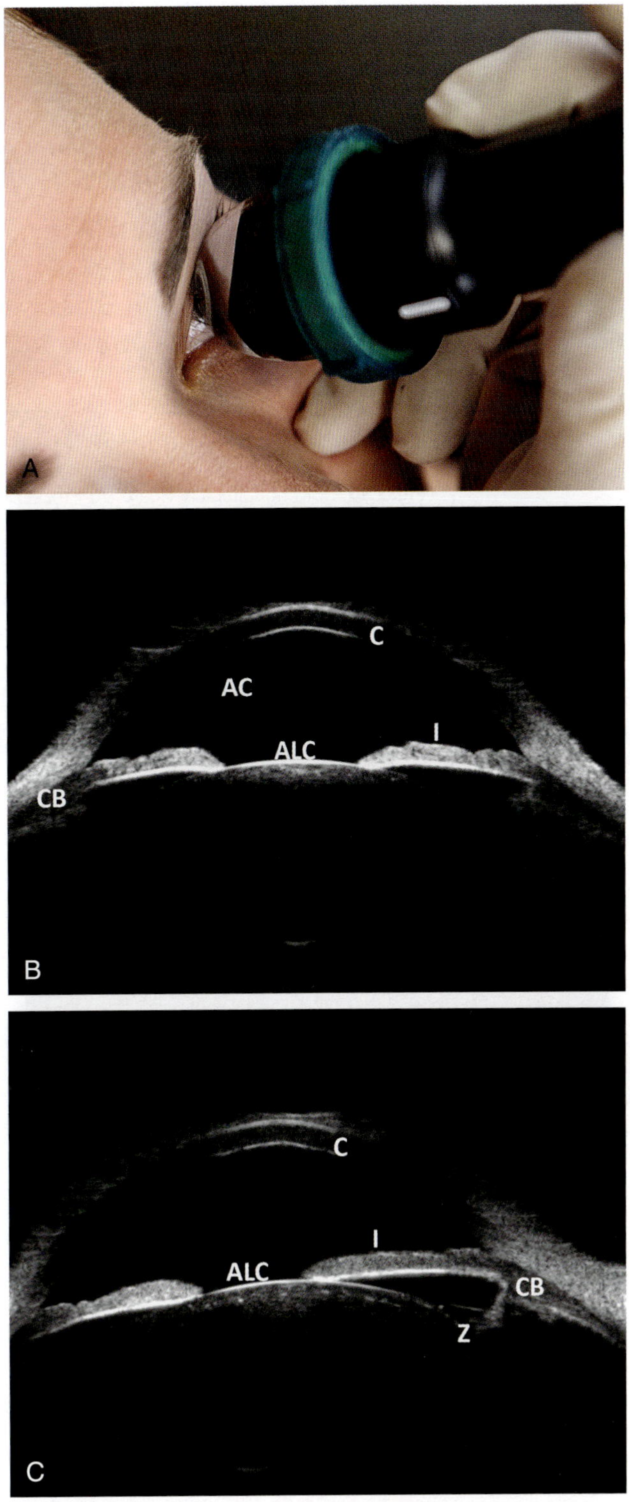

• **Fig. 2.29** UBM axial scan. **(A)** Probe placement on the center of the cornea. **(B)** The corresponding sonogram shows the axial view of the anterior segment. *ALC*, Anterior lens capsule; *AC*, anterior chamber; *CB*, ciliary body; *C*, cornea; *I*, iris; *Z*, zonules. **(C)** Axial scan is slightly inclined to assess the zonules.

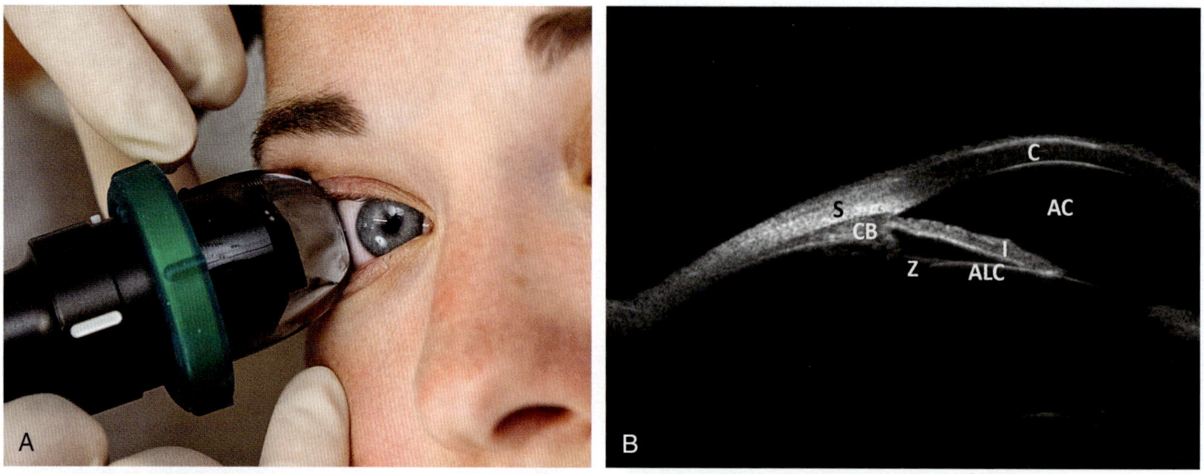

• **Fig. 2.30** UBM Longitudinal Scan. **(A)** Probe placed on the corneoscleral limbus to scan the temporal meridian. The patient looks slightly at the opposite meridian. **(B)** The corresponding sonogram shows the anteroposterior extension of the temporal meridian. *AC*, Anterior chamber; *ALC*, anterior lens capsule; *C*, cornea; *CB*, ciliary body; *I*, iris; *S*, sclera *Z*, zonules.

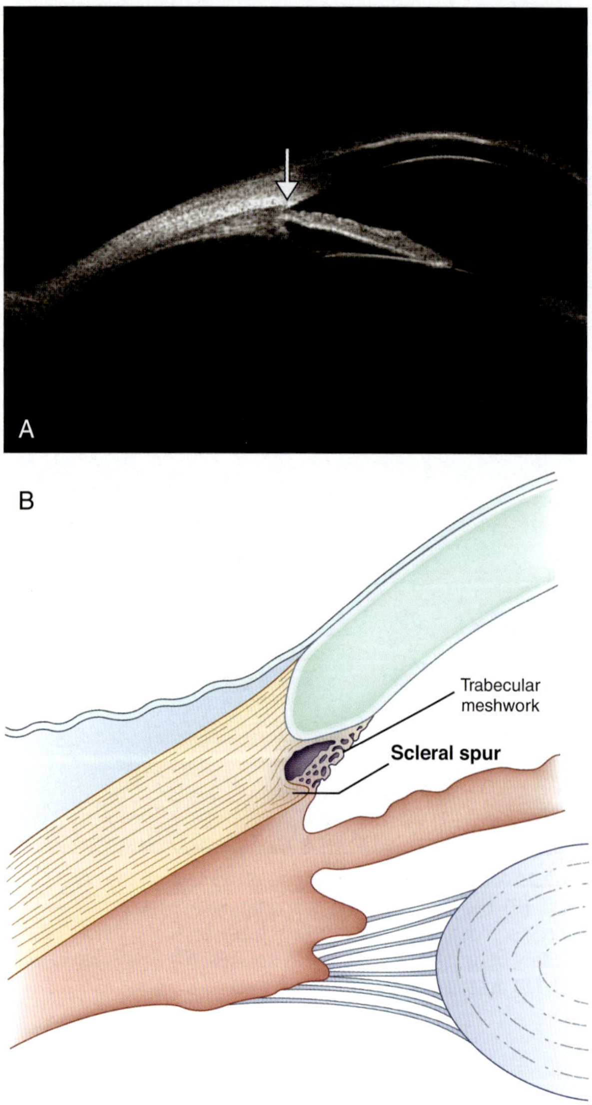

• **Fig. 2.31** UBM Longitudinal Scan to Assess the Anterior Chamber Angle. **(A)** The scleral spur (*arrow*) marks the posterior border of the trabecular meshwork. **(B)** Schematic diagram of the angle showing the anterior chamber angle structures.

The instruments display an area of better resolution, usually demarcated by a line or two parallel lines. Moving the probe up and down positions the object of interest in this zone.

Standard Labeling of Ophthalmic Ultrasound Images

The main purpose of labeling a sonogram is to identify the area of interest and communicate how it was obtained through transducer orientation. This information provides a means for communication from one operator to another, from sonographer to image interpreter, and from one site or institution to another.

The sonograms are labeled according to the eye region where the sound beam is aimed.

A recommended format of label should contain the following:

1. Laterality: OD (*ocular dexter*) for the right eye and OS (*ocular sinister*) for the left eye.
2. Scanning plane:
   a. Transverse scan: the resulting sonogram should be labeled with the clock hour centered in the sonogram, followed by the region. **P**, posterior (the region just as the nerve is touched); **PE**, posterior to the equator; **EP**, equator posterior (just behind the equator); **E**, equator (just anterior to the rectus muscle insertion; **EA**, anterior to the equator; **O,** ora serrata; **CB**, ciliary body; **AX**, optic axis (Fig. 2.33).
      Example: 9E indicates the sound beam centered at the 9 o'clock meridian at the region of the equator using a transverse scan.
   b. Longitudinal scan: the sonogram is labeled with the abbreviation L (longitudinal), adding the clock hour of the meridian scanned.
      Example: L12 indicates the 12 o'clock meridian using a longitudinal scan.

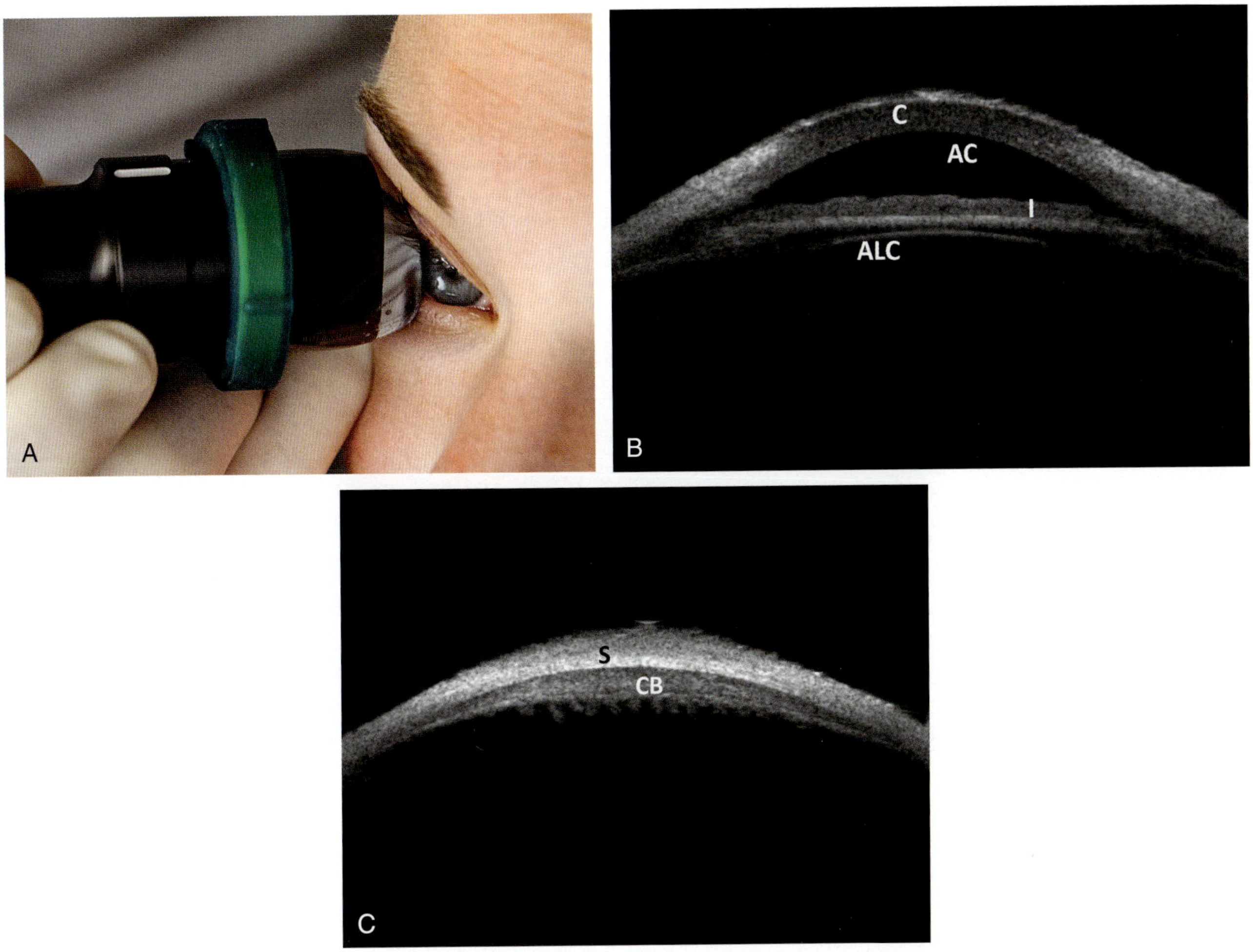

• **Fig. 2.32** UBM Transverse Scan. **(A)** The probe is placed parallel to the limbus. **(B)** Transverse section at the level of the anterior chamber. **(C)** Transverse section slightly posterior to the limbus. *AC*, Anterior chamber; *ALC*, anterior lens capsule; *C*, cornea; *CB*, ciliary body; *I*, iris; *S*, sclera.

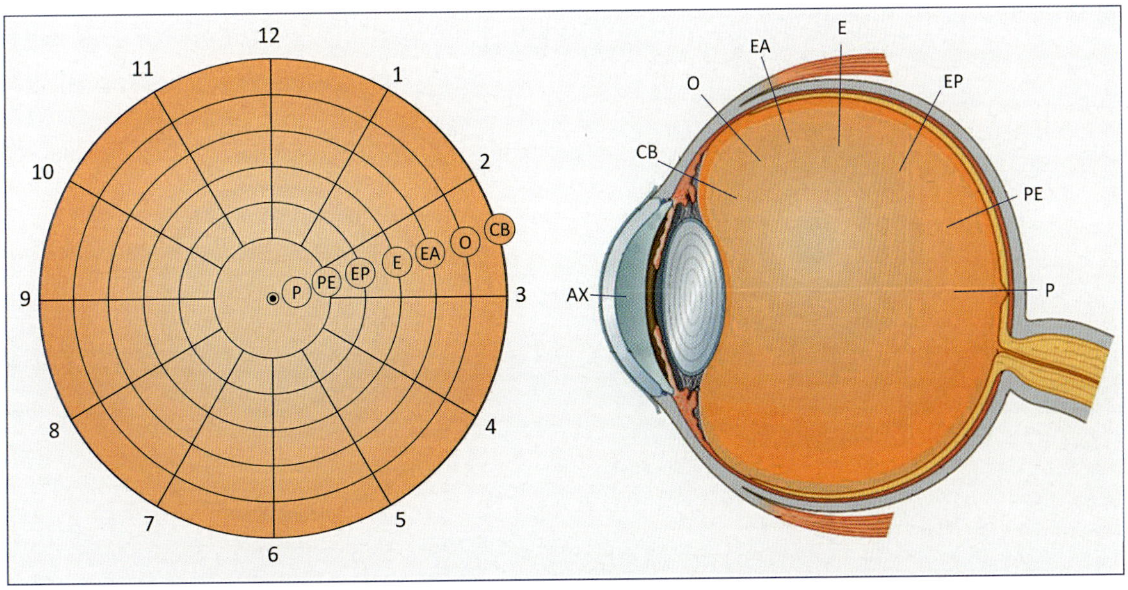

• **Fig. 2.33** Labeling an Ophthalmic Sonogram. Fundus diagram and axial horizontal section of the eye show the fundus regions.

References

1. Ossoinig KC. Standardized echography: basic principles, clinical applications, and results. *Int Ophthalmol Clin*. 1979;19:127–210.
2. Pavlin CJ, Harasiewicz K, Sherar MD, Foster FS. Clinical use of ultrasound biomicroscopy. *Ophthalmology*. 1991;98:287–295.
3. Allemann N, Coleman DJ, Pavlin CJ, Huang D. Imaging the anterior segment: high-frequency ultrasound and anterior segment OCT. *J Ophthalmol*. 2013:398715.
4. Guthoff RF, Labriola LT, Stachs O. Diagnostic ophthalmic ultrasound. In: Ryan SJ, ed. *Retina*. 5th ed. Elsevier; 2013.
5. Byrne SF. Standardized echography of the eye and orbit. *Neuroradiology*. 1986;28(5–6):618–640.
6. Garcia JP. *Dynamic Ophthalmic Ultrasonography*. Lippincott Williams & Wilkins; 2009.
7. Dutton JJ, Byrne SF, Proia AD. *Diagnostic Atlas of Orbital Diseases*. WB Saunders Company; 2000.

3

The Normal Globe and Orbit

CAMILE FREITAS TONIN AND NORMA ALLEMANN

The normal human eye can be studied using ocular ultrasound to access the intraocular structures through three scanning strategies: axial, longitudinal, and transversal, and all must be used during the routine examination.[1] The anatomical correspondence of the eye is easily recognized in the image recorded on the ultrasound, respecting the already standardized orientation of the probe marker for adequate definition of what is above and below the image window (ultrasound).[2]

Some exam techniques can be used to obtain ocular ultrasound images: contact techniques, through the eyelids (transpalpebral) or direct (corneal touch), both using conductive gel; and immersion techniques, using an immersion cup filled with saline solution. In this last modality, distancing the probe from the eyeball allows structures from the anterior segment to appear in the image window.

Normal Adult Eye

The normal adult eye has a well-delimited posterior contour and is normally spherical.

When using the contact technique in B-scan ultrasound, the anterior segment is observed in a low-resolution area of the ultrasound (Fig. 3.1).

The normal lens appears as a well-defined, ecolucent oval structure. The posterior capsule is always evident in the phakic eye, regardless of the transparency of the structure. The crescent-shaped center of the posterior lens capsule is hyperreflective and, generally, best demonstrated in relation to the periphery of the lens.

The vitreous body of the normal eye is ecolucent, which creates an acoustic void in the cavity, with no identification of A-scan mode peaks.

The posterior ocular wall comprises of three layers, and the B-scan mode usually allows differentiation between two of them: the retinochoroidal layer and the sclera.

The optic nerve appears as a conical-shaped acoustic shadow placed posterior to the ocular wall.[3]

An axial B-scan of a normal eye shows aligned echoes from the cornea, anterior and posterior lens capsules, vitreous, posterior ocular wall, and orbital fat.

A longitudinal B-scan demonstrates one slice of the eye, allowing the observation of the posterior ocular wall at that meridian, from the optic nerve to the periphery.

Axial Scan

The normal adult eye is best measured when the B-scan and C-vectors are perfectly aligned. Measurements of the axial length of the eye are taken using axial scans.

In axial scans, the anterior surface of the cornea is poorly defined due to its proximity to the ultrasound probe when using contact techniques. The crystalline lens must be aligned with the optic nerve for adequate positioning of the C vector and must occupy the center of the ultrasound. The approximate measurement of the anteroposterior diameter of the globe can be taken in both A- and B-scans using contact or immersion techniques (Figs. 3.2 and 3.3, video 3.1).

The mean adult values for axial length are 22–25 mm.[4,5]

- Contact Technique

  When using contact technique, the first best-defined structure is the posterior lens capsules aligned with the sound beam for 100% reflections (echoes) (Figs. 3.1 and 3.2).

  The evaluation of the iris, anterior chamber angle, posterior chamber, and zonular ligaments remain at low resolution when using the 10 MHz probes. However, variation is possible depending on the ultrasound machines used.
- Immersion Technique

  Immersion technique is used to distance the cornea and anterior segment structures from the probe, utilizing a scleral shell with saline solution.

When using immersion technique, the distinction between the two corneal surfaces (anterior and posterior) is possible, and the echoes appear as two high-amplitude peaks in A-scan mode ultrasound (Fig. 3.3 and video 3.1).

Longitudinal Scan

The longitudinal scan evaluates a specific meridian from the optic disc to the periphery of the posterior ocular wall, placed in the ultrasound from the bottom to the top,

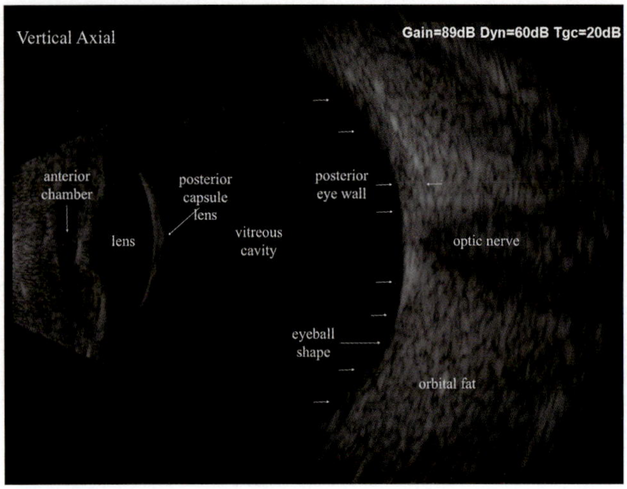

• **Fig. 3.1** Morphological globe analysis of the normal adult eye. 10 MHz B-scan ultrasound, vertical axial scan, transpalpebral contact technique. On the ultrasound, it is possible to identify the anterior segment in a low-resolution area (anterior chamber). The contour of the posterior eye wall is normally spherical (*horizontal arrows pointing right*). The normal lens appears as a well-defined, ecolucent oval structure. The posterior capsule is always evident in the phakic eye, regardless of the transparency of the structure. The crescent-shaped center of the posterior lens capsule is hyperreflective and generally best demonstrated in relation to the periphery of the lens. The vitreous body of the normal eye is ecolucent, on A-scan mode peaks identified, which creates an acoustic void in the cavity. The posterior ocular wall (*horizontal arrow pointing left*) can be identified on ultrasound as two layers: retinochoroidal layer and sclera. The optic nerve appears as a conical-shaped acoustic shadow. The orbital fat is highly reflective.

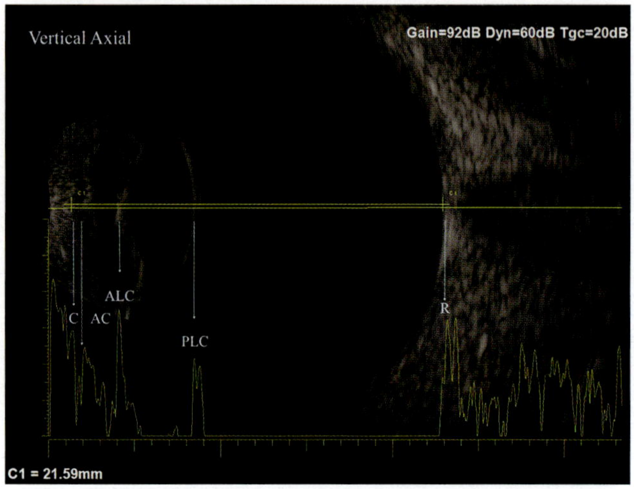

• **Fig. 3.2** Measurement of the axial length of the normal adult eye using B-mode guided biometry. 10 MHz B-scan ultrasound, vertical axial scan, transpalpebral contact technique. The anterior surface of the cornea is poorly defined due to its proximity to the ultrasound probe. The crystalline lens must be aligned with the optic nerve for adequate positioning of the C-vector and must occupy the center of the ultrasound. The approximate measurement of the anteroposterior diameter of the globe can be taken in both A- and B-scans. Along the C-vector, peaks of variable amplitude are recorded according to the structure present in the sound beam: *C*. cornea (presumed); *AC*, anterior chamber; *ALC*, anterior lens capsule; *PLC*, posterior lens capsule; *R*, retina. The axial measurement is measured from the anterior echo of the cornea to the retina. The approximate axial length value in the example is 21.59 mm.

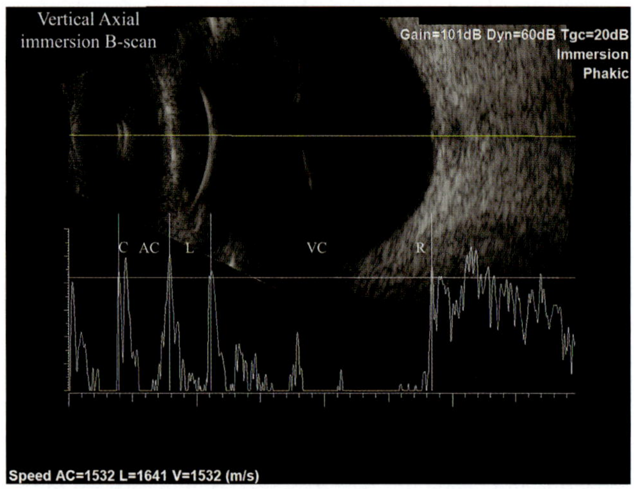

• **Fig. 3.3** Measurement of axial length of the normal adult eye using B-mode guided biometry. 10 MHz B-scan ultrasound, vertical axial scan, immersion technique. Using immersion, the distinction between the two corneal peaks (anterior and posterior) is possible, appearing as two high-amplitude peaks observed in A-mode (C). Here, four vectors are available in A-mode, whose editing must coincide with mode B: *C*, cornea; *AC*, anterior chamber; *L*, lens; *VC*, vitreous cavity; *R*, retina. The axial measurement obtained is 24.57 mm.

respectively. Therefore, the optic nerve and the periphery of the eye wall occupy the edges of the image window and can hardly be together in the same ultrasound. The normal optic disc follows the smooth profile of the eye wall. All meridians look the same and must be correctly identified according to the meridian evaluated in clock hours (e.g., 1 o'clock longitudinal and 2 o'clock longitudinal).

Using the longitudinal scan, when the probe is positioned to evaluate the anterior portion of the ocular wall, it is possible to image part of the anterior chamber angle, as well as the iris and ciliary body. This is possible under maximal excursion of the eye and forward angulation of the transducer/probe (Fig. 3.4 and video 3.2). A posterior acoustic shadowing artifact is typically observed at the periphery of the posterior eye wall.

For better analysis, the posterior ocular wall can be divided in posterior pole, equator, and periphery (Fig. 3.4). This clinical correlation makes it easier to locate structures and injuries, especially in serial examinations.

On ocular ultrasound, the ocular wall appears as a homogeneous band of hyperreflectivity, with two hyperreflective peaks: the retinal profile and the sclera, respectively. It is only possible to evaluate the retina in isolation if it is detached or if there is subretinal fluid accumulation.

The four rectus muscles are accessed in both longitudinal and transverse scans with some peculiarities: the muscular insertion is generally analyzed in longitudinal scans and is hyporeflective with a linear appearance. The muscular belly portion of a normal extrinsic muscle has medium reflectivity and can be better defined in transverse scans. To measure the thickness of the muscle, transverse scans are taken moving the probe along the path of the muscle to better identify

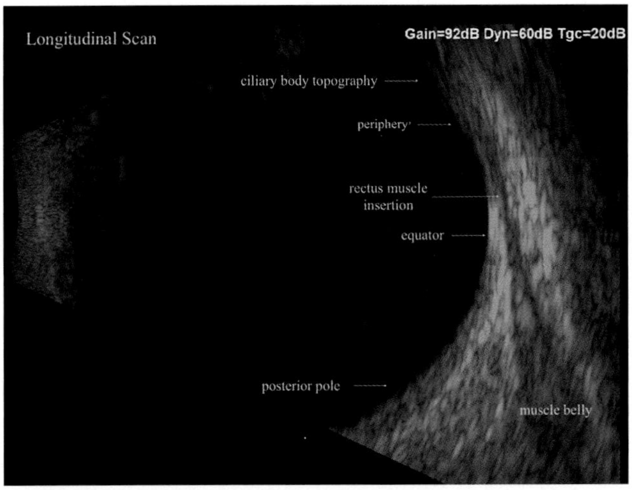

• **Fig. 3.4** Posterior ocular wall of the normal adult eye. 10 MHz B-scan ultrasound, longitudinal scan, transpalpebral contact technique. For a better analysis, the clinical nomenclature that divides the posterior ocular wall in posterior pole, equator, and periphery can be used. The ocular wall appears as a homogeneous band of hyperreflectivity, with the retinal profile being the first hyperreflective peak after the posterior capsule and anterior to the sclera. It is only possible to evaluate the retinal leaflet once it has become detached or in the presence of subretinal fluid. The rectus muscle accessed in longitudinal scan presents the muscular insertion as a hypo-reflective linear structure. The reflectivity of the muscle belly is moderate. Due to the opening of sound analysis if the periphery of the eye wall is the object of study, the optic nerve may not be present in the image window, as shown in the figure.

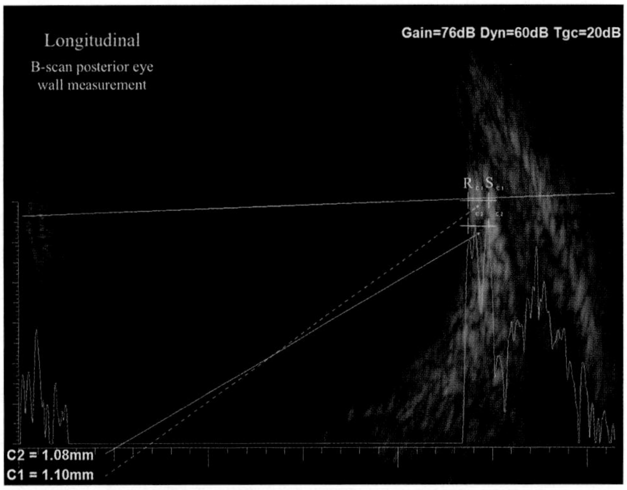

• **Fig. 3.5** Posterior ocular wall of the normal adult eye. 10 MHz B-scan ultrasound, longitudinal scan, transpalpebral contact technique. It is essential to maintain a low gain of the device enough to delimit the posterior profile of the wall, corresponding to the sclera, facilitating its distinction from the orbital contents, which are hyperreflective on ultrasound. A posterior ocular wall measurement of around 1.5 mm can be considered normal. The measurement obtained in B-scan is 1.10 mm and using the reference of A-scan peaks (anterior surface or the retina and transition sclera/orbital fat) is 1.08 mm.

the muscle sheath, which presents a higher reflectivity and is used as a reference to take the measurements.

It is extremely important that the gain of the device is low enough to delimit the posterior profile of the wall, corresponding to the sclera, facilitating its distinction from the orbital contents, which are hyperreflective on ultrasound (Fig. 3.5). Cross-sectional scans often allow this analysis more easily while at the periphery of the ultrasound images, the eye wall is poorly defined, making it difficult to evaluate properly. A posterior ocular wall measurement of around 1.5 mm can be considered normal, and values lower than 1 mm or greater than 2 mm are observed in myopic and hyperopic eyes, respectively.[6]

Degeneration of the vitreous body is a physiological phenomenon that accompanies human aging. The vitreous opacities that are observed during this process in the normal eye appear in ultrasound as hyporeflective interfaces or echoes with different shapes, such as points, lines, and mobile circles in small quantities and sparse in the vitreous cavity.[7,8] The study of the vitreous body is static and kinetic, seeking to quantify and qualify the echoes identified in all meridians (scanning the eye in 360 degrees). The movement is always carried out, keeping the meridian under evaluation and fixing the probe. The opacities formed are mobile, following the characteristic high mobility of the vitreous body with post-movement.

Detachment of the posterior hyaloid and collapse of the vitreous body occur as a natural evolution of the normal degeneration process of the vitreous body. The detached posterior hyaloid is a tenuous, mobile, hyporeflective membrane, separated but maintaining proximity from the posterior ocular wall except at the periphery, where the vitreous base remains attached (Fig. 3.5 and video 3.3). It is extremely important to evaluate the relationship of vitreous echoes to the retinal interface due to the possibility of anomalous adhesions considered sites of attention in serial evaluations.

Normal Pediatric Eye

The eye of the infant has different proportions of intraocular structures, usually the anterior chamber depth and the axial length are smaller, and the crystalline lens appears to be more spherical.[9]

Before birth, a prenatal ultrasound examination considers the age of the fetus to determine if the ocular axial length is in the normal range.

The mean axial length of a full-term newborn eye measures 16–18 mm.[10,11]

Growth in ocular axial length is observed every month in the first years, and there are tables of normal measurements of different populations for reference.[9]

Premature infants may present a different progression of axial length growth; the age of birth has to be adjusted before comparing to the reference table of normal standards for growth in the axial length of a child's eye.[12]

Preterm infants, even without retinopathy of prematurity, have a shorter axial length in comparison to full-term infants. Authors suggest that the axial length in eyes of preterm infants does not reach the same value as that of eyes of full-term ones.[12]

Symmetry should always be evaluated. The evaluation of axial length in infants can be done using B-mode biometry or A-scan biometry (Fig. 3.6). A-scan biometry under immersion is considered the most reliable for serial evaluation of ocular growth in infants.

Pathologic conditions such as retinopathy of prematurity, malformations, development of congenital cataract, or congenital glaucoma may influence the rate of growth of the axial length.

Ocular growth is generally influenced by several potential factors.[13] Axial length at birth is, on average, 0.24 mm larger for males than for females (Fig. 3.7). Correlations of axial length to anthropometric parameters such as birth weight, and orbitofacial parameters such as head circumference, are suggested.[13]

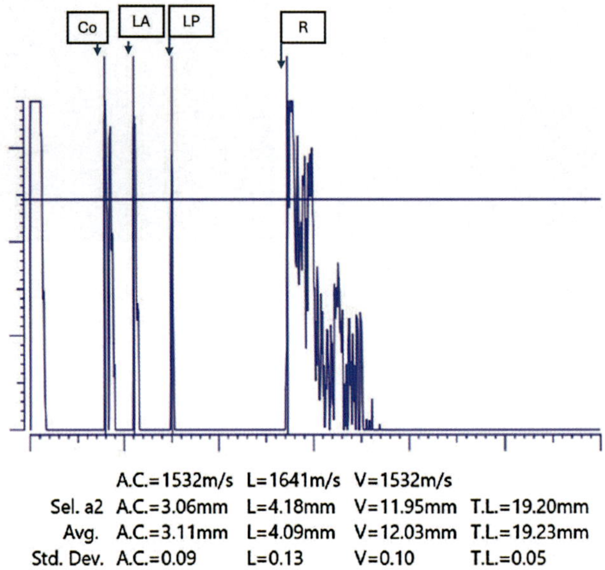

• **Fig. 3.6** A-scan biometry, immersion biometry, 3-month-old male infant. A-scan demonstrates the anterior surface of the cornea (Co), anterior and posterior lens capsules (LA and LP), and retina (R), allowing to measure following average distances: ACD, anterior chamber depth (average AC = 3.11 mm); L, lens thickness (L = 4.09 mm); V, vitreous cavity depth (V = 12.03 mm) and average total axial length (TL = 19.23 mm). 10 MHz B-scan ultrasound, vertical axial scan, immersion technique. Using immersion technique, a coupling media allows distancing the eye from the ultrasound probe, thereby allowing access to image the anterior segment.

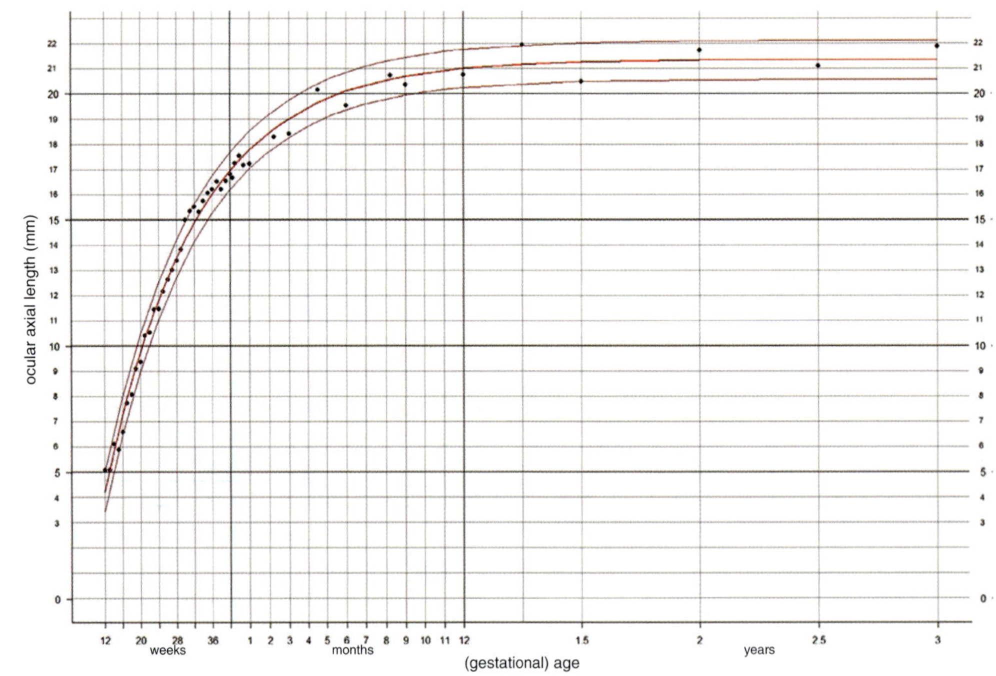

• **Fig. 3.7** Growth curve for ocular axial length (x-axis in mm) from 12 weeks of gestation up to 3 years old (y-axis). The thick red center line depicts mean axial length; the upper and lower red lines indicate 90% of all values. (From Groot ALW, Lissenberg-Witte BI, van Rijn LJ, Hartong DT. Meta-analysis of ocular axial length in newborns and infants up to 3 years of age. Surv Ophthalmol. 2022 Mar-Apr;67(2):342-352). doi: 10.1016/j.survophthal.2021.05.010.)

References

1. Silverman RH. Focused ultrasound in ophthalmology. *Clin Ophthalmol.* 2016;10:1865–1875.
2. Lorente-Ramos RM, Armán JA, Muñoz-Hernández A, Gómez JM, de la Torre SB. US of the eye made easy: a comprehensive how-to review with ophthalmoscopic correlation. *Radiographics.* 2012;32(5):E175–E200.
3. Papalini EP. Optic nerve: measure the diameter of its sheath to detect intracranial hypertension. *Rev Bras Oftalmol.* 2018;77(2):68–71.
4. Ganesh D, Lin SR. Global metrics on ocular biometry: representative averages and standard deviations across ten countries from four continents. *Eye (Lond).* 2023;37(3):511–515.
5. Sorsby A, Leary GA, Richards MJ, Chaston J. Ultrasonographic measurement of the components of ocular refraction in life: 2. Clinical procedures: ultrasonographic measurements compared with phakometric measurements in a series of 140 eyes. *Vision Res.* 1963;3(11-12):499–505.
6. Guthoff R, Berger RW, Draeger J. Measurements of ocular coat dimensions by means of combined A- and B-scan ultrasonography. *Ophthalmic Res.* 1984;16(6):289–291.
7. Petrash JM. Aging and age-related diseases of the ocular lens and vitreous body. *Invest Ophthalmol Vis Sci.* 2013;54(14): ORSF54–9.
8. Lumi X, Hawlina M, Glavač D, et al. Ageing of the vitreous: from acute onset floaters and flashes to retinal detachment. *Ageing Res Rev.* 2015;21:71–77.
9. Jin P, Li M, He X, et al. Anterior-chamber angle and axial length measurements in normal chinese children. *J Glaucoma.* 2016;25(8):692–697.
10. Blomdahl S. Ultrasonic measurements of the eye in the newborn infant. *Acta Ophthalmol (Copenh).* 1979;57(6):1048–1056.
11. Fledelius HC, Christensen AC. Reappraisal of the human ocular growth curve in fetal life, infancy, and early childhood. *Br J Ophthalmol.* 1996;80(10):918–921.
12. Zha Y, Zhu G, Zhuang J, Zheng H, Cai J, Feng W. Axial length and ocular development of premature infants without ROP. *J Ophthalmol.* 2017;2017:6823965.
13. Groot ALW, Lissenberg-Witte BI, van Rijn LJ, Hartong DT. Meta-analysis of ocular axial length in newborns and infants up to 3 years of age. *Surv Ophthalmol.* 2022;67(2):342–352.

4

Vitreoretinal Disorders

BERNADETE AYRES AND MARK W. JOHNSON

The vitreous gel, retina, choroid, sclera, and optic nerve comprise a posterior segment unit that preserves the anatomic integrity and physiological functions of the eye. The functional stability of the posterior segment can be disrupted by a wide variety of pathologic conditions such as vitreous hemorrhage, penetrating globe trauma, endophthalmitis, vitreoretinal traction, retinal detachment, and uveal effusion. Although complete ophthalmic examination with dilated ophthalmoscopy and multimodal imaging is typically sufficient to thoroughly assess the posterior segment, media opacification precludes the use of conventional biomicroscopy and imaging modalities. In this scenario, ultrasound is an essential tool. A comprehensive and standardized echographic evaluation allows the clinician to identify abnormalities, formulate a differential diagnosis, and develop a treatment plan for many important disorders of the posterior segment.

Vitreous Humor

Vitreous Syneresis

This degenerative condition occurs with aging but can be precocious in myopia, inflammatory states, and after ocular trauma or surgery. The strands of syneretic vitreous collagen are detected with B-scan ultrasonography as multiple, dispersed, mobile, low-reflective dot-dashes signals.

CASE

A 67-year-old woman with myopia presented with a floaters complaint. B-scan ultrasound demonstrated mildly dense, dispersed vitreous opacities, and attached retina (Fig. 4.1 and sonogram Video 4.1).

Vitreous Hemorrhage

Vitreous hemorrhage (VH) is an urgent ophthalmic condition that may cause an abrupt decrease in visual acuity and often develops as a complication of underlying disease. The annual incidence of VH is approximately seven cases per 100,000 population. Proliferative diabetic retinopathy, vitreous detachment with or without a retinal tear, and ocular trauma are the most common causes of VH. Patients with acute VH complain of visual haze, floaters, and the perception of shadows.[1]

Evaluation of vitreoretinal diseases in eyes with fundus-obscuring VH often presents a diagnostic challenge. Ultrasound is the gold standard ancillary test to identify the etiology as well as the characteristics of the hemorrhage. Findings on A- and B-scan ultrasonography depend on the severity and duration of the hemorrhage. In acute VH, scattered, mobile low-reflective dots and dashes echo sources are observed in the vitreous cavity. In subacute to chronic VH, the blood organizes into membranous and clump formations exhibiting higher reflectivity. Additionally, the vitreous mobility declines slightly as the age of the hemorrhage increases. When evaluating VH it is critical to perform a systematic B-scan ultrasonography examination of all quadrants, especially in the periphery to rule out retinal tears.

CASE

A 58-year-old man with a history of lattice degeneration presented with a complaint of new floaters. The ophthalmic evaluation revealed vitreous hemorrhage (Fig. 4.2).

CASE

A 68-year-old man with a history of exudative age-related macular degeneration presented with vitreous hemorrhage (Fig. 4.3).

The sedimentation property of red blood cells often causes VH to settle in the inferior quadrant, resulting in a pseudomembrane that can mimic a retinal detachment. Careful observation of dynamic ultrasonography will disclose that pseudo-membranes discontinue as they extend superiorly.

CASE

A 40-year-old man with a history of proliferative diabetic retinopathy presented with a complaint of floaters. Indirect ophthalmoscopy revealed diffuse vitreous hemorrhage (Fig. 4.4).

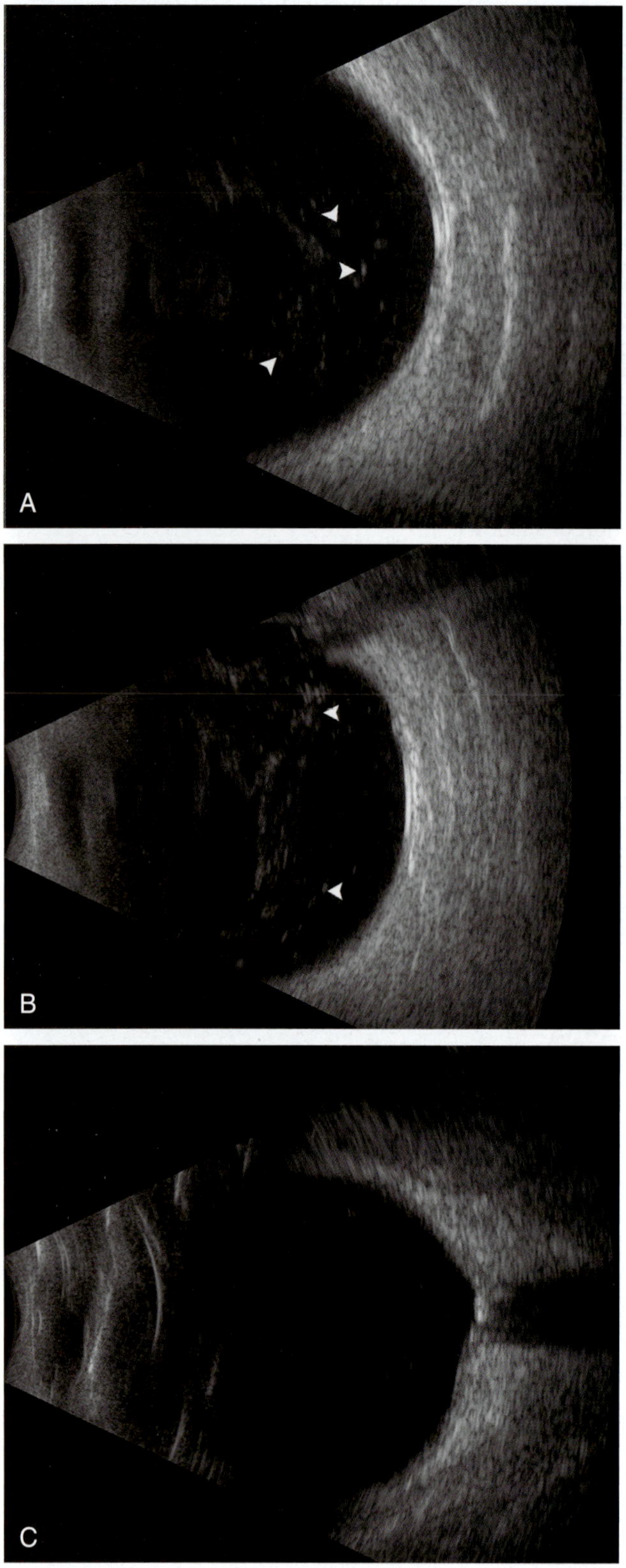

• **Fig. 4.1** Vitreous Syneresis. **(A)** Transverse, **(B)** longitudinal, and **(C)** axial B-scans show mildly dense, dispersed vitreous opacities (*arrowheads*) in the myopic eye.

The biochemical metabolism of blood in the vitreous gel differs from that of blood in the subhyaloid space. Subvitreal blood usually remains dispersed and low-reflective over time.

CASE

A 71-year-old man with a history of proliferative diabetic retinopathy and no view of the fundus because of vitreous hemorrhage was referred for ultrasound evaluation (Fig. 4.5 and sonogram Video 4.2).

Typically, VH is homogeneously scattered in the vitreous cavity; however, in some cases, the blood can be largely confined to a localized area such as overlying the optic disc in Terson syndrome or avulsed optic nerve.

CASE

A 51-year-old man was referred to a retina clinic complaining of a decrease in visual acuity, which occurred after he underwent surgery for a ruptured cerebral aneurysm (Fig. 4.6).

TEACHING POINTS

The sonographic characteristics of the vitreous hemorrhage coupled with clinical history allow precise diagnosis of etiology of the bleeding.

The differential diagnosis of vitreous hemorrhage includes:

- Inflammatory/infectious conditions causing vitritis such as panuveitis or endophthalmitis.
- Primary central nervous system lymphoma masquerading as chronic vitreous hemorrhage.

Ultrasound evaluation should be performed at the early presentation of the vitreous hemorrhage to rule out a retinal tear and retinal detachment.

A serial follow-up exam for clearance of the vitreous hemorrhage should be performed using the same gain setting and comparing the same area.

Asteroid Hyalosis

Asteroid hyalosis is a relatively uncommon, mostly unilateral, age-related vitreous condition occurring with greater frequency in men than in women. It has no significant association with systemic diseases.[2] The asteroid bodies consist of lipid-containing calcium surrounded by a network of fibrils. In most cases, patients are asymptomatic or minimally symptomatic. On slit-lamp examination, the asteroid bodies appear as white to yellow-white, small, round to oval opacities suspended fairly evenly throughout the vitreous body.

On B-scan ultrasonography, asteroid hyalosis is characterized by diffuse or focally aggregated bright point-like echo sources with positive aftermovement. Typically, an echo-free zone is observed between the calcium soap clusters and the posterior hyaloid or ocular wall. On A-scan examination, the asteroid bodies produce multiple medium- to high-amplitude spikes in the vitreous space.

CASE

A 53-year-old woman presented with decreased vision and a dense cataract. An ultrasound exam revealed a unilateral asteroid hyalosis (Fig. 4.7 and sonogram Video 4.3)

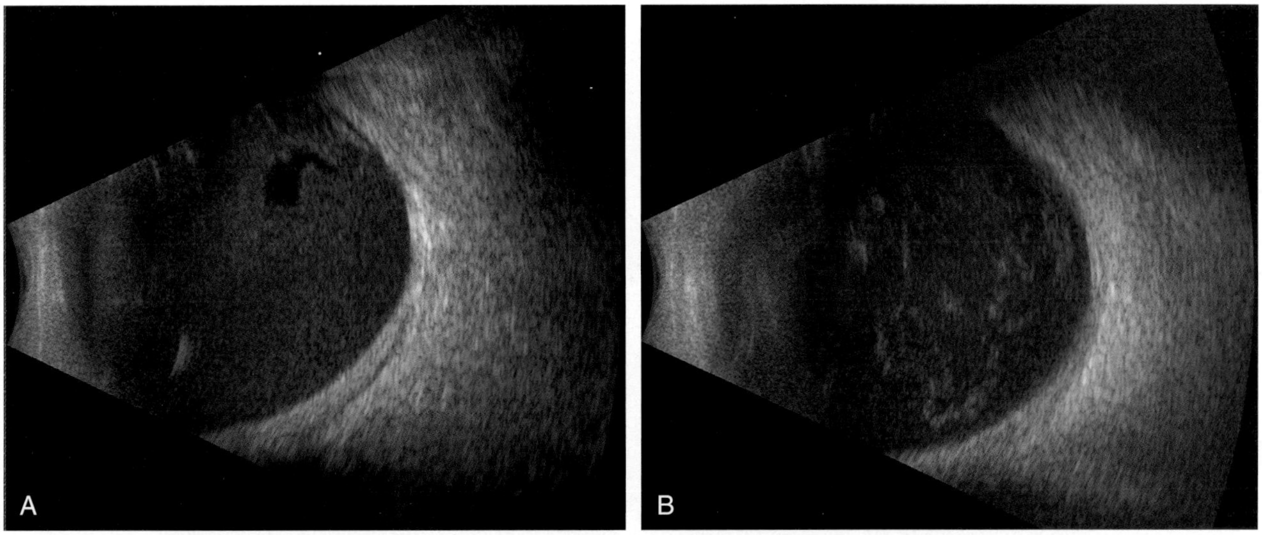

• **Fig. 4.2** Vitreous Hemorrhage. **(A)** Longitudinal B-scan ultrasound displays dense, homogeneously dispersed vitreous opacities in case of recent vitreous hemorrhage. **(B)** Follow-up ultrasound examination displays higher-reflective clump and membrane-like formations in case of subacute vitreous hemorrhage.

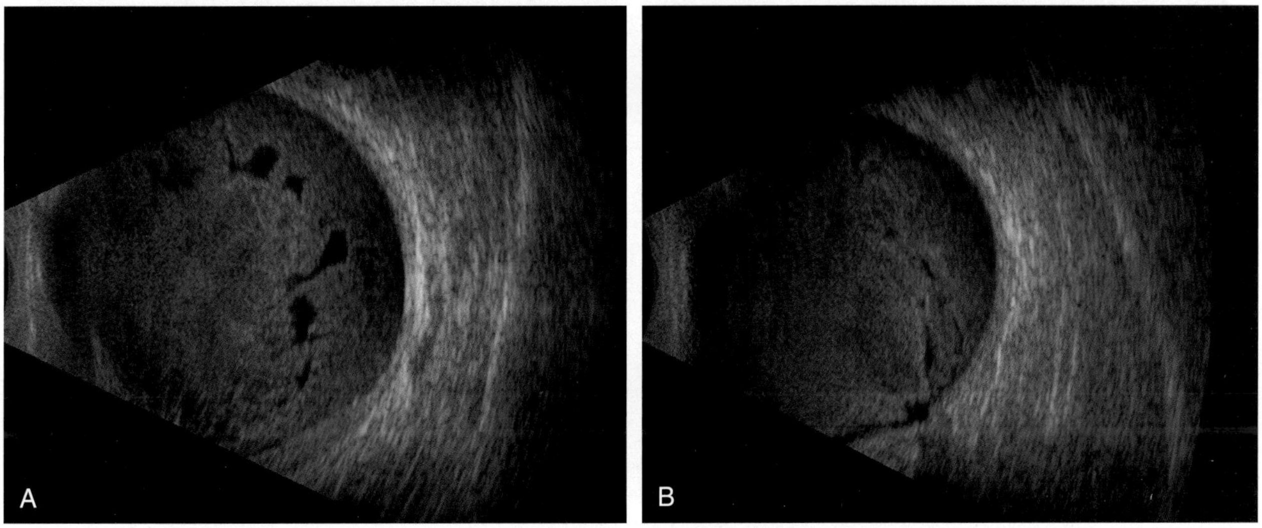

• **Fig. 4.3** Vitreous Hemorrhage. **(A)** Transverse and **(B)** longitudinal B-scans show dense, diffuse vitreous hemorrhage contouring low-reflective liquefied pockets in the vitreous gel.

Posterior Vitreous Detachment

Posterior vitreous detachment (PVD) is commonly defined as a separation between the posterior vitreous cortex and the internal limiting membrane of the retina. PVD is the culmination of aging changes in the vitreous and can occur earlier in life in eyes with myopia, inflammatory disease, retinal vascular diseases, and following trauma or cataract surgery. Age-related PVD typically begins as a shallow, localized separation of the hyaloid from the perifoveal retina and progresses slowly over months or years until it separates from the optic disc margin to produce the signs and symptoms of a Weiss ring.[3] As the PVD evolves, it may cause traction at points of firm vitreoretinal adhesion in the posterior pole or fundus periphery and thereby induce a variety of serious pathologic events at the vitreoretinal interface.

Total Posterior Vitreous Detachment

When the vitreous is completely detached from the internal limiting membrane of the retina, the posterior vitreous face appears as a thin, smooth, concave membrane located at a variable distance from the ocular coats on B-scan ultrasonography. A high gain setting is used to image the low echogenicity of the posterior vitreous face. As the gain is diminished, the brightness of the posterior hyaloid membrane attenuates. On kinetic examination, the posterior hyaloid displays intense wave-like aftermovement.

CASE

A 59-year-old man presented with vitreous hemorrhage for 11 days. B-scan ultrasound evaluation revealed hemorrhagic total posterior vitreous detachment (Fig. 4.8 and sonogram Video 4.4).

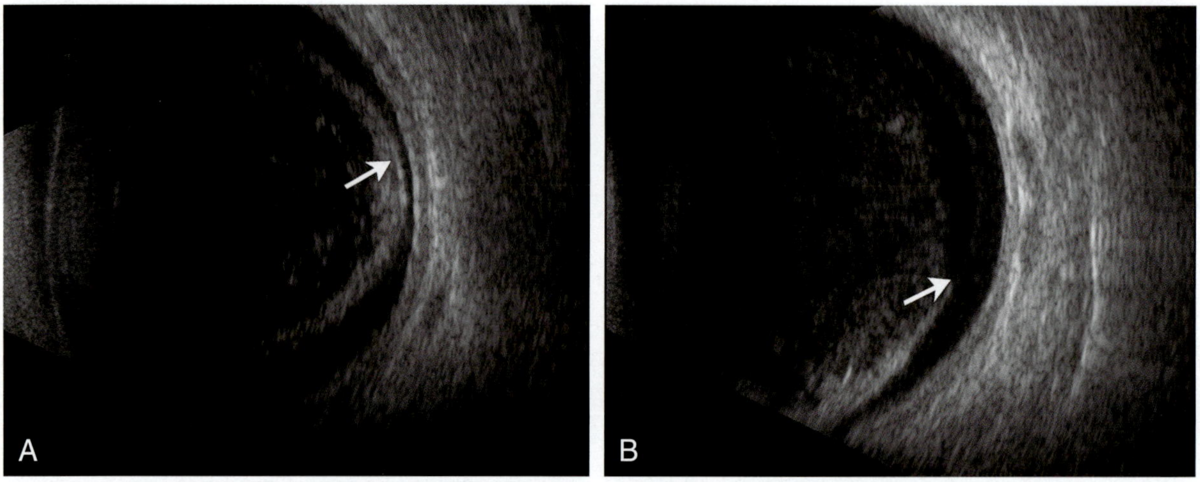

• **Fig. 4.4** Layered Vitreous Hemorrhage. **(A)** Transverse B-scan ultrasound through the inferior quadrant shows layered vitreous hemorrhage resembling a retinal membrane (*arrow*). **(B)** Transverse B-scan ultrasound through the nasal aspect of the globe shows progressive thinning and discontinuation (*arrow*) of the membrane in the superior region of the ultrasonography.

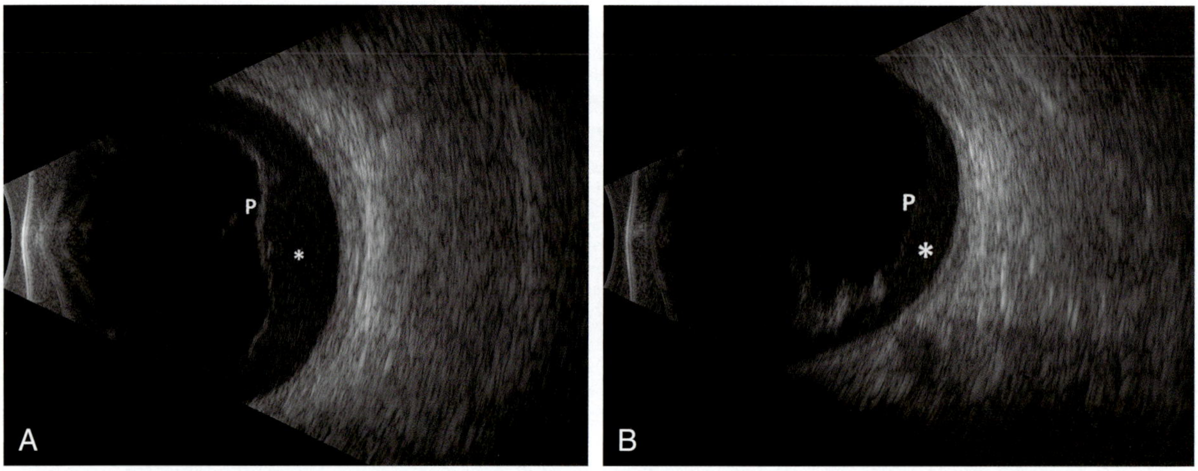

• **Fig. 4.5** Subhyaloid Hemorrhage. **(A)** Transverse and **(B)** longitudinal B-scans demonstrate dense, homogeneously dispersed subhyaloid hemorrhage without clot formation (*asterisk*). The blood collection is outlined anteriorly by a posterior vitreous detachment (P).

CASE

A 71-year-old man underwent preoperative ultrasound examination of an eye with a dense cataract. A total posterior vitreous detachment was detected (Fig. 4.9 and sonogram Video 4.5).

Partial Posterior Vitreous Detachment

Incomplete PVD may adopt different configurations, such as incomplete peripheral PVD and incomplete posterior PVD. Anomalous adhesions between the posterior vitreous face and the retinal surface are commonly found in pathologic retinal conditions such as proliferative retinal vascular diseases, inflammatory disorders, lattice degeneration, and hereditary vitreoretinopathies. And in otherwise normal eyes, sites of especially firm vitreoretinal adhesion can be found at the fovea, along retinal vessels, at the optic disc margin, and at the vitreous base. Thus, as partial PVD evolves, it can exert traction at various vitreoretinal adhesion sites and cause complications such as macular hole, vitreomacular traction, vitreopapillary traction, vitreous hemorrhage, retinal tear, and retinal detachment.[3–4]

B-scan ultrasonography can demonstrate sites of vitreoretinal adhesion and estimate the associated traction on the retina. A funnel-shaped partial PVD with vitreopapillary adhesion can sometimes mimic a retinal detachment. Topographic, quantitative, and kinetic techniques, outlined in Table 4.1, should be used to differentiate detached posterior vitreous cortex from detached retina or detached choroid. This can be more challenging in the presence of long-standing vitreous hemorrhage, which usually forms membranes of medium echogenicity. B-scan ultrasonographic examination demonstrates multiple hemorrhagic vitreal membranes delimited by a partial or total posterior vitreous detachment.

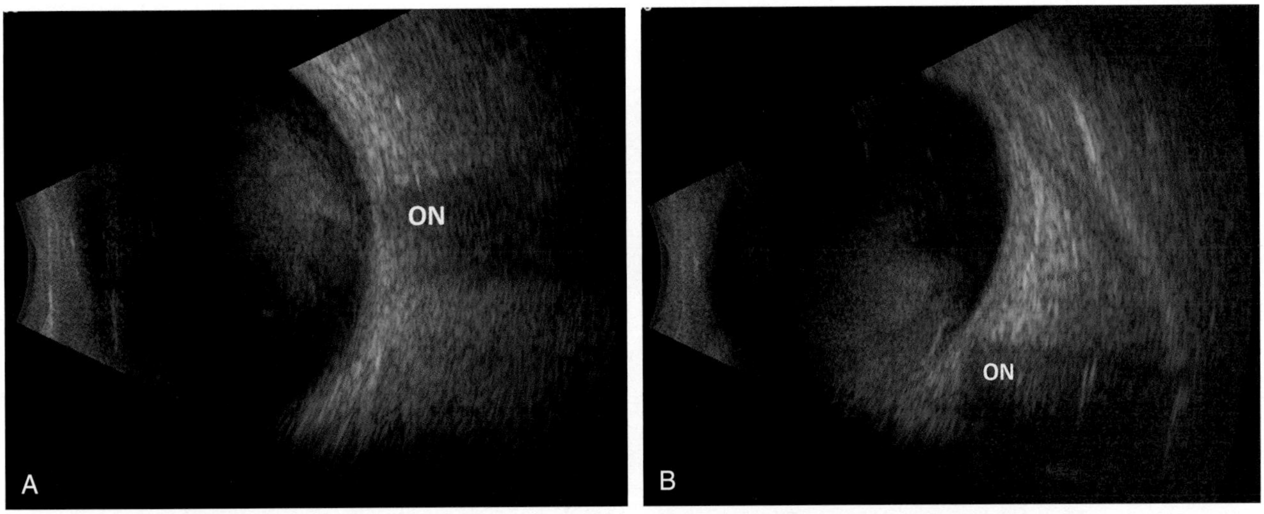

• **Fig. 4.6** Vitreous Hemorrhage in a patient with Terson syndrome. **(A)** Transverse and **(B)** longitudinal B-scans display a vitreous hemorrhage concentrated near the optic disc. *ON*, Optic nerve.

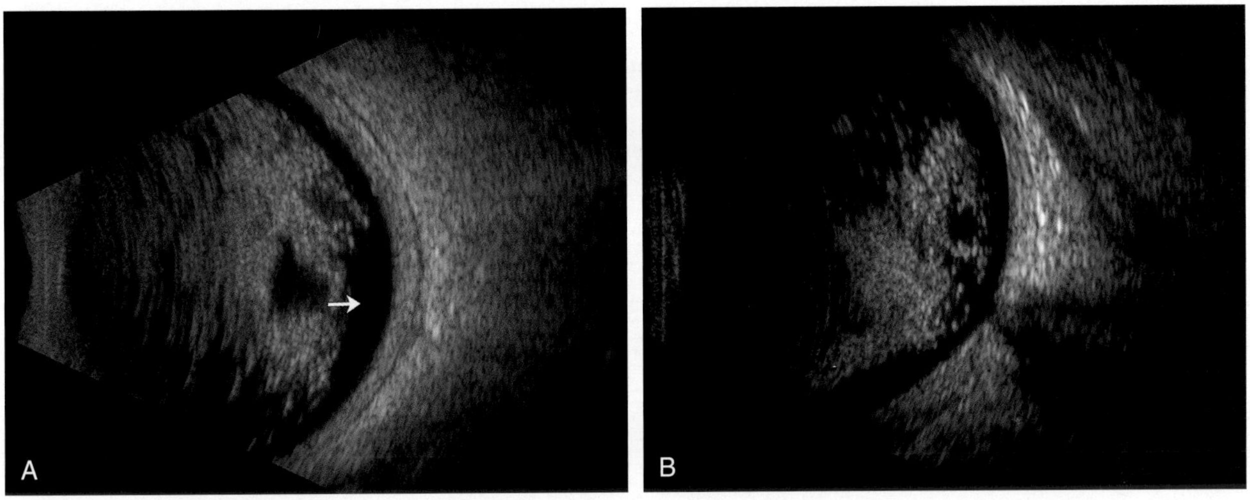

• **Fig. 4.7** Asteroid Hyalosis. **(A)** Transverse B-scan shows diffuse bright point-like echoes in the vitreous cavity with an echo-free zone (*arrow*) next to the ocular wall. **(B)** Longitudinal B-scan at low gain setting shows that the echoes remain highly reflective.

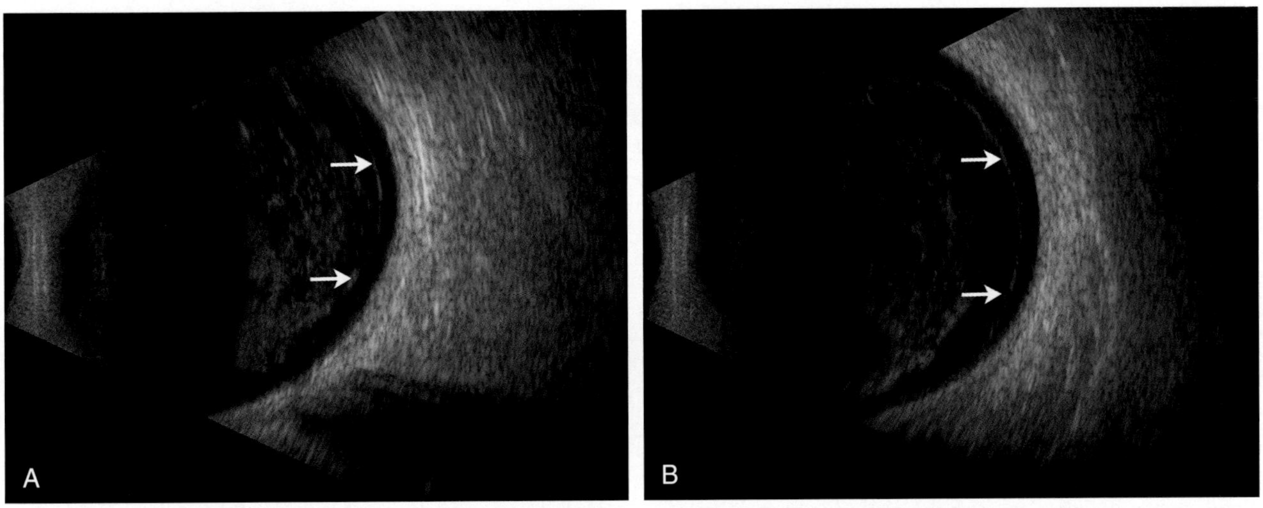

• **Fig. 4.8** Total Posterior Vitreous Detachment. **(A)** Longitudinal B-scan ultrasound showing a vitreous hemorrhage with membranous and clump formations and a posterior hyaloid membrane (*arrows*) completely detached from the retina surface. **(B)** Transverse B-scan ultrasound displays a low-medium reflective, smooth hyaloid membrane (*arrows*).

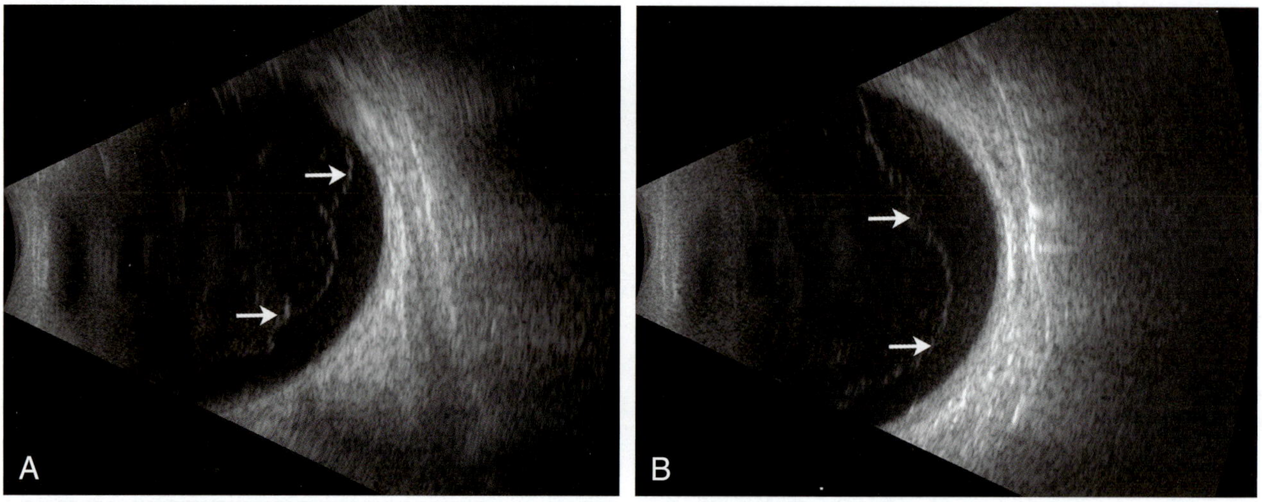

• **Fig. 4.9** Total Posterior Vitreous Detachment. **(A)** Longitudinal and **(B)** transverse B-scans at high gain show a low-reflective posterior vitreous cortex (*arrows*) completely detached from the retinal surface.

TABLE 4.1 Acoustic Characteristics of Posterior Vitreous Detachment, Retinal Detachment, and Choroidal Detachment

Acoustic Characteristic	Posterior Vitreous Detachment	Retinal Detachment	Choroidal Detachment
Shape	Smooth, open funnel	Smooth or folded, open or closed funnel	Smooth dome
Reflectivity	Majority: low-medium	Hyperreflective	Hyperreflective
Peripheral and disc insertions	Ora serrata Edge of optic disc	Ora serrata Center of optic disc	Ciliary body Posterior pole (not at the disc)
Aftermovement	Majority:wave-like, undulating	Shaky	Jiggly or none
Persistence in low gain	Disappears	Persists	Persists
Blood flow along	Absent	Present	Present

CASE

A 56-year-old man with proliferative diabetic retinopathy and vitreous hemorrhage was referred for echographic evaluation that demonstrated a partial posterior vitreous detachment (Fig. 4.10 and sonogram Video 4.6).

In most cases, the biomicroscopic diagnosis of a posterior vitreous detachment, retinal detachment, or choroidal detachment is straightforward. However, in some instances, the ophthalmoscopic appearance of a membrane can be atypical and ultrasonographic characteristics (Table 4.1) can be helpful in differentiating the entities.

Vitreomacular Traction

B-scan ultrasound at a high gain setting can demonstrate focal or broad adhesion of the hyaloid membrane to the macular region associated with separation of the posterior vitreous cortex in other areas of the posterior or peripheral fundus.

CASE

A 64-year-old woman presented with a history of panuveitis and no fundus view secondary to haze vitreous. Vitreomacular traction was diagnosed on B-scan (Fig. 4.11 and sonogram Video 4.7).

Vitreoschisis

A split of the posterior vitreous cortex can occur during vitreoretinal separation, especially in proliferative retinopathy and intermediate or posterior uveitis. On B-scan ultrasound, the inner wall of vitreoschisis presents low or medium reflectivity and undulating aftermovement, similar to that of the posterior hyaloid. The outer wall of the vitreoschisis cavity corresponds to a partial thickness cortical vitreous layer, which can be adherent or separated from the internal limiting membrane of the retina.[5] Typically, this layer becomes echographically visible as it organizes into a fibroglial epiretinal membrane.

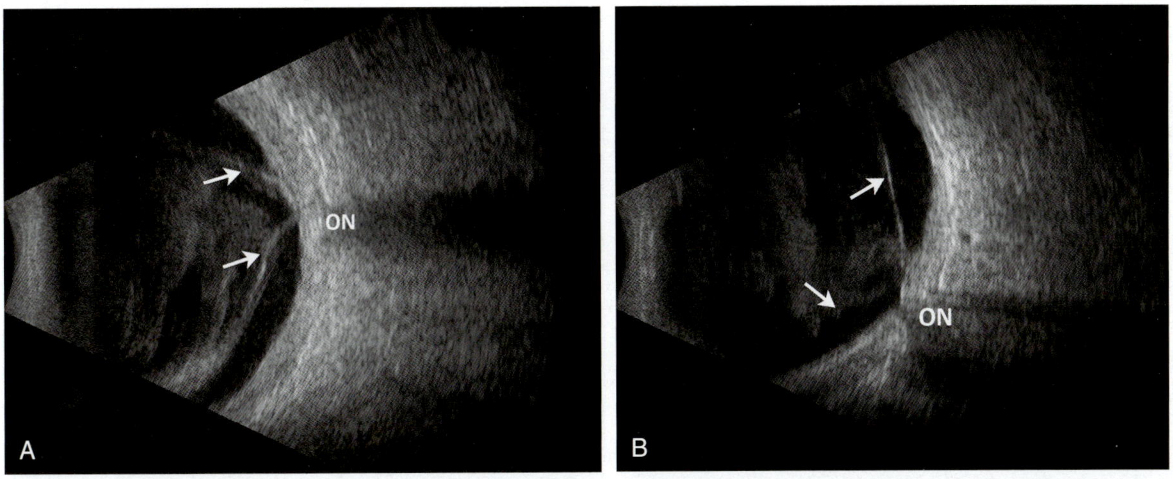

• **Fig. 4.10** Partial Posterior Vitreous Detachment. **(A)** Transverse and **(B)** longitudinal B-scans aimed at the posterior pole display a funnel-shaped partial posterior vitreous detachment (*arrows*) with focal adhesion to the retinal surface in the area of the optic nerve (ON).

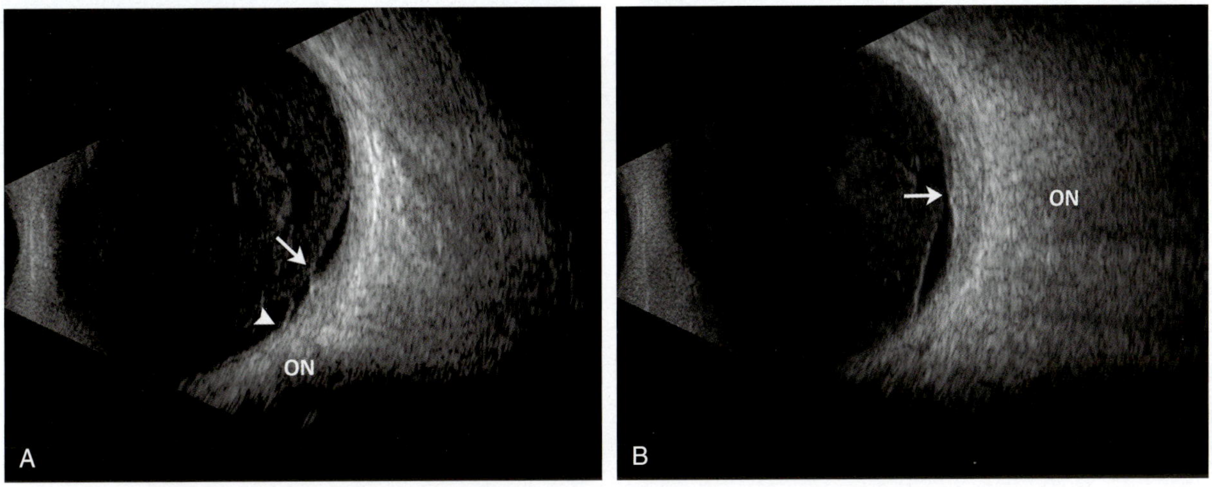

• **Fig. 4.11** Vitreomacular Traction. **(A)** Longitudinal and **(B)** transverse B-scans showing dispersed, moderately dense vitreous opacities and partial posterior vitreous detachment with vitreomacular adhesion causing mild retinal traction (*arrow*). Vitreopapillary adhesion (*arrowhead*) is also apparent. *ON*, Optic nerve.

CASE

A 26-year-old man with a history of granulomatous panuveitis presented for an annual follow-up visit. B-scan ultrasonography identified vitreoschisis (Fig. 4.12 and sonogram Video 4.8).

TEACHING POINTS

PVD typically displays a wave-like aftermovement on B-scan.

Transverse and longitudinal B-scan ultrasound imaging the optic nerve can characterize the pattern of the PVD as total or partial.

Identifying PVD status may assist in the decision-making process regarding the optimal surgical technique for retinal detachment repair.

In proliferative retinopathy, ultrasound is essential to monitor the severity of the vitreoretinal adhesions and the status of the retina.

Retina

Retinal Tears

Prevention of retinal detachment is critically dependent on the early detection of retinal breaks. The most common morphologies of retinal breaks induced by vitreoretinal traction are horseshoe (flap) tears and operculated tears. Retinal tears are usually located at the posterior margin of the vitreous base (near the equator) and are most common in the superotemporal followed by the superonasal quadrants.

B-scan ultrasonography is a helpful diagnostic imaging modality for the detection of retinal breaks. Echographically, a horseshoe retinal tear appears as a hyperechoic flap arising from the retinal layer. In almost all cases, the flap is adherent to the posterior vitreous cortex. An operculated tear appears as a small hyperreflective membrane disconnected from the retinal layer and overlying a retinal defect. A high sensitivity gain setting

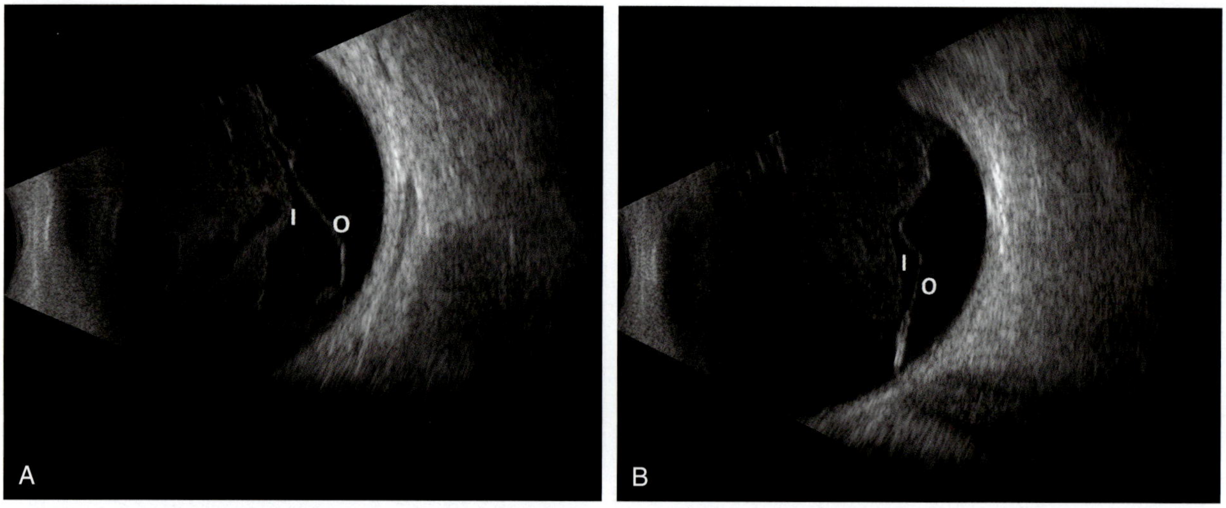

• **Fig. 4.12** Vitreoschisis. **(A)** Transverse and **(B)** longitudinal B-scans of posterior vitreous detachment with vitreopapillary adhesion and a splitting of the posterior vitreous cortex (vitreoschisis). *I*, Inner wall; *O*, outer wall.

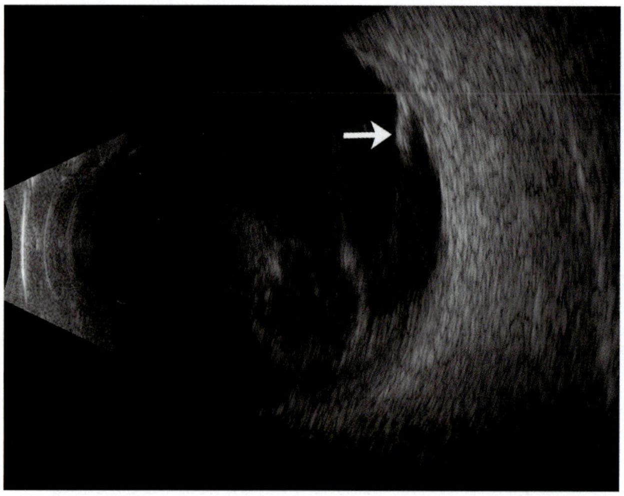

• **Fig. 4.13** Retinal Tear. Longitudinal B-scan ultrasound demonstrates a peripheral hyperechoic flap (*arrow*) adherent to the fundus and to the posterior hyaloid membrane.

should be employed to screen the fundus. Once a suspected break is detected, transverse, longitudinal, and kinetic studies should be used to determine its location and mobility. All quadrants must be screened, given the possibility of multiple breaks. When available, a high-frequency 20 MHz probe can be used to help clarify questionable images. On A-scan ultrasound, horseshoe tears and operculated tears exhibit highly reflective spikes.

In acute posterior vitreous detachment complicated by vitreous hemorrhage, if no retinal tear or detachment is found initially, patients are often followed with frequent visits and ultrasonographic examination. In this situation, the absence of a detectable retinal tear on B-scan ultrasound examination does not rule-out the presence of an occult retinal break.

CASE

A 46-year-old man presented to the clinic complaining of floaters and flashes. Ophthalmologic examination showed vitreous hemorrhage and a possible peripheral retinal tear (Fig. 4.13 and sonogram Video 4.9).

CASE

A 56-year-old woman with no remarkable systemic history presented with a complaint of floaters. Ophthalmoscopy revealed vitreous hemorrhage and a peripheral retinal break (Fig. 4.14).

CASE

A 55-year-old healthy woman presented with acute painless decreased vision. She had experienced floaters and flashes a few days earlier. Dilated fundus examination revealed vitreous hemorrhage. An ultrasound examination detected a peripheral retinal tear (Fig. 4.15 and sonogram Video 4.10).

TEACHING POINTS

Patients who present with symptoms of sensation of flashing light (photopsia) and/or persistent floaters should be suspected of having a retinal tear.

Retinal tears are frequently located on the vitreous base area, ranging from the equator to the ora serrata. Ultrasound scanning must extend to the far periphery to rule out a tear.

Retinal Detachment

Retinal detachment (RD) is a potentially blinding condition that typically requires prompt diagnosis and urgent intervention to prevent irreversible vision loss. Almost all retinal detachments can be categorized into one of the following four types: 1) *rhegmatogenous* RD occurs as a result of a retinal break; 2) *traction* RD develops when vitreoretinal adhesions or contractile membranes pull the retina off of the eye wall; 3) *exudative* RD, also called serous RD, develops secondary to retinal or choroidal vascular leakage (such as that occurring with retinal or choroidal vascular diseases, tumors, or inflammation); and 4) *combined tractional and rhegmatogenous* RD.[6]

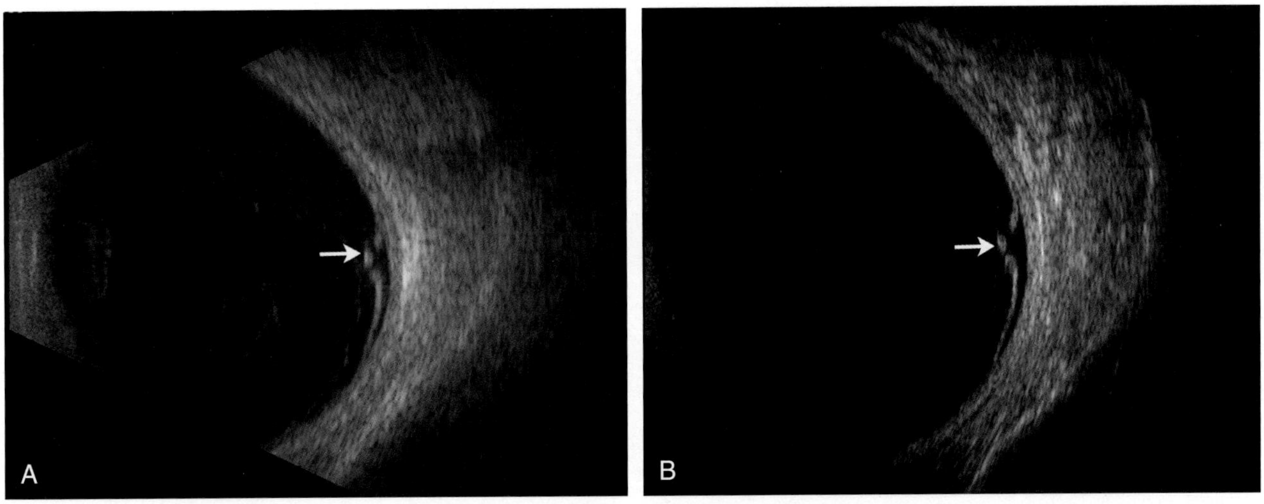

• **Fig. 4.14** Operculated Retinal Tear. Transverse B-scans through the peripheral fundus with 10 MHz **(A)** and 20 MHz **(B)** probes demonstrate an avulsed fragment of retinal tissue on the posterior hyaloid (arrow) overlying a focal retinal defect. There is localized subretinal fluid around the break.

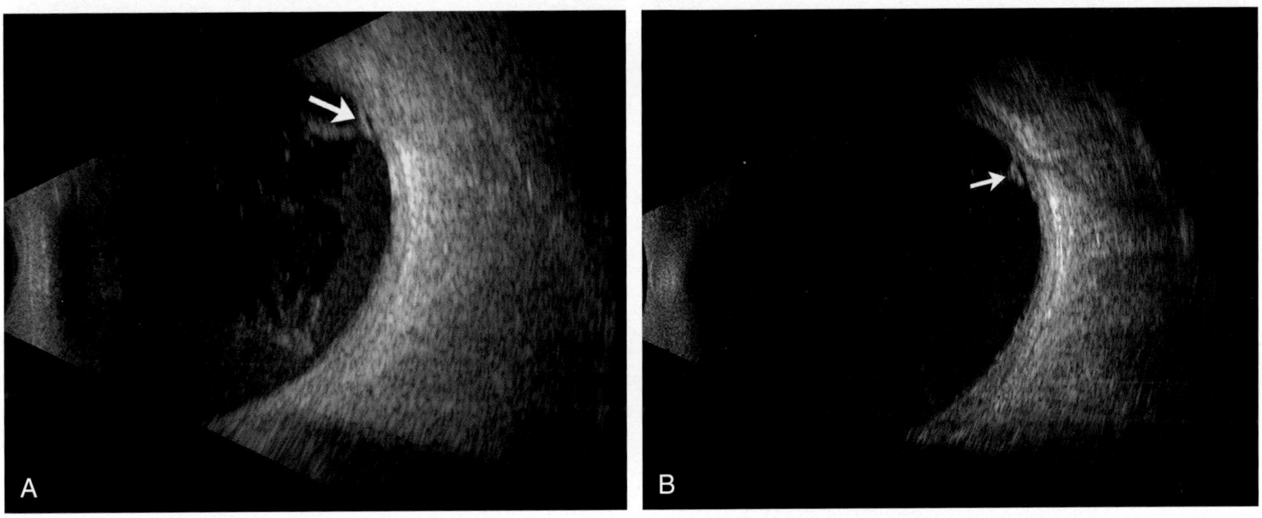

• **Fig. 4.15** Horseshoe Retinal Tear. **(A)** Longitudinal B-scan ultrasound with 10-MHz probe shows a peripheral retinal tear (*arrow*) and sub-hyaloid hemorrhage. **(B)** Same peripheral retinal tear (*arrow*) imaged with 20-MHz probe.

On B-scan ultrasonography, a detached retina typically appears as a distinctly bright, continuous membrane. On dynamic examination, the retina typically exhibits a shaky aftermovement. An A-scan ultrasound aimed perpendicular to a retinal membrane displays a 100% high, single spike at tissue sensitivity. A vertical trembling motion of the spike can be observed at a reduced gain setting.[7]

CASE

A 60-year-old man was evaluated for floaters, followed by dramatically decreased vision related to a total retinal detachment (Fig. 4.16 and sonogram Video 4.11).

Once an RD or suspected RD has been detected, B-scan topographic, quantitative, and kinetic techniques are performed to assess involved fundus meridians, membrane configuration, membrane reflectivity, vitreoretinal adhesions, peripheral and optic disc insertions, the status of subretinal space, macular involvement, and membrane mobility.

Retinal detachments vary widely in extent and may be localized, extensive, or total. A total RD usually has a funnel shape, which can be opened, closed, or somewhere in between. An extensive or total RD usually inserts into the optic disc posteriorly and extends to the ora serrata anteriorly. There may be cyst formation, subretinal proteinaceous particles, and even focal or diffuse retinal calcification in long-standing RD.[8]

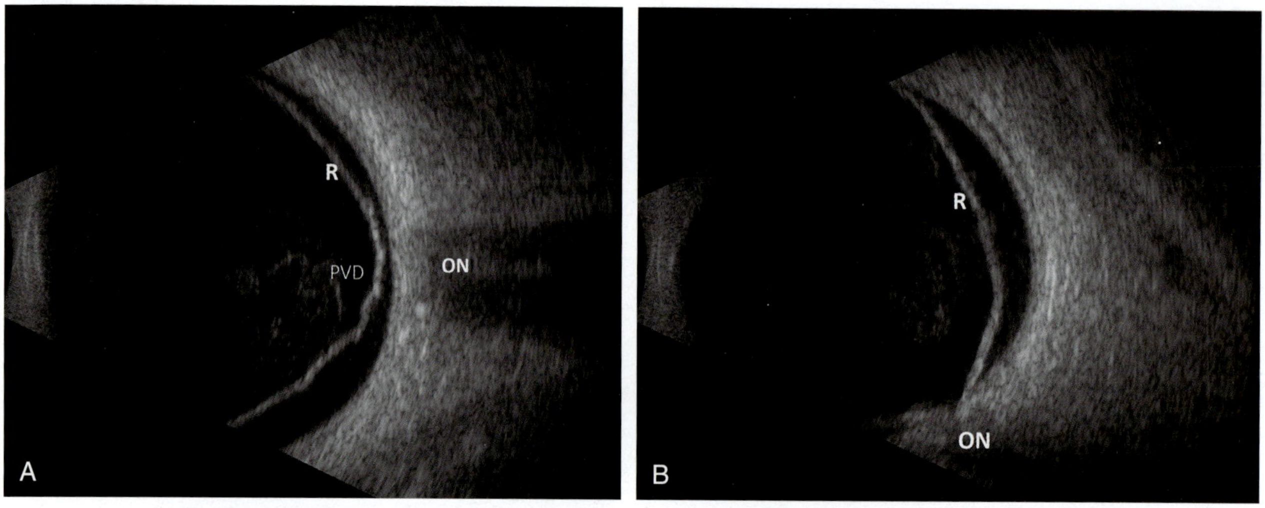

• **Fig. 4.16** Total Retinal Detachment. **(A)** Transverse B-scan ultrasound shows a highly reflective continuous membrane consistent with retinal detachment (R). Note a posterior vitreous detachment (PVD) located anteriorly to the detached retina. **(B)** Longitudinal B-scan ultrasound demonstrates the posterior insertion of the detached retina into the optic nerve (ON).

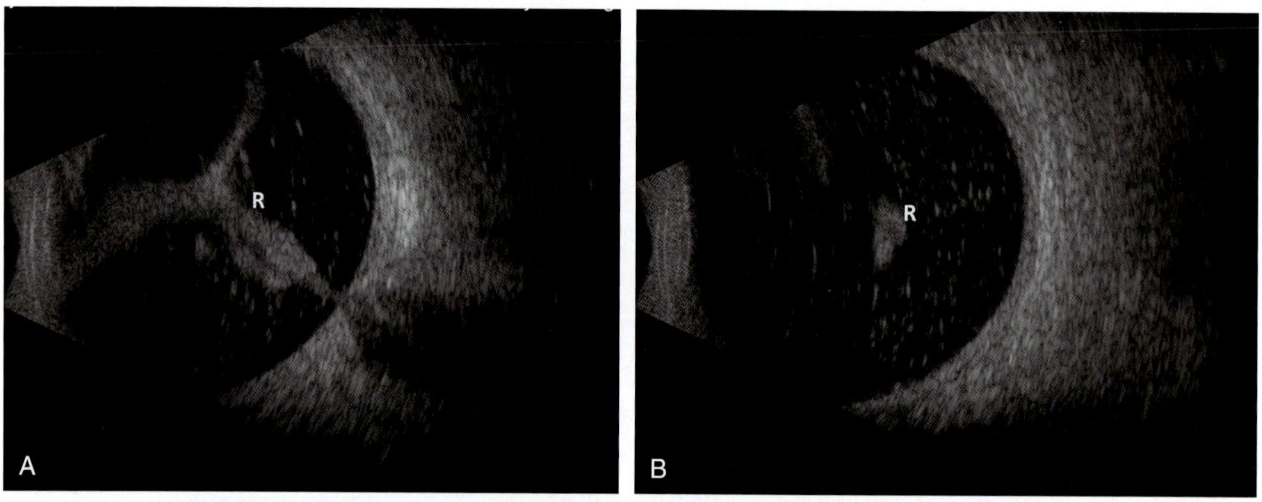

• **Fig. 4.17** Long-standing Closed Funnel-Shaped Total Retinal Detachment (R) with Subretinal Opacities in **(A)** longitudinal and **(B)** transverse views.

CASE

A 60-year-old woman with a history of choroidal melanoma and retinopathy following radiation treatment presented with retinal detachment (Fig. 4.17).

CASE

A 40-year-old woman with a history of ocular trauma and chronic retinal detachment presented with a blind, painful eye. Ophthalmoscopy of the posterior pole was not possible, and B-scan ultrasound evaluation disclosed a retinal detachment with dense subretinal opacities (Fig. 4.18 and sonogram Video 4.12).

CASE

A 40-year-old man presented to the clinic with a long-standing traumatic retinal detachment (Fig. 4.19 and sonogram Video 4.13).

Rhegmatogenous Retinal Detachment

In rhegmatogenous retinal detachment, the detached retina has a convex configuration, often with corrugations and shaky aftermovement. The subretinal space usually is acoustically clear. Retinal breaks are commonly located at or anterior to the fundus equator or in the region of the ora serrata. Rhegmatogenous RD originating from the posterior pole is uncommon. Vitreous gel is typically seen to be adherent to the flaps of any associated tears.

CASE

A 62-year-old healthy man was referred to the retina clinic with a diagnosis of vitreous hemorrhage and retinal detachment. Ultrasound evaluation revealed the rhegmatogenous nature of the retinal detachment (Fig. 4.20 and sonogram Video 4.14).

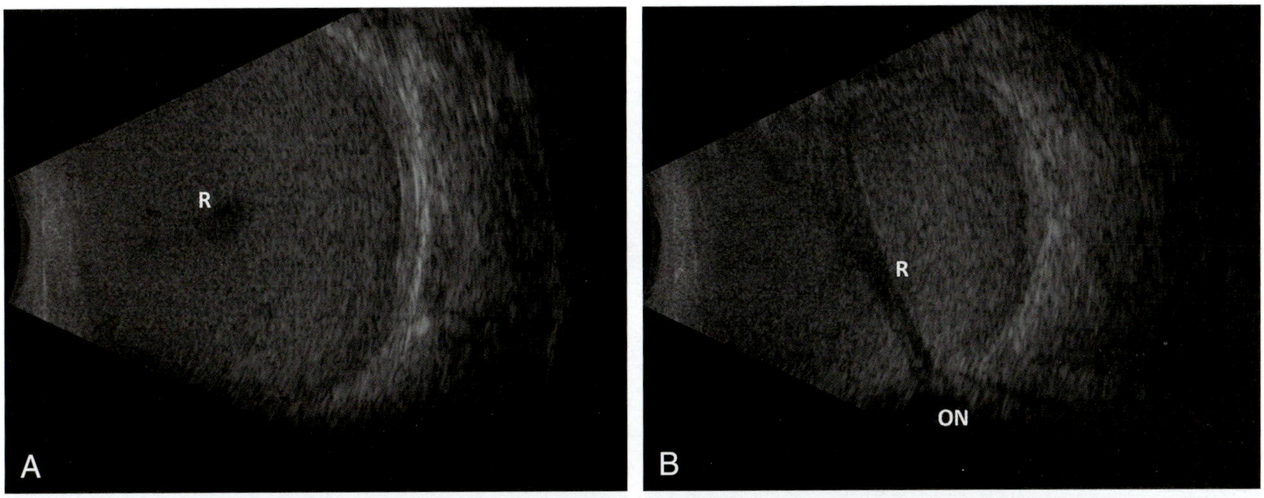

• **Fig. 4.18** Echolucent Closed Funnel Retinal Detachment with Dense Subretinal Opacities. **(A)** Transverse B-scan ultrasound at medium-high gain setting shows an echolucent circle (R) in the vitreous cavity. **(B)** A longitudinal B-scan ultrasound shows the funnel configuration of a retinal detachment (R) inserting in the optic nerve (ON). The dense opacities surrounding the retina create a retinal reversed image.

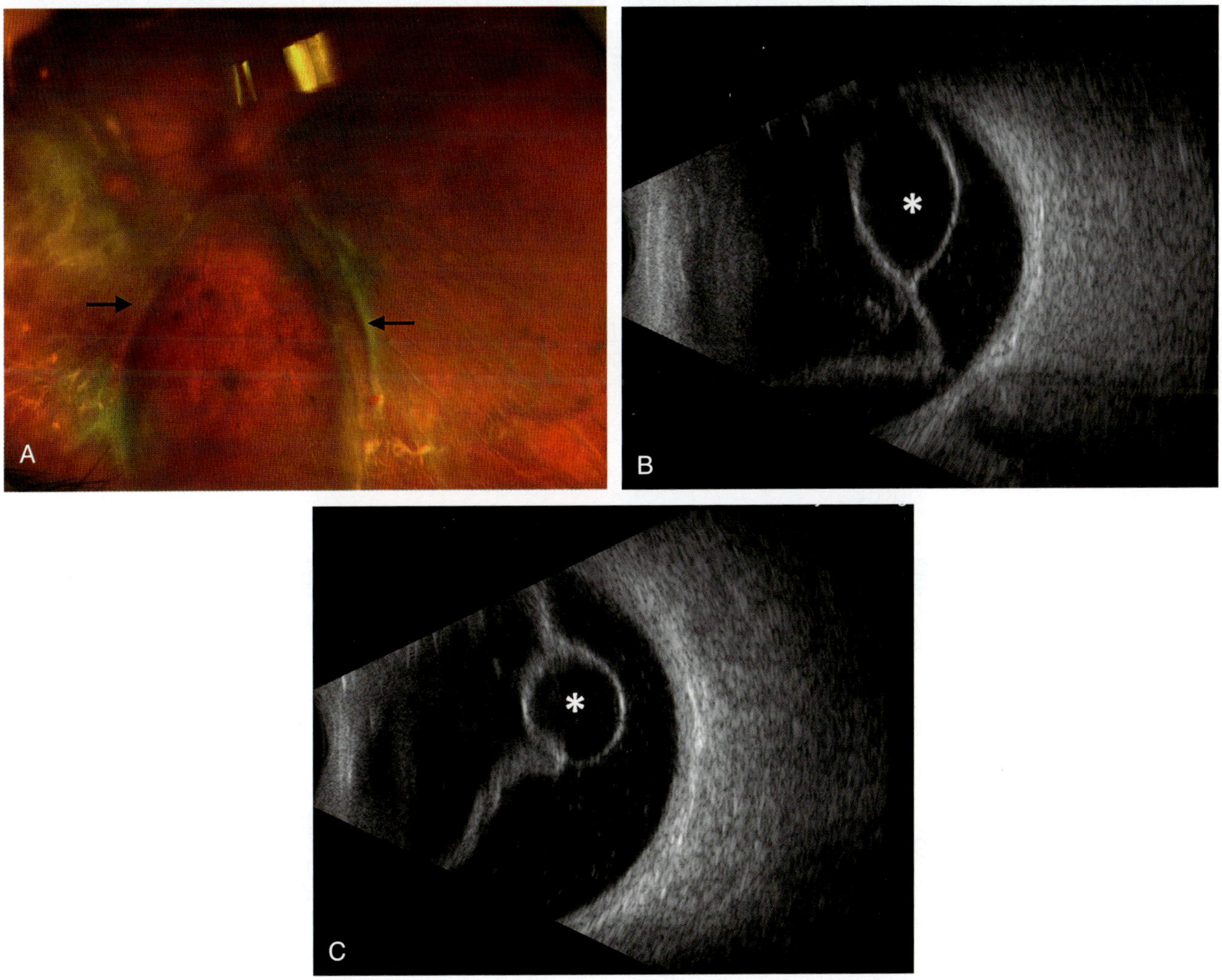

• **Fig. 4.19** Long-standing Retinal Detachment with Retinal Cyst. **(A)** Wide-field fundus photography showing total retinal detachment with a large retinal cyst (*arrows*). **(B)** Longitudinal and **(C)** transverse B-scans display a chronic, open funnel total retinal detachment with a large retinal cyst (*asterisk*) and subretinal opacities.

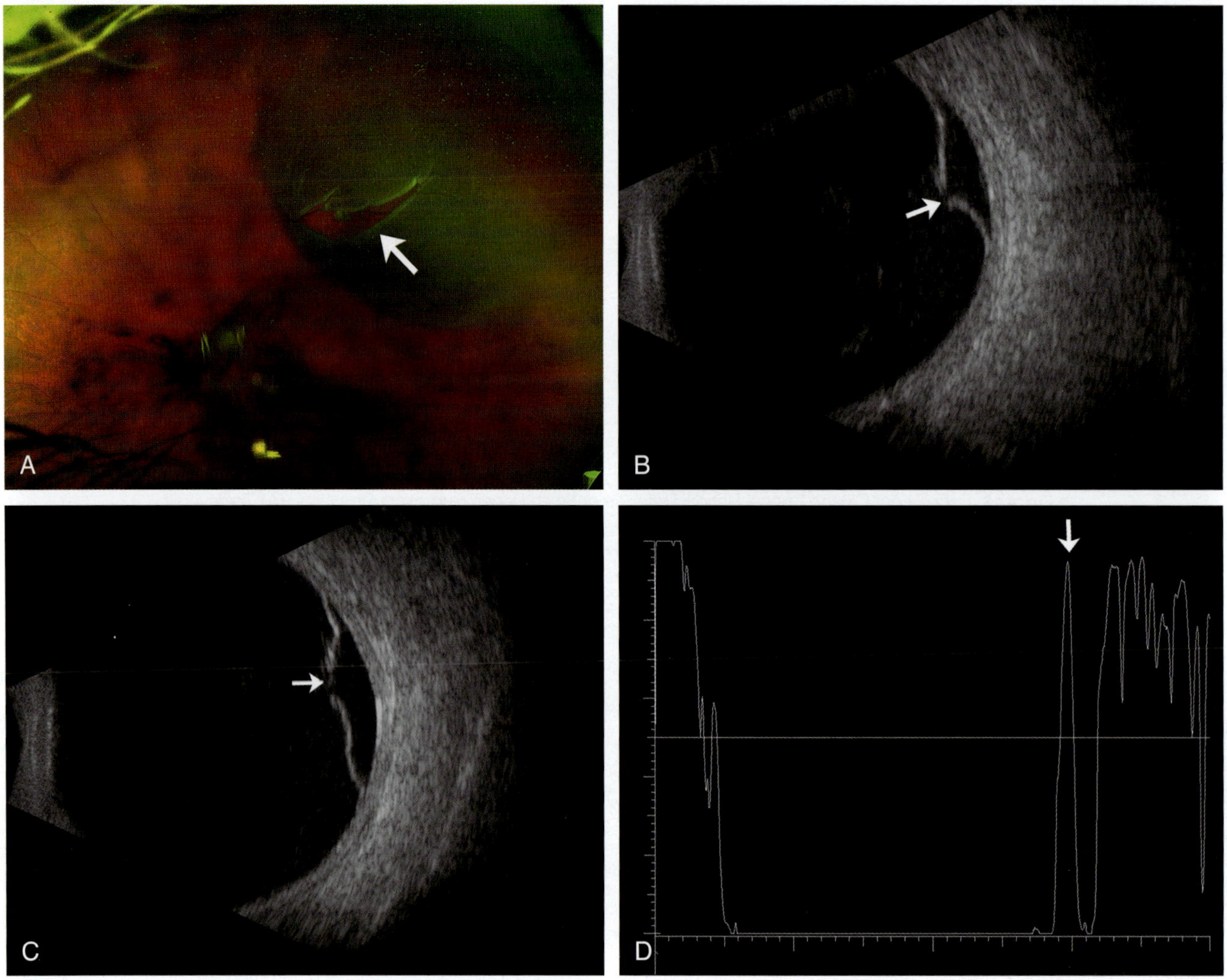

• **Fig. 4.20** Rhegmatogenous Retinal Detachment. **(A)** Color fundus photography shows a retinal tear (*arrow*) and retinal detachment superiorly. **(B)** Longitudinal and **(C)** transverse B-scans show a break (*arrow*) in the localized midperipheral retinal detachment. There is adhesion of the posterior vitreous cortex at the edge of the retinal break and a moderately dense hemorrhage beneath the posterior hyaloid (subhyaloid hemorrhage). A-scan **(D)** displays a 100% high, single-peaked spike produced by the detached retina (*arrow*).

CASE

A 15-year-old girl with a history of lattice degeneration presented for urgent evaluation for floaters. Past ocular history was significant for retinal tear in the fellow eye. Fundus and ultrasound examinations showed retinal detachment with retinal tear (Fig. 4.21 and sonogram Video 4.15).

CASE

A 26-year-old man with a history of ocular trauma was evaluated for retinal detachment. Ultrasonography demonstrated retinal detachment secondary to retinal dialysis (Fig. 4.22).

Rhegmatogenous Retinal Detachment Secondary to Retinal Dialysis

Retinal dialysis is a tear of the retina from its insertion at the ora serrata. Most retinal dialyses result from blunt trauma. The retinal detachments caused by retinal dialyses typically progress slowly and are only shallowly elevated. Longitudinal B-scan is the most useful view for assessing the peripheral retina in such cases.

Traction Retinal Detachment

Traction RDs are commonly seen in proliferative retinal vascular diseases such as diabetic retinopathy, sickle cell retinopathy, and retinopathy of prematurity. They can also develop as a complication of proliferative vitreoretinopathy after penetrating ocular trauma.

B-scan ultrasound can demonstrate the retinal traction caused by partial PVD and proliferative membranes on the retinal surface. Traction retinal detachment often has

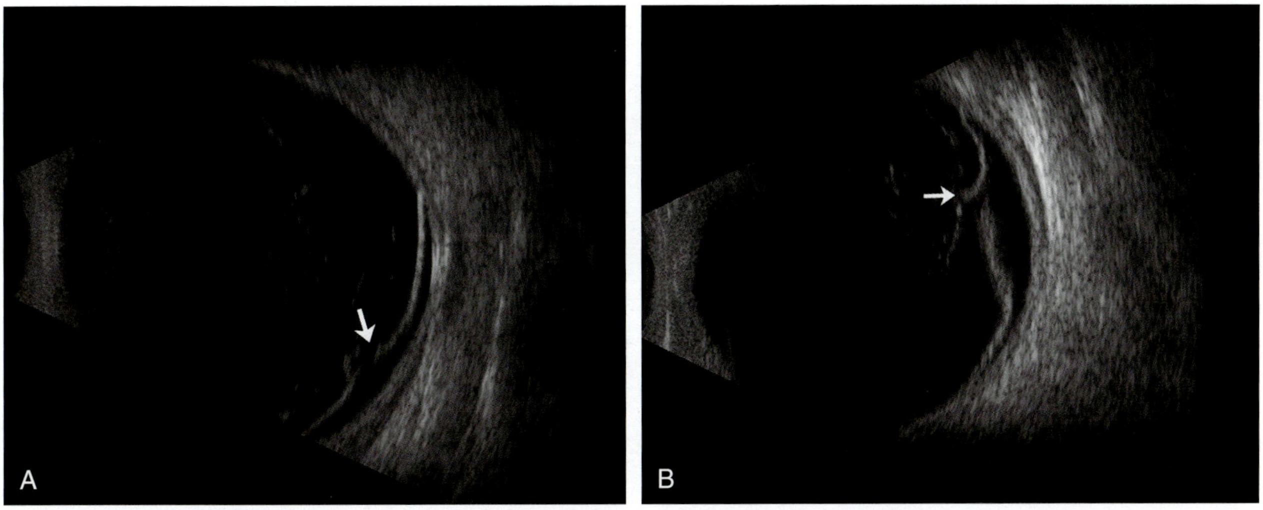

• **Fig. 4.21** Rhegmatogenous Retinal Detachment. **(A)** Transverse and **(B)** longitudinal B-scans show shallow retinal detachment with a retinal tear (*arrow*). A focal discontinuity in the detached retina is seen at the tear site, which is attached to a low reflective hyaloid membrane.

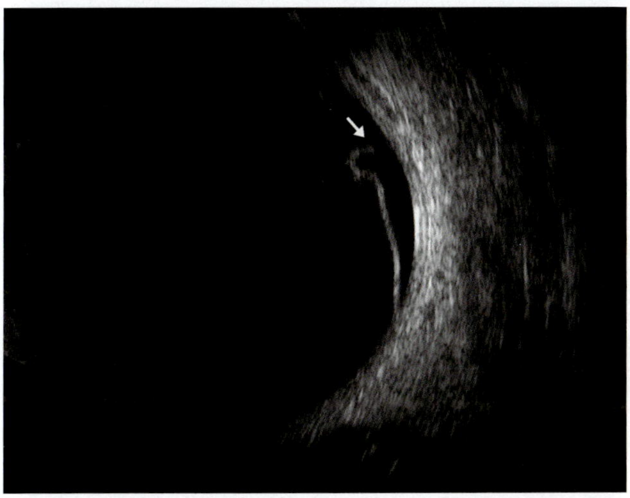

• **Fig. 4.22** Rhegmatogenous Retinal Detachment Secondary to Retinal Dialysis. Longitudinal B-scan shows a shallow retinal detachment with a discontinuity (*arrow*) of the retina at its peripheral insertion (dialysis).

a concave surface, is free of retinal breaks and localized in extent, and shows minimal retinal mobility. The detached retina may be elevated by a narrow vitreoretinal adhesion causing a tent-like pattern, or by a broad vitreoretinal adhesion causing a table-top pattern. The subretinal space can be anechoic or contain opacities in cases of subretinal hemorrhage.

In proliferative diabetic retinopathy, there is fibrovascular tissue at the interface between the posterior vitreous cortex and retina. The contraction of this complex can cause substantial vitreoretinal traction and consequent RD. Initially, the retina is typically elevated along the temporal vascular arcades, but with progression the traction RD may extend into the retinal periphery and/or macular area. Furthermore, traction RD in the far periphery can result from anterior hyaloidal fibrovascular proliferation, a severe postoperative complication occurring after vitrectomy or extracapsular cataract extraction.[9–10] In sickle cell retinopathy, the traction RD also tends to occur in the periphery.

CASE

A 50-year-old man with a history of type 2 diabetes mellitus presented with decreased visual acuity, vitreous hemorrhage, and no fundus view. Sonographic features were consistent with traction retinal detachment (Fig. 4.23 and sonogram Video 4.16).

CASE

A 49-year-old with a history of type 2 diabetes mellitus was referred for a sonographic evaluation of traction retinal detachment (Fig. 4.24 and sonogram Video 4.17).

Exudative (Serous) Retinal Detachment

Exudative (serous) RD occurs when fluid leaking from choroidal or retinal vessels enters the subretinal space. The abnormal leakage may be caused by inflammation, infiltration by malignant cells, or retinal or choroidal vascular diseases. Exudative RD can therefore be associated with such disorders as Harada's disease, posterior scleritis, choroidal melanoma, metastatic choroidal tumors, Coat's disease, nanophthalmic or idiopathic uveal effusion, age-related macular degeneration, idiopathic central serous chorioretinopathy, and pregnancy-induced hypertension.[11]

On B-scan ultrasonographic examination, exudative retinal detachment is characterized by a bullous, convex

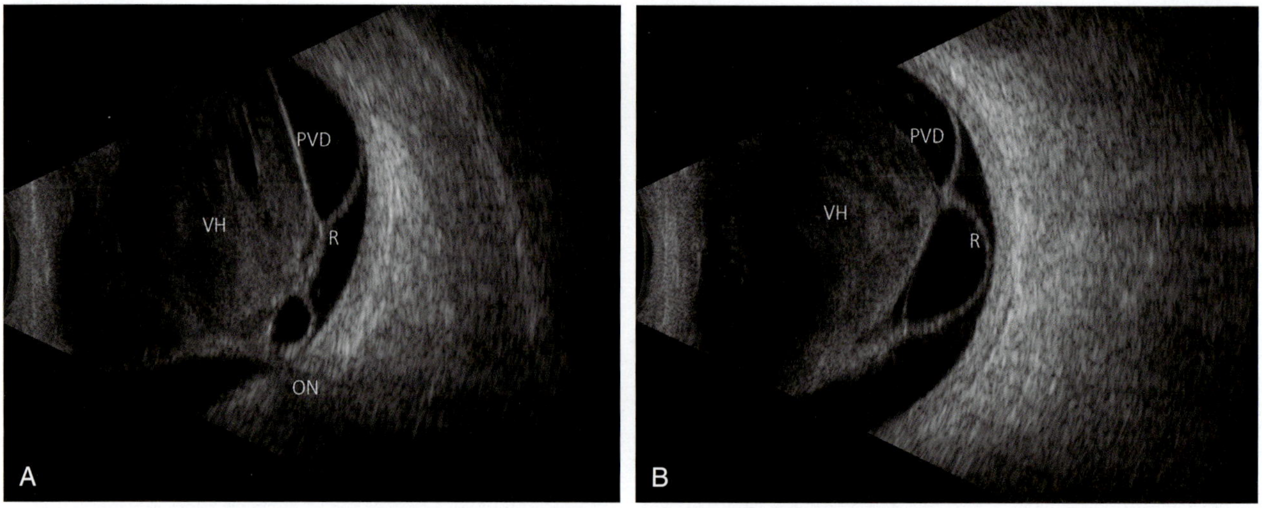

• **Fig. 4.23** Traction Retinal Detachment. **(A)** Longitudinal and **(B)** transverse B-scans display a fibrovascular membrane on the posterior vitreous surface pulling the retina **(R)** off the back wall of the eye. *VH*, Vitreous hemorrhage; *PVD*, posterior vitreous detachment; *ON*, optic nerve.

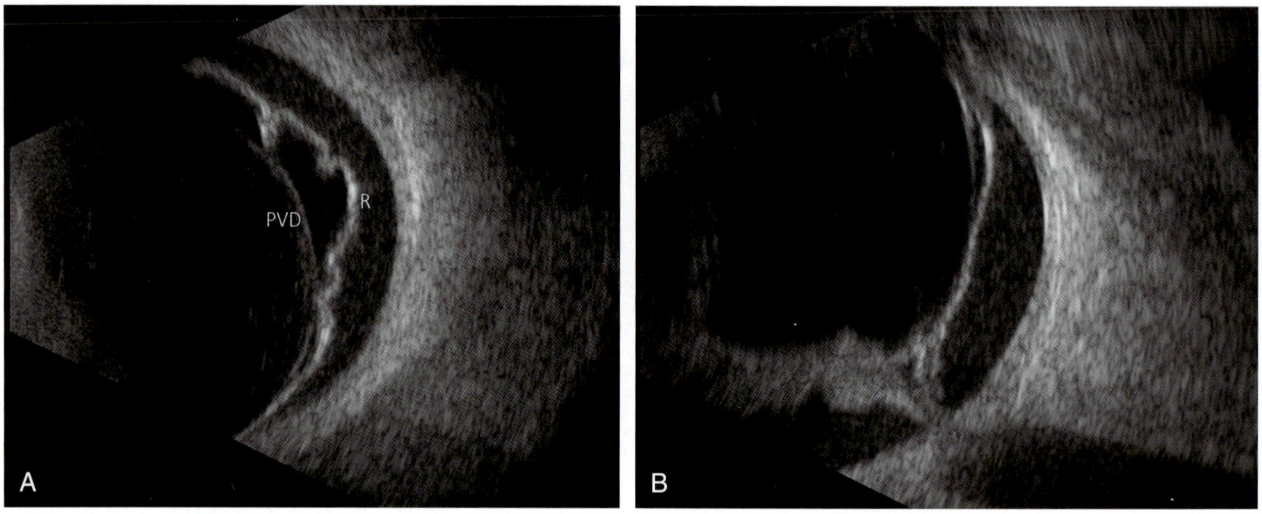

• **Fig. 4.24** Traction Retinal Detachment. **(A)** Transverse B-scan ultrasound shows posterior vitreous detachment (PVD) with multifocal vitreoretinal adhesions giving rise to traction retinal detachment (R). **(B)** Longitudinal B-scan ultrasound shows a total retinal detachment with a closed funnel posteriorly and subretinal opacities consistent with subretinal hemorrhage.

elevated membrane with a smooth or slightly folded surface. The detached retina is mobile and shows the phenomenon of "shifting fluid," wherein the extent of subretinal fluid changes with alterations in eye position. For example, in the upright position, gravity causes the subretinal fluid to accumulate under the inferior retina, but upon adopting a supine position the fluid shifts posteriorly.

CASE

A 53-year-old woman was diagnosed with panuveitis and was evaluated for multilobulated serous retinal detachment (Fig. 4.25) and anterior chamber inflammatory cells.

TEACHING POINTS

Topographic and kinetic techniques detect a detached retina as a uniformly thick, folded membrane with shaky aftermovement.

A total RD usually has a typical funnel shape (open or closed), inserted into the optic disc posteriorly and at the ora serrata anteriorly.

Sonographic characterization of RD can demonstrate breaks (rhegmatogenous RD), vitreoretinal traction (tractional RD), or inflammatory, neoplastic, or vascular conditions (exudative RD).

Longitudinal and transverse approaches scanning the temporal posterior pole define the macular involvement in RD; macula-on or macula-off.

Sonographic features of long-standing, chronic RD are retinal cysts, subretinal lipid particles, or focal or diffuse retinal calcification. These features can help guide the urgency of surgical repair.

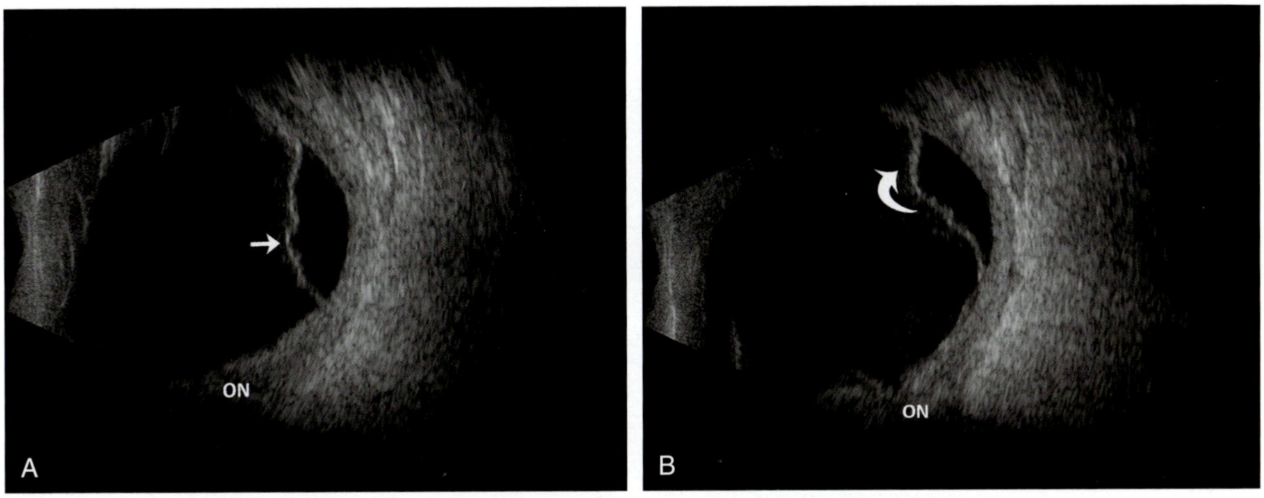

• **Fig. 4.25** Exudative Retinal Detachment. **(A)** Longitudinal B-scan ultrasound aimed inferiorly reveals convex serous retinal detachment (*arrow*) in the supine position. **(B)** In the upright position, the subretinal fluid shifts to a more peripheral region of the inferior fundus (*curved arrow*). *ON*, Optic nerve.

Choroidal Neovascularization and Disciform Process

Choroidal neovascularization (CNV) consists of fibrovascular tissue growth beneath the neurosensory retina. The vessels may lie between the choroid and retinal pigment epithelium (RPE) or between the RPE and the sensory retina. CNV may cause the following complications: hemorrhagic RPE detachment, serous and hemorrhagic retinal detachment, vitreous hemorrhage, and subretinal scarring, also termed disciform scarring.

CNV may develop in a variety of pathologic conditions. Age-related macular degeneration is the most common cause. Other entities include ocular histoplasmosis, myopic maculopathy, angioid streaks, pachychoroid spectrum disorders and choroidal rupture.

Ultrasound imaging can demonstrate a lesion located in the macular area or less commonly in the periphery with an irregular, slightly lobulated surface or dome-shaped contour. The internal structure is usually irregular, and the internal reflectivity varies according to its contents. Serous fluid or fresh hemorrhage produces low reflectivity, while older organized hemorrhage and fibrovascular scar produce high reflectivity. Eventually, the blood or blood products can migrate through the retina into the vitreous cavity generating massive vitreous opacification. Since these lesions can mimic intraocular tumors, close follow-up with serial ultrasound evaluations will demonstrate decreasing thickness of the disciform process.

CASE

An 86-year-old woman with a history of age-related macular degeneration presented with worsening vision in the left eye. Fundus examination revealed a disciform scar in the right eye and poor visualization in the left eye due to dense vitreous hemorrhage (Fig. 4.26 and sonogram Video 4.18).

Retinal Pigment Epithelial Detachment

Detachment of the RPE occurs between the basal lamina of the RPE and Bruch's membrane, and the etiology can be classified into the following categories: inflammatory, infiltrative, serous, fibrovascular, hemorrhagic, and serous. Pigment epithelial detachments are most often associated with age-related macular degeneration, polypoidal choroidal vasculopathy, and central serous choroidopathy. However, they can also be associated with a spectrum of inflammatory, infectious, neoplastic, iatrogenic, and idiopathic disorders of the RPE and choroid.[12]

On B-scan ultrasonography, retinal pigment epithelial detachment appears as a localized hyperreflective, thick, dome-shaped membrane with a smooth surface and sharply demarcated borders. The content of the sub-RPE space can be serous fluid, hemorrhage, fibrovascular scar, or inflammatory or neoplastic cellular infiltrate.

CASE

An 82-year-old woman with a history of wet age-related macular degeneration, presented to the clinic with vision deterioration. Fundus examination revealed a large central disciform scar with overlying fluid and areas of atrophy (Fig. 4.27).

CASE

A 69-year-old man with a history of exudative age-related macular degeneration presented with dense vitreous hemorrhage and no fundus view. Sonographic features were consistent with hemorrhagic retinal pigment epithelial detachment (Fig. 4.28).

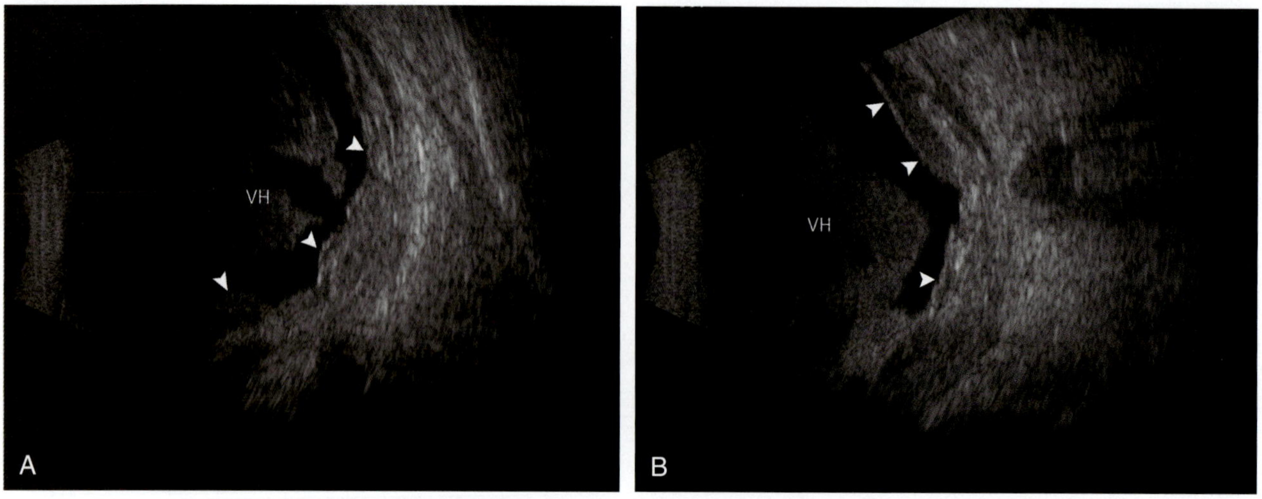

• **Fig. 4.26** Disciform Process. **(A)** Longitudinal and **(B)** transverse B-scans through the temporal posterior pole demonstrate dense vitreous hemorrhage (VH) associated with an extensive, lobulated, irregularly structured hemorrhagic disciform lesion (*arrowheads*).

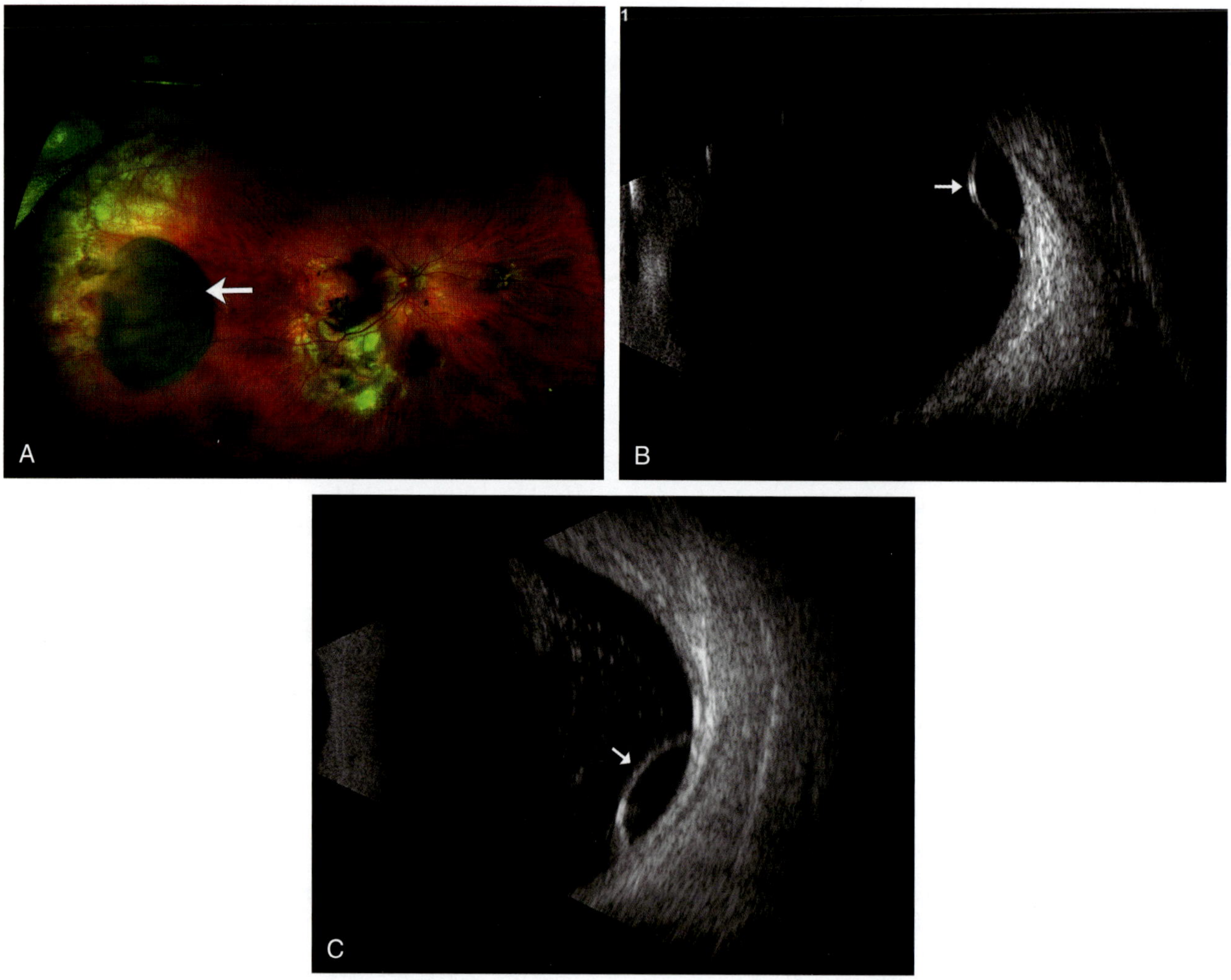

• **Fig. 4.27** Retinal Pigment Epithelial Detachment. **(A)** Wide-field fundus photograph demonstrates a central disciform scar and a temporal pigment epithelium detachment (*arrow*). **(B)** Longitudinal and **(C)** transverse B-scans showing a pigment epithelium detachment as a dome-shaped membrane with smooth surface and sharply demarcated insertion (*arrow*).

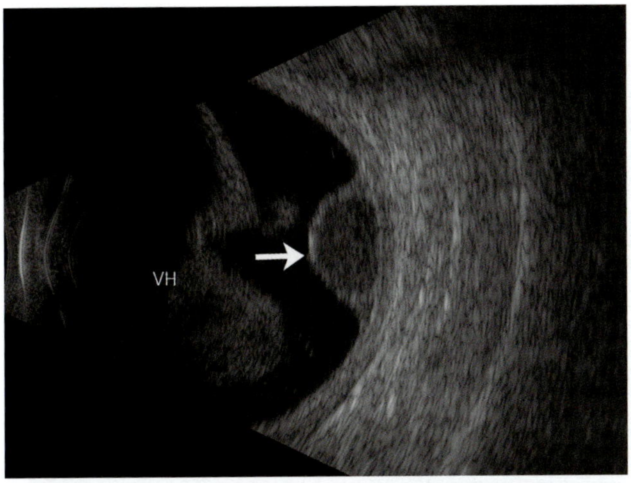

• **Fig. 4.28** Hemorrhagic Retinal Pigment Epithelial Detachment. Transverse B-scan ultrasound through macular area displays dense vitreous hemorrhage (VH) with a posterior vitreous detachment and hemorrhagic pigment epithelial detachment (*arrow*).

Degenerative Retinoschisis

Degenerative retinoschisis (RS) is defined as a splitting of the neurosensory retina into inner and outer layers. Clinically, RS presents as a smooth, transparent or translucent, peripheral elevation with immobile fluid that does not collapse with scleral depression.[13] Degenerative RS is an age-related condition, typically located in the temporal quadrants; however, it can be seen anywhere in the retina, and most patients have bilateral involvement.

On B-scan ultrasound, RS appears as a shallowly-elevated or dome-shaped, smooth, thin, peripheral membrane located anterior to the equator. On A-scan ultrasound, RS presents a high-amplitude single-peaked spike.

CASE

A 70-year-old woman with a history of narrow-angle glaucoma was referred by a glaucoma specialist to evaluate a bilateral peripheral fundus membrane. Dilated fundus biomicroscopy revealed bilateral peripheral retinoschisis (Fig. 4.29).

It is important to differentiate RS from retinal detachment. Scleral depression in conjunction with ultrasound observation is valuable to distinguish RS from retinal detachment; in contrast to retinal detachment, scleral indentation fails to collapse the fluid cavity in retinoschisis.[14]

CASE

A 59-year-old asymptomatic man presented for routine examination. Dilated fundus examination revealed bilateral peripheral retinoschisis (Fig. 4.30 and sonogram Video 4.19).

A high-resolution B-scan ultrasound can be used reliably to differentiate between RS and RD.15 On B-scan with 20 MHz high-resolution probe, RS generates a single hyperreflective continuous line (Fig. 4.31A), while RD generates two hyperreflective lines (Fig. 4.31B).

Schisis-Detachment

Schisis-detachment is seen only in cases of retinoschisis. It is always associated with a break in the outer retinal layer, which allows fluid in the retinoschisis cavity to access the subretinal space.[16] Patients with schisis-detachment are usually asymptomatic.

On B-scan ultrasound, schisis-detachment appears as a dome shaped, smooth peripheral membrane located

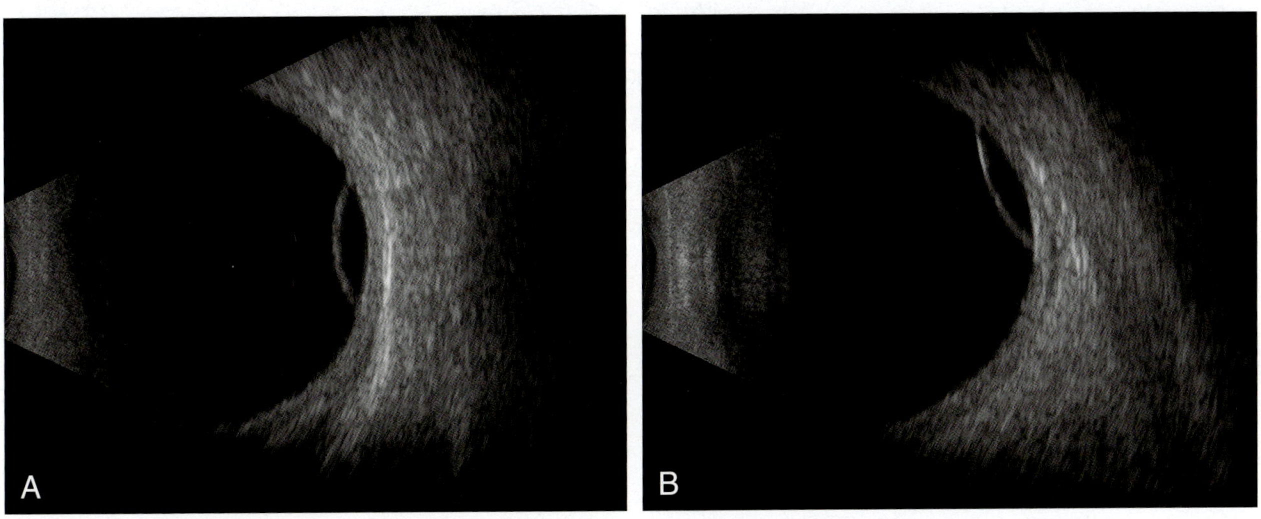

• **Fig. 4.29** Degenerative Retinoschisis. **(A)** Transverse B-scan ultrasound through the peripheral aspect of the fundus displays a smooth, dome-shaped, thin membrane. **(B)** Longitudinal B-scan ultrasound displays the peripheral location of the retinoschisis.

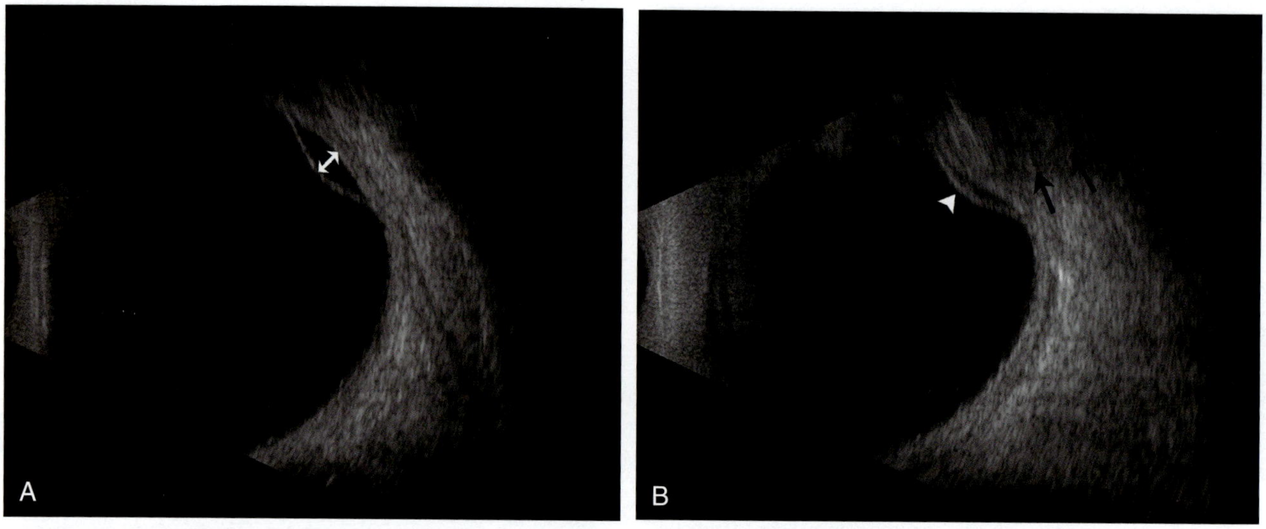

• **Fig. 4.30** Scleral Indentation in Retinoschisis. **(A)** Longitudinal B-scan ultrasound of a retinoschisis cavity located in the fundus periphery (*connected arrows*). **(B)** Scleral depression is performed over the area of retinoschisis. The distance between the retinoschisis and sclera decreases slightly but does not flatten completely with indentation (*arrowhead*). Shadow area from the depressor on extraocular space (*arrows*).

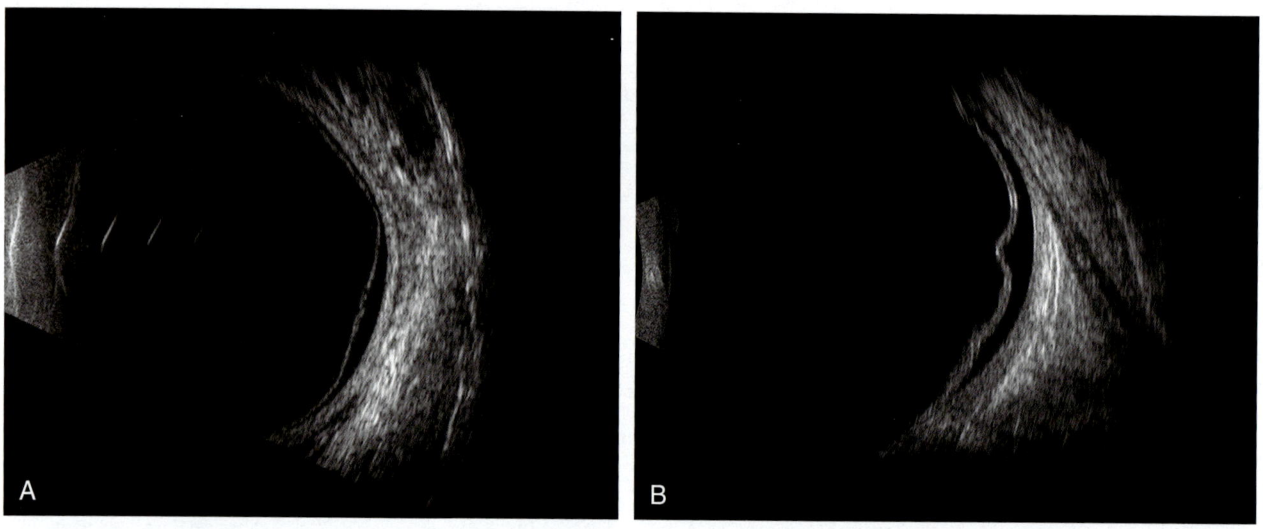

• **Fig. 4.31** **(A)** Retinoschisis imaged with a 20 MHz B-scan probe shows a single hyperreflective line. **(B)** Retinal detachment imaged with a 20 MHz B-scan probe typically appears as double highly reflective lines.

anterior to the equator with a hole in the outer retinal layer that is also elevated from the retinal pigment epithelium.

CASE

A 73-year-old man was referred for evaluation of a choroidal nevus at the posterior pole. On ultrasound assessment, a peripheral, temporal schisis-detachment (Fig. 4.32 and sonogram Video 4.20) was incidentally discovered.

TEACHING POINTS

Bilaterality is a typical characteristic of retinoschisis; therefore, the fellow eye always needs to be investigated.

B-scan ultrasound with simultaneous scleral depression can be used to differentiate retinoschisis from retinal detachment. With depression, the retina flattens as subretinal fluid is pushed through the retinal breaks into the vitreous cavity. Retinoschisis will not flatten fully.

While uncomplicated retinoschisis, with no associated outer retinal layer breaks, usually is a benign process, schisis detachment can progress to symptomatic retinal detachment that requires intervention.

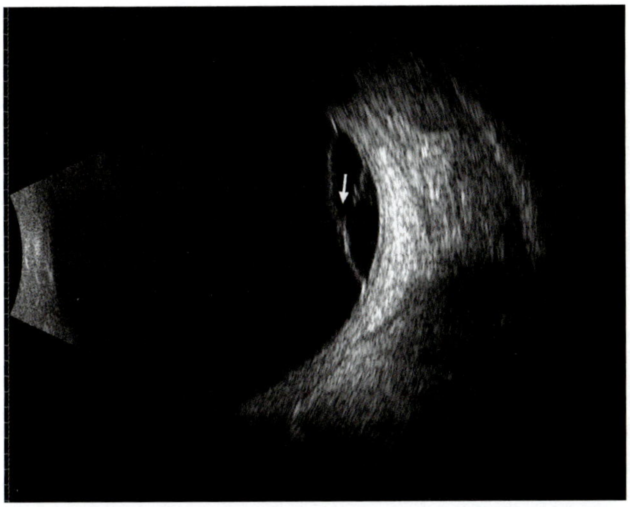

• **Fig. 4.32** Schisis-Detachment. Longitudinal B-scan ultrasound shows a localized peripheral schisis-detachment with hole (*arrow*) in the outer retinal layer and detachment of the neurosensory retina at the posterior aspect of the lesion.

Macular Edema

Fluid leakage in the macular area can accumulate in the subretinal space or in the retina. There are diverse causes of macular edema, including uveitic or postoperative inflammation, retinal vascular disease (such as diabetic retinopathy and retinal vein occlusion), central serous retinopathy, choroidal neovascularization, adverse drug effects, tractional conditions, and retinal dystrophies such as retinitis pigmentosa.

On B-scan ultrasonography, macular edema appears as a focal, highly reflective, slightly elevated membrane just temporal to the optic disc.

CASE

Macular edema. A 62-year-old man with uveitis associated with multiple sclerosis presented urgently with a complaint of decreased vision. Ophthalmoscopic evaluation revealed inflammatory cells in the anterior chamber, vitritis, and macular edema (Fig. 4.33 and sonogram Video 4.21).

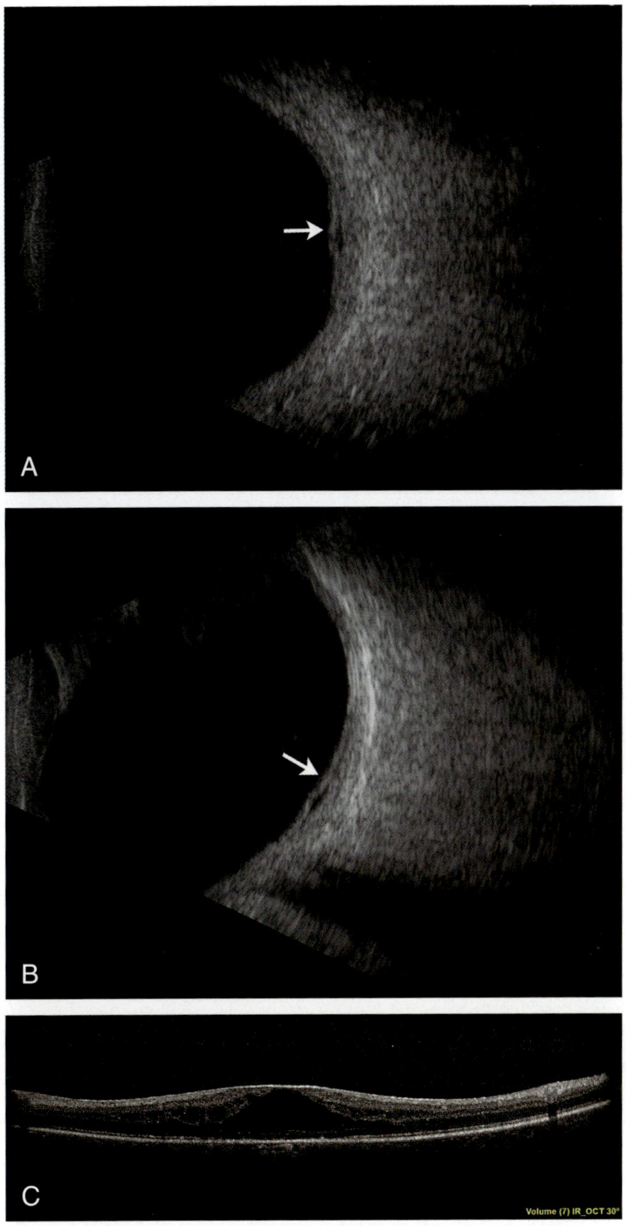

• **Fig. 4.33** Macular Edema. **(A)** Vertical transverse B-scan, **(B)** longitudinal B-scan, and **(C)** spectral-domain OCT through macular area demonstrating focal edema.

CASE

A 52-year-old woman was evaluated for blurred vision of 6 months' duration and signs of intraocular inflammation. A routine systemic workup for uveitis was negative. The patient underwent uveal biopsy, and histopathology revealed sarcoid uveitis (Fig. 4.34).

Choroid

Choroidal Thickening

The normal choroid is thickest (0.25 mm) at the posterior pole and gradually thins anteriorly (0.10 mm). Choroidal thickening, either localized or diffuse, can occur in several ocular conditions and be associated with inflammation, vascular disease, neoplasia, scleropathy, and hypotony, among others.

Choroidal Detachment

Choroidal detachment (CD), choroidal effusion, ciliochoroidal detachment, and ciliochoroidal effusion are terms that have been used interchangeably to define an

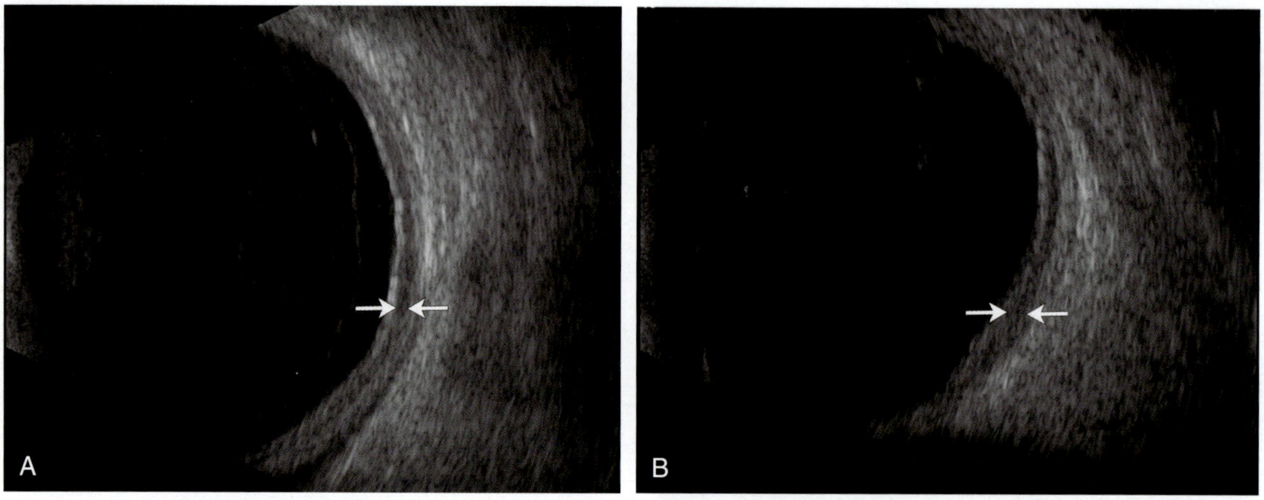

• **Fig. 4.34** Inflammatory Choroidal Thickening. **(A)** Transverse and **(B)** longitudinal B-scans show diffuse choroidal thickening (*arrows*) in a patient with sarcoid uveitis.

TABLE 4.2 Classification and Causes of Choroidal Detachment

Classification	Causes
Inflammatory	Trauma and intraocular surgery Uveitis Scleritis
Hydrostatic	Hypotony and wound leak Rhegmatogenous retinal detachment Drug-induced Increased uveal venous pressure (e.g., AV fistulas, Valsalva, pulmonary hypertension, etc.)
Uveal effusion syndrome	Hypermetropic or nanophthalmic Idiopathic

abnormal collection of fluid in the outer layers of the choroid or suprachoroidal space. As shown in Table 4.2, choroidal detachment (CD) is typically associated with hypotony, increased uveal venous pressure, inflammation, scleral abnormalities, or some combination of these factors.

With respect to size, CDs can vary from small, localized areas to massive involvement of all quadrants. Choroidal detachment can be restricted to the periphery or can extend to the posterior pole. The height of elevation can be shallow or bullous. In severe cases of massive elevation, retina-to-retina apposition occurs in the center of the vitreous cavity, a variant termed appositional or "kissing" choroidal detachment. The nature of the fluid in the suprachoroidal space can be serous or hemorrhagic.

On B-scan ultrasound, CD typically presents as a thick, smooth, dome-shaped, hyperreflective membrane. A longitudinal view is the best approach to assess the extent of the detachment. The peripheral insertion extends anterior to the ora serrata and is continuous anteriorly with some degree of ciliary body detachment. Bullous CD extending to the posterior pole has a sharp posterior insertion adjacent to but never into the optic disc. Extensive CDs involving more than two quadrants show a typical scalloped appearance on transverse scans. On dynamic examination, CDs may or may not show jiggly aftermovement. On A-scan ultrasound, a detached choroid presents a steeply rising, double-peaked wide spike.

CASE

A 78-year-old man with choroidal effusion, likely idiopathic, underwent ultrasound evaluation showing serous choroidal elevation involving all quadrants (Fig. 4.35 and sonogram Video 4.22).

In bullous or even moderately elevated serous CDs, a distinct band can often be observed in the suprachoroidal space, extending from the posterior face of the choroid to the sclera. This band may represent a stretched vortex vein or a transcleral ciliary nerve.

CASE

An 88-year-old man presented with a choroidal "mass" after cataract surgery. Ultrasound revealed the serous nature of a localized choroidal effusion (Fig. 4.36).

CASE

A 68-year-old man with a history of lung adenocarcinoma presented with bilateral bullous choroidal detachment (Fig. 4.37) following monoclonal antibody therapy.

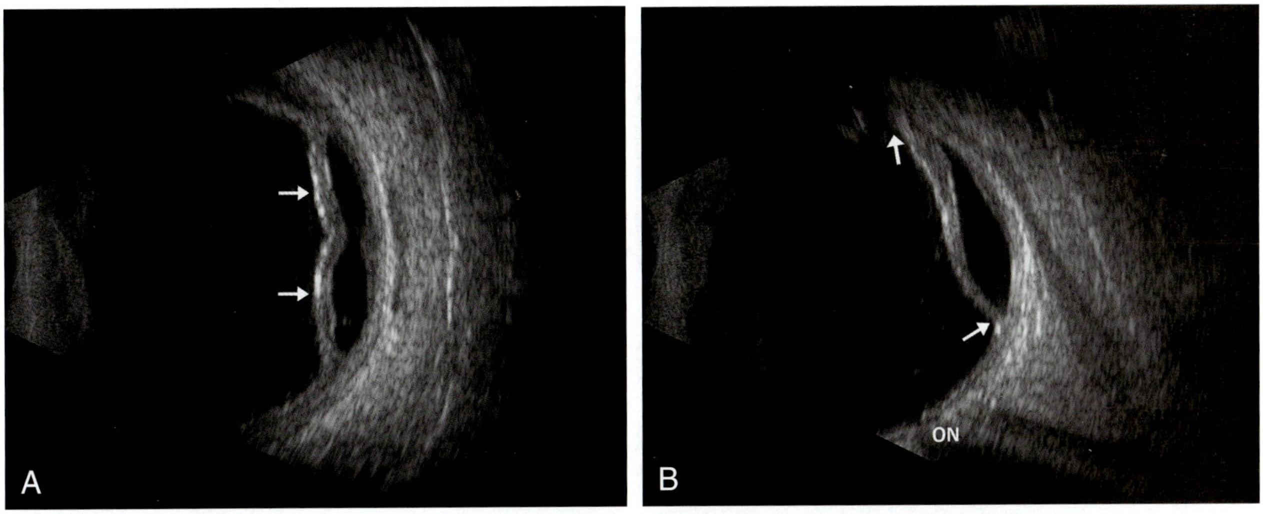

• **Fig. 4.35** Choroidal Effusion. **(A)** Transverse B-scan ultrasound shows the choroid separated from the sclera along with the retinal layer, appearing as a smooth, highly reflective membrane with multiple, scalloped insertions (*arrows*). The suprachoroidal space is anechoic, indicating the serous nature of the process. **(B)** A longitudinal view demonstrates the posterior insertion of the detached choroid near the optic nerve (ON) and the anterior insertion extending to the region of the ciliary body (*arrows*).

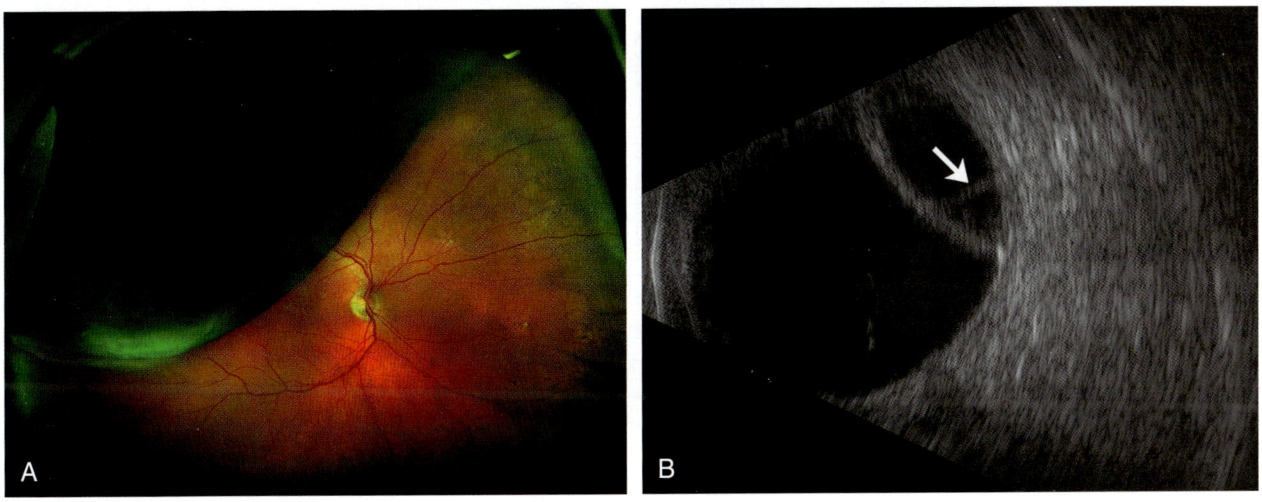

• **Fig. 4.36** Serous Choroidal Detachment. **(A)** Wide-field fundus photography shows choroidal elevation superiorly. **(B)** Longitudinal B-scan ultrasound image of serous choroidal detachment with a band in the suprachoroidal space (*arrow*).

In suprachoroidal hemorrhage, the appearance and mobility of the opacities in the suprachoroidal space vary over time. On initial evaluation, fresh clots appear as high-reflective, solid-appearing masses with irregular internal structure and irregular shape. In subsequent visits as the clots liquefy, the opacities become more dispersed, homogeneous, hypoechoic, and mobile.[17]

CASE

89-year-old man presented with severe vision loss after a penetrating corneal transplant. Ultrasound showed appositional hemorrhagic choroidal detachment (Fig. 4.38 and sonogram Video 4.23).

CASE

A 60-year-old man presented with loss of vision and hyphema following blunt trauma. Ultrasound demonstrated focal cyclodialysis and shallow ciliochoroidal detachment extending for 360° (Fig. 4.39 and sonogram Video 4.24).

TEACHING POINTS

Monitoring the liquefaction of the blood in suprachoroidal hemorrhage can be achieved with serial follow-up B-scans, which facilitate planning the appropriate time for surgical drainage of the hemorrhagic material.

Regressing choroidal detachment shows decreasing elevation and may become more mobile and folded, mimicking retinal detachment. The observation of peripheral insertion anterior to the ora serrata, and posterior insertion outside of the optic disc, aides in the diagnosis of choroidal detachment.

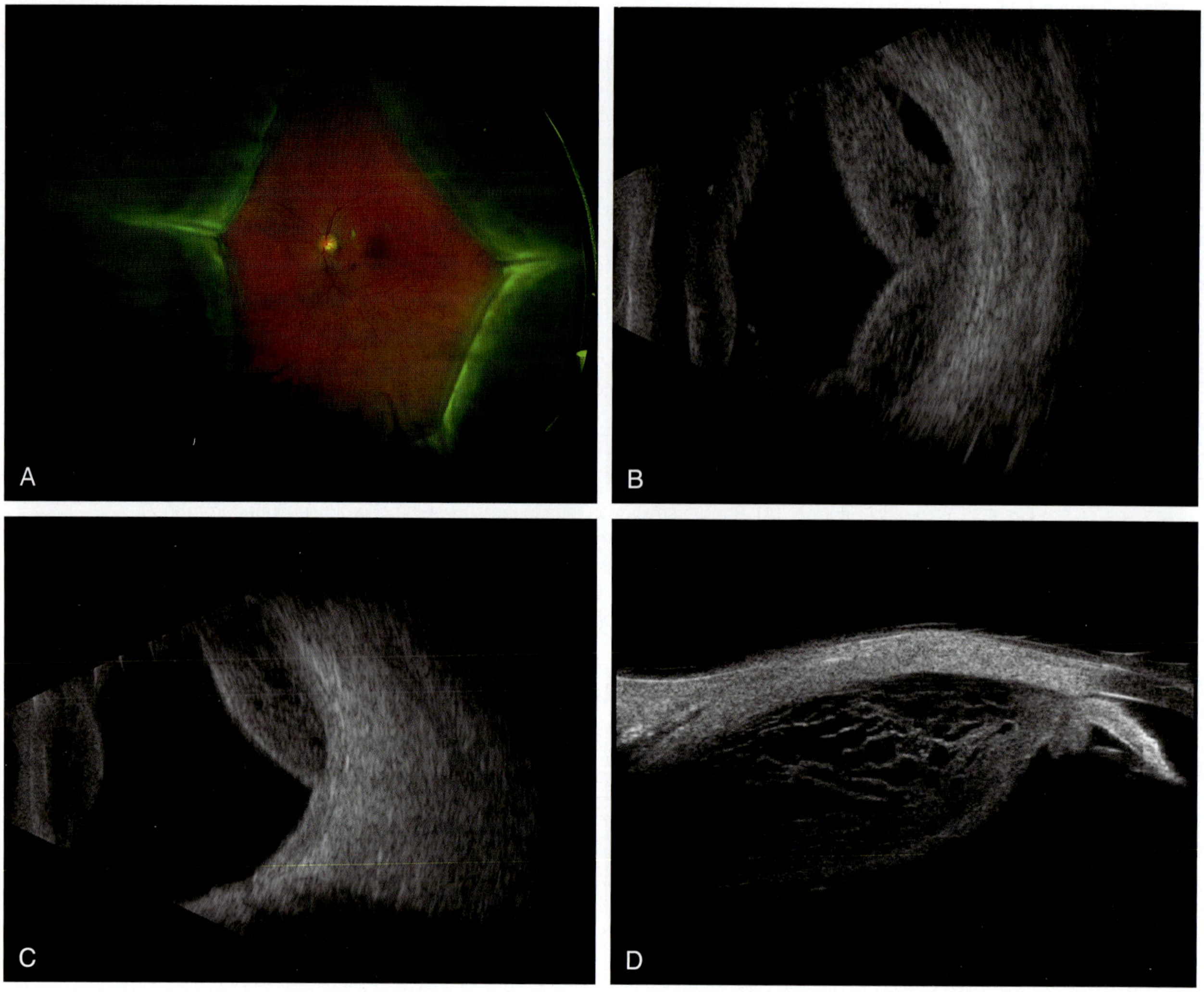

• **Fig. 4.37** Drug-Induced Choroidal Effusion. **(A)** Wide-field fundus photography shows bullous choroidal elevations involving all quadrants. B-scan in **(B)** transverse and **(C)** longitudinal views demonstrates drug-induced choroidal effusion. **(D)** Ultrasound biomicroscopy shows the anterior extension of the massive edema in the supraciliary space.

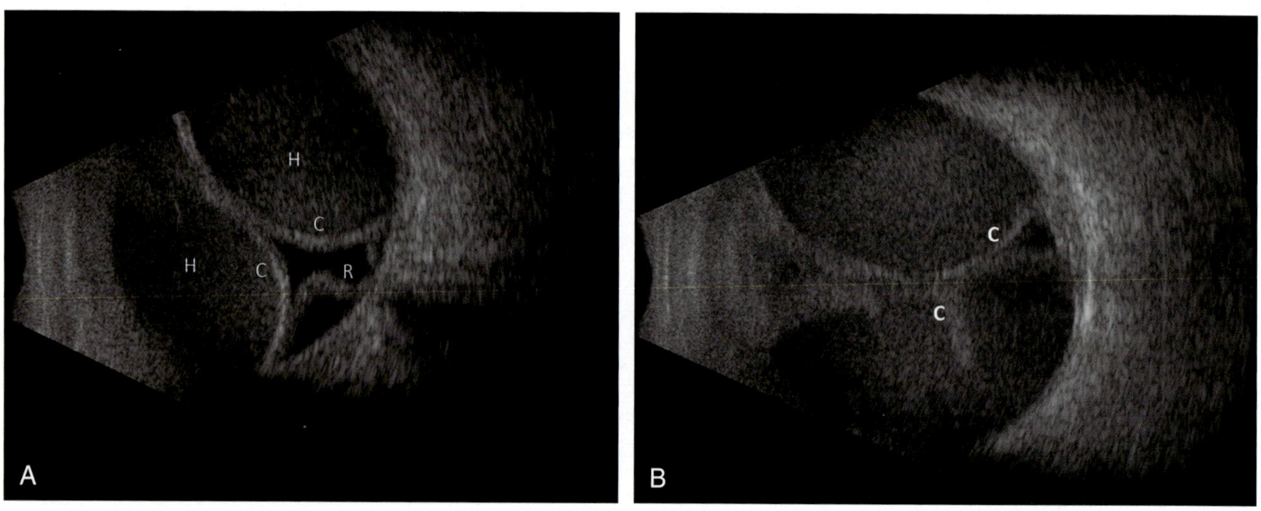

• **Fig. 4.38** Hemorrhagic Choroidal Detachment. **(A)** Longitudinal and **(B)** transverse B-scans show a bullous, appositional ("kissing") hemorrhagic choroidal detachment. The blood (H) in the suprachoroidal space has a fluid appearance with dense and homogeneously dispersed opacities. *R*, Retina; *C*, choroid.

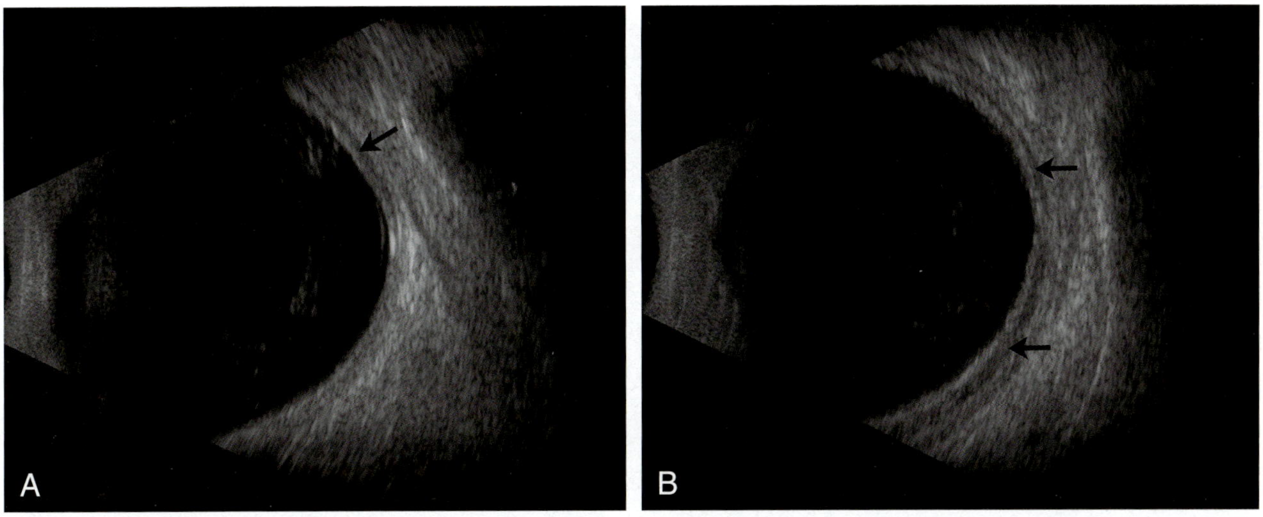

• **Fig. 4.39** Shallow Ciliochoroidal Detachment. **(A)** Longitudinal B-scan ultrasound demonstrates slight elevation of the choroid extending anteriorly (*arrow*). **(B)** A transverse B-scan ultrasound of the fundus periphery demonstrates a smooth thick annular membrane (arrows).

Retinochoroidal Coloboma

Ocular colobomas are thought to arise from errors in embryogenesis involving impaired closure of the optic fissure. The colobomatous defect can involve the cornea, lens, optic nerve, and uvea, usually located inferiorly. Retinochoroidal colobomas can vary from minor defects in the equatorial region that do not interfere with the vision to large cavitations involving the disc and macula and causing severe vision impairment.

Increased relative coloboma excavation (ratio of colobomas depth to axial length) and the presence of a retrobulbar cyst are associated with increased risk of retinal detachment and severe visual impairment.[18]

Histologically, the retinal pigment epithelium is absent in the area of coloboma but is usually hyperplastic at the edges, the neural retina is atrophic, the choroid is partially or completely absent, and the sclera may be thin or distended.

On B-scan ultrasound, a retinochoroidal coloboma is characterized by an excavated area with a thin retinochoroidal layer and hyperreflective base. The transition from the normally structured fundus to colobomatous fundus is well delineated by B-scan ultrasound.

CASE

An 84-year-old woman presented with progressive deterioration of vision. She was found to have a retinochoroidal coloboma with an associated visual field defect (Fig. 4.40).

Sclera

The high reflectivity of the normal anterior sclera is distinct from the adjacent less-reflective episcleral, ciliary body, and corneal tissues on UBM examination. The sclera is thinnest immediately posterior to the insertions of the rectus muscles.

The posterior sclera can be assessed on B-scan using axial, transverse, and longitudinal scans. The sclera is thickest in the region surrounding the optic disc. A potential space, the sub-Tenon's space, separates the outer surface of the sclera from the orbital fat and can be distended by inflammatory, neoplastic, or hemorrhagic infiltrates.

Senile Scleral Plaque

Senile scleral plaques are well-circumscribed, slate-grey, oblong areas within the sclera found posterior to the limbus and anterior to the insertions of the horizontal rectus muscles. Senile scleral plaques are asymptomatic, often bilateral, and most frequently seen in persons older than 70 years. Histopathology demonstrates calcium deposition and decreased scleral cellularity.[19]

CASE

A 78-year-old man was referred for ultrasound evaluation for vitreous hemorrhage of unclear etiology. B-scan ultrasound examination showed mild vitreous opacities and the incidental finding of a senile scleral plaque (Fig. 4.41 and sonogram Video 4.25) in the nasal periphery.

Scleral Infolding

Severe ocular hypotony can cause the scleral wall to collapse inward, resulting in choroid and retina redundancy which results in chorioretinal folding. The anteroposterior diameter of the eye shortens. Hypotony may occur after ocular inflammation, trauma, or surgery.

CASE

A 45-year-old man presented urgently for evaluation of hypotony and choroidal detachment following bleb-associated endophthalmitis and vitrectomy. Ultrasound examination disclosed choroidal detachment and severe scleral infolding (Fig. 4.42).

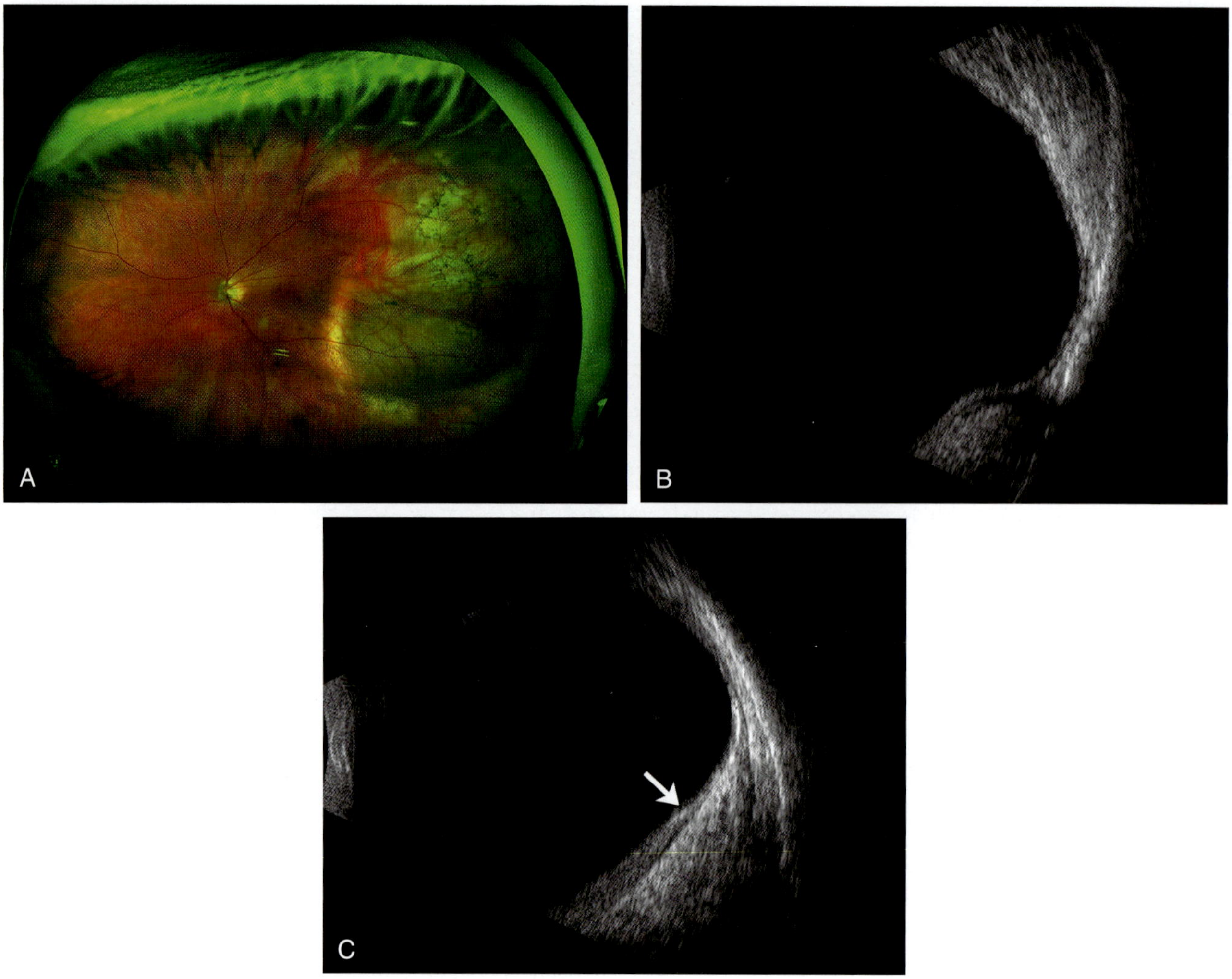

• **Fig. 4.40** Retinochoroidal coloboma. **(A)** Wide-field fundus photography shows a choroidal coloboma temporal to the macular area. **(B)** Transverse view displaying an outward bulging of the sclera with thin retinochoroidal layer. **(C)** The longitudinal view displays a well-demarcated transition from the normally structured fundus to the colobomatous fundus (*arrow*).

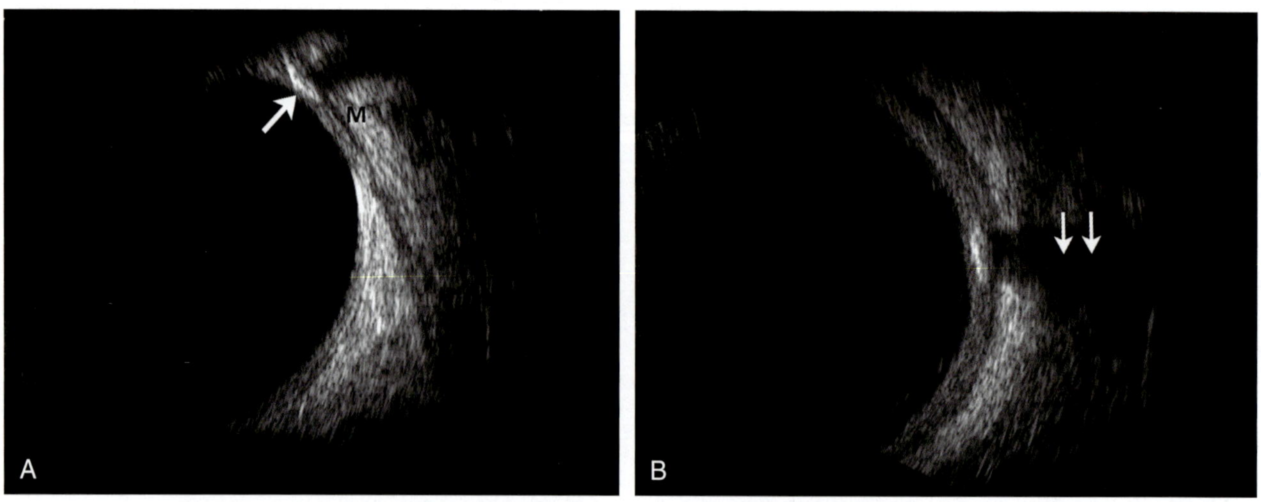

• **Fig. 4.41** Senile Scleral Plaque. **(A)** Longitudinal view of senile scleral plaque (*arrow*) localized anterior to the insertion of a horizontal extraocular muscle (M). **(B)** Transverse view aimed anteriorly demonstrates a focal calcification of the ocular coats causing shadowing of orbital tissue (double arrow).

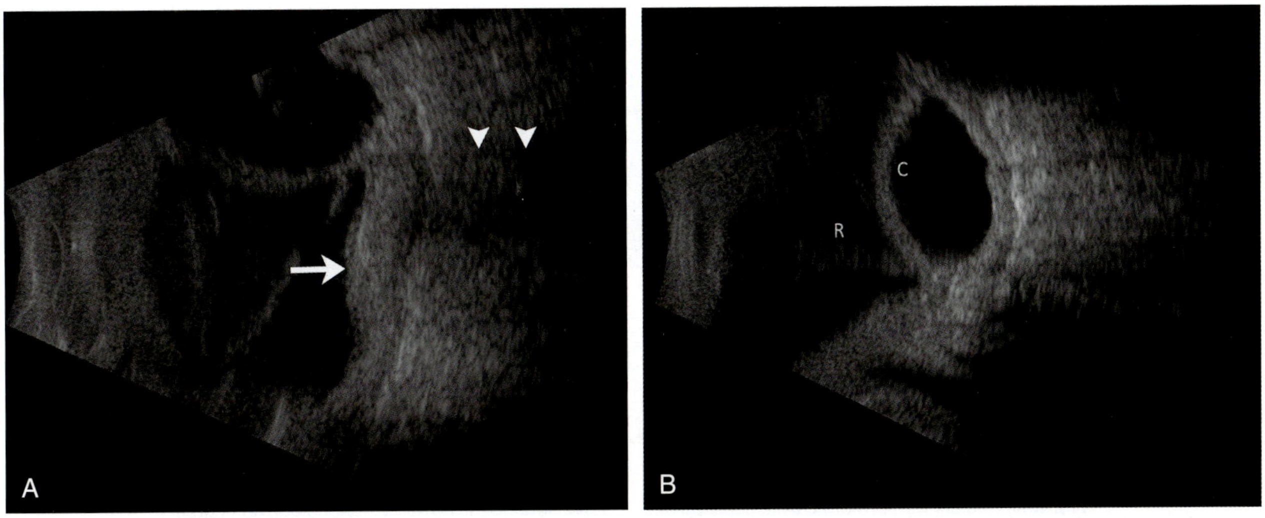

• **Fig. 4.42** Scleral Infolding. **(A)** Transverse view of scleral folds (*arrow*). The folded sclera is highly reflective, causing shadowing of adjacent orbital tissue (*arrowheads*). **(B)** The longitudinal view shows irregular posterior contour of the globe with scleral folds. *C*, Choroid; *R*, retina.

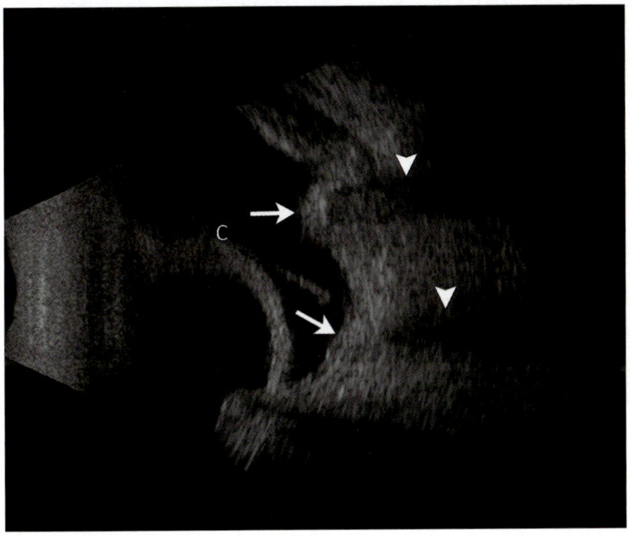

• **Fig. 4.43** Scleral Infolding. Longitudinal B-scan ultrasound displays scleral folds (*arrows*) with orbital shadowing (*arrowheads*). *C*, Detached choroid.

CASE

A 39-year-old woman presented with hypotony following a corneal transplant, presumably due to a wound leak. An ultrasound examination with minimal pressure on the globe showed a collapsed globe with marked scleral folds (Fig. 4.43).

Posterior Staphyloma

Posterior staphyloma is present most commonly in eyes with pathologic myopia and is defined as an outpouching of the wall of the eye that has a radius of curvature that is less than the surrounding curvature of the wall of the eye. Posterior staphyloma is usually located at the temporal edge of the optic disc and may involve the macula. Other less frequent patterns are: peripapillary, inferior, and nasal.[20]

Axial B-scan ultrasonography using horizontal, vertical, or oblique orientation at medium gain setting can be performed to demonstrate a posterior staphyloma's location, depth, and width.

CASE

A 77-year-old man with cone-rod dystrophy was referred for ultrasound evaluation of the posterior contour of the globe for retinal implant placement. B-scan ultrasound detected a juxtapapillary temporal outpouching of the eye wall (Fig. 4.44).

Post-Surgical Morphologic Changes

Scleral Buckling

Scleral buckling is an effective surgical technique for repairing rhegmatogenous retinal detachment and involves suturing a buckling element to the external scleral surface (explant) or placing it within a dissected scleral pocket (implant). Elements composed of solid silicone rubber are currently employed in most cases. The major patterns of scleral buckling are: circumferential (encircling or segmental) and radial.

The peripheral scleral indentation can be imaged with a longitudinal B-scan ultrasound. The interface of the episclera/buckle is high-reflective, with an echolucent band corresponding to the interior of the buckle and shadowing of the orbital tissue posterior to it. Transverse B-scan sonography of all quadrants is used to evaluate the extent of the buckling.

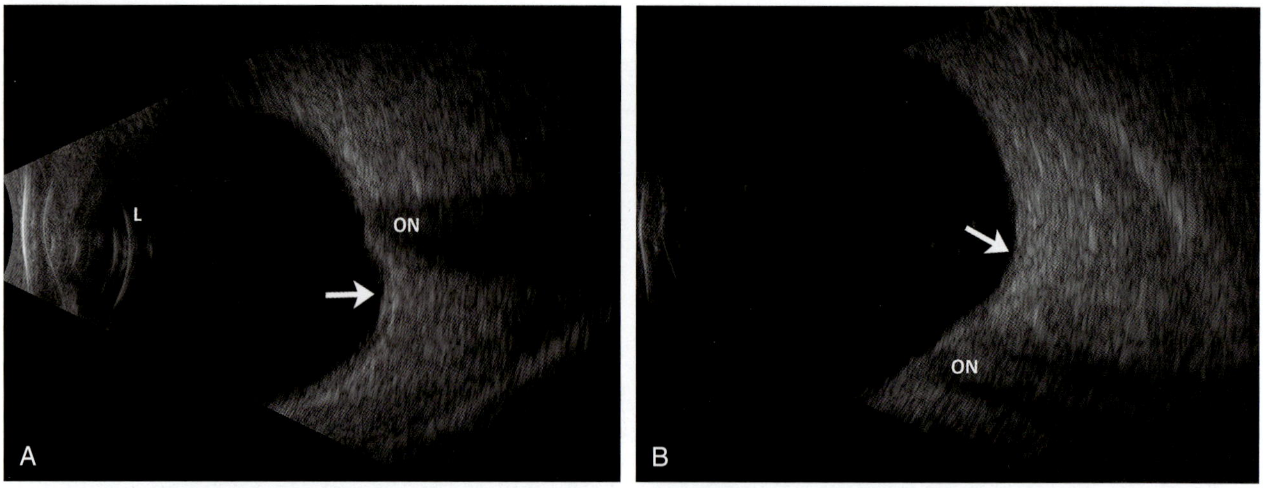

• **Fig. 4.44** Posterior Staphyloma. **(A)** Horizontal axial B-scan ultrasound shows posterior staphyloma temporal to the optic disc (*arrow*). **(B)** Longitudinal B-scan ultrasound aimed at the macular meridian shows outpouching of the posterior eye wall (*arrow*). *L*, Posterior lens capsule; *ON*, optic nerve.

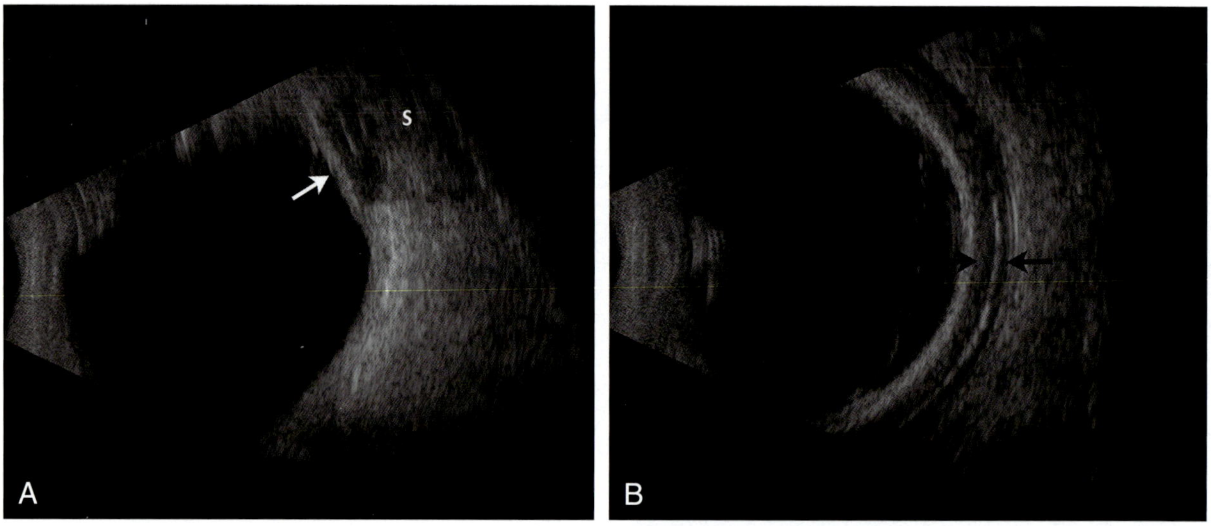

• **Fig. 4.45** Encircling Circumferential Scleral Buckle. **(A)** Longitudinal B-scan ultrasound shows a peripheral scleral indentation induced by the scleral buckle (*arrow*) and shadowing of the orbital tissue (S). **(B)** Transverse B-scan ultrasound aimed at the peripheral fundus shows an encircling circumferential buckle (*arrows*).

CASE

An 83-year-old man presented with a history of a scleral buckling procedure for rhegmatogenous retinal detachment 28 years earlier (Fig. 4.45 and sonogram Video 4.26).

CASE

A 30-year-old man with a history of buckling surgery using a segmental silicone sponge was evaluated with B-scan ultrasound (Fig. 4.46).

Silicone Oil

Silicone oil is an effective retinal tamponade used in repairing complex retinal detachment. However, the presence of silicone oil precludes reliable sonographic evaluation. Silicone oil-filled eyes produce an apparent "lengthening" of the eye because the velocity of sound transmission is slower in silicone oil than in vitreous gel.

CASE

An 84-year-old with a history of vitrectomy and silicone oil tamponade for retinal detachment presented with corneal opacity precluding assessment of the posterior segment. B-scan ultrasound showed an enlarged globe and marked sound attenuation (Fig. 4.47).

Following silicone oil removal with vitrectomy, remnant oil droplets appear as multiple point-like bright echoes floating in the vitreous cavity on B-scan ultrasound.

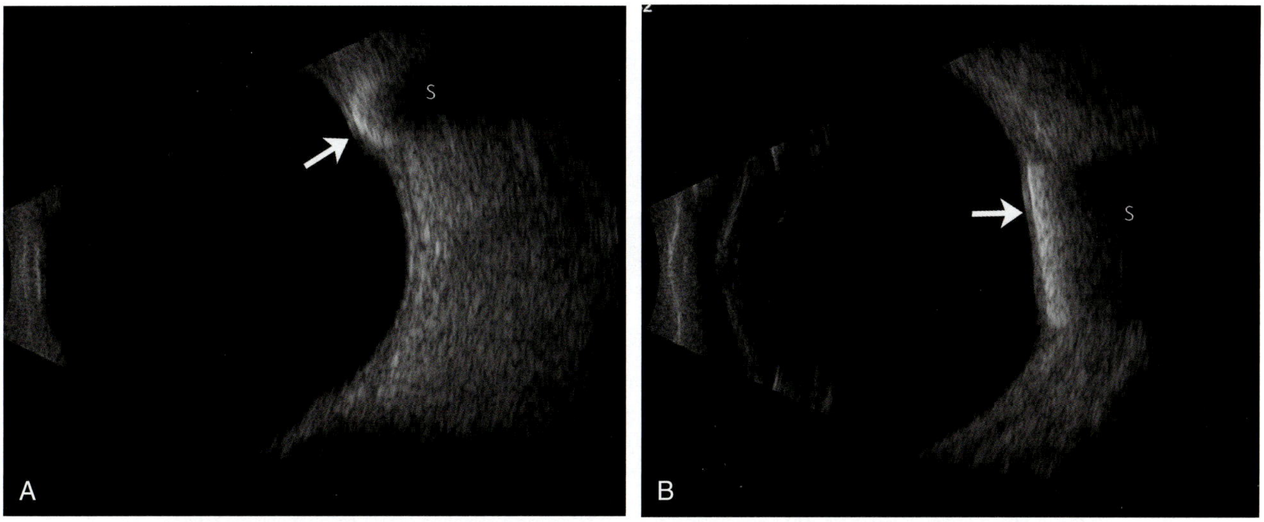

• **Fig. 4.46** Segmental Scleral Buckle. B-scan ultrasound with **(A)** longitudinal and **(B)** transverse approaches demonstrate a segmental circumferential scleral silicone sponge (*arrow*) producing a mild indentation of the peripheral ocular wall and marked posterior shadowing (S).

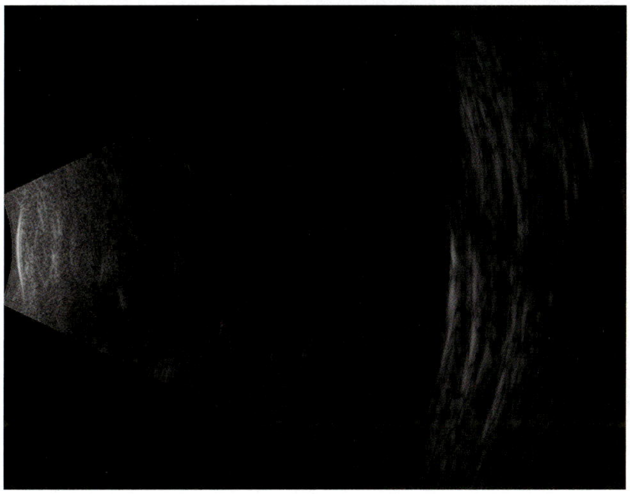

• **Fig. 4.47** Silicone Oil Filling the Eye precludes reliable sonographic imaging of the fundus. Artifact of axial elongation and attenuation.

CASE

A 37-year-old man with a history of retinal detachment surgery with scleral buckling combined with vitrectomy and silicone oil tamponade. Following stable retinal reattachment, he underwent removal of silicone oil. B-scan ultrasound examination disclosed retinal attachment and remnant silicone oil droplets in the vitreous cavity (Fig. 4.48 and sonogram Video 4.27).

Perfluorocarbon Liquid

Perfluorocarbon liquid is used as an intraoperative temporary vitreous substitute in complicated retinal detachment repair. Retained droplets of intravitreal perfluorocarbon are well tolerated and are imaged on ultrasound as high reflective particles followed by reverberation artifacts, adherent to the retinal surface.

CASE

A 55-year-old man presented for cataract evaluation. His past ocular history was significant for retinal detachment repair surgery. B-scan ultrasound examination revealed an attached retina and a residual bubble of perfluorocarbon adherent to the retinal surface (Fig. 4.49 and sonogram Video 4.28).

Intraocular Gas

In retinal detachment surgery, an intraocular gas bubble flattens the retina by providing internal tamponade. At the gas-tissues interface, almost all the incident ultrasound signal is reflected, precluding a view of structures posterior to the bubble. The dissolution of the intraocular gas can take many weeks and depends on the volume, concentration, and type of gas injected. When approximately 50% of the gas volume has been absorbed, the patient can be examined by ultrasound in an upright position with the neck flexed, allowing partial evaluation of the posterior pole.

CASE

A 66-year-old man underwent pars plana vitrectomy and internal limiting membrane peeling with gas tamponade. Three days after surgery, he underwent B-scan ultrasound examination for dense vitreous hemorrhage (Fig. 4.50 and sonogram Video 4.29).

Post-Vitrectomy

In vitrectomized eyes, the remnant of anterior vitreous gel (the vitreous skirt) can be imaged using ultrasound. On a transverse view, the vitreous skirt appears as a hyperechoic membrane extending circumferentially in all quadrants in the pre-equatorial region. The truncated hyaloid appears as a short membrane attached to the peripheral retina with a free edge on longitudinal views. Moreover, with recurrent vitreous

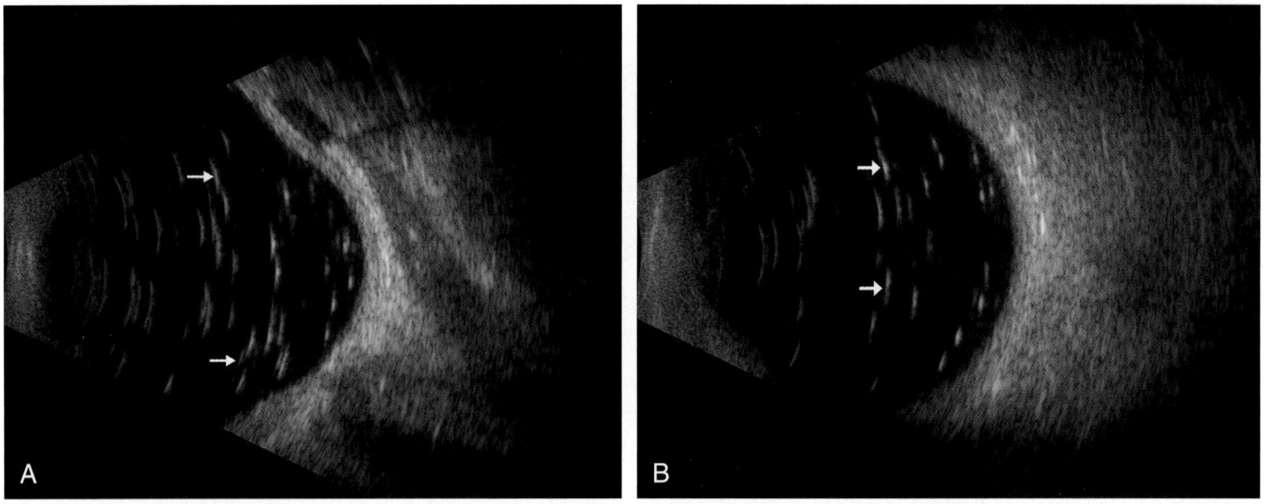

• **Fig. 4.48** Silicone Oil Droplets. **(A)** Longitudinal and **(B)** transverse B-scans display mobile, highly reflective echoes (*arrows*) dispersed in the vitreous cavity.

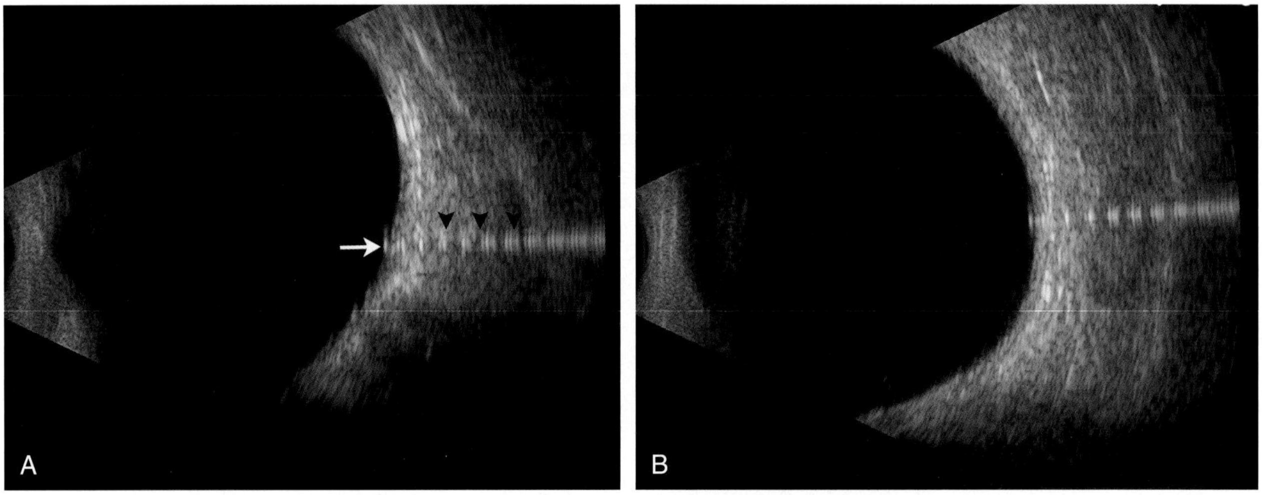

• **Fig. 4.49** Retained Perfluorocarbon. **(A)** Longitudinal and **(B)** transverse B-scans show a hyperechoic focal signal (*arrow*) on the retina surface with a comet-tail reverberation artifact (*arrowheads*) typical of retained of perfluorocarbon.

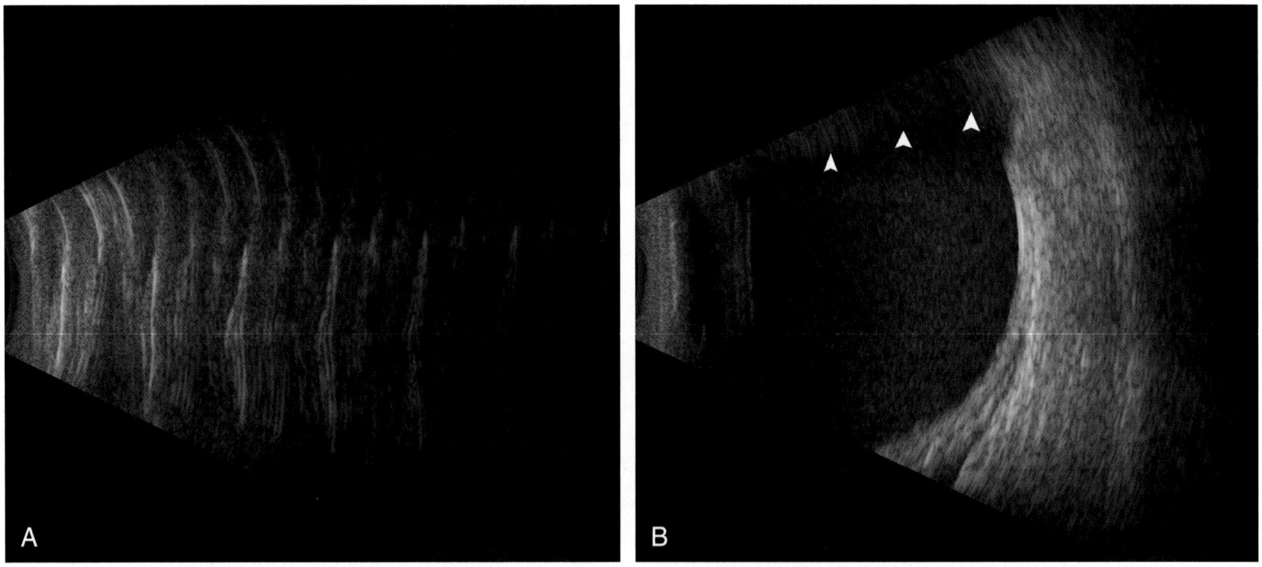

• **Fig. 4.50** Intraocular Gas. **(A)** Transverse B-scan ultrasound with the patient in supine position shows bright linear reverberation artifacts of the sound waves in a gaseous medium. **(B)** With the patient in an upright position, the gas bubble is located in the superior vitreous cavity (*arrowheads*), allowing partial fundus examination with transverse B-scanning.

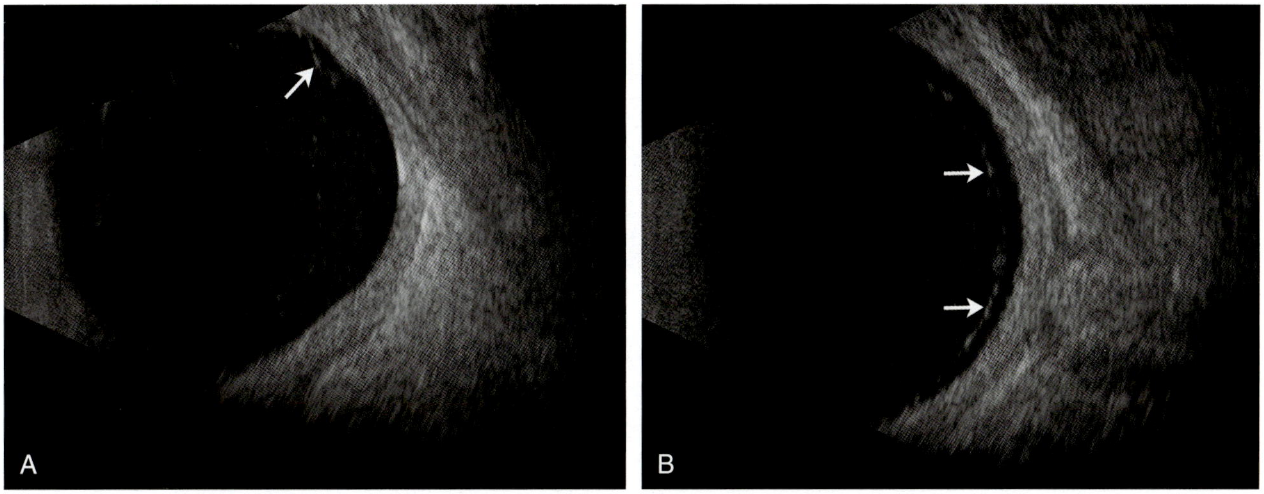

• **Fig. 4.51** Vitreous Skirt. **(A)** Longitudinal B-scan ultrasound shows moderately dense vitreous hemorrhage and a remnant of the vitreous gel ("vitreous skirt") in the far periphery (*arrow*). **(B)** Transverse B-scan ultrasound through the peripheral aspect of the fundus shows the circumferential extension of the vitreous skirt.

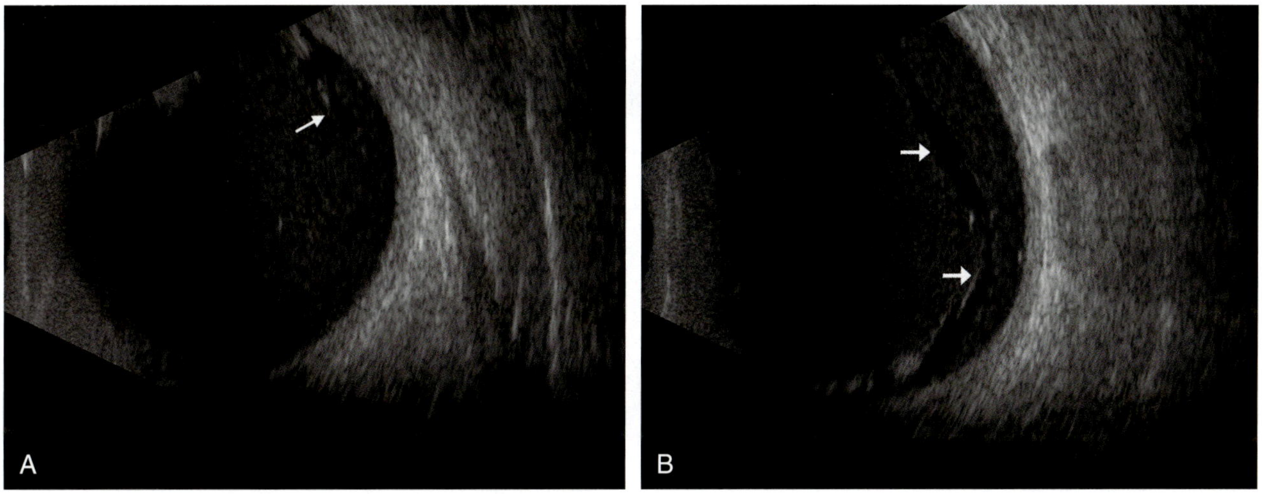

• **Fig. 4.52** Vitreous Skirt. **(A)** Longitudinal and **(B)** transverse B-scans display dense vitreous hemorrhage with a peripheral vitreous membrane (skirt) (*arrow*).

hemorrhage in vitrectomized eyes, the blood remains homogeneously dispersed throughout the vitreous cavity (without clot formation) and shows slow, spontaneous motion (convection movement).

CASE

A 63-year-old woman with a history of proliferative diabetic retinopathy and vitrectomy surgery presented with recurrent vitreous hemorrhage (Fig. 4.51 and sonogram Video 4.30).

CASE

A 79-year-old man with a history of intraocular lens exchange and anterior vitrectomy presented with vitreous hemorrhage and no view of the fundus. B-scan ultrasound examination disclosed flat retina, vitreous hemorrhage, and a peripheral vitreous skirt (Fig. 4.52 and sonogram Video 4.31).

Retinal Prosthesis

One of the components of a retinal prosthesis, the electrode array, is surgically tacked onto the retina surface in the macular area, allowing the electrical charges to stimulate the underlying retina. The array provides a highly reflective surface and causes acoustic shadowing of the underlying macula, precluding ultrasound from assessing changes in this area.

CASE

A 70-year-old man with end-stage retinitis pigmentosa underwent an uncomplicated Argus II retinal prosthesis implantation. After five years, the patient had improved visual functional and a well-positioned electrode array on the retinal surface (Fig. 4.53).

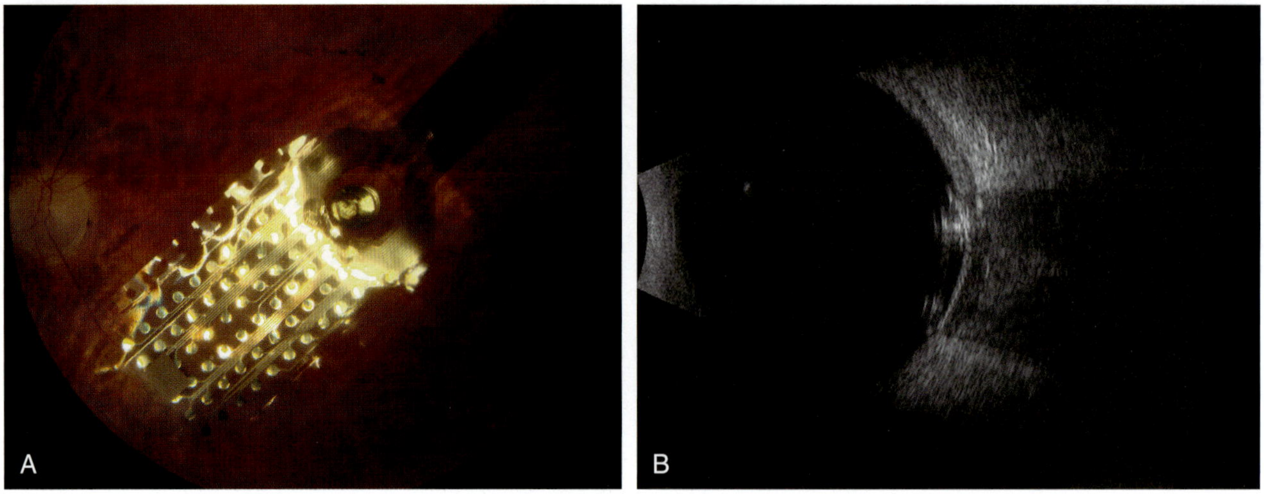

• **Fig. 4.53** Retinal Prosthesis. **(A)** Fundus photo shows a well-positioned electrode array resting on the macula in a patient with retinitis pigmentosa. **(B)** Transverse B-scan ultrasound shows retinal prosthesis electrode array over the macula.

References

1. Spraul CW, Grossniklaus HE. Vitreous hemorrhage. *Surv Ophthalmol.* 1997;42:3–39.
2. Mitchell P, Wang MY, Wang JJ. Asteroid hyalosis in an older population: the Blue Mountains Eye Study. *Ophthalmic Epidemiol.* 2003;10:331–335.
3. Johnson MW. Posterior vitreous detachment: evolution and complications of its early stages. *Am J Ophthalmol.* 2010;149:371–382.
4. Carrero JL. Incomplete posterior vitreous detachment: prevalence and clinical relevance. *Am J Ophthalmol.* 2012;153(3):497–503.
5. Chu TG, Lopez PF, Cano MR, et al. Posterior vitreoschisis. An echographic finding in proliferative diabetic retinopathy. *Ophthalmology.* 1996;103:315–322.
6. Hay A, Landers M. Types of pathogenetic mechanisms of retinal detachment. In: Ryan SJ, ed. *Retina.* (Vol. 3). 3rd ed. Mosby; 2000 :1971.
7. Blumenkranz MS, Byrne SF. Standardized echography (ultrasonography) for the detection and characterization of retinal detachment. *Ophthalmology.* 1982;89:821–831.
8. DiBernardo C, Greenberg E. The retina. *Opthalmic Ultrasound, a Diagnostic Atlas.* 2nd ed. Thieme; 2007:40.
9. Lewis H, Abrams GW, Williams GA. Anterior hyaloidal fibrovascular proliferation after diabetic vitrectomy. *Am J Ophthalmol.* 1987;104:607–613.
10. Ulbig MR, Hykin PG, Foss AJ, Schwartz SD, Hamilton PA. Anterior hyaloidal fibrovascular proliferation after extracapsular cataract extraction in diabetic eyes. *Am J Ophthalmol.* 1993;115:321–326.
11. Shah DN, Al-Moujahed A, Newcomb CW, et al. Exudative retinal detachment in ocular inflammatory diseases: risk and predictive factors. *Am J Ophthalmol.* 2020;218:279–287.
12. Zayit-Soudry S, Moroz I, Loewenstein A. Retinal pigment epithelial detachment. *Surv Ophthalmol.* 2007;52(3):227–243.
13. Banda HK, Shah A, Shah GK. Application of wide-field infrared reflectance imaging in retinoschisis, retinal detachments, and schisis detachments. *Int J Retina Vitreous.* 2019;5(Suppl 1):42.
14. Boldt HC, Brown DM, McGeorge AJ. Echographic diagnosis of degenerative retinoschisis facilitated by scleral indentation. *Am J Ophthalmol.* 1994;118:123–124.
15. Agarwal A, Fan S, Invernizzi A, et al. Characterization of retinal structure and diagnosis of peripheral acquired retinoschisis using high-resolution ultrasound B-scan. *Graefes Arch Clin Exp Ophthalmol.* 2016;254:69–75.
16. Rachitskaya AV, Yuan A, Singh RP, Sears JE, Schachat AP. Optical coherence tomography of outer retinal holes in senile retinoschisis and schisis-detachment. *Br J Ophthalmol.* 2017;101:445–448.
17. Chu TG, Green RL. Suprachoroidal hemorrhage. *Surv Ophthalmol.* 1999;43:471–486.
18. Venincasa VD, Modi YS, Aziz HA, et al. Clinical and echographic features of retinochoroidal and optic nerve Colobomas. *Invest Ophthalmol Vis Sci.* 2015;56:3615–3620.
19. Scroggs MW, Klintworth GK. Senile scleral plaques: a histopathologic study using energy-dispersive x-ray microanalysis. *Hum Pathol.* 1991;22:557–562.
20. Ohno-Matsui K, Alkabes M, Salinas C, et al. Features of posterior staphylomas analyzed in wide-field fundus images in patients with unilateral and bilateral pathologic myopia. *Retina.* 2017;37:477–486.

5

Intraocular Inflammation

BERNADETE AYRES, THERESE SASSALOS, AND THIRAN JAYASUNDERA

Uveitis is defined as inflammation of the uveal tract, the iris, the ciliary body, and the choroid. Inflammation of these structures is frequently accompanied by the involvement of the surrounding tissues, including the cornea, sclera, vitreous, retina, and optic nerve.

The intraocular inflammation may be classified based on the onset and course: *acute, subacute, chronic,* and *recurrent*; on the anatomical involvement: *anterior, intermediate, posterior,* and *panuveitis*; on the pathologic etiology: *granulomatous* and *non-granulomatous*; or based on the etiologic mechanism: *traumatic, immunologic, infectious,* and *masquerade.*

Ultrasound is a reliable tool for assessing intraocular inflammation and is essential in differentiating the possible diagnosis. In addition, ultrasound can detect the extension of the inflammatory process and monitor the course of the disease and response to therapy.

Evaluation of the inflammatory involvement of the iris, ciliary body, and anterior vitreous, along with the anterior chamber and the posterior chamber, can be done with Ultrasound Biomicroscopy (UBM).

The inflammatory changes in the anterior segment characterized by UBM are the presence of keratic precipitates (Fig. 5.1), cells or membrane-like exudates in the anterior chamber, iris thickening or iris atrophy, ciliary body thickening, and cyclitic membrane.[1,2]

Intermediate uveitis is characterized by inflammation that primarily affects the pars plana (Fig. 5.2), anterior vitreous, and peripheral retina with inflammatory collections. Snowballs are whitish focal collections of inflammatory cells and exudate, usually most numerous in the inferior vitreous. Snowbanks (Fig. 5.3) are gray-white fibrovascular exudative plaque, most frequently found inferiorly along the pars plana and ora serrata. Mild anterior uveitis can co-occur, and a cystoid macular edema is often seen in intermediate uveitis.

The vitreous opacities can be characterized by an aggregate of inflammatory cells, strands, or membranes. These opacities can be diffusely dispersed or confined to a specific area of the vitreous. Follow-up exams should be performed to assess the worsening or improvement of the inflammation. Although there is no accurate method to quantify the vitreous haze with ultrasound,[3] the examiner can grade the density of the vitreous haze as follows: clear vitreous; mildly dense; moderately dense (Fig. 5.4 and Video 5.1); severely dense. A serial exam (Fig. 5.5) must be performed using the same gain level and aiming at the same area.

Posterior vitreous detachment, either total or partial (Fig. 5.6 and Video 5.2), is a frequent finding in long-standing vitreous inflammation. The detached hyaloid can be thickened and covered by inflammatory precipitates. Posterior vitreoschisis, a splitting of the cortical vitreous, occasionally is seen in chronic processes.

Choroidal lesions are common in posterior inflammatory diseases. Increased choroidal thickening (Fig. 5.7) can be detected by ultrasound as a sign of choroidal or retinochoroidal inflammation. The appearance of choroiditis can vary greatly. It can be focal or diffuse, discreet, or severely thickened.

Retinal changes can be associated with several ocular inflammatory processes and present a variation in extent and height. Macular edema (Fig. 5.8 and Video 5.3) is a common retinal finding in patients with uveitis. Ultrasound is useful in differentiating rhegmatogenous and exudative retinal detachment (Fig. 5.9) based on the shifting of fluid (see Fig. 4.25), which is more characteristic of an exudative retinal detachment.

The optic nerve may be affected in uveitis. Ultrasound can be used to demonstrate optic disc elevation in cases of papillitis (Fig. 5.10).

Distinct Inflammatory Disorders of the Eye

Scleritis

Scleritis is an inflammatory disorder involving the sclera. It is most common in women in their fourth to sixth decades of life and is often associated with underlying systemic disease. Based on the anatomic site of inflammation, scleritis can be classified as an anterior and posterior disease.

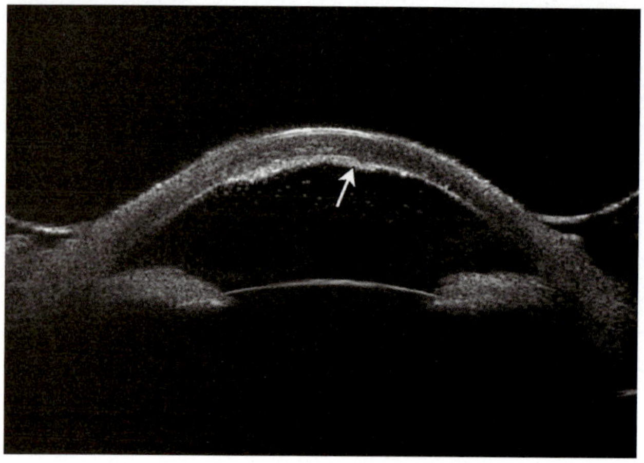

• **Fig. 5.1** Anterior Uveitis. UBM image of keratic precipitates (*arrow*) and inflammatory cells in the anterior chamber in herpes simplex keratouveitis.

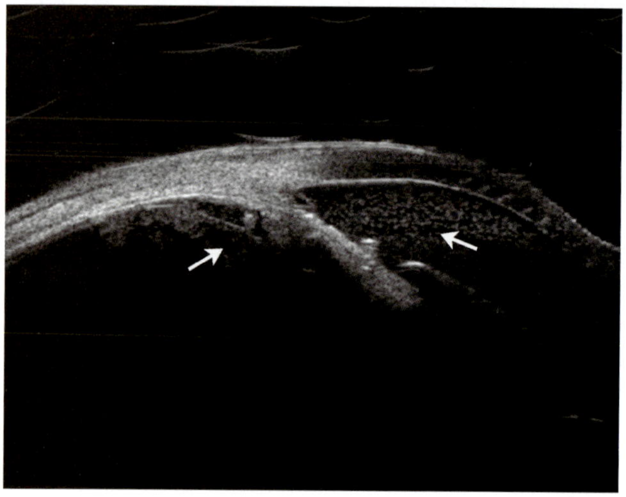

• **Fig. 5.2** Intermediate Uveitis. UBM longitudinal scan showing dense inflammatory cells (*arrows*) in the anterior chamber and mild opacities overlying the pars plana.

Anterior Scleritis

Anterior uveitis has been subdivided into diffuse, nodular, necrotizing with inflammation, and necrotizing without inflammation. Pain and redness are the cardinal signs.

UBM enables the visualization of distinct features of anterior scleritis. Nodular anterior scleritis is clearly identified as a well-circumscribed, nonhomogeneous, low reflective scleral thickening (Fig. 5.11). The overlying episclera and underlying ciliary body are usually inflamed. Diffuse anterior scleritis involves either a segment of the globe or the entire anterior scleral and is characterized by low reflective scleral thickening with a molted appearance. The healing of the necrotic scleral area is displayed as scleral thinning on UBM.[4]

CASE

A 54-year-old female presented with nodular anterior scleritis in the left eye (Fig. 5.11 and Video 5.4). Her rheumatologic and microbial workup were negative.

Episcleritis Versus Scleritis

UBM is a valuable tool to differentiate episcleritis from scleritis. In Episcleritis, UBM can demonstrate a conjunctival and episcleral thickening with an intact sclera.

CASE

A 60-year-old female presented with nodular episcleritis (Fig. 5.12 and Video 5.5). A laboratory workup revealed elevated serum rheumatoid factor.

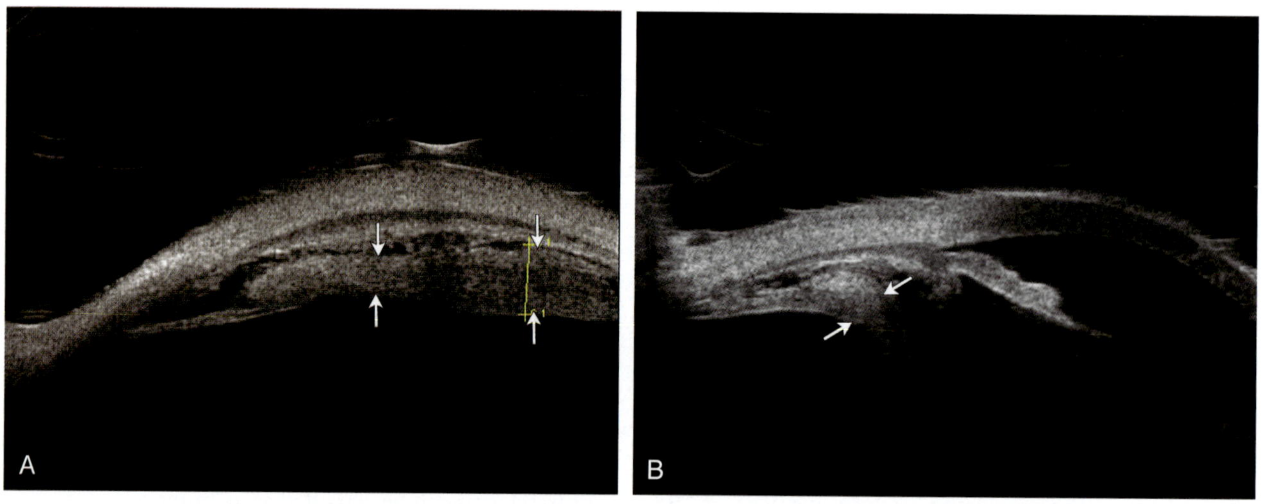

• **Fig. 5.3** Intermediate Uveitis and Snowbank Formation. **(A)** Transverse and **(B)** longitudinal UBM scans through the inferior quadrant show condensation of inflammatory cells and debris along the pars plana forming a snowbank (*arrows*).

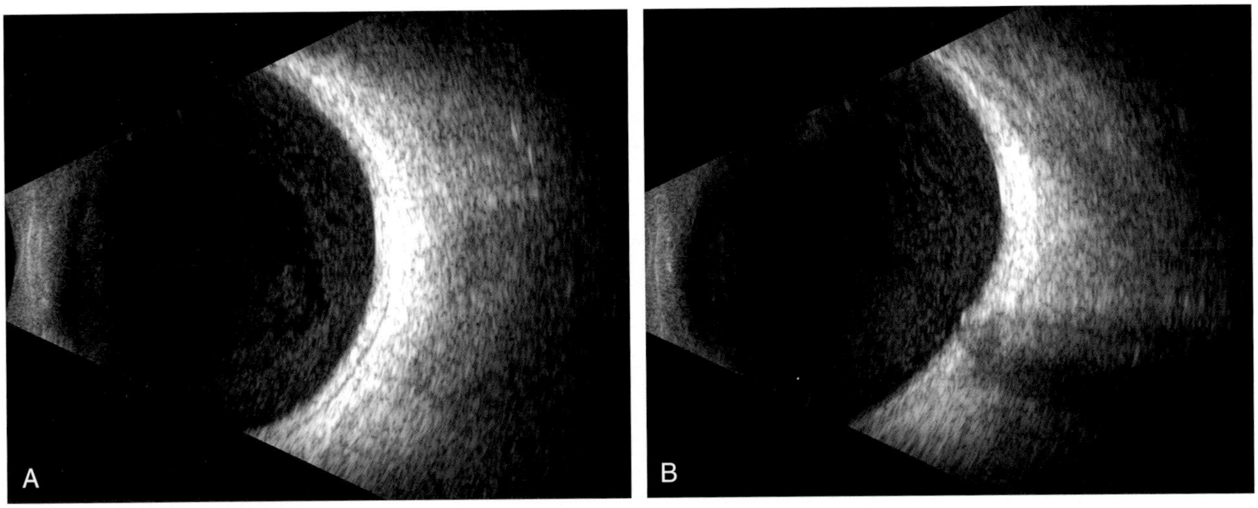

• **Fig. 5.4** Vitreous Opacities in Panuveitis. **(A)** Transverse and **(B)** longitudinal B-scans display moderately dense, dot-like vitreous opacities in a 23-year-old female with panuveitis.

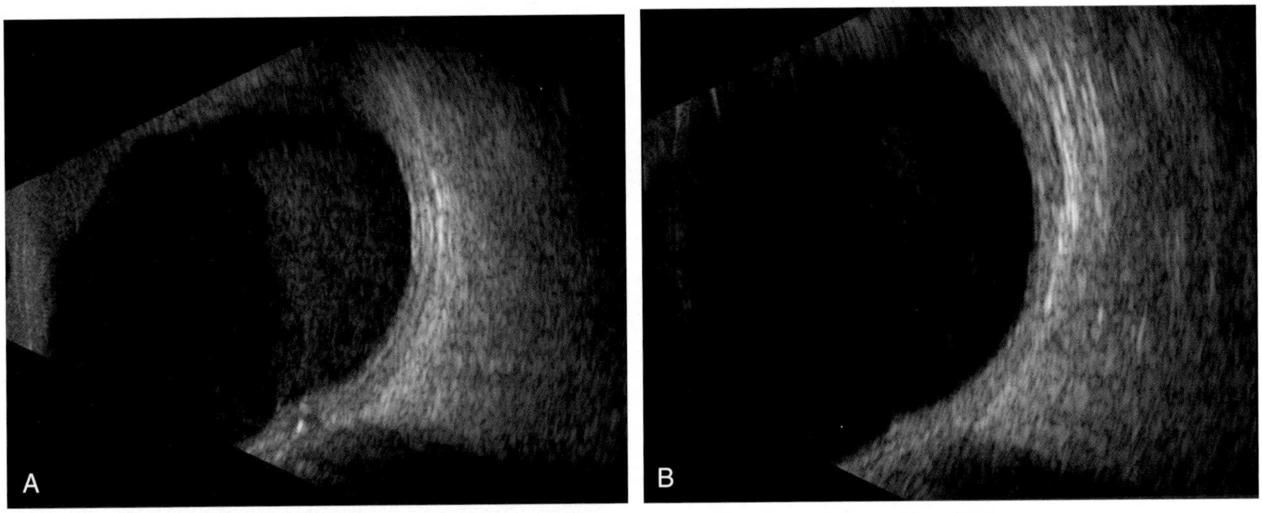

• **Fig. 5.5** Sequential Ultrasound. B-scan exams of a 19-year-old male with panuveitis under immunosuppressive therapy demonstrate decreasing density of the vitreous cells. **(A)** Initial visit and **(B)** follow-up exam using the same gain level and aiming at the same area.

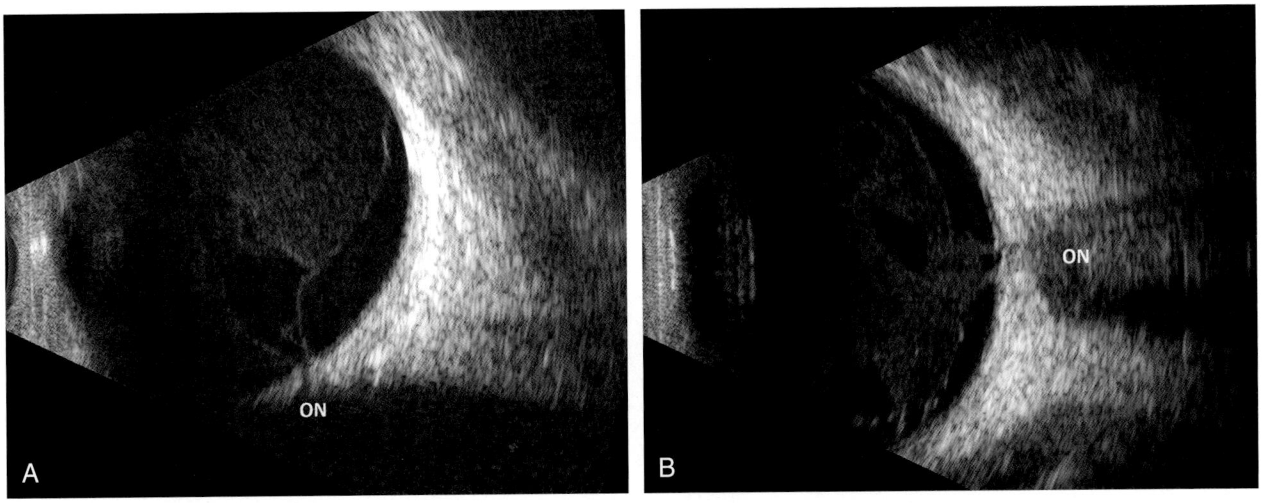

• **Fig. 5.6** Posterior Vitreous Detachment. **(A)** Longitudinal and **(B)** transverse B-scans of a partial posterior vitreous detachment in a 38-year-old female with sarcoid uveitis. The posterior hyaloid remains attached to the edge of the optic disc. *ON*, Optic nerve.

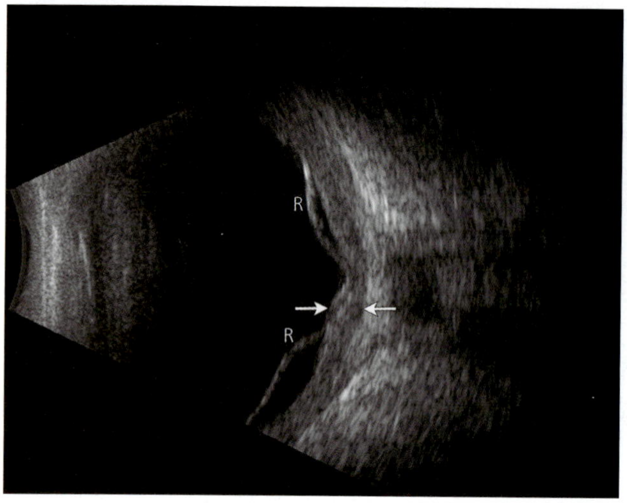

• **Fig. 5.7** Choroidal Thickening. Transverse B-scan through the posterior pole demonstrates diffuse choroidal thickening (*arrows*) and shallow exudative retinal detachment (R) in an 18-year-old female with panuveitis.

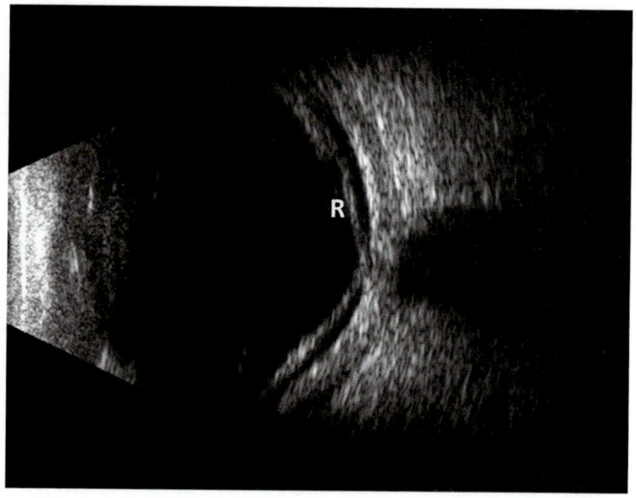

• **Fig. 5.9** Exudative Retinal Detachment. Transverse B-scan at optic disc area showing shallow exudative retinal detachment (R) and diffuse choroidal thickening in a 25-year-old patient with panuveitis associated with juvenile rheumatoid arthritis.

Posterior Scleritis

Posterior scleritis is defined as inflammation of the sclera posterior to the ora serrata. Pain is the most common symptom. It may occur in focal or diffuse forms and can be associated with retinochoroidal thickening, exudative retinal detachment, or choroidal effusion.

Some tumors, such as choroidal melanoma, can masquerade posterior scleritis, lymphoma, and metastatic carcinoma.

On B-scan ultrasonography, posterior scleritis is characterized by homogeneous, highly reflective thickening of the sclera with an adjacent low reflective widening of the sub-Tenon's space corresponding to edema or inflammatory infiltration. In diffuse posterior scleritis involving

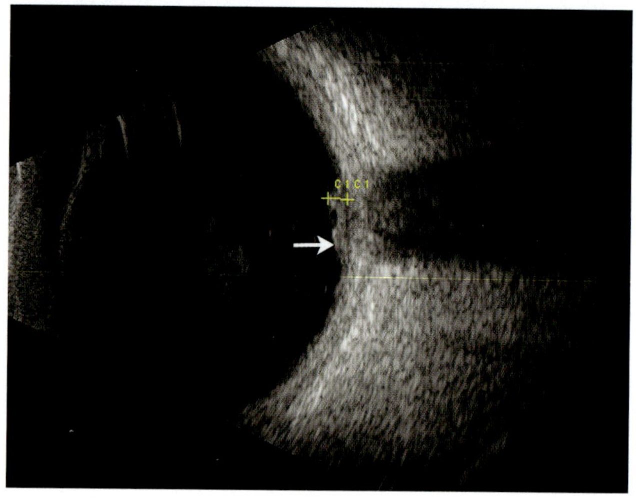

• **Fig. 5.10** Papillitis. Transverse B-scan through the optic nerve demonstrates an optic disc swelling (*arrow*) in a 65-year-old woman with panuveitis.

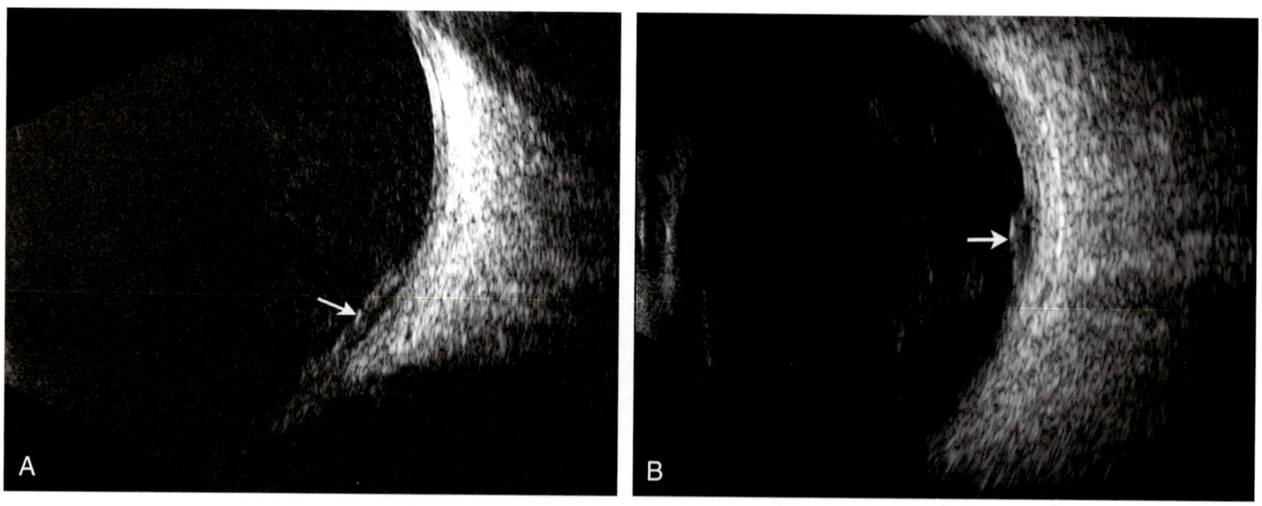

• **Fig. 5.8** Macular Edema. **(A)** Longitudinal and **(B)** transverse vertical B-scans through the macula showing macular edema (*arrow*) in a 16-year-old girl with a history of posterior uveitis presented with ocular pain when tapering prednisone.

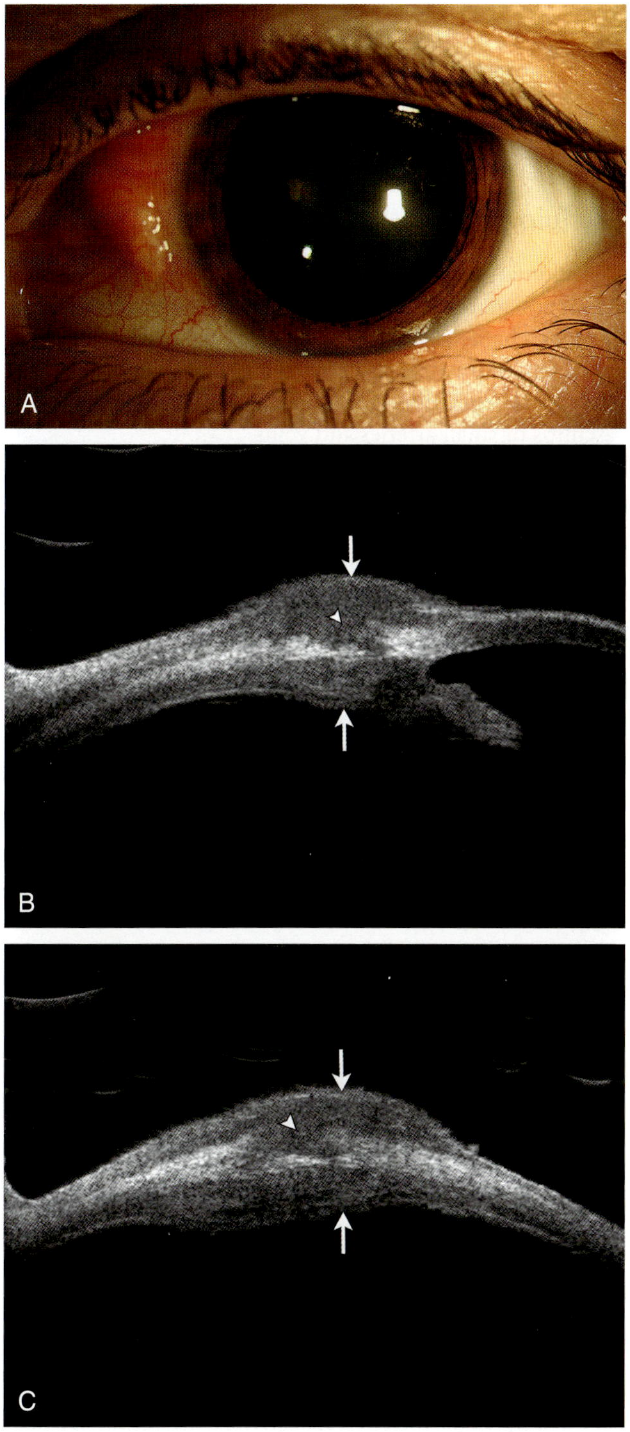

• **Fig. 5.11** Anterior Nodular Scleritis. **(A)** Clinical picture of nodular scleritis demonstrates focal scleral injection and a subconjunctival nodule at nasal limbus. UBM **(B)** longitudinal and **(C)** transverse scans show nodular, low reflective lesion involving the episclera, sclera, and ciliary body (*arrows*). Note a focal discontinuity in the scleral layer (*arrowhead*), a sign of scleral inflammation.

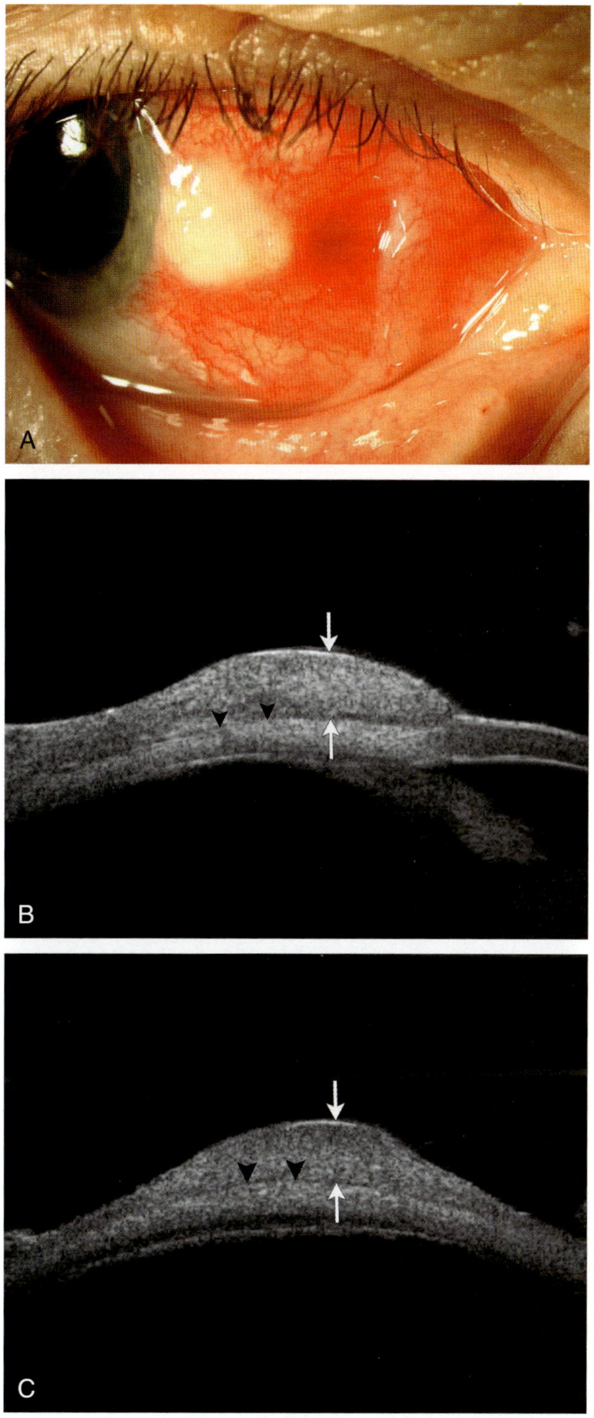

• **Fig. 5.12** Nodular Episcleritis. **(A)** Clinical picture of episcleritis showing avascular node surrounded by dilated episcleral vessels. UBM images in **(B)** longitudinal and **(C)** transverse positions display a conjunctival and episcleral nodular lesion (*arrows*) with no involvement of the underlying sclera (*arrowheads*).

the peripapillary area, the distended sub-Tenon's space around the optic nerve produces a "T-sign" (Fig. 5.13). In some cases, the inflammatory process extends to a contiguous extraocular muscle insertion, and a low reflective tendon enlargement can be noted.[5]

CASE

A 76-year-old female presented with rapidly worsening ocular pain, conjunctival chemosis, and scleral injection. Ultrasonography examination revealed posterior scleritis (Fig. 5.13). Laboratory workup was negative for infectious processes.

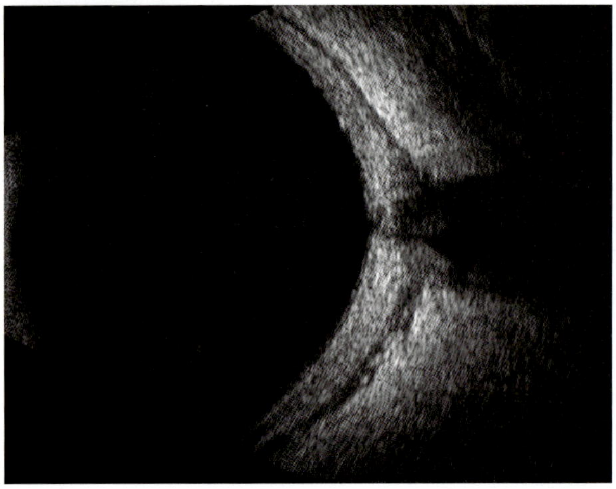

• **Fig. 5.13** Posterior Scleritis. Transverse B-scan showing highly reflective scleral thickening involving the posterior pole and distended sub-Tenon's space around the optic nerve producing a "T-sign."

CASE

A 76-year-old female with rheumatoid arthritis presented with recurrent bilateral diffuse posterior scleritis (Fig. 5.14 and Video 5.6).

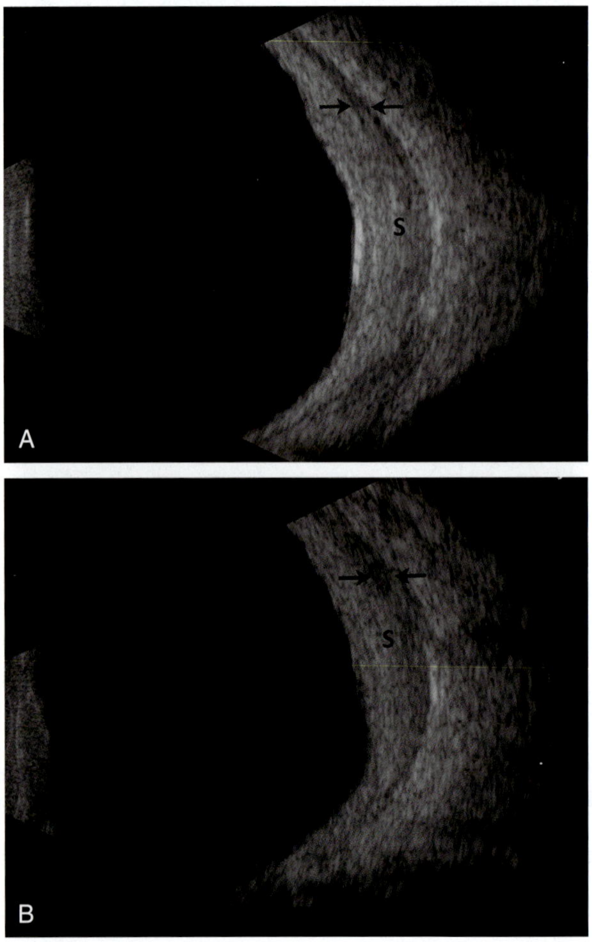

• **Fig. 5.14** Posterior Scleritis. **(A)** Transverse and **(B)** longitudinal B-scan show homogeneous highly reflective thickened sclera (S) with an adjacent low reflective widening of the sub-Tenon's space (*arrows*).

TEACHING POINTS

In posterior scleritis, B-scan ultrasonography can reveal a "T-sign" indicative of fluid accumulation at the sub-Tenon's space accompanied by enhancive scleral thickness.

Granulomatosis With Polyangiitis

Granulomatosis with polyangiitis, formerly known as Wegener's granulomatosis, is a multisystem autoimmune disorder characterized by the classic triad of necrotizing granulomatous vasculitis of the upper and lower respiratory tract, focal segmental glomerulonephritis, and necrotizing vasculitis of small arteries and veins.

Ocular involvement includes granulomatous orbital mass, uveitis, scleritis, and retinitis.

Anterior scleritis of any type, particularly diffuse anterior or necrotizing disease, with or without peripheral ulcerative keratitis can be related to granulomatosis with polyangiitis.[6] Posterior scleritis has also been reported.[7]

CASE

A 47-year-old female with a clinical history of granulomatosis with polyangiitis, in use of prednisone and methotrexate, presented with decreased vision and severe pain in the left eye. Slit lamp biomicroscopy revealed mild scleral injection. Fundus examination revealed retinal folds temporally. B-scan ultrasound exam revealed evidence of posterior scleritis (Fig. 5.15).

Sarcoidosis

Sarcoidosis is a systemic inflammatory disorder with unknown etiology. It affects many organs, including the eye, and is characterized by noncaseating granulomas. Ocular involvement in sarcoidosis includes acute nongranulomatous or chronic granulomatous iridocyclitis, vitritis, choroidal granuloma, retinal vasculitis, optic disc granuloma, and papilledema. The definitive diagnosis of sarcoidosis requires biopsy and histopathological exam; however, specific laboratory and imaging tests can support a presumed or probable diagnosis.[8]

Ultrasonography can be a useful tool for evaluation of sarcoid uveitis. UBM can show unilateral or bilateral, diffuse, or nodular thickening of the ciliary body with medium to medium-high internal reflectivity.[9] Posterior segment B-scan can demonstrate vitreous and subhyaloid opacities and focal or diffuse, medium reflective choroidal thickening. Other echographic features include exudative retinal detachment and optic disc elevation.

CASE

A 52-year-old Caucasian woman presented with painless decreased vision in the right eye for eight months with signs of panuveitis. Laboratory and systemic imaging workups were negative. Ultrasound exam revealed uveal thickening and shallow exudative retinal detachment (Fig. 5.16 and Video 5.7). Ciliary body incisional biopsy and histopathology exam demonstrated sarcoidosis.

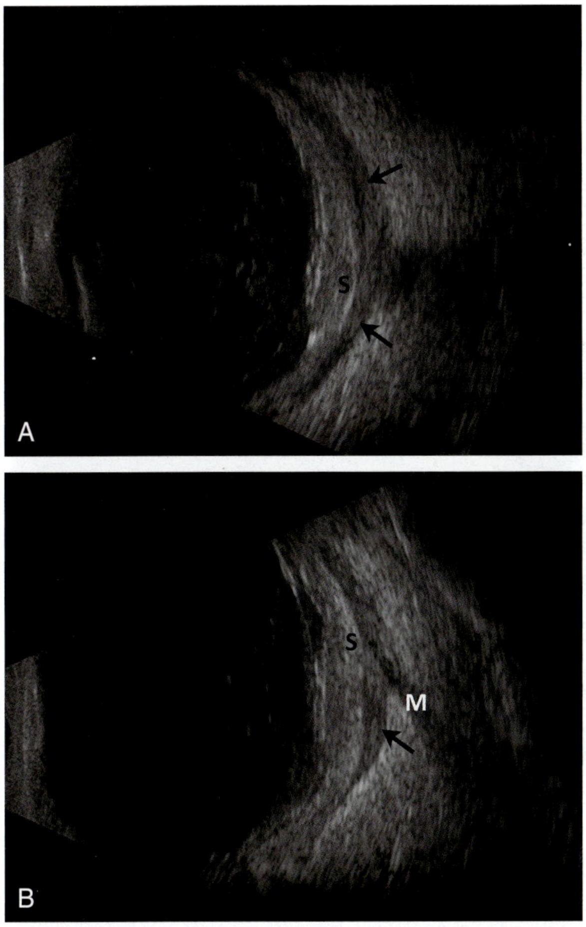

• **Fig. 5.15** Granulomatosis with Polyangiitis. **(A)** Transverse and **(B)** longitudinal B-scans shows vitritis, a highly reflective massive thickened posterior sclera (S) with a minimally elevated retina, fluid in the sub-Tenon's space (*arrow*), and thickening of the tendon of an adjacent rectus muscle (M).

CASE

A 12-year-old African-American boy presented with unilateral anterior uveitis and a mass located in the angle inferiorly (Fig. 5.17). Histopathological exam of the mass demonstrated granulomatous inflammation most consistent with sarcoidosis.

CASE

An 81-year-old Caucasian man presented with bilateral panuveitis (Fig. 5.18) and bilateral hilar lymphadenopathy on a chest CT scan. A ciliary body biopsy was performed and resulted in a diagnosis of sarcoidosis.

Vogt-Koyanagi-Harada Syndrome

Vogt-Koyanagi-Harada Syndrome (VKH) is an idiopathic multisystem inflammatory disease that consists of bilateral granulomatous panuveitis variably associated with vitiligo, alopecia, poliosis, auditory dysfunction, and central nervous system damage. The disease is most common in the third to fifth decades of life but can affect all age groups, including the pediatric population.

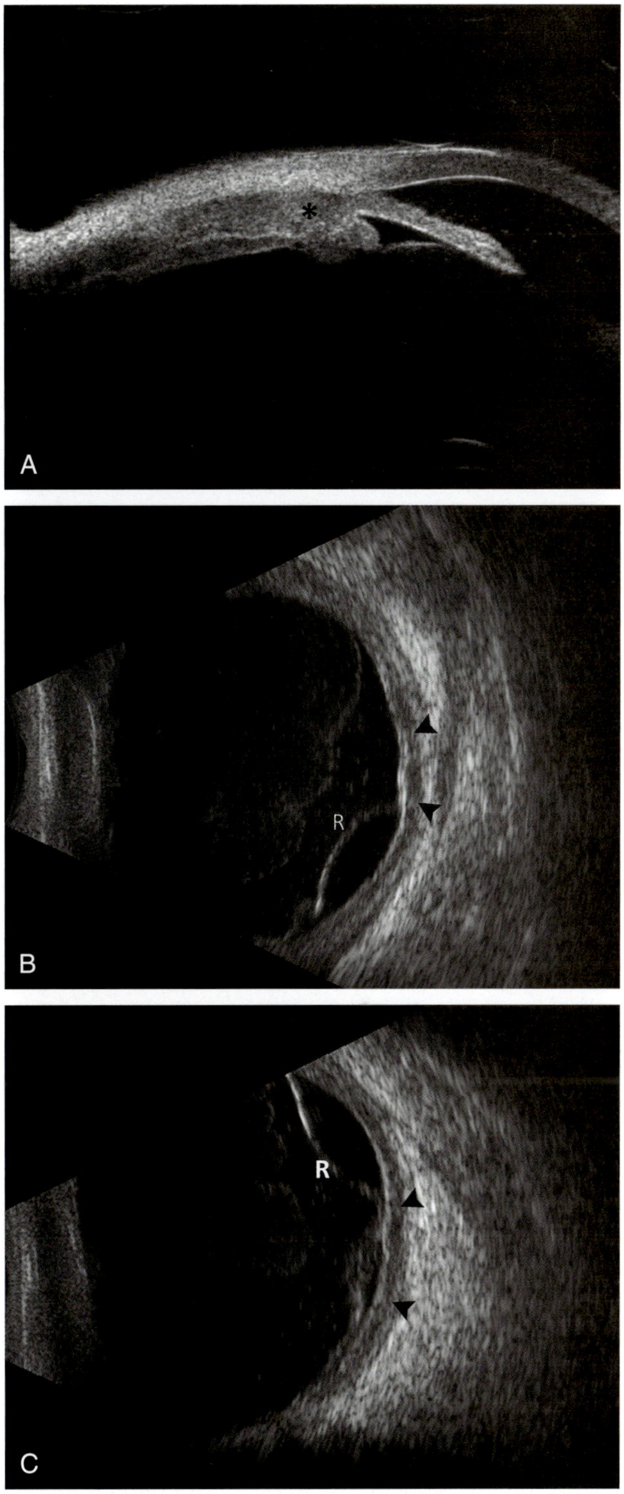

• **Fig. 5.16** Sarcoid Uveitis. **(A)** Ultrasound biomicroscopy in radial section showing moderately dense dispersed opacities in the anterior chamber and medium-highly reflective thickening of the ciliary body (asterisk). **(B)** Transverse and **(C)** longitudinal B-scan ultrasound showing vitritis, exudative retinal detachment (R), and medium reflective diffuse choroidal thickening (*arrowheads*).

VKH evolves in phases, classified as a prodromal, uveitic, convalescent, and chronic/recurrent. The acute ocular or

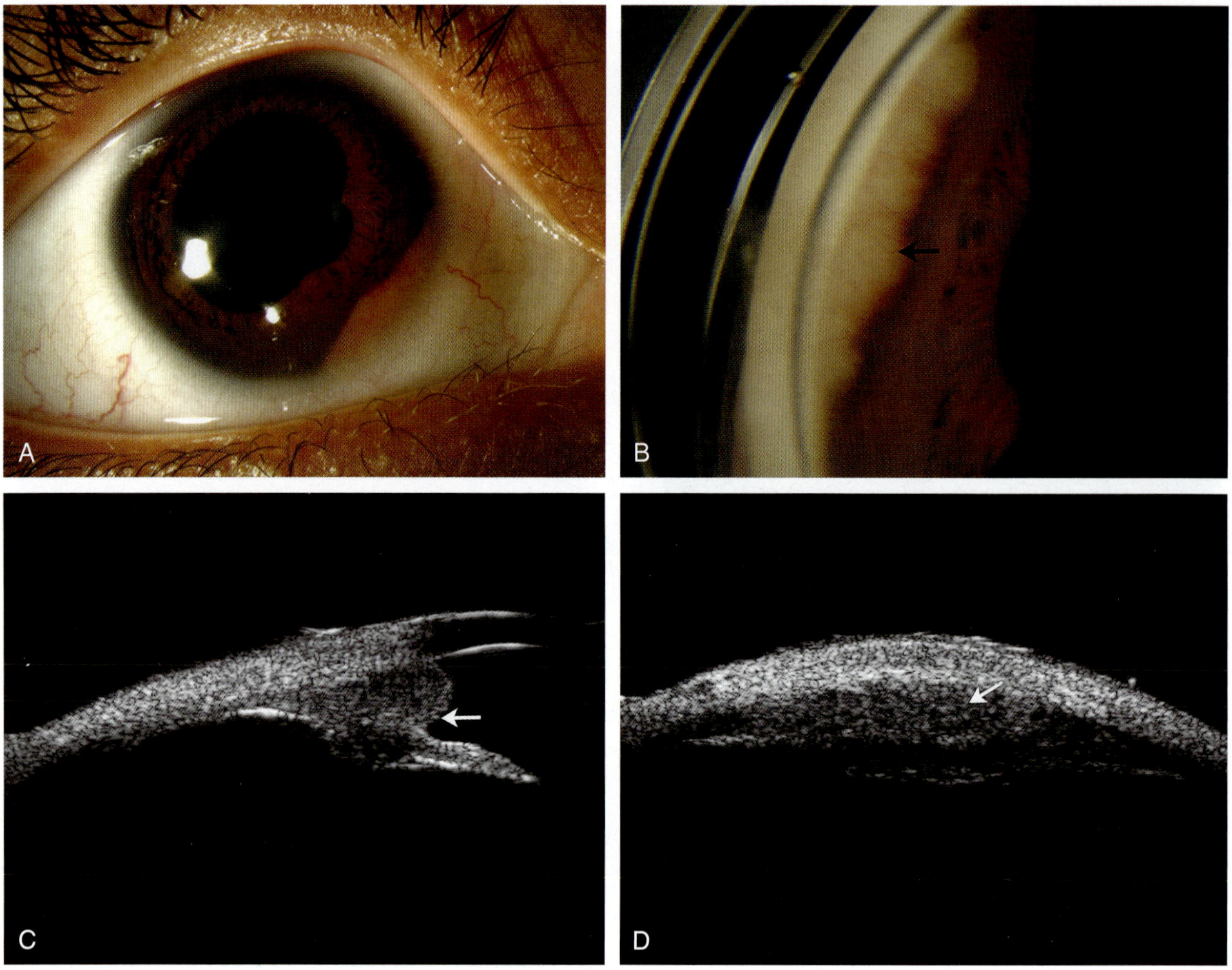

• **Fig. 5.17** Sarcoid Uveitis. **(A)** Anterior segment picture and **(B)** gonioscopy picture show a nodular lesion at the angle (*arrow*) with superficial vascularization. **(C)** UBM longitudinal and **(D)** transverse views show a homogeneous, medium reflective thickening of the ciliary body (*arrow*) and root of the iris.

uveitic phase is characterized by anterior and posterior uveitis, exudative retinal detachment, swollen optic disc, vitritis, anterior chamber cells, and keratic precipitates. Swelling of the ciliary body may displace the lens-iris diaphragm forward and shallow the anterior chamber, which can lead to angle closure.

A- and B-scan ultrasonography can reveal low to medium reflective uveal thickening, shallowly elevated multiple serous retinal detachments, vitreous opacities, and thickening of the sclera or episclera.[10]

Ultrasound biomicroscopy performed in the uveitic phase can show low reflective thickening of the ciliary body and shallow anterior chamber. Some patients show ciliochoroidal detachment and angle-closure.[11]

CASE

A 35-year-old male presented with bilateral decreased vision, symptoms of meningismus, and bilateral serous detachments with intervening areas of attached retina (Fig. 5.19).

Sympathetic Ophthalmia

Sympathetic ophthalmia (SO) is a bilateral granulomatous uveitis that usually occurs following an inciting penetrating injury or surgery to one or both eyes. Therefore, penetrating trauma to one eye (the exciting eye) will result in an inflammatory response not only in that eye but also in the fellow eye (the sympathizing eye). The time to development of SO varies from 2 weeks to 50 years, with approximately 90% of patients developing the disease within 1 year of injury.[12]

Patients typically present with bilateral acute granulomatous anterior uveitis with mutton-fat keratic precipitates. The posterior segment involvement can be characterized by vitritis, retinal vasculitis, choroiditis, papillitis, and serous retinal detachment. White-yellowish lesions can be seen at the peripheral fundus of patients with SO (Dalen-Fuchs nodules).

The diagnosis of SO is usually based on the history and clinical signs of intraocular inflammation. Ultrasound can be adjunct to support the diagnosis and monitor the response to treatment.

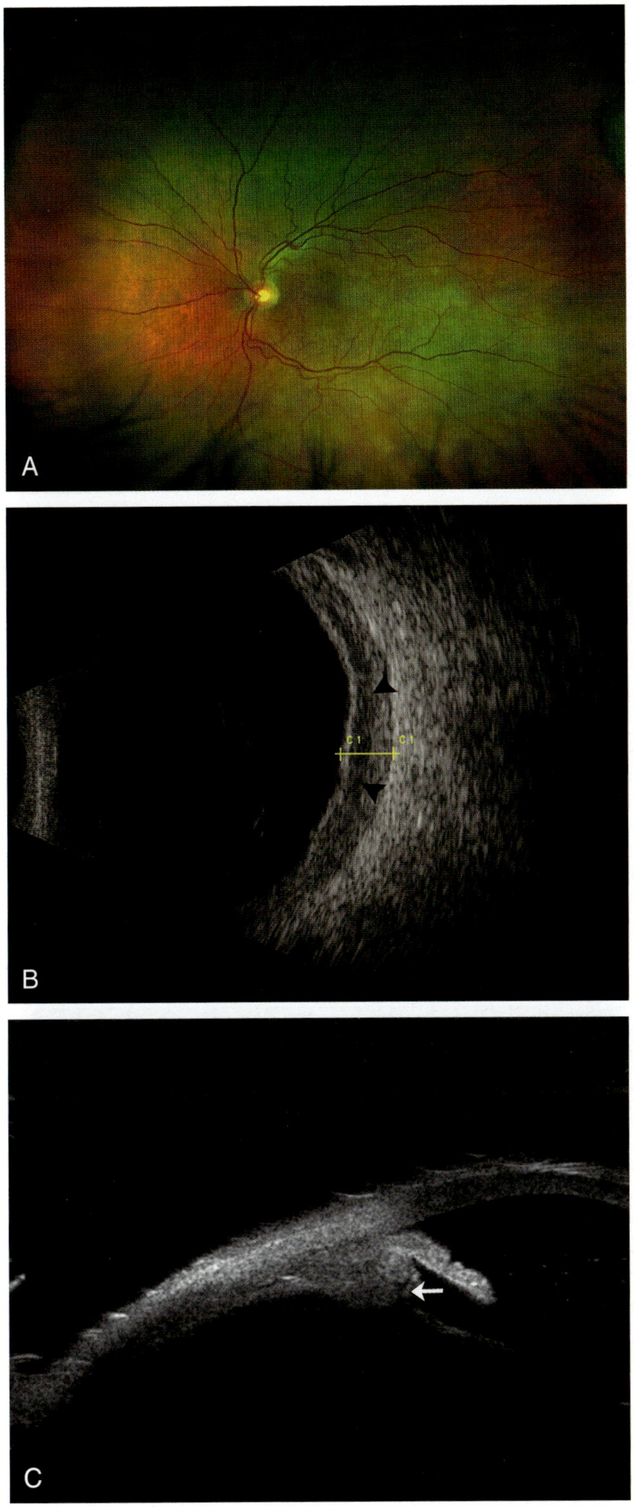

• **Fig. 5.18** Sarcoid Uveitis. **(A)** Widefield fundus photography of left eye showing exudative retinal detachment inferiorly. **(B)** B-scan in transverse view showing moderately dense, dispersed vitreous opacities, posterior vitreous detachment, and marked medium reflective diffuse choroidal thickening (*arrowheads*). **(C)** Ultrasound biomicroscopy, radial section temporally showing mildly dense, dispersed opacities in the anterior chamber and moderate thickening of the ciliary body (*arrow*).

CASE

A 10-year-old boy had a diagnosis of sympathetic ophthalmia in the right eye (Fig. 5.20) 2 months after an episode of ocular-penetrating injury with a retained intraocular foreign body in the left eye.

Ocular Tuberculosis

Uveitis is the most common manifestation of ocular tuberculosis and can encompass the anterior segment, posterior segment, or both.[13] Scleritis can present concomitantly with uveitis.

The presumptive diagnosis of ocular tuberculosis is established by positive QuantiFERON-TB and tuberculin skin tests. Laboratory and imaging workups rule out pulmonary and systemic tuberculosis as well as other possible etiologies.

The disseminated form of tuberculosis-related uveitis is the most common, presented with multiple well-circumscribed yellow whitish retinochoroidal lesions dispersed at the posterior pole. Focal uveitis, also termed *tuberculoma*, is the next common clinical presentation. The mass is typically elevated and may be accompanied by an overlying retinal detachment.

B-scan ultrasonography can demonstrate the typical findings of uveitis, such as vitreous opacities and uveal thickening, which can be diffuse or localized. Exudative retinal detachment and optic disc elevation (papillitis) can also occur.

A ciliary body or choroidal tuberculoma should be differentiated from intraocular tumors or infective abscesses.

CASE

A 31-year-old healthy female presented with a macular amelanotic choroidal mass. Systemic workup revealed a positive QuantiFERON-TB Gold test without evidence for extraocular involvement by CT-imaging. She was diagnosed with a presumptive choroidal tuberculoma (Fig. 5.21).

CASE

A 23-year-old African female with a history of decreased vision was referred to evaluate fundus mass in the right eye. Fundos examination revealed moderate cells in the vitreous and a yellowish ciliochoroidal mass inferiorly. Extensive workup for uveitis was negative except for the QuantiFERON-TB Gold test. Ultrasonography examination revealed ciliary body granuloma and vitritis (Fig. 5.22 and Video 5.8).

Endophthalmitis

Infectious endophthalmitis is a vision-threatening condition that may occur after intraocular surgery, accidental ocular injury, or endogenous infection. Ultrasonographic evaluation should be performed if significant media opacity prevents a good view of the fundus. Echographic features, in combination with clinical presentation, aid in the diagnosis and influence clinical decision making.

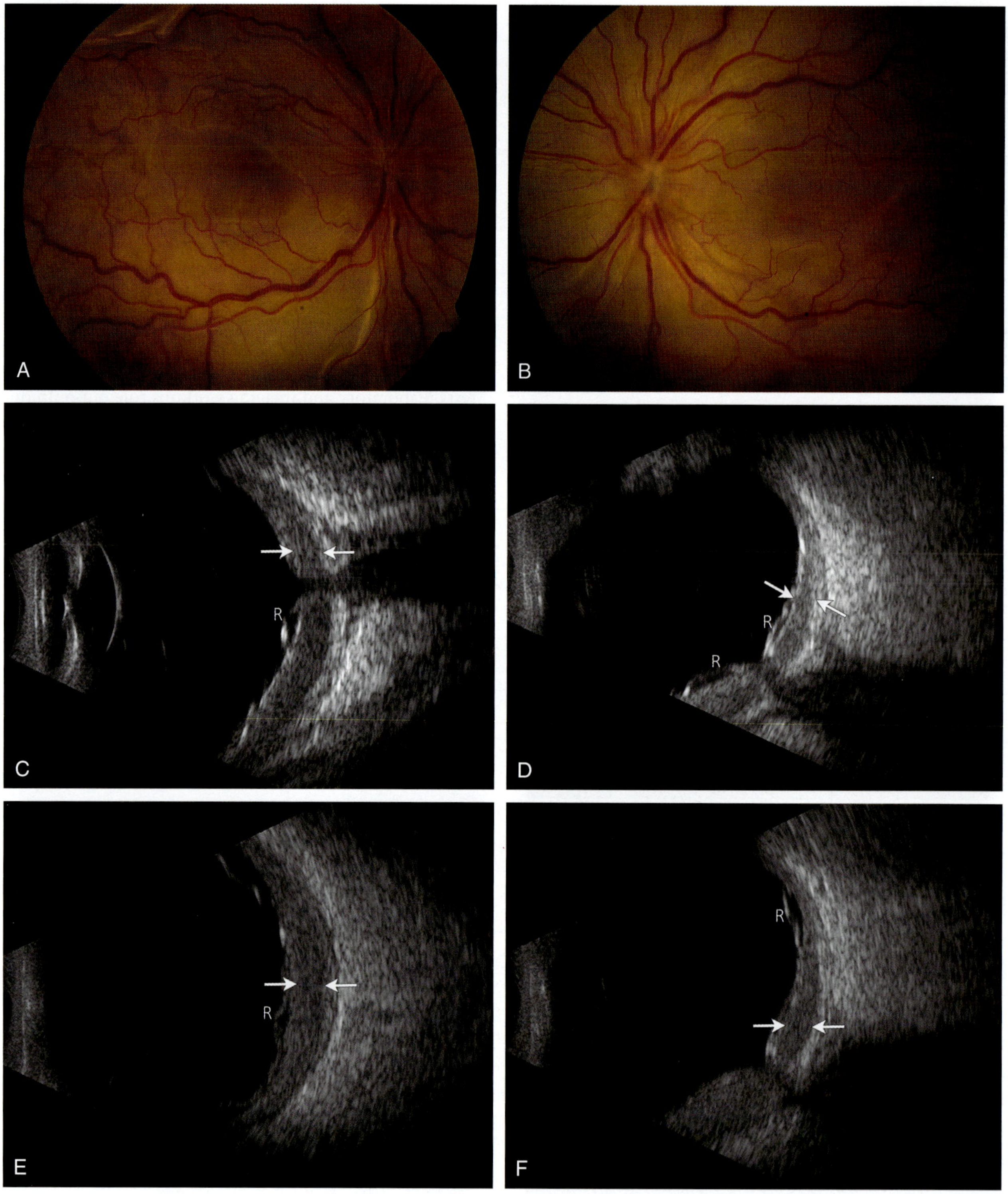

• **Fig. 5.19** Vogt-Koyanagi-Harada Syndrome**.** Fundus photos of the right and **(A)** left eye **(B)** display serous detachment with discontinuous areas of attached retina and optic disc edema. B-scans through the posterior pole of the right eye **(C** and **D)** and left eye **(E** and **F)** demonstrate low reflective choroidal thickening (*arrows*) with shallow, discontinuous, serous retinal detachment (R).

Echographic features reported to be associated with endophthalmitis include vitreous opacities, either dot-like or membranous, posterior vitreous detachment, subhyaloid opacities, retinal detachment, subretinal opacities, retinochoroidal thickening, choroidal detachment, and orbital inflammation.[14–16]

As a first step, the ultrasound exam must proceed to assess the uninvolved eye using a high gain set to compare

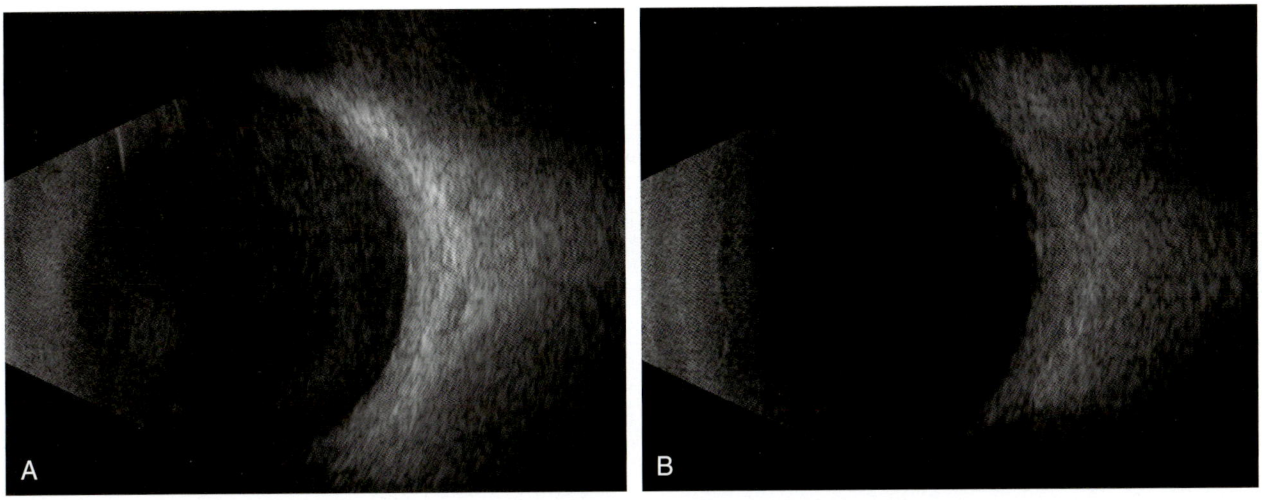

• **Fig. 5.20** Sympathetic Ophthalmia. **(A)** Transverse B-scan at high gain demonstrates moderately dense dispersed vitreous opacities. **(B)** Transverse B-scan at decreased gain aimed at posterior pole demonstrates thickening of the ocular coats and optic disc elevation.

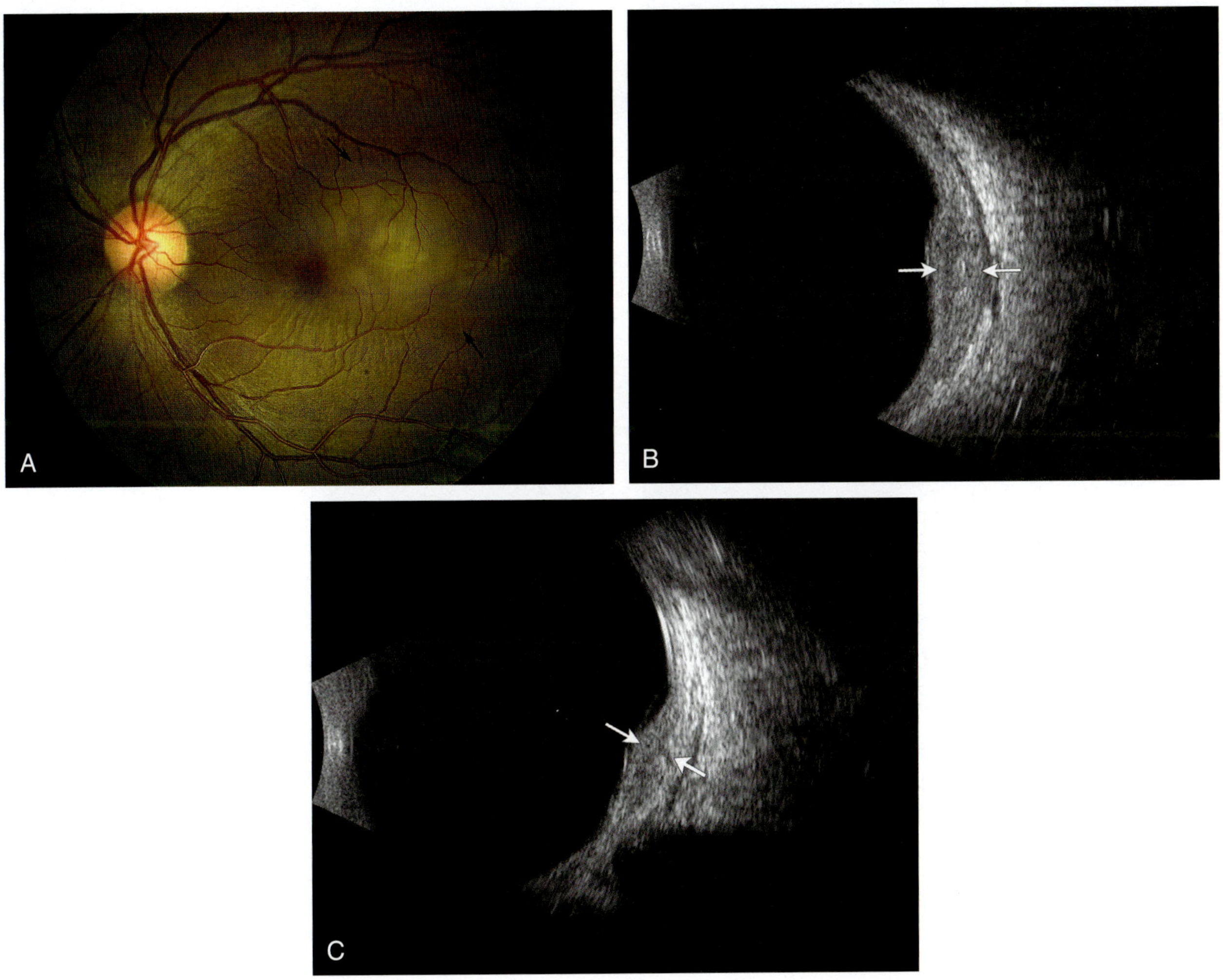

• **Fig. 5.21** Ocular Tuberculosis. **(A)** Fundus photography showing an amelanotic mass (*arrows*) in the superotemporal aspect of the macula. **(B)** Transverse B-scan showing a dome-shaped medium to highly reflective tuberculoma involving all the coats of the eye (*arrows*) associated with mild widening of the sub-Tenon's space **(C)** Longitudinal B-scan showing tuberculoma located at the posterior pole (*arrows*) with subretinal fluid at the apex of the lesion.

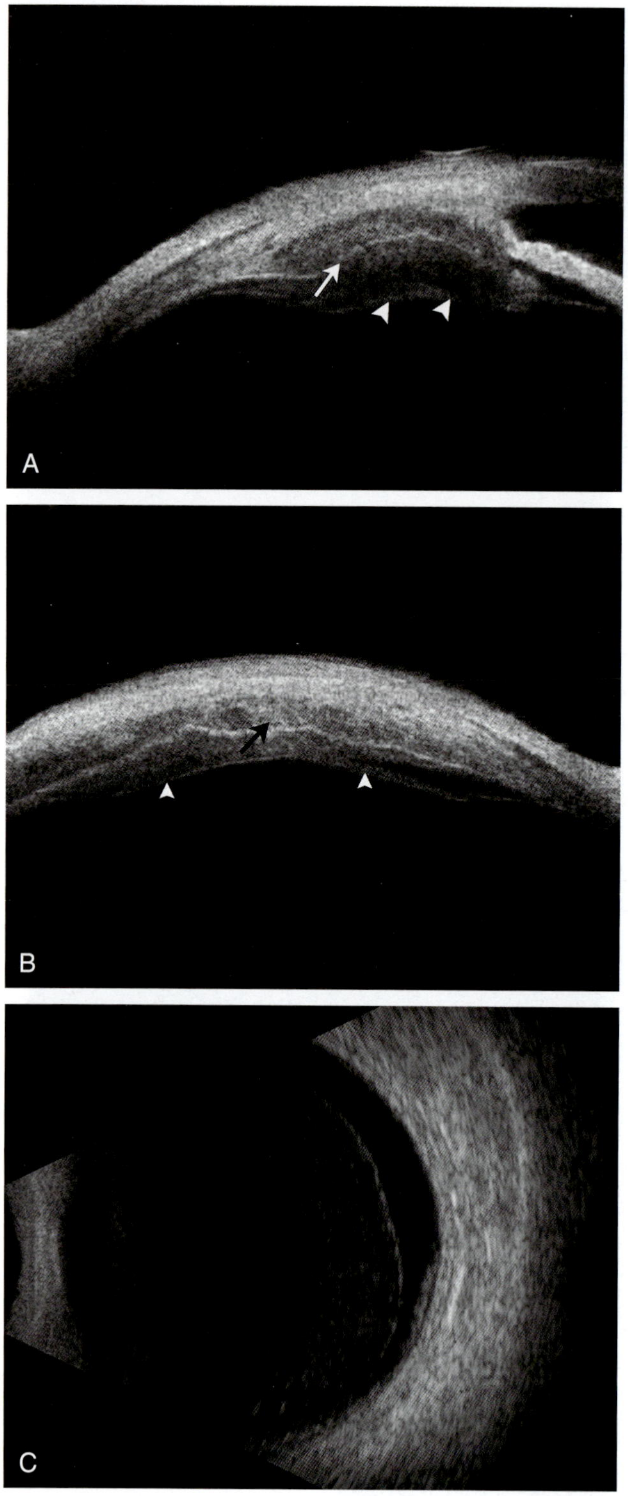

• **Fig. 5.22** Ocular Tuberculosis. **(A)** UBM longitudinal and **(B)** transverse view showing thickening of the ciliary body (*arrow*) and overlying aggregates of inflammatory cells composing a snowbank formation (*arrowheads*). **(C)** Posterior segment B-scan shows moderately dense vitritis and posterior vitreous detachment.

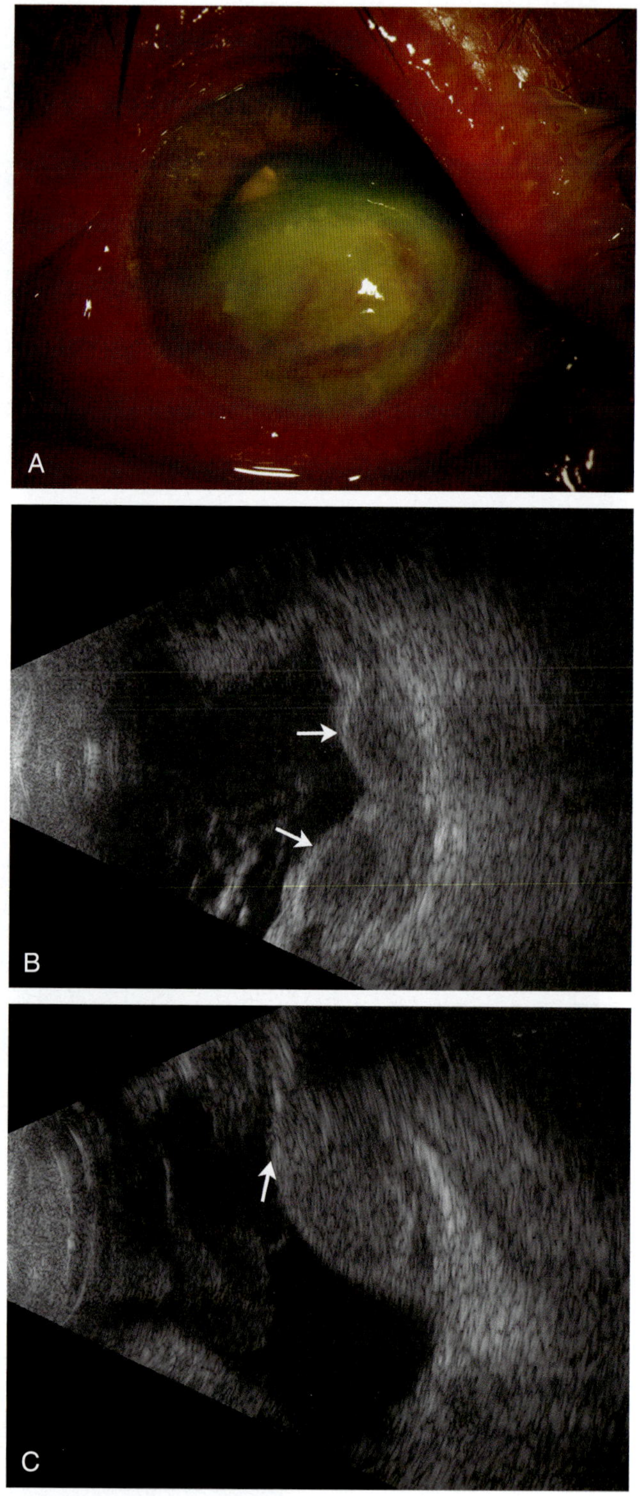

• **Fig. 5.23** Endophthalmitis. **(A)** Clinical picture showing corneal ulcer inferiorly. **(B)** Transverse B-scan shows moderately dense membranous vitreous opacities and extensive non-serous choroidal elevation (*arrows*). **(C)** Longitudinal B-scan shows the extension of the choroidal elevation posterior to the equator (*arrow*).

with the features of the affected eye. The density of the vitreous opacities is graded as mild, moderate, and dense. Moderate and dense dispersed opacities and vitreal membrane formations are more likely to be found in endophthalmitis. Some patients can show posterior vitreous detachment with thickened posterior hyaloid. Moreover, retinal detachment and choroidal detachment are associated with a worse visual prognosis.[16]

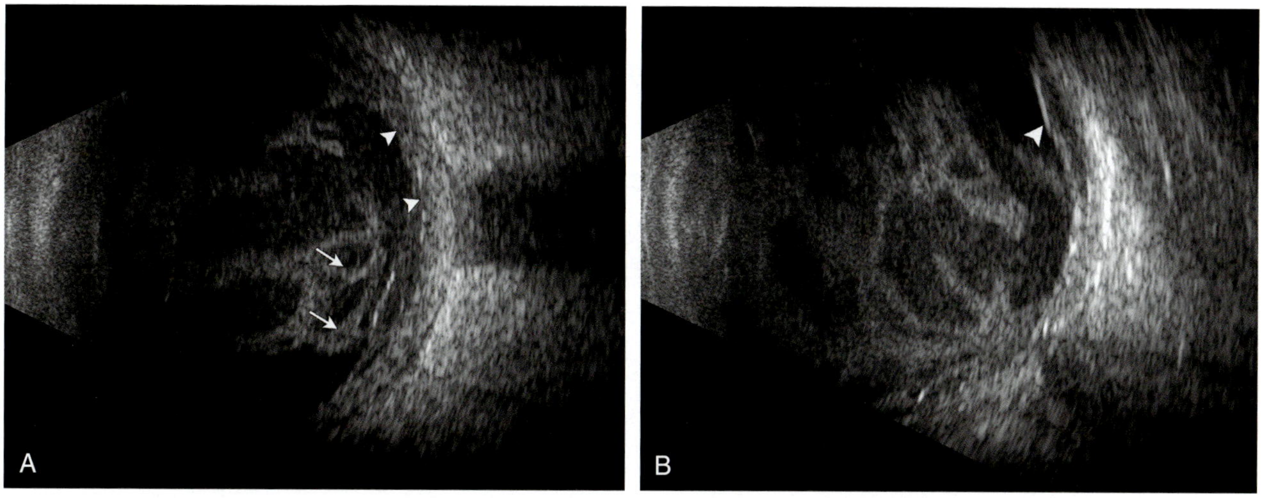

• **Fig. 5.24** Endophthalmitis. **(A)** Transverse B-scan of bacterial endophthalmitis demonstrates dense, predominately membranous vitreous opacities (*arrows*) and diffuse choroidal thickening (*arrowheads*) involving the posterior pole. **(B)** Longitudinal view displays a choroidal elevation extending anteriorly to the ciliary body (*arrowhead*).

CASE

A 73-year-old woman presented with a Staphylococcus aureus corneal ulcer that progressed to culture-positive endophthalmitis had an ultrasound evaluation (Fig. 5.23).

CASE

A 77-year-old male presented with ocular pain and decreased vision after a corneal transplant. An ophthalmic exam revealed hypopyon and vitreous haze. Ultrasound findings were consistent with endophthalmitis (Fig. 5.24 and Video 5.9). Vitreous tap culture was positive for Gram-positive bacteria.

TEACHING POINTS

Moderate and dense dispersed and membranous vitreous opacities are significantly more likely to be found on ultrasound exam in the endophthalmitis. In addition, choroidal thickening or retinal detachment should raise concerns for endophthalmitis.

Suspected cases should be monitored carefully with serial ultrasound exams to detect the worsening or improvement of the disorder.

Uveitis-Glaucoma-Hyphema Syndrome

Uveitis-glaucoma-hyphema syndrome (UGH syndrome) is a rare condition caused by the mechanical trauma of a malpositioned intraocular lens over adjacent structures (iris, ciliary body, iridocorneal angle), leading to a spectrum of iris transillumination defect, microhyphema, and pigmentary dispersion, concomitant with elevated intraocular pressure. The syndrome occurs most commonly with iris-supported anterior chamber intraocular lenses and less frequently with posterior chamber intraocular lenses, either sulcus-fixated or in-the-bag placed lenses.[17] Rarely, UGH syndrome can be associated with iris prosthesis, glaucoma implant, capsular tension ring, and Soemmering ring.

Ultrasound biomicroscopy is a helpful tool to evaluate intraocular lens position, especially in areas inaccessible to slit-lamp biomicroscopy. The horizontal and vertical axial scans assess the inclination of the optic body of the lens and the plane position of the haptics. The longitudinal scan through the angle region is used to assess the contact of the haptics to the uveal tissue. A swinging flashlight test, back and forth in the contralateral eye, can be performed to stimulate iris movement in the examined eye; the examiner should detect if there is rubbing of the lens implant or its haptics while keeping the probe steady. Occasionally, the diagnosis of UGH syndrome cannot be excluded with an examination performed in a standard supine position; therefore, additional scans should be performed in sitting and head-down positions.

CASE

A 67-year-old male with a history of cataract surgery, anterior vitrectomy, and lens implant in the sulcus in the right eye presenting a complaint of foreign body sensation. A slit lamp biomicroscopy exam revealed ciliary injection. An ultrasound exam was requested to evaluate the intraocular lens implant position (Fig. 5.25 and Video 5.10).

CASE

A 55-year-old male presented with late-onset UGH syndrome caused by a Soemmering's ring 6 years after cataract extraction and lens implant. Slit lamp biomicroscopy revealed trace cells in the anterior chamber and iris transillumination defect inferiorly. Ultrasound biomicroscopy exam was consistent with UGH syndrome secondary to Soemmering's ring (Fig. 5.26 and Video 5.11).

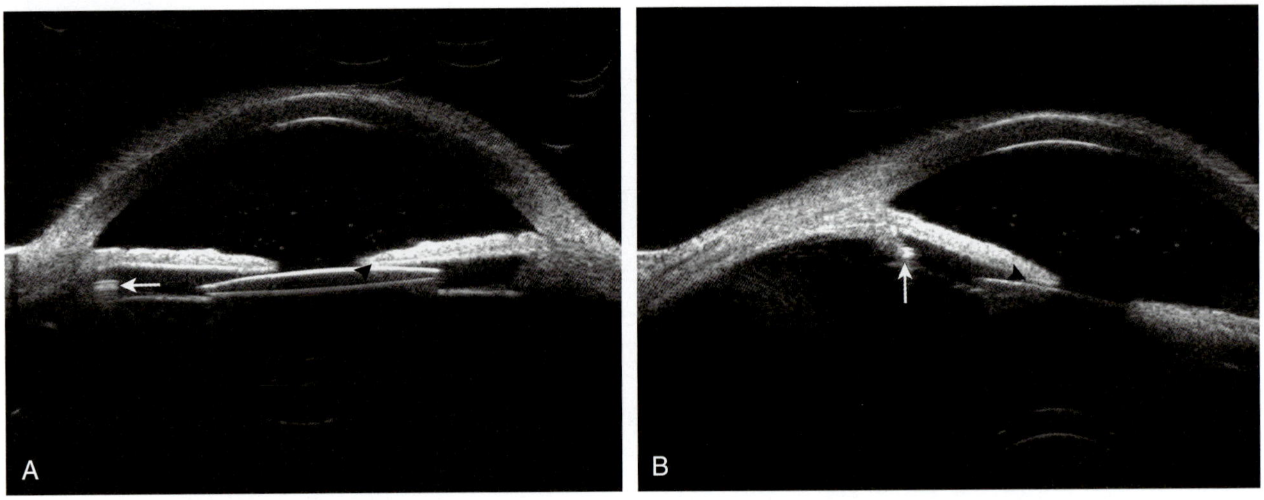

• **Fig. 5.25** Uveitis-Glaucoma-Hyphema Syndrome. UBM horizontal axial **(A)** and longitudinal **(B)** scans show dispersed opacities in the anterior chamber, a posterior chamber intraocular lens implant in contact with the posterior surface of the iris (*arrowhead*), and a haptic in the sulcus (*arrow*). The implant is slightly tilted and outside the capsular bag.

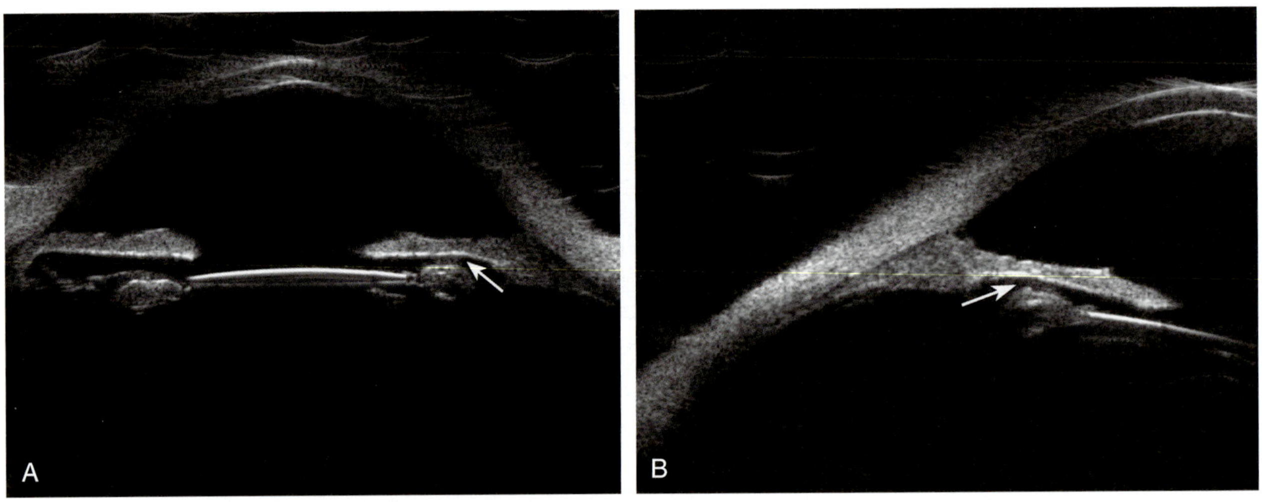

• **Fig. 5.26** Uveitis-glaucoma-hyphema syndrome. **(A)** UBM vertical axial displays a posterior chamber intraocular lens implant surrounded by a prominent Soemmering's ring touching the iris inferiorly (*arrow*). Note the slight anterior deviation of the pigmented epithelium line. **(B)** UBM longitudinal view of an Soemmering's ring-iris touch.

TEACHING POINTS

Ultrasound biomicroscopy can accurately assess the intraocular lens position. The axial scan displays the optic body of the lens, while the longitudinal scan is appropriate for evaluating the haptics position.

References

1. Tran VT, LeHoang P, Herbort CP. Value of high-frequency ultrasound bomicroscopy in uveitis. *Eye (Lond)*. 2001;15:23–30.
2. Peizeng Y, Qianli M, Xiangkun H, Hongyan Z, Li W, Kijlstra A. Longitudinal study of anterior segment inflammation by ultrasound biomicroscopy in patients with acute anterior uveitis. *Acta Ophthalmol*. 2009;87:211–215.
3. Liu X, Hui BT, Way C, et al. Noninvasive Instrument-based tests for detecting and measuring vitreous inflammation in uveitis: a systematic review. *Ocul Immunol Inflamm*. 2020;6:1–12.
4. Zur D, Neudorfer M, Shulman S, Rosenblatt A, Habot-Wilner Z. High-resolution ultrasound biomicroscopy as an adjunctive diagnostic tool for anterior scleral inflammatory disease. *Acta Ophthalmol*. 2016;9:e384–e389.
5. McCluskey PJ, Watson PG, Lightman S, Haybittle J, Restori M, Branley M. Posterior scleritis: clinical features, systemic associations, and outcome in a large series of patients. *Ophthalmology*. 1999;106:2380–2386.
6. Cocho L, Gonzalez-Gonzalez LA, Molina-Prat N, Doctor P, Sainz-de-la-Maza M, Foster CS. Scleritis in patients with granulomatosis with polyangiitis (Wegener). *Br J Ophthalmol*. 2016;100:1062–1065.
7. Sandhu RK, Adams T, Sibley C, Suhler EB, Kim DH. Granulomatosis with polyangiitis (gpa) presenting with frosted branch angiitis. *Retin Cases Brief Rep*. 2016;10:249–251.
8. Mochizuki M, Smith JR, Takase H, et al. Revised criteria of international workshop on ocular sarcoidosis (IWOS) for the diagnosis of ocular sarcoidosis. *Br J Ophthalmol*. 2019;103:1418–1422.

9. Teo HMT, Elner SG, Sassalos TMP, Elner VM, Demirci H. Ciliary body mass as a feature of ocular sarcoidosis. *JAMA Ophthalmol.* 2020;138:300–304.
10. Forster DJ, Cano MR, Green RL, Rao NA. Echographic features of the Vogt-Koyanagi-Harada syndrome. *Arch Ophthalmol.* 1990;108:1421–1426.
11. Wada S, Kohno T, Yanagihara N, et al. Ultrasound biomicroscopic study of ciliary body changes in the post-treatment phase of Vogt-Koyanagi-Harada disease. *Br J Ophthalmol.* 2002;86:1374–1379.
12. Sen HN, Nussenblatt RB. Sympathetic ophthalmia: what have we learned? *Am J Ophthalmol.* 2009;148:632–633.
13. Dalvin LA, Smith WM. Intraocular manifestations of mycobacterium tuberculosis: a review of the literature. *J Clin Tuberc Other Mycobact Dis.* 2017;7:13–21.
14. Dacey MP, Valencia M, Lee MB, et al. Echographic findings in infectious endophthalmitis. *Arch Ophthalmol.* 1994;112:1325–1333.
15. Rachitskaya AV, Flynn HW Jr, Fisher YL, Ayres B. Correlation between baseline echographic features of endophthalmitis, microbiological isolates, and visual outcomes. *Clin Ophthalmol.* 2013;7:779–785.
16. Christopher KL, Hood CT, Mian SI, Ayres B. Endophthalmitis in advanced microbial keratitis: risk factors and examination findings. *Cornea.* 2020;39:1096–1101.
17. Zhang L, Hood CT, Vrabec JP, Cullen AL, Parrish EA, Moroi SE. Mechanisms for in-the-bag uveitis-glaucoma-hyphema syndrome. *J Cataract Refract Surg.* 2014;40:490–492.

6 Glaucoma

BERNADETE AYRES AND SAYOKO MOROI

Imaging plays a critical role in the diagnosis and management of glaucoma. The different ultrasound modalities show different additive diagnostic purposes for glaucoma specialists. A-scan biometry can define the axial ocular length in glaucomatous patients; eyes that are hyperopic or nanophthalmic are more likely to have angle closure, while myopic eyes are more susceptible to open-angle glaucoma. Lower-frequency B-scan ultrasound is suitable to evaluate choroidal effusion and is indispensable to estimated optic disc cupping in cases of opaque media. Ultrasound biomicroscopy (UBM) can objectively qualify and quantify various diagnostic parameters for assessing the anterior chamber.

Assessment of Anterior Segment

UBM provides a high-resolution, accurate, and reproducible qualitative evaluation of the anterior segment and quantitative measurements of the camerular angle and achieves visualization of structures posterior to the iris.[1–2] The common anterior imaging parameters are illustrated in Fig. 6.1 and described in Table 6.1.

The UBM exam is performed with the patient supine, fixing a point in the ceiling under standard low-room illumination, using axial and longitudinal scans. A systematic exam of the anterior segment using UBM should observe the following:

- Detection of inflammatory or hemorrhagic opacities, lens remnants, intraocular foreign body, and extension of synechiae in the anterior chamber
- Measurement of the anterior chamber depth (ACD). The ACD is measured as the perpendicular distance from the center of the corneal endothelial surface to the anterior lens surface, using the pupillary margins as a guide
- Assessment of the lens-iris diaphragm plan
- Centralization and location of the intraocular lens implant in pseudophakic patients
- Measurement of sulcus-to-sulcus diameter
- Measurement of ciliary process to ciliary process distance (diameter)
- Identification of the scleral spur
- Evaluation of the angle opening. Qualitative and quantitative assessment of the angle
- Evaluation of the iris, shape, thickness, and insertion. Iris insertion is classified into the following categories: basal iris insertion, defined as the iris insertion located near the base of the ciliary body; middle iris insertion, defined as the iris insertion located around the middle portion of the ciliary body; apical iris insertion, defined as the iris inserted toward the apex of the ciliary body
- Evaluation of the ciliary body, shape, and thickness
- Localization of the ciliary processes in relation to the scleral spur
- Aperture of the ciliary sulcus
- Iris-lens contact distance

The scleral spur (Figs. 6.2 and 6.3 and Videos 6.1 and 6.2) is the landmark for assessing the parameters of the angle region. On UBM the scleral spur is localized by following the sclera (highly reflective) and ciliary body (low reflective) interfaces until it intersects a line project along the corneal endothelium. The trabecular meshwork lies anterior to the scleral spur for about 500 μm.

TEACHING POINTS

- The scleral spur is identified in the ultrasound biomicroscopy (UBM) image as a protrusion of the sclera into the anterior chamber, which can be traced from the line of attachment between the ciliary body and scleral tissue at the irido-scleral corneal junction.
- TIP: Use a longitudinal approach and medium gain setting and place the probe at the corneoscleral limbus as perpendicular as possible to the angle. Move the probe delicately forward–back and left–right to focus the scleral spur better.

Pupillary Block

In the pupillary block, there is a relative resistance to the passage of the aqueous humor between the iris and the lens resulting in an increase in anterior bowing of the iris (iris bombe) with the shallow peripheral anterior chamber and iridotrabecular contact. The angle may be closed or narrow/occludable.

CASE

A 55-year-old man with a history of uveitis presented with ocular pain and increased intraocular pressure. The ophthalmic exam showed pupillary seclusion, causing extreme anterior bowing of the iris and angle-closure (Fig. 6.4).

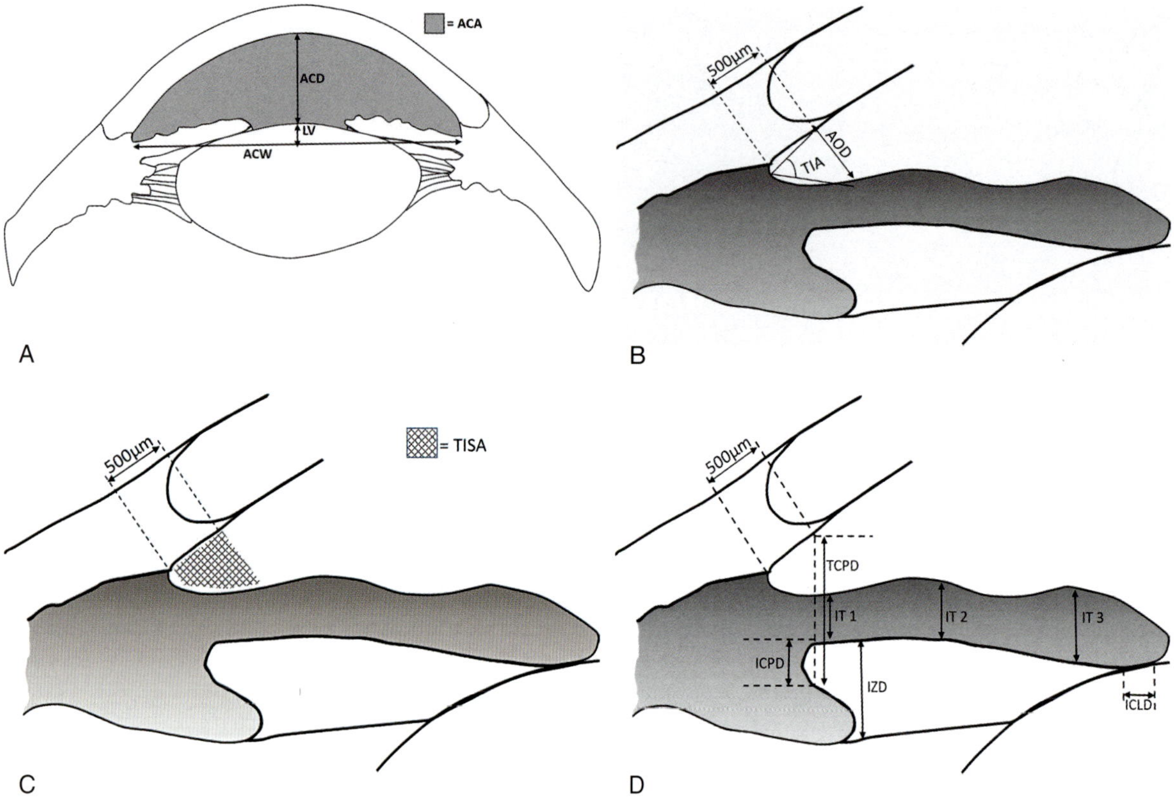

• **Fig. 6.1** Parameters for quantitative measurement of the anterior segment with UBM, described in Table 6.1. **(A)** *ACA*, Anterior chamber area; *ACD*, anterior chamber depth; *ACW*, anterior chamber width; *LV*, lens vault. **(B)** *AOD*, Angle opening distance; *TIA*, trabecular-iris angle. **(C)** *TISA*, Trabecular iris surface area. **(D)** *ICPD*, Iris-ciliary process distance or sulcus ciliaris; *IZD*, Iris-zonule distance; *ILCD*, Iris-lens contact distance; *IT*, Iris thickness; *TCPD*, trabecular-ciliary process distance.

TABLE 6.1 Parameters for Quantitative Measurement of Anterior Segment with UBM

Anterior Chamber Depth (ACD)	Perpendicular Distance from the Center of the Corneal Endothelial Surface to the Anterior Lens Surface
Anterior chamber area (ACA)	Cross-sectional area of the anterior chamber bordered by the posterior surface of the cornea, the anterior surface of the iris, and the anterior surface of the lens within the pupil
Lens vault (LV)	Perpendicular distance between the anterior pole of the crystalline lens and the horizontal line joining the two scleral spurs
Anterior chamber width (ACW)	Sclera spur-to-scleral spur distance
Trabecular-iris angle (TIA)	Angle formed from angle recess to 500 µm from the scleral spur on trabecular meshwork and perpendicular on the surface of iris
Angle opening distance (AOD)	Distance between the trabecular meshwork and the iris at 500 µm from the scleral spur
Trabecular iris surface area (TISA)	Area bounded anteriorly by the AOD, posteriorly by a line drawn from the scleral spur perpendicular to the plane of the inner scleral wall to the opposing iris, superiorly by the inner corneoscleral wall and inferiorly by the iris surface
Iris thickness 1 (IT 1)	Iris thickness at 500 µm anterior to the scleral spur
Iris thickness 2 (IT 2)	Iris thickness at 2 mm from the iris root
Iris thickness 3 (IT 3)	Maximum iris thickness near the pupillary margin
Trabecular-ciliary process distance (TCPD)	Distance between the trabecular meshwork and ciliary process at 500 µm anterior to the scleral spur
Iris-ciliary process distance (ICPD) or sulcus ciliaris	Distance between the iris pigment epithelium and ciliary process along the line of TCPD
Iris-zonule distance (IZD)	Distance between the iris pigmented epithelium and the first visible zonule. Corresponds to the posterior chamber depth
Iris-lens contact distance (ILCD)	Measured along the iris pigment pigmented epithelium from the pupillary margin to the point where the anterior lens surface leaves the iris

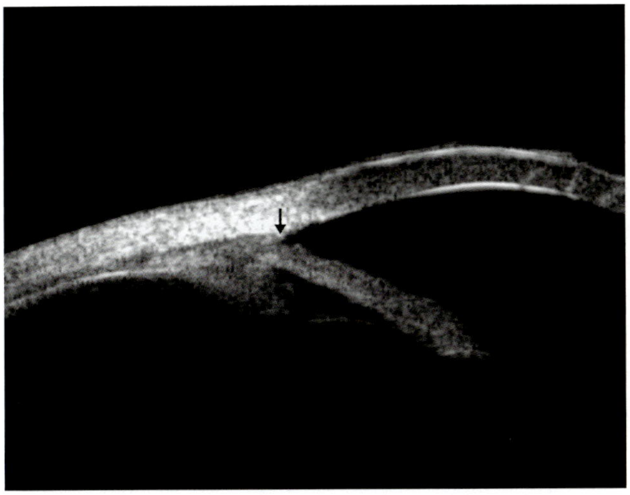

• **Fig. 6.2** Scleral spur. Longitudinal view on UBM with the probe placed at the limbus, perpendicular to the angle displaying the scleral spur (*arrow*) and open angle.

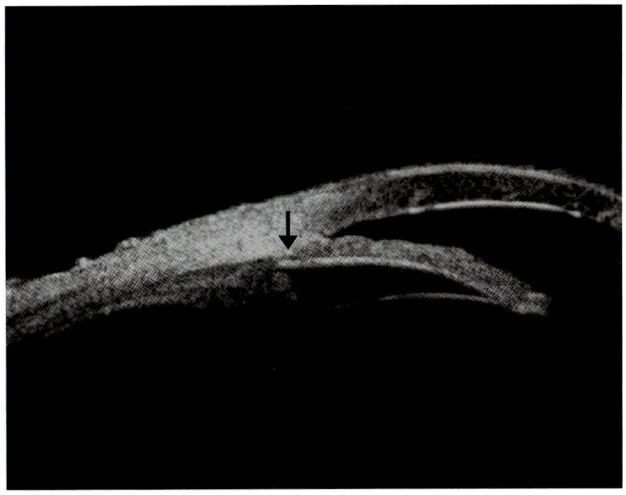

• **Fig. 6.3** Scleral spur. Longitudinal view on UBM displaying the scleral spur (*arrow*) and angle closure.

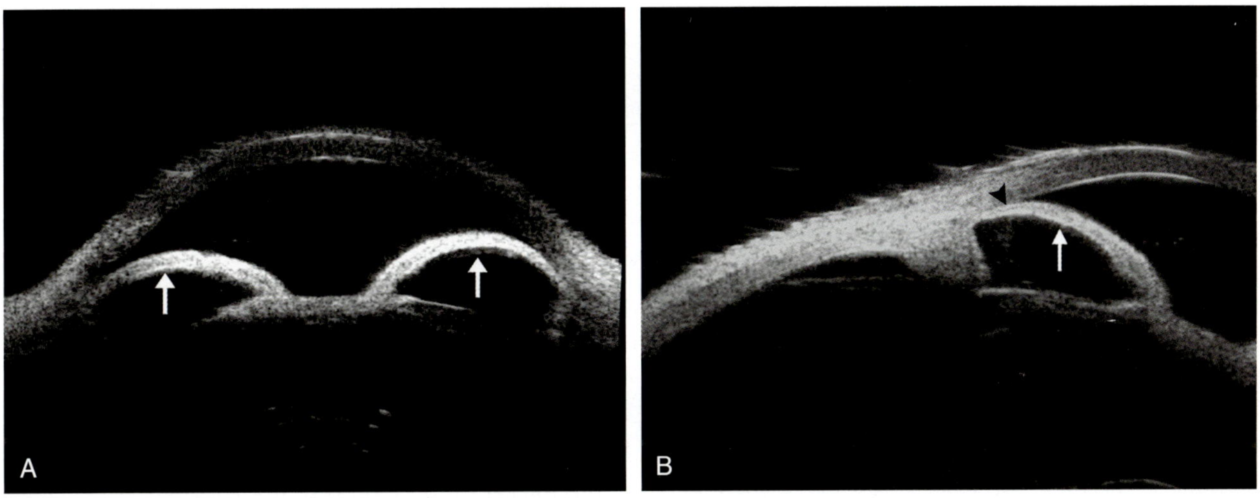

• **Fig. 6.4** Pupillary block. **(A)** UBM horizontal axial and **(B)** longitudinal scans show a shallow peripheral anterior chamber, which is deep centrally, iris bombe (*arrow*), and angle closure (*arrowhead*).

CASE

A 57-year-old woman with a history of retinal detachment repair and cataract extraction with an intraocular lens implant presented with decreased vision, elevated intraocular pressure, and anterior bowing of the iris (Fig. 6.5 and Video 6.3).

CASE

A 44-year-old woman presented with ocular pain and elevated intraocular pressure 6 days after cataract surgery. The slit-lamp exam showed iris bombe and a fibrin membrane covering the pupil. The patient underwent Nd:YAG laser membranectomy with regression of the bombe and angle opening (Fig. 6.6).

TEACHING POINTS

UBM Features of Pupillary Block

- Anterior bowing of the iris
- Shallow peripheral anterior chamber
- Apposition of the iris to the trabecular meshwork
- Open ciliary sulcus
- Shallow anterior chamber in the contralateral eye

The flattening of the iris profile after iridotomy confirms the pupillary block mechanism.

Pupillary block glaucoma may commonly occur secondary to:

- Phacomorphic glaucoma due to cataractous lens intumescence
- Aphakia with pupillary obstruction or synechiae to anterior hyaloid surface
- Pseudophakia with dislocated anterior or posterior intraocular lens or pupillary capture by intraocular lens implant.

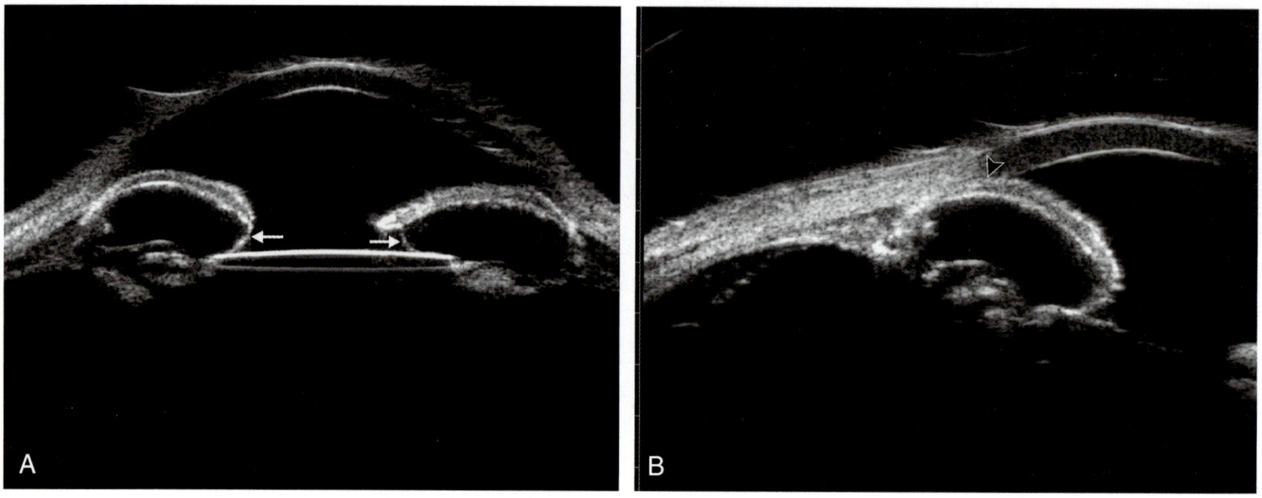

• **Fig. 6.5** Pupillary block. **(A)** UBM horizontal axial view demonstrates anterior bowing of the iris and posterior synechiae to the edge of the anterior lens capsule (*arrows*). **(B)** UBM longitudinal view demonstrates angle closure (*arrowhead*) in a pupillary block.

Plateau Iris

Plateau iris configuration is defined as an occludable angle with a flat iris, a relatively deep central anterior chamber, and anteriorly rotated ciliary processes with a narrow ciliary sulcus. The anteriorly positioned ciliary processes mechanically push the iris root against the trabecular meshwork. *Plateau iris syndrome* describes angle closure (spontaneous, in the dark, or after dilation) despite patent iridotomy.[3]

CASE

A 45-year-old man presented with elevated intraocular pressure, angle closure, and bilateral laser peripheral iridotomy. Gonioscopy revealed bilateral appositional angle closure with no peripheral anterior synechiae (Fig. 6.7).

CASE

A 57-year-old woman presented to the emergency service complaining of severe headache, ocular pain, and blurred vision. She was found to have pressure in the 70s and angle closure. The patient received acetazolamide orally and anterior chamber paracentesis with decreased intraocular pressure and significantly improved symptoms. UBM evaluation demonstrated angle closure with plateau iris configuration (Fig. 6.8 and Video 6.4).

CASE

A 74-year-old woman presented for cataract evaluation and was diagnosed with glaucoma suspect, based on large optic disc cupping in both eyes. She had intraocular pressures within normal limits and angle closure on gonioscopy and underwent peripheral laser iridotomy (Fig. 6.9 and Video 6.5).

TEACHING POINTS

Qualitative diagnostic criteria on UBM for plateau iris configuration:

- Anterior rotation of the ciliary body with anterior displacement of the adjacent iris
- Steep rise of the iris root
- Flat central iris plane
- Narrow or absent ciliary sulcus
- Iridotrabecular contact

Phacomorphic Glaucoma

Phacomorphic glaucoma is acute angle-closure glaucoma precipitated by an intumescent cataractous lens. The iris is displaced anteriorly, and the swollen lens increases a relative pupillary block. In this setting, the contralateral eye has a deeper anterior chamber.

CASE

A 74-year-old woman presented with a decreased vision in her right eye for 1 year. A slit-lamp exam showed a dense, intumescent cataract, a shallow anterior chamber in the right eye, and a deeper anterior chamber in the fellow eye (Fig. 6.10).

Malignant Glaucoma

Malignant glaucoma, also called aqueous misdirection or ciliary block glaucoma, describes secondary glaucoma presenting a shallow or flat anterior chamber, angle closure, and elevated intraocular pressure in a patient with peripheral iridectomy and normal posterior segment anatomy. The phenomenon commonly follows intraocular surgery.

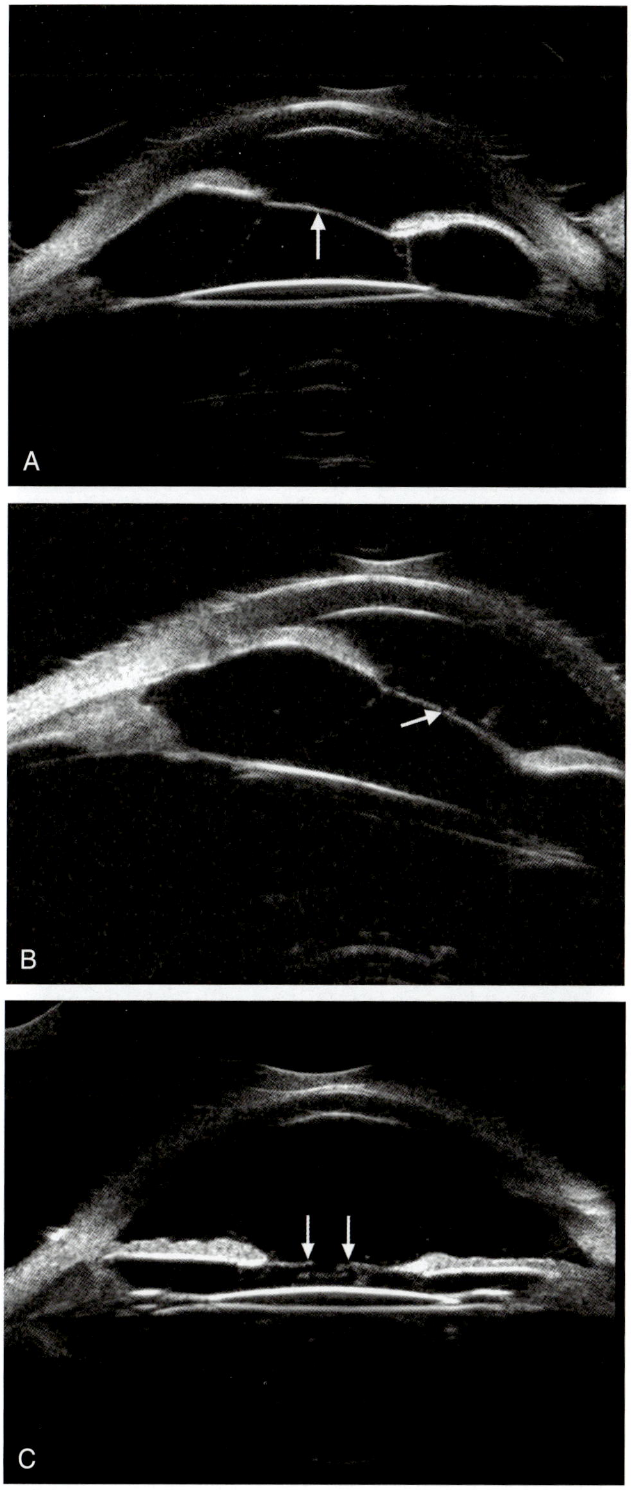

• **Fig. 6.6** Fibrin membrane pupillary block glaucoma. **(A)** UBM horizontal axial and **(B)** longitudinal scans show a shallow anterior chamber, angle closure, and a thin fibrin membrane (*arrow*) across the pupil in a pseudophakic eye. **(C)** UBM exam after Nd:YAG membranectomy shows ruptured fibrin membrane (*arrows*), deepening of the anterior chamber, and opening of the angle.

UBM can demonstrate central and peripheral flattening of the anterior chamber, anterior displacement of the crystalline lens or intraocular lens implant, and anterior rotation of the ciliary body pushing the iris. Occasionally, a minimal amount of fluid can be detected in the supraciliary space. B-scan ultrasound can help differentiate malignant glaucoma from choroidal effusion and suprachoroidal hemorrhage.[4,5]

CASE

An 80-year-old woman with a past ocular history of cataract surgery and intraocular lens implant presented with sharp ocular pain, decreased vision, and elevated intraocular pressure. The biomicroscopy revealed an absent peripheral anterior chamber and a shallow central anterior chamber. Clinical and imaging diagnosis was consistent with malignant glaucoma. The patient underwent Nd:YAG laser capsulotomy/hyaloidotomy with a deepening of the anterior chamber and angle opening (Fig. 6.11).

CASE

An 88-year-old woman was referred for evaluation of uncontrolled intraocular pressure despite medical therapy and YAG laser iridotomy (Fig. 6.12).

Pigment Dispersion Syndrome and Pigmentary Glaucoma

Pigment dispersion syndrome is a bilateral condition where posterior bowing of the iris results in the rubbing of the pigment epithelium against bundles of zonules, releasing pigments throughout the anterior segment. The clinical presentation of pigment dispersion syndrome is characterized by pigments on the corneal endothelium arranged vertically (Krukenberg spindle), dense pigmentation of the trabecular meshwork, and midperiphery transillumination defects of the iris. Intraocular pressure elevation in pigmentary glaucoma occurs as a consequence of overload of pigment in the trabecular meshwork. Over time, chronic pigment release can lead to elevated intraocular pressure and frank pigmentary glaucoma.

UBM has been used to demonstrate the midperiphery iris concavity, iridozonular contact, and wide region of apposition of the iris against to the anterior lens capsule, especially during blinking or accommodation, creating a "reverse" pupillary bock.[6,7]

CASE

A 32-year-old man presented with a history of iris transillumination. Intraocular pressure was 16 mmHg in the right eye and 14 mmHG in the left eye. Slit-lamp examination revealed pigments in the corneal endothelium arranged vertically in both eyes. Gonioscopy revealed a hyperpigmented trabecular meshwork. UBM showed a concave iris configuration (Fig. 6.13).

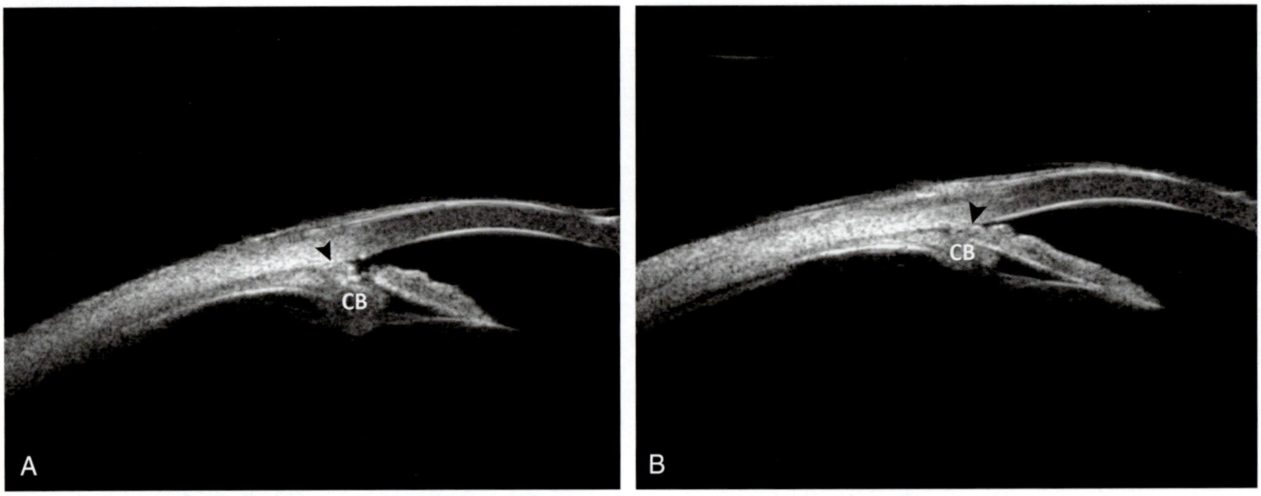

• **Fig. 6.7** **(A)** Plateau iris configuration. UBM longitudinal sections display an angle closure (*arrowhead*) despite peripheral iridotomy. **(B)** The iris is flat, and the ciliary body is anteriorly displaced, pushing the iris root against the trabecular meshwork. *CB*, Ciliary body.

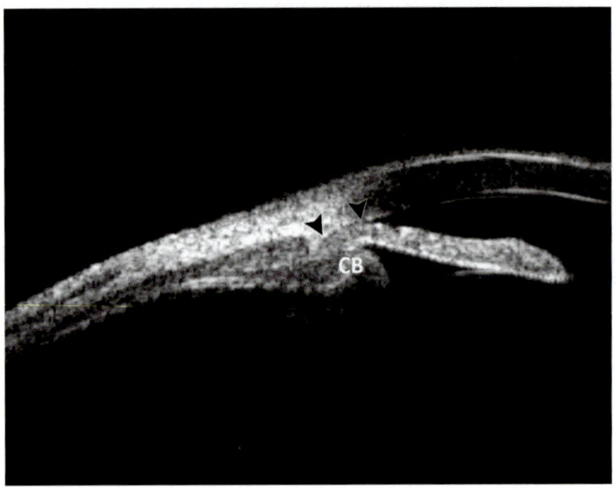

• **Fig. 6.8** UBM longitudinal scan displays a shallow anterior chamber, angle closure (*arrowheads*), a straight profile of the iris, and anterior rotation of the ciliary body. *CB*, Ciliary body.

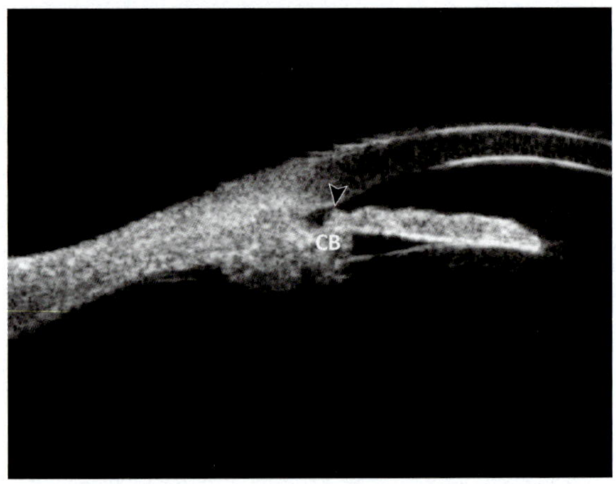

• **Fig. 6.9** UBM longitudinal view showing angle-closure (*arrowhead*) in plateau iris configuration. The iris is inserted at the apex of the ciliary processes. *CB*, Ciliary body.

TEACHING POINTS

Clinical Features of Pigment Dispersion Syndrome

- Usually asymptomatic or mild discomfort
- Spindle-shaped deposition of pigment on the corneal endothelium (Krukenberg spindle)
- A slightly concave midperipheral iris
- Iris transillumination

UBM Findings

- Concave iris configuration
- Increased iridolenticular contact area
- Increased iris posterior bowing during accommodation

Cyclodialysis

Cyclodialysis describes the disinsertion of the longitudinal muscle of the ciliary body from the scleral spur, which results in a cleft, allowing direct communication between the anterior chamber and the supraciliary space. Blunt trauma is the most common cause, followed by iatrogenic surgical complications. Clinical findings at presentation include hypotony, shallow anterior chamber, macular edema, optic disc edema, corneal edema, and blurred vision. Ultrasound biomicroscopy can accurately diagnose the presence and extension of a cyclodialysis and the associated suprachoroidal effusion.[8,9] The exam should be performed with minimal probe pressure, using a longitudinal scan to screen all meridians.

CASE

A 41-year-old woman with pigmentary glaucoma, status post trabeculoplasty, and later goniotomy, presented for evaluation hypotony. Intraocular pressure was 3 mmHg, and biomicroscopy demonstrated a shallow anterior chamber. Fundus examination showed a full optic disc, macular folds, tortuous vasculature, and chorioretinal folds. UBM demonstrated cyclodialysis extending from 2 o'clock to 4 o'clock and supraciliary effusion (Fig. 6.14 and Video 6.6).

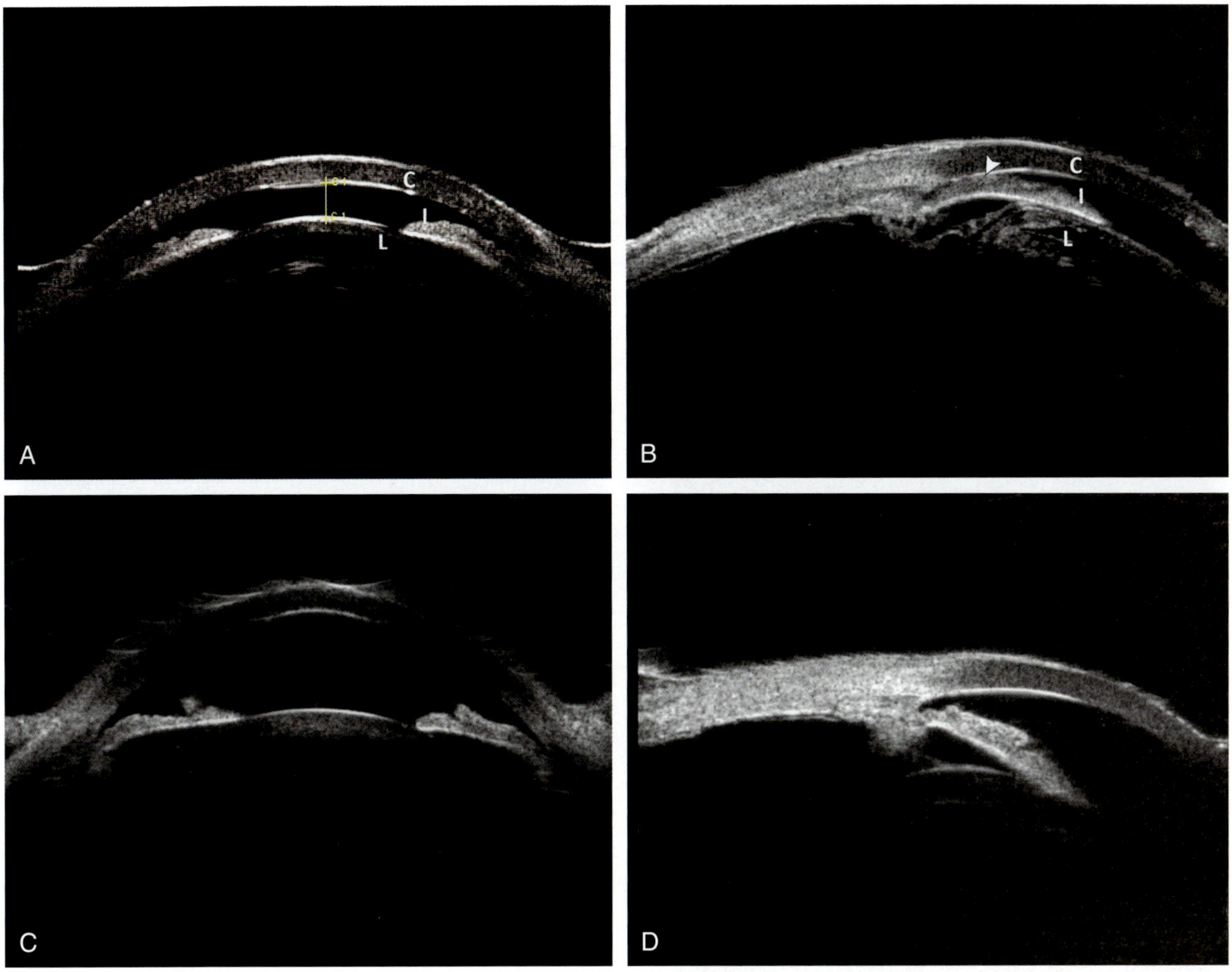

• **Fig. 6.10** Phacomorphic glaucoma. UBM echograms of phacomorphic glaucoma. **(A)** The axial view of the right eye shows a shallow anterior chamber and anterior displacement of the iris and crystalline lens. **(B)** The longitudinal view shows an angle closure (*arrowhead*), cataractous lens, and ciliary processes positioned at the level of the scleral spur. **(C–D)** Comparative UBM echograms of the fellow eye show a deeper anterior chamber and open angle. *C*, Cornea; *I*, iris; *L*, lens.

CASE

A 51-year-old woman with a history of blunt trauma and angle recession had goniotomy, trabeculectomy, and cataract extraction with intraocular lens implant and was referred for evaluation of ocular hypotony and cyclodialysis (Fig. 6.15).

TEACHING POINTS

- Most cases of cyclodialysis are caused by blunt trauma.
- Ocular hypotony is a leading sign of cyclodialysis.
- The UBM exam for diagnosis of cyclodialysis is better conducted using a longitudinal approach and a soft water-filled probe cover. Soften probe cover by removing some fluid.
- The cleft region is usually obvious from the displacement of the iris in the same direction.
- Scan all meridians to determine the extension of the cyclodialysis and future exam comparison.

Drug-Induced Angle-Closure Glaucoma

Numerous systemic and topical drugs can induce acute angle-closure glaucoma including adrenergic agonists, anticholinergics, cholinergics, sulfonamides, supplements, and serotonergic medications. The resulting acute glaucoma occurs unilaterally or bilaterally. Typically, the patient complains of nausea, blurred vision, and severe ocular pain. The ophthalmic exam can reveal myopic shift, closure of the trabecular meshwork, shallow central anterior chamber, and elevated intraocular pressure.[10,11] On UBM exam, supraciliary effusion with forwarding displacement of the lens-iris diaphragm can be demonstrated.[12]

CASE

A 31-year-old female presented to the emergency room complaining of bilateral blurred vision. Her systemic medications include Topiramate 25 mg twice a day. An ophthalmic exam disclosed elevated intraocular pressure and a shallow anterior chamber in both eyes (Fig. 6.16). Six days after the discontinuity of the Topiramate, there was a resolution of the process.

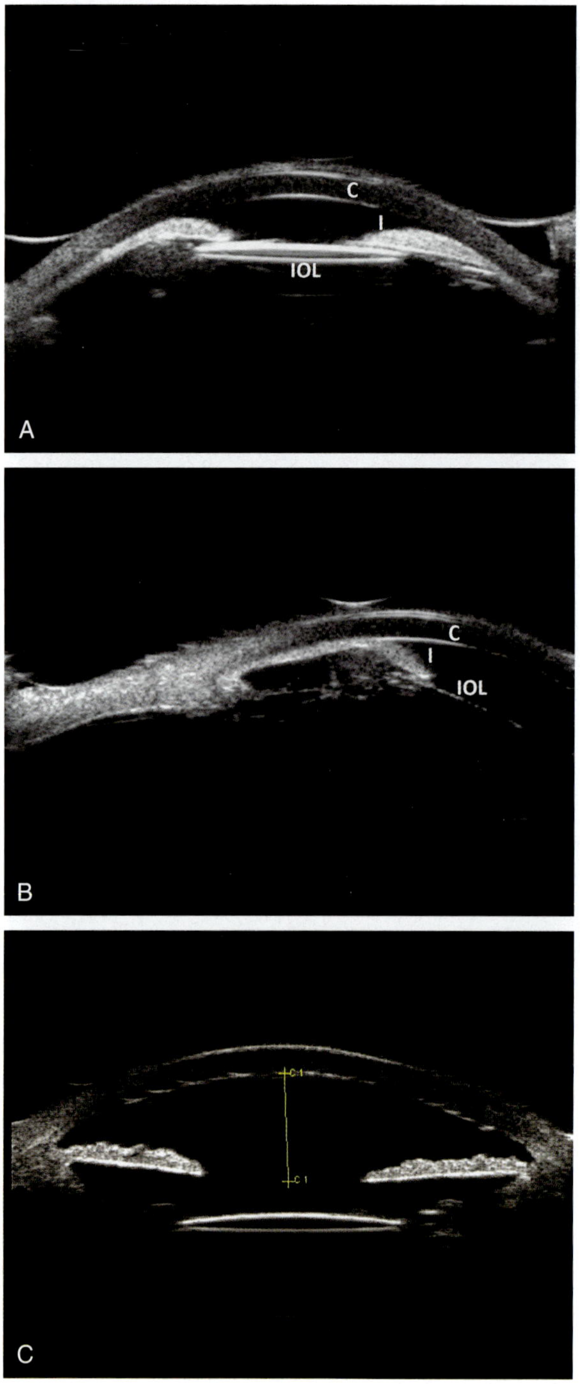

• **Fig. 6.11** Pseudophakic malignant glaucoma. **(A)** UBM axial and **(B)** longitudinal views show anterior displacement of the iris-lens diaphragm, shallow anterior chamber, and angle closure. **(C)** UBM axial view after Nd:YAG laser for disruption of the lens capsule and anterior hyaloid face demonstrated deepening of the anterior chamber and angle opening. *C*, Cornea; *IOL*, intraocular lens implant; *I*, iris.

TEACHING POINTS

UBM can show ciliary body edema, and supraciliary effusion with forward displacement of the lens-iris diaphragm in cases of drug-induced angle-closure glaucoma.

Systemic medications are known to increase the risk of angle-closure glaucoma:

- Sulfonamides: topiramate, acetazolamide, methazolamide
- Diuretics: hydrochlorothiazide and indapamide
- Serotonin-norepinephrine reuptake inhibitor: venlafaxine

Angle-Closure Secondary to Primary Cysts of the Iris Pigment Epithelium

Primary iris pigment epithelium cysts occur spontaneously and are defined as epithelial-lined structures that arise in the posterior iris layer. They can be in any region between the pupillary margin to the iridociliary sulcus. They can occur as single, more common, or multiple cysts.[13] Occasionally, angle-closure glaucoma may develop when multiple cysts involve an extensive circumferential area. On UBM, the iris pigment epithelium cysts characteristically have thin walls and anechoic contents.[14]

CASE

A 37-year-old man was referred for bilateral elevated intraocular pressure and angle closure. A biomicroscopy exam revealed anterior bowing of the iris in all quadrants in both eyes. UBM exam revealed anterior bowing of the iris and multiple cysts of iris pigment epithelium, causing angle closure for 360° in both eyes (Fig. 6.17).

TEACHING POINTS

- Peripheral iris pigment epithelium cysts are characterized by anterior and peripheral bowing of the iris.
- The differential diagnosis of primary iris cysts should be made with solid lesions such as melanoma, medulloepithelioma, pigment epithelium adenoma, and metastases.
- Angle-closure glaucoma associated with multiple peripheral ciliary cysts occurs when angular involvement is more than 180°.

Glaucoma Associated With Nanophthalmos

Nanophthalmos is defined as a small eye without other ocular or systemic malformations. The nanophthalmic eye has several anatomic characteristics, such as short axial length, shallow anterior chamber depth, forward displacement of the lens, anteriorly rotated ciliary body, small ciliary ring diameter, and thick sclera. Nanophthalmos has an increased risk of having a chronic, painless type of angle-closure glaucoma in middle age due to the natural increase in the lens size.[15,16]

CASE

A 68-year-old woman had chronic angle-closure glaucoma. Ultrasound evaluation revealed anatomic features of nanophthalmos. The patient underwent Nd:YAG laser iridotomy and hyaloidotomy resulting in the deepening of the anterior chamber and angle opening (Fig. 6.18).

Suprachoroidal Hemorrhage

Suprachoroidal hemorrhage, either intraoperative or delayed, is rare but a severe complication of intraocular surgery. Angle-closure glaucoma can be secondary to anterior

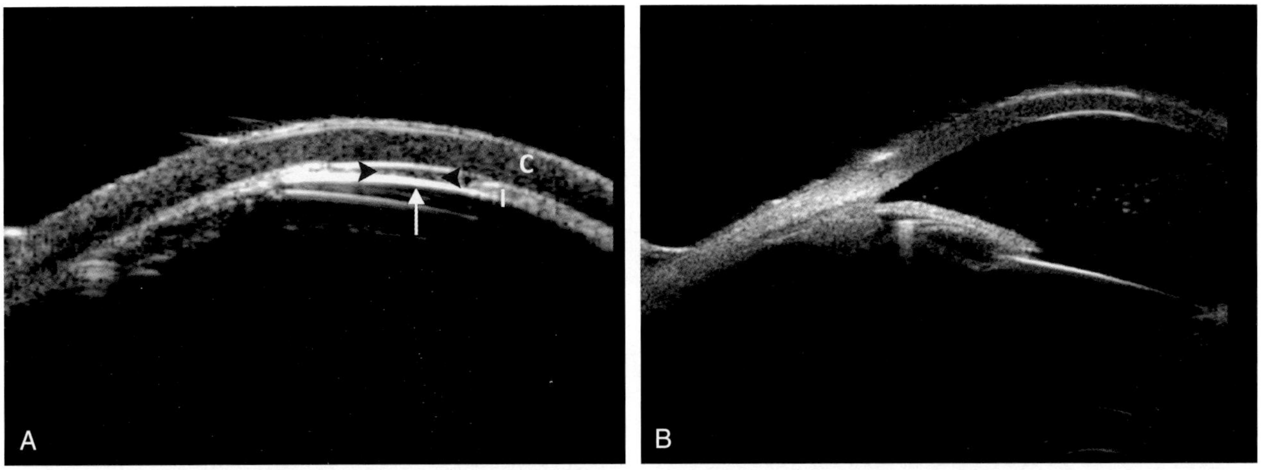

• **Fig. 6.12** Malignant glaucoma. **(A)** UBM axial scan demonstrates a marked anterior displacement of the intraocular lens implant (*arrow*) and a flat anterior chamber with complete iris apposition to the cornea (*arrowheads*). **(B)** UBM exam after combined vitrectomy and goniosynechiolysis demonstrates reposition of the iris-lens diaphragm. *C*, Cornea; *I*, iris.

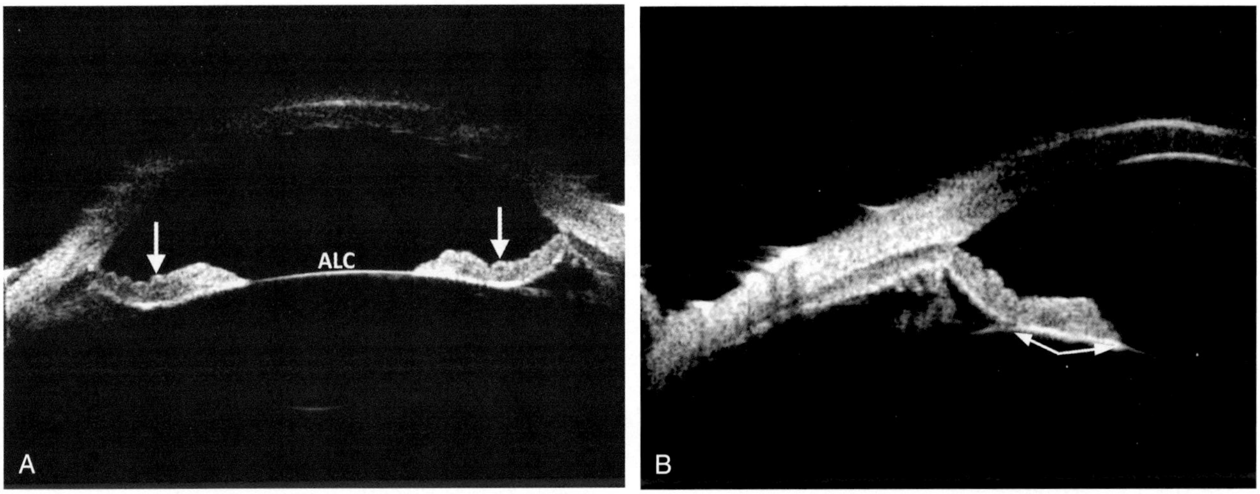

• **Fig. 6.13** Pigment dispersion syndrome. **(A)** UBM in axial view displays a deep anterior chamber and marked posterior bowing of the iris (*arrow*). **(B)** The longitudinal view displays an open angle and wide area of iris-lens contact distance (*connected arrows*); the zonule is likely in contact with the iris pigmented epithelium. *ALC*, Anterior lens capsule.

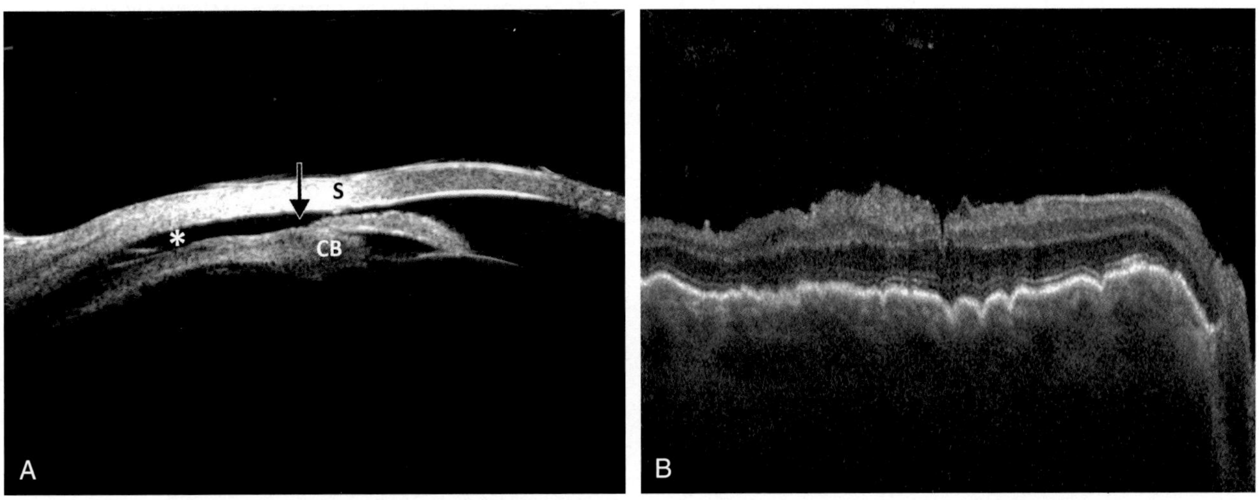

• **Fig. 6.14** Cyclodialysis. **(A)** UBM longitudinal scan demonstrates an anteriorly rotated, disinserted ciliary body from the sclera (*arrow*) and supraciliary fluid (*asterisk*). **(B)** Optical coherence tomography demonstrating hypotony maculopathy in case of cyclodialysis.

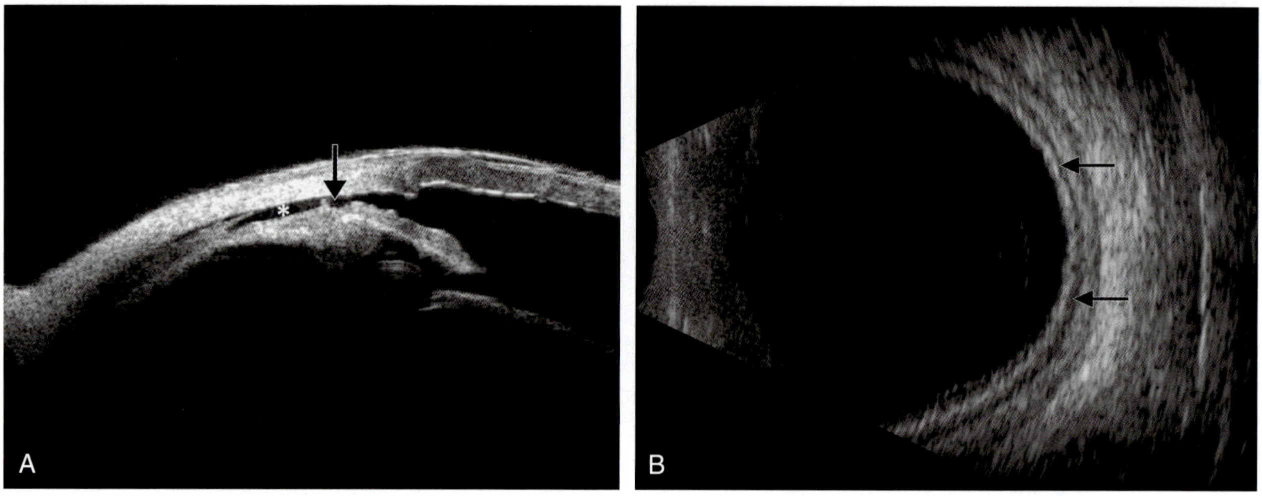

• **Fig. 6.15** Cyclodialysis. **(A)** UBM longitudinal view demonstrates a disinserted ciliary body (*arrow*) and fluid in the supraciliary space extending to the suprachoroidal space (*asterisk*). B-scan transverse view, aimed at the far periphery, shows shallow ciliochoroidal effusion (*arrows*).

movement of the lens-iris diaphragm during suprachoroidal hemorrhage.

CASE

A 66-year-old man with a visually significant cataract underwent phacoemulsification surgery with an intraocular lens implant. On the third week post-surgery, the patient developed uncontrolled elevated intraocular pressure and underwent trabeculectomy. One week later, the patient presented with ocular pain, and the intraocular pressure remained elevated. Slit-lamp examination indicated a shallow anterior chamber and angle closure (Fig. 6.19).

Glaucoma Surgeries

When pharmacologic and laser treatment fails to control intraocular pressure (IOP), incisional surgery such as trabeculectomy, trabeculotomy, glaucoma drainage device implantation, or trabecular meshwork bypass is required to control the IOP. B-scan ultrasound and UBM are useful to evaluate post-operative anatomic changes in the anterior chamber and devices' position, patency, and function.

Trabeculectomy

Trabeculectomy has been widely employed as a treatment for glaucoma. The outcome of this surgery depends on the formation of a functioning shunt, termed *filtration bleb*, to enable the egress of aqueous from the eye. The morphology of the bleb and route of the aqueous under the scleral flap can be visualized using UBM.

Using a longitudinal scan, UBM can image the following features:

- Bleb height
- The thickness of the bleb wall
- Internal reflectivity of the bleb (bleb cavity)
- Presence of cystic spaces within the bleb or bleb wall
- Scleral flap apposition to underlying sclera
- Route under the scleral flap and patency of the internal ostium

The height of the bleb is measured from the highest point on the bleb to the longest line from the outer surface of the sclera. A functional bleb typically presents tall or moderated height, thick wall, low to medium internal reflectivity, internal cysts, visible route, and non-obstructed ostium.[17,18]

CASE

A 72-year-old woman with a history of primary open-angle glaucoma underwent trabeculectomy with mitomycin C resulting in successful controlled intraocular pressure (Fig. 6.20).

Microinvasive Glaucoma Surgery (MIGS)

These modalities target physiologic outflow pathways or optimize previously utilized glaucoma surgical methods to deliver safety, efficacy, and individualized care to the patient. Based on anatomical location as well as method of intraocular pressure reduction MIGS techniques can be classified in Schlemm's canal, suprachoroidal or subconjunctival MIGS.[19]

Trabeculotomy

Trabeculotomy lowers intraocular pressure by improving the flow of aqueous through Schlemm's canal without bleb formation. Gonioscopy-assisted transluminal trabeculotomy is a novel MIGS with an ab interno approach for circumferential trabeculotomy.[20]

On UBM, the trabecular leaflet resulting after the procedure is identified as a thin membrane inserted at the posterior zone of the unroofed trabecular meshwork.[21]

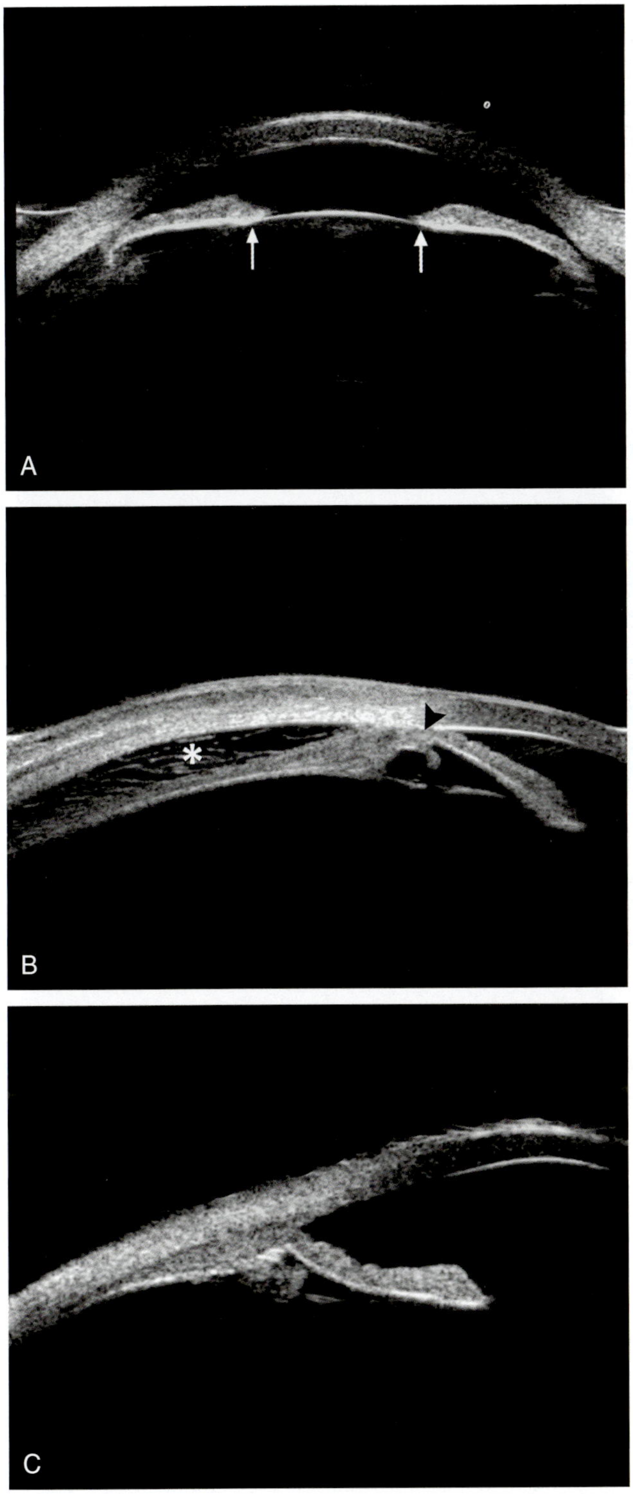

• **Fig. 6.16** Drug-induced angle closure. **(A)** UBM axial view showing forward displacement of the lens-iris diaphragm (*arrows*) and shallow anterior chamber. **(B)** Longitudinal view showing angle closure (arrowhead) and fluid in the supraciliary space (*asterisk*). **(C)** Longitudinal UBM 6 days after cessation of the inciting medication shows a deepening of the anterior chamber, resolution of the uveal effusion, and angle opening.

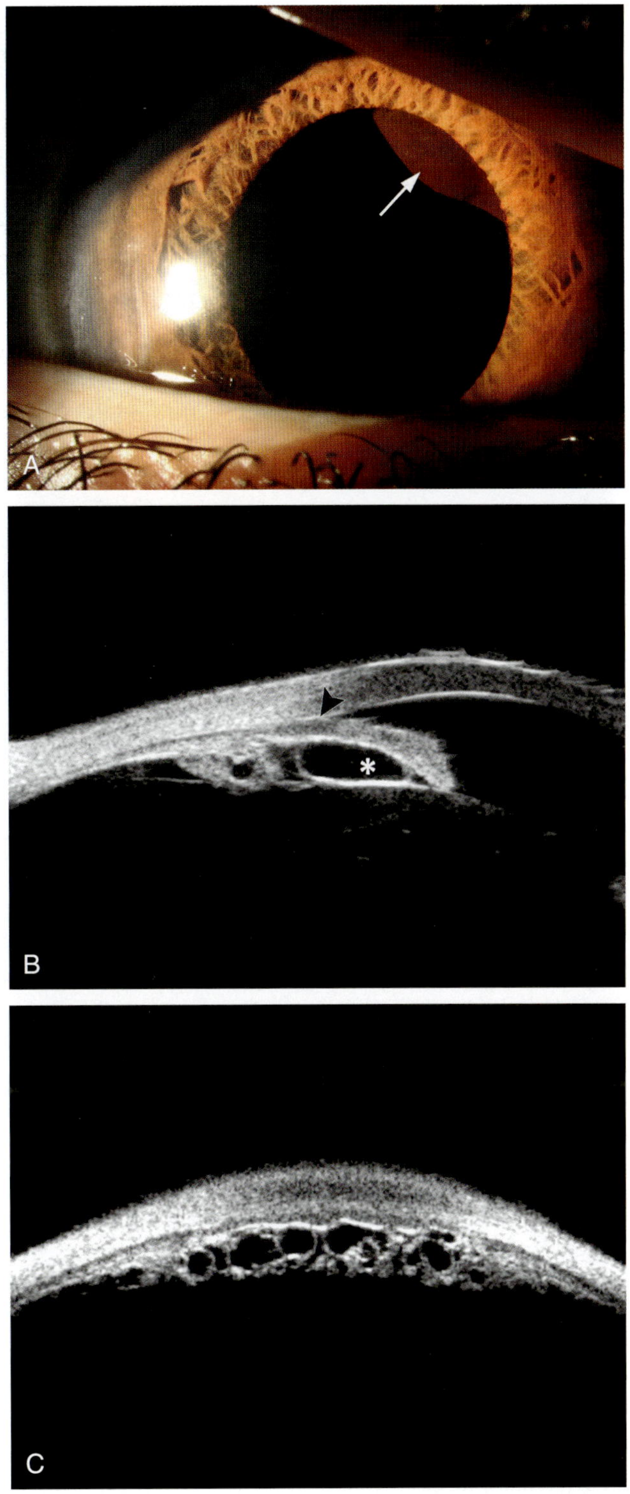

• **Fig. 6.17** Primary cyst of the iris pigment epithelium. **(A)** Slit-lamp photo of a retroiridal pigment epithelium cyst (*arrow*). **(B)** UBM longitudinal view showing a large, pigmented epithelium cyst (*asterisk*) displacing the iris anteriorly and closing the angle (*arrowhead*). **(C)** UBM in transverse view shows multiple cysts over a wide area.

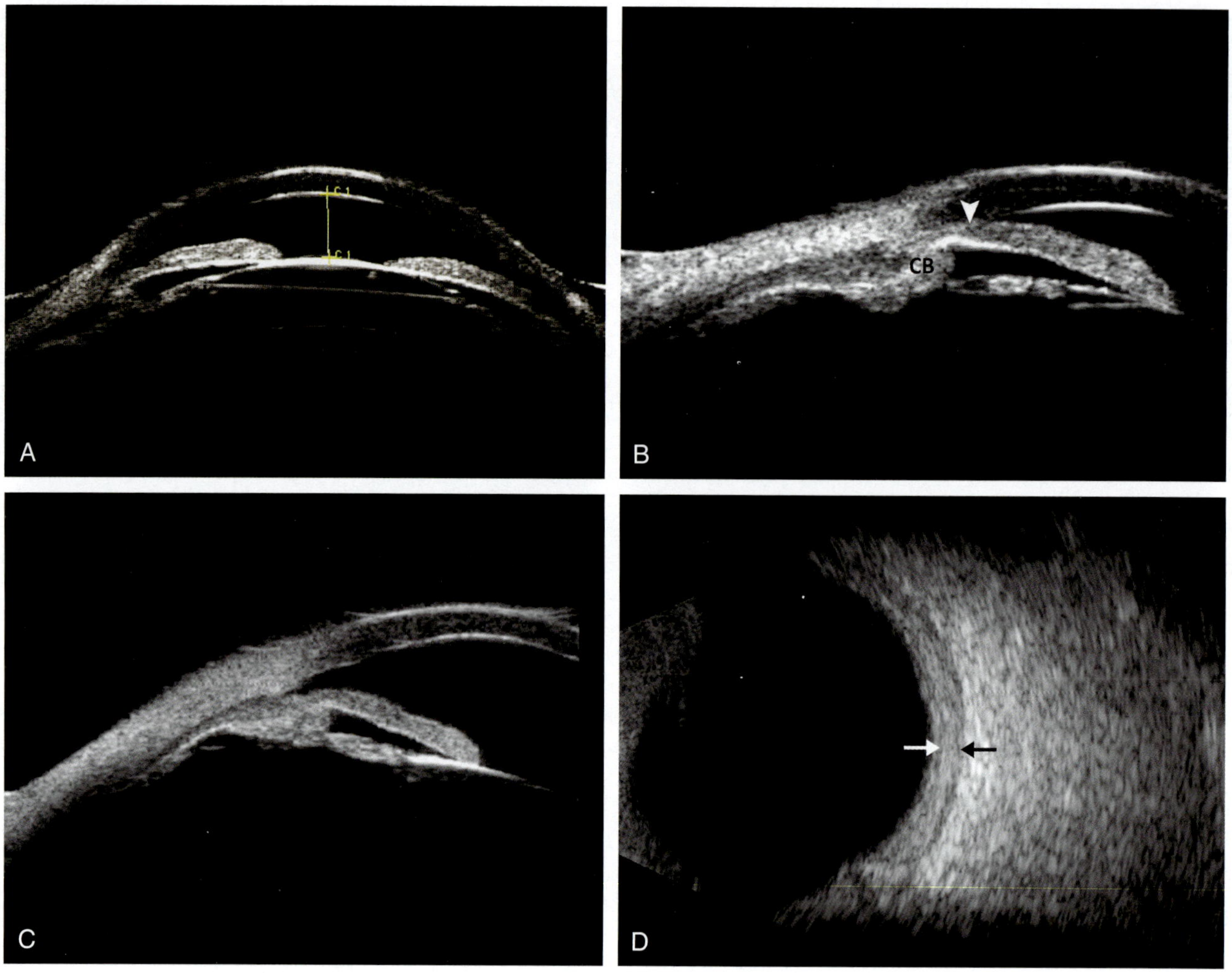

• **Fig. 6.18** Nanophthalmos. **(A)** UBM axial and **(B)** longitudinal scans in nanophthalmos show a shallow anterior chamber, forward displacement of iris-lens implant diaphragm, angle-closure (*arrowhead*), and anterior rotation of the ciliary body. **(C)** Deepening of the anterior chamber and angle opening after Nd:YAG laser iridotomy and hyaloidotomy. **(D)** B-scan ultrasound in nanophthalmic eye showing thickened sclera and choroid (*arrows*). *CB*, Ciliary body.

CASE

A 49-year-old woman with primary open-glaucoma and 30 mmHg intraocular pressure, despite maximum-tolerated medical therapy, underwent gonioscopy-assisted transluminal trabeculotomy (Fig. 6.21).

MIGS devices

Hydrus Microstent

The Hydrus microstent is 8 mm in length with a 290 micron lumen, with three windows placed in Schlemm's canal, and functions as a trabecular meshwork bypass stent. It is made of nitinol, a flexible, biocompatible titanium and nickel alloy.

CASE

A 44-year-old woman with primary open-angle glaucoma and subluxated lens underwent phacoemulsification with an intraocular lens implant and Hydrus microbypass stent insertion (Fig. 6.22 and Video 6.7).

Xen Gel Stent

Xen Gel Stent is 6 mm long with a 45 micron lumen implant made from porcine gelatin. The stent drains aqueous fluid from the anterior chamber to the subconjunctival space.

CASE

An 83-year-old woman with refractory primary open-angle glaucoma had successfully implanted a XEN gel stent. The inserter was introduced into the anterior chamber and, under indirect gonioscopic guidance, was implanted into the superonasal angle. The stent emerged in the superonasal subconjunctival space (Fig. 6.23 and Video 6.8).

Glaucoma Drainage Device

Glaucoma drainage devices create alternate aqueous pathways by channeling aqueous from the anterior chamber through a long tube to an equatorial plate that promotes bleb formation.

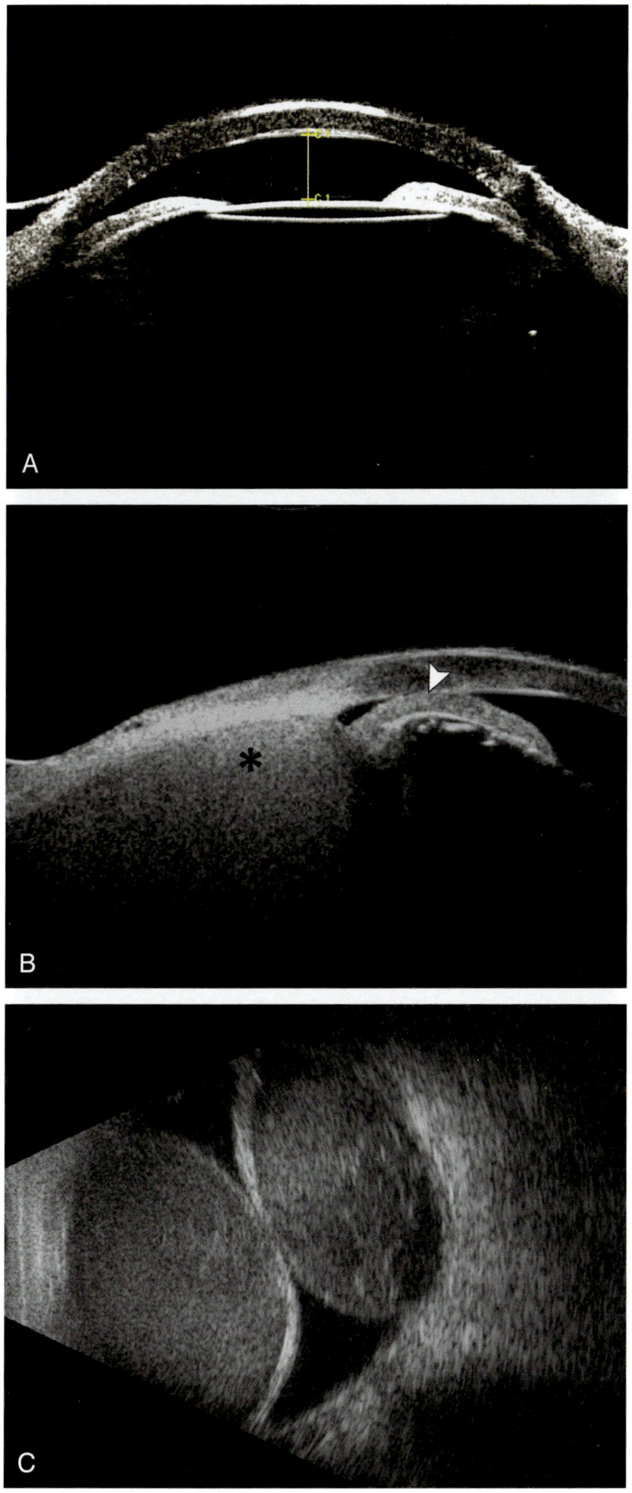

• **Fig. 6.19** Suprachoroidal hemorrhage. **(A)** UBM axial approach demonstrates a shallow anterior chamber and anterior displacement of the iris-lens diaphragm. **(B)** UBM longitudinal approach demonstrates angle closure (*arrowhead*) and massive hemorrhage in the supraciliary space (*asterisk*). **(C)** Bullous, appositional hemorrhagic choroidal detachment on longitudinal B-scan.

Currently, these devices are available in different sizes, materials, and designs with the presence or absence of a pressure-regulating valve. All devices consist of a silicone rubber tube connected to an endplate. Most glaucoma implants are placed in the superotemporal quadrant. The tube is most often placed in the anterior chamber; however, the tube may also be placed in the ciliary sulcus in a pseudophakic eye or in the pars plana in a vitrectomized eye.

Displacement and obstruction of the tube can be detected with UBM, and the best approach is the longitudinal scan. The tube is identified as multiple parallel lines extending from the anterior chamber or sulcus area to the suprascleral space.[22]

On B-scan, the plate of the glaucoma drainage device is identified as two parallel, hyperreflective lines in the extrascleral space, usually superotemporally. If fluid is present in a bleb, it will be seen as an echolucent area underlying or overlying the plate. The amount of fluid around the plate can be evaluated with B-scan to assess the patency/function of the device. Flattening of the sclera under the plate is characteristic of moderate and large blebs.[23,24]

CASE

A 65-year-old male with a history of central retinal vein occlusion and subsequent neovascular glaucoma had a glaucoma drainage device implanted with successful IOP control (Fig. 6.24).

Glaucoma Drainage Device Tube Obstruction

CASE

A 76-year-old man with a history of poorly controlled primary open-angle glaucoma had a glaucoma valve implanted with the tube placed into the ciliary sulcus presented with high intraocular pressure at 3 weeks postoperatively (Fig. 6.25 and Video 6.9).

Evaluation of Fluid Bleb Surrounding a Glaucoma Drainage Device Plate

CASE

A 90-year-old woman with a history of uveitic glaucoma had a drainage device inserted with satisfactory intraocular pressure lowering. B-scan ultrasound demonstrated moderate fluid surrounding the plate (Fig. 6.26 and Video 6.10).

TEACHING POINTS

Patency of the Glaucoma Drainage Device

- If the fluid is present in a bleb, it will be seen as an echolucency area underlying and/or overlying the plate that indents or flattens the sclera.
- Elevated IOP after surgery results from blockage of the tube tip, blockage within the glaucoma drainage device, or bleb encapsulation.
- Lack of fluid around the plate associated with elevated intraocular pressure suggests a nonpatent glaucoma drainage device.
- Presence of fluid around the plate with elevated intraocular pressure is suggestive of bleb encapsulation.

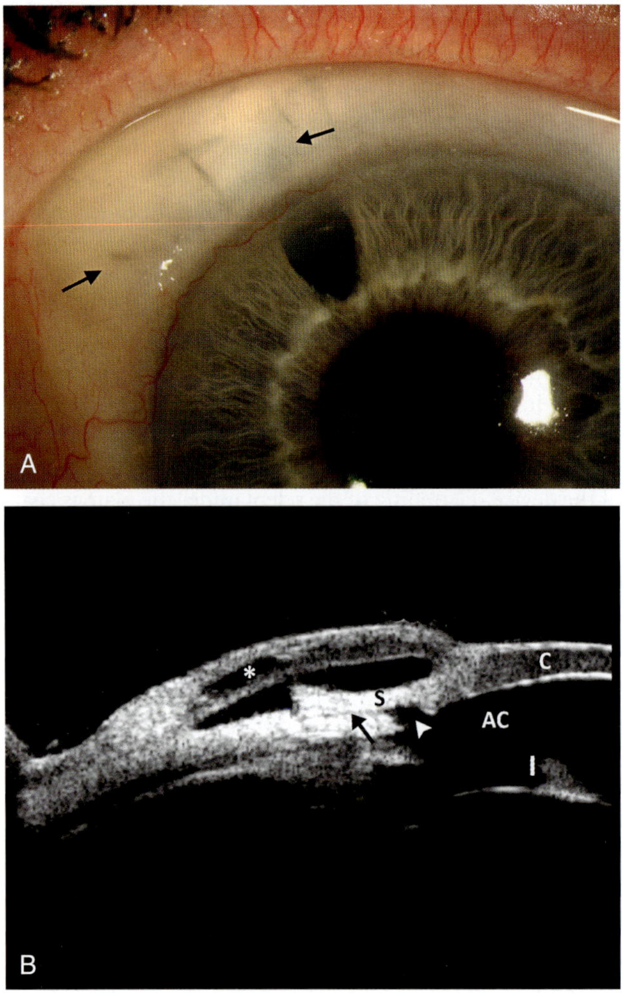

• **Fig. 6.20** Trabeculectomy. **(A)** Slit-lamp photo of an elevated, broad diffuse, juxtalimbal bleb with an avascular central zone (*arrows*). **(B)** UBM longitudinal scan demonstrates a moderately elevated bleb with a thick wall and low reflective intrableb cavity. There is a cystic space within the wall (*asterisk*). The sclerectomy ostium (*arrowhead*) is open, and the aqueous route (*arrow*) is visible. *AC*, Anterior chamber; *C*, cornea; *I*, Iridectomy *S*, scleral flap.

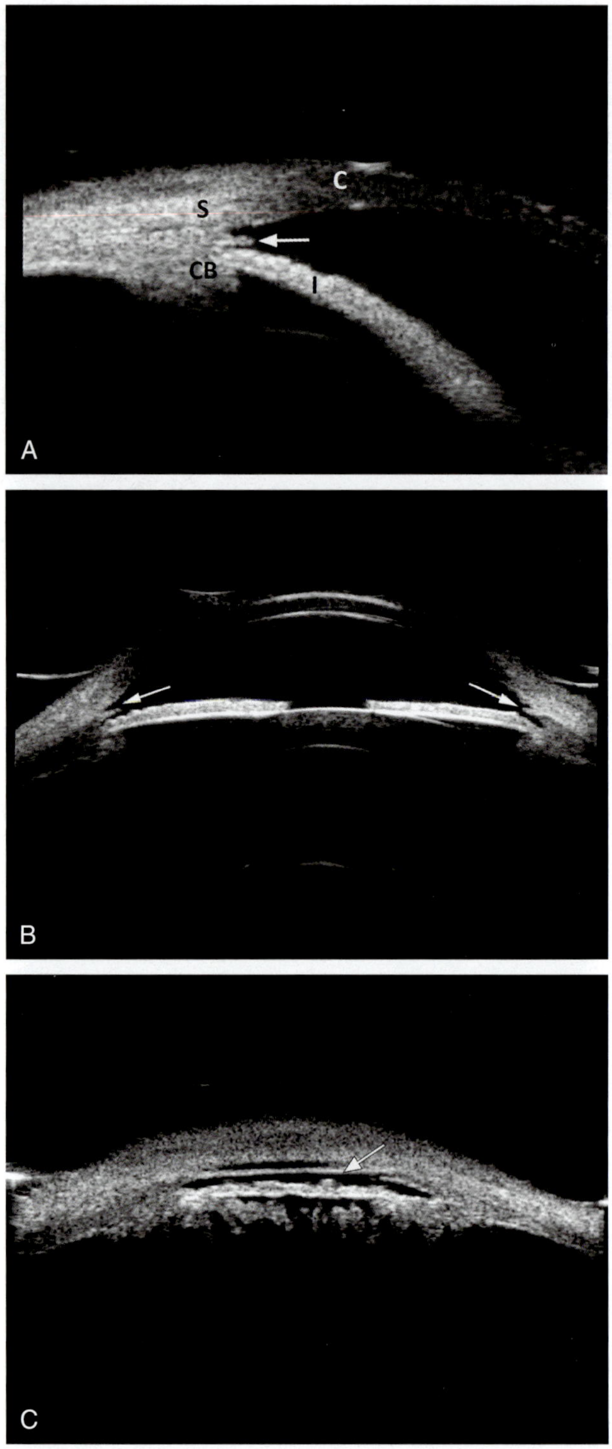

• **Fig. 6.21** Trabeculotomy. UBM images of the opening of the inner wall of the Schlemm's canal with the formation of a trabecular meshwork leaflet. **(A)** Longitudinal and **(B)** axial views display focal stump membrane (*arrow*) corresponding to the unroofed trabecular meshwork leaflet. **(C)** The transverse view displays a circumferential unroofed trabecular meshwork leaflet (*arrow*). *AC*, Anterior chamber; *C*; cornea; *CB*, ciliary body; *I*, iris; *S*, sclera.

Evaluation of Optic Disc Cupping With B-Scan

Ophthalmic B-scan ultrasound can help in evaluating the cup-to-disc ratio in glaucomatous patients and is essential in patients with opaque media. The role of echography in assessing the optic disc cupping has been previously investigated and showed a strong correlation with fundus biomicroscopy and optical coherence tomography.[25] The optic disc is best assessed using a transverse approach aimed at the nasal region with the probe placed on the temporal limbus, using a medium-gain set. Moreover, a longitudinal 12 o'clock is useful to evaluate the vertical elongation of the cup. Careful examination of the peripapillary region assists in the differentiation of pseudo-glaucomatous cupping in the set of thickening of the retinochoroidal layer around the optic disc.

CASE

A 48-year-old woman with a history of angle-closure glaucoma presented with a cup-to-disc ratio of 0.8 on fundus biomicroscopy (Fig. 6.27 and Video 6.11).

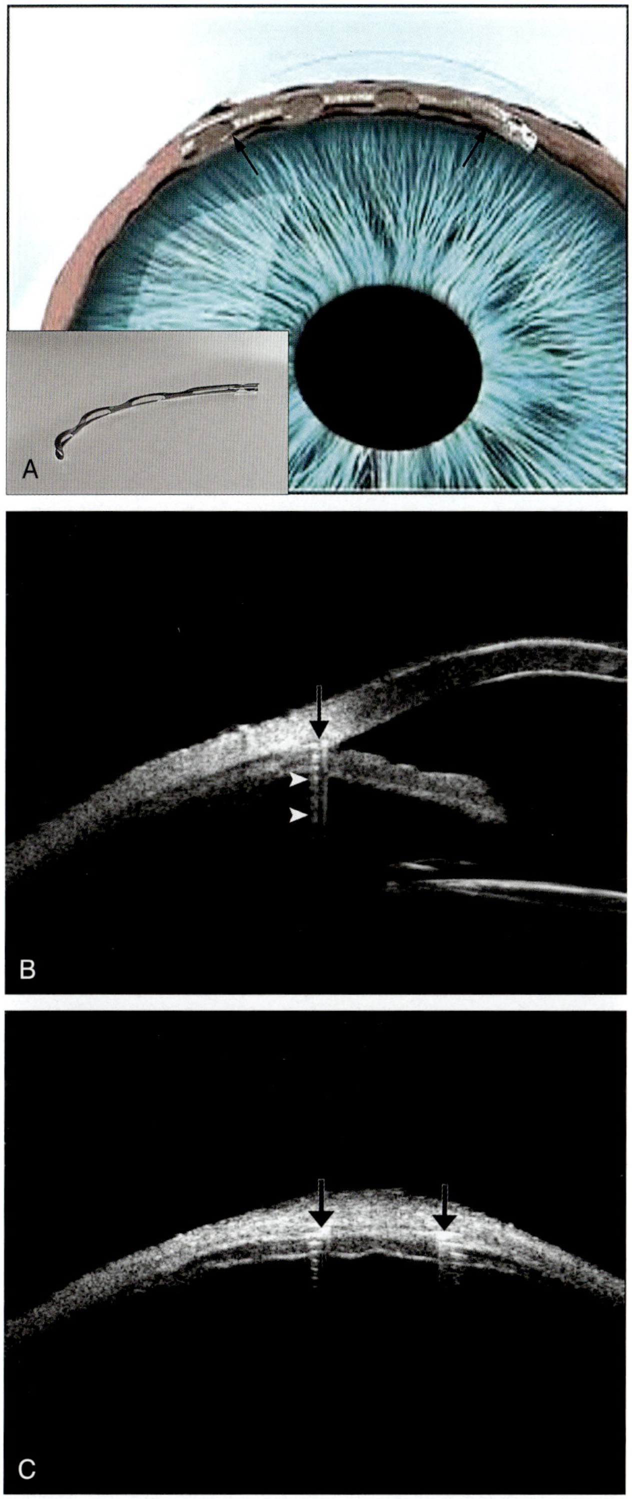

• **Fig. 6.22** **(A)** Hydrus microstent (*arrows*). **(B)** UBM longitudinal view showing a properly positioned Hydrus microstent (*arrow*) at the Schlemm's canal producing multiple reverberations signals (*arrowheads*). **(C)** Transverse section of the microstent (*arrows*) at the level of the Schlemm's canal.

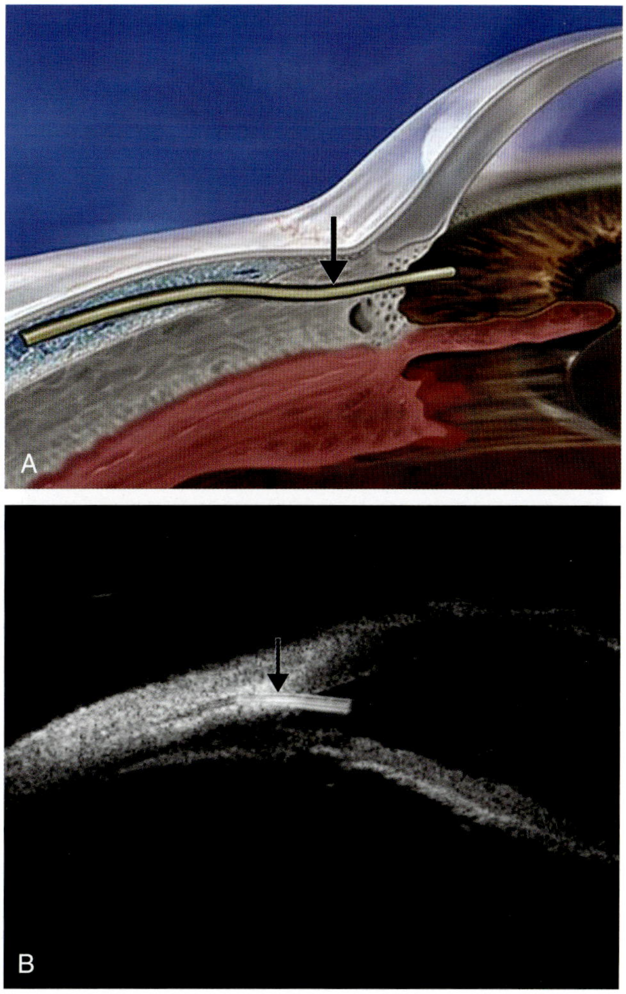

• **Fig. 6.23** XEN Gel Stent. **(A)** The microstent (*arrow*) implant accesses the subconjunctival space. **(B)** UBM longitudinal view of a XEN Gel Stent (*arrow*) extending from the anterior chamber to the subconjunctival space, inserted just above the scleral spur.

TEACHING POINTS

- Patients with opaque media-like dense cataracts or corneal opacity with an uncertain visual prognosis would benefit from ultrasonic optic cup evaluation, especially in those cases where extensive glaucomatous damage is suspected.
- A transverse vertical scan aimed at the nasal region is the best approach to evaluate the vertical diameter of the optic disc cup. The gain is set at the minimum necessary to get the best resolution of the optic disc.
- Elongation of the vertical cup diameter and the presence of optic disc asymmetry are indicative of glaucoma. Comparison with the fellow eye assists in the distinction.

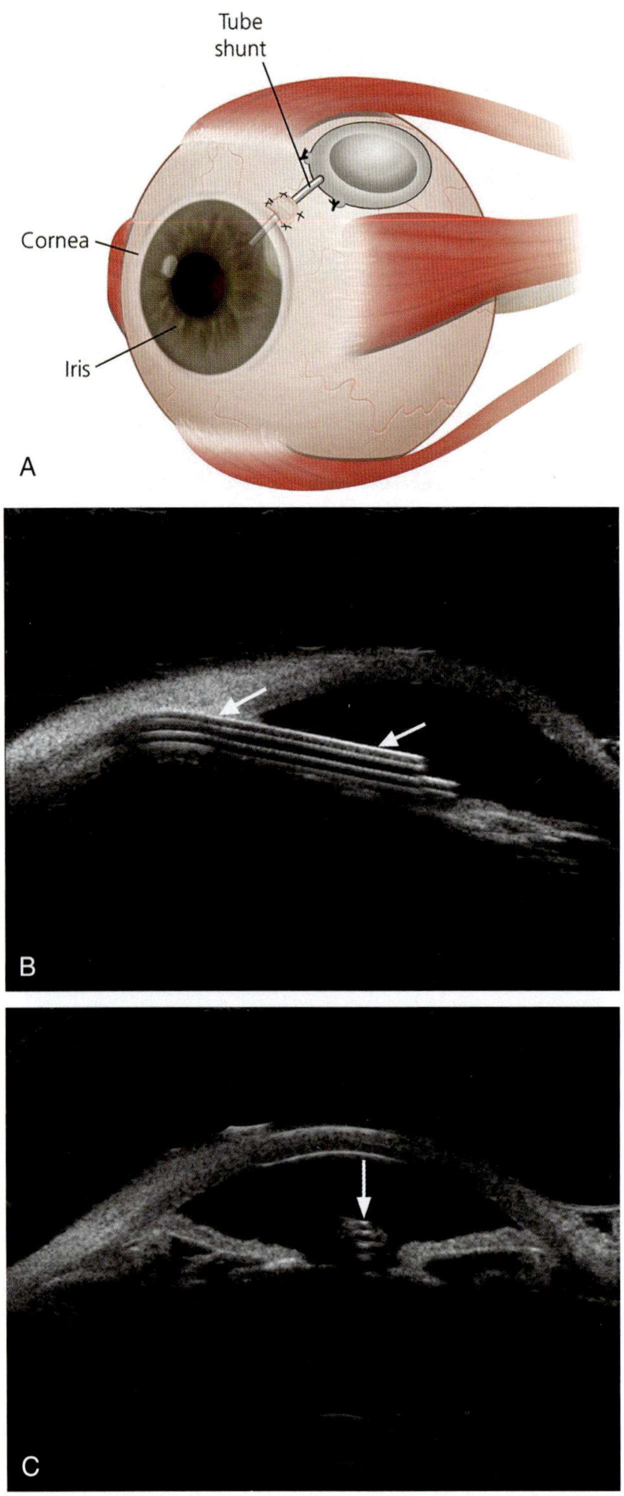

• **Fig. 6.24** Glaucoma drainage device. **(A)** Glaucoma shunt implant. **(B)** UBM longitudinal scan shows a non-obstructed tube of a glaucoma implant extending from the suprascleral space to the anterior chamber (*arrows*). **(C)** Transverse section at the tip of the tube (*arrow*) in the anterior chamber. (From a from the ophthalmic assistant, Harold Stein, Chapter 25, figure 25.49).

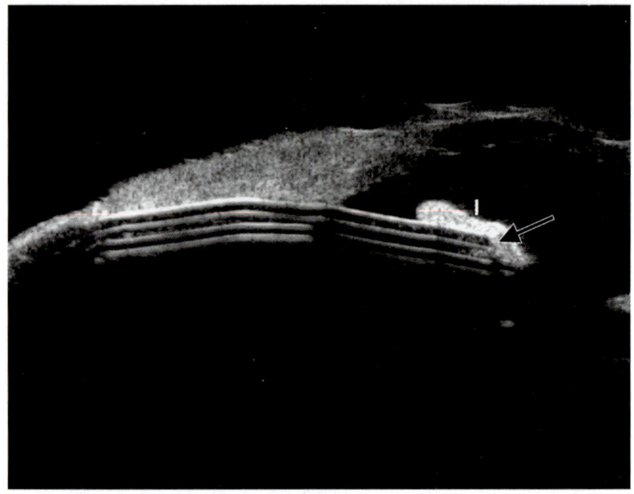

• **Fig. 6.25** Glaucoma drainage device tube obstruction. Longitudinal view UBM demonstrates a sulcus-placed tube (*arrow*) with the tip occluded by iris tissue. *I*, Iris.

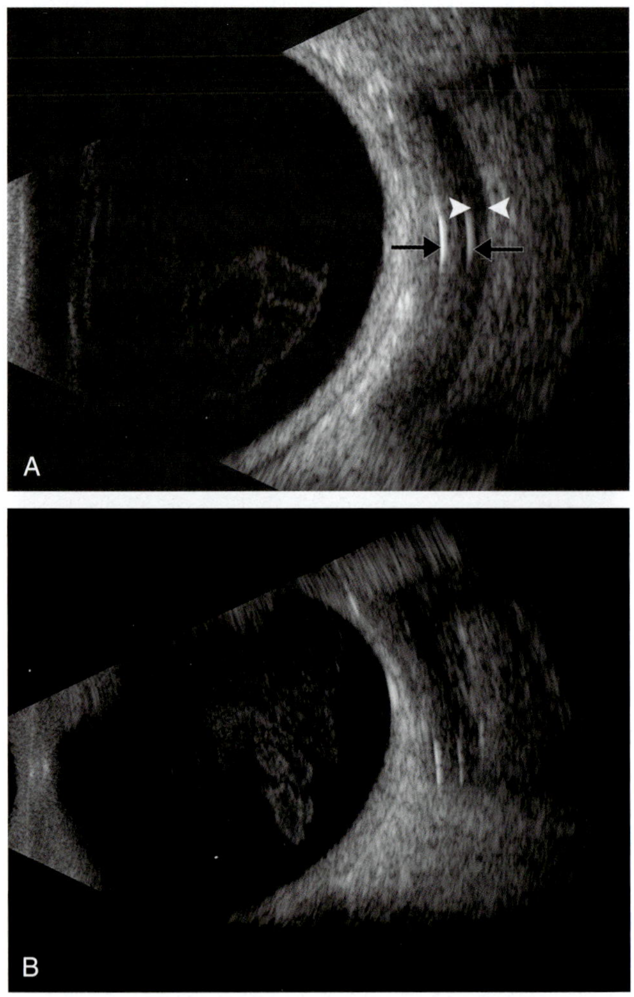

• **Fig. 6.26** Fluid bleb surrounding a glaucoma drainage device plate. **(A)** Transverse B-scan shows an echolucent fluid bleb (*arrowheads*) overlying a highly reflective plate (*arrows*). **(B)** Longitudinal view B-scan ultrasound shows the midperipheral location of the implant.

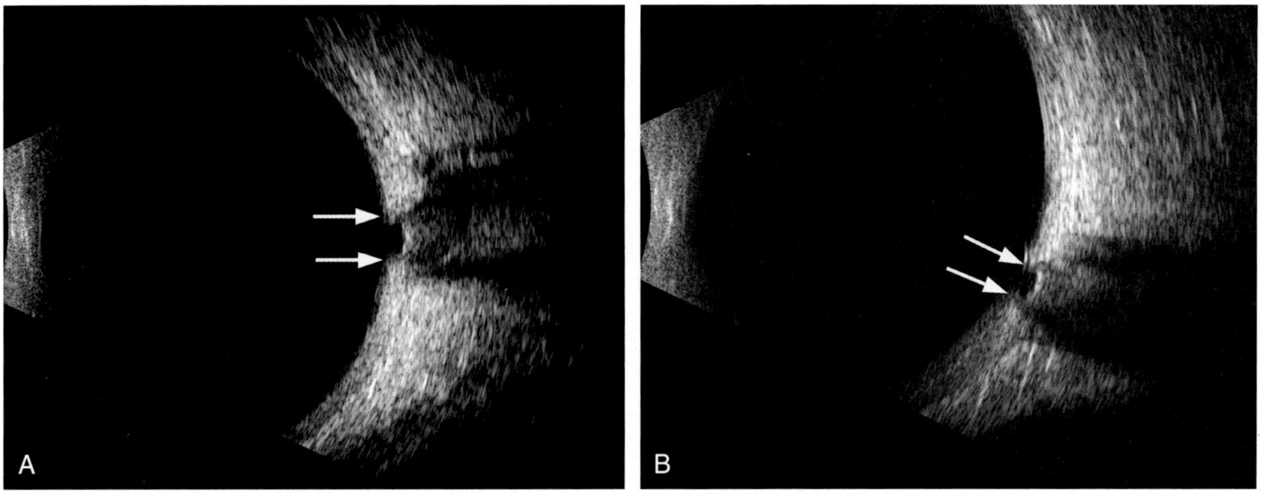

• **Fig. 6.27** Optic disc cupping. **(A)** B-scan ultrasound transverse and **(B)** longitudinal view showing large glaucomatous optic disc cupping (*arrows*).

References

1. Ishikawa H, Liebmann JM, Ritch R. Quantitative assessment of the anterior segment using ultrasound biomicroscopy. *Curr Opin Ophthalmol.* 2000;11:133–139.
2. Chansangpetch S, Rojanapongpun P, Lin SC. Anterior segment imaging for angle closure. *Am J Ophthalmol.* 2018;188:16–29.
3. Mansoori T, Sarvepally VK, Balakrishna N. Plateau Iris in primary angle closure glaucoma: an ultrasound biomicroscopy study. *J Glaucoma.* 2016;25:82–86.
4. Trope GE, Pavlin CJ, Bau A, Baumal CR, Foster FS. Malignant glaucoma. Clinical and ultrasound biomicroscopic features. *Ophthalmology.* 1994;101:1030–1035.
5. Balekudaru S, Choudhari NS, Rewri P, et al. Surgical management of malignant glaucoma: a retrospective analysis of fifty-eight eyes. *Eye (Lond).* 2017;31:947–955.
6. Potash SD, Tello C, Liebmann J, Ritch R. Ultrasound biomicroscopy in pigment dispersion syndrome. *Ophthalmology.* 1994;101:332–339.
7. Mora P, Sangermani C, Ghirardini S, Carta A, Ungaro N, Gandolfi S. Ultrasound biomicroscopy and iris pigment dispersion: a case–control study. *Br J Ophthalmol.* 2010;94:428–432.
8. Gentile RC, Pavlin CJ, Liebmann JM, et al. Diagnosis of traumatic cyclodialysis by ultrasound biomicroscopy. *Ophthalmic Surg Lasers.* 1996;27:97–105.
9. Hwang JM, Ahn K, Kim C, Park KA, Kee C. Ultrasonic biomicroscopic evaluation of cyclodialysis before and after direct cyclopexy. *Arch Ophthalmol.* 2008;126:1222–1225.
10. Murphy RM, Bakir B, O'Brien C, Wiggs JL, Pasquale LR. Drug-induced bilateral secondary angle-closure glaucoma: a literature synthesis. *J Glaucoma.* 2016;25:99–105.
11. Yang MC, Lin KY. Drug-induced Acute Angle-closure glaucoma: a review. *J Curr Glaucoma Pract.* 2019:104–109.
12. Aref AA, Sayyad FE, Ayres B. Lee RK Acute bilateral angle closure glaucoma induced by methazolamide. *Clin Ophthalmol.* 2013;7:279–282.
13. Lois N, Shields CL, Shields JA, Mercado G. Primary cysts of the iris pigment epithelium. Clinical features and natural course in 234 patients. *Ophthalmology.* 1998;105:1879–1885.
14. Ayres B, Allemann N, Nakanami C, Adan C. Cistos primários do epitélio pigmentar da íris e corpo ciliar: aspectos de biomicroscopia ultra-sônica. *Arq Bras Oftalmol.* 2000;63:337–343.
15. Carricondo PC, Andrade T, Prasov L, Ayres BM, Moroi SE. Nanophthalmos: a review of the clinical spectrum and genetics. *J Ophthalmol.* 2018;2018:2735465.
16. Guo C, Zhao Z, Zhang D, et al. Anterior Segment Features in Nanophthalmos With Secondary Chronic Angle Closure Glaucoma: an ultrasound biomicroscopy study. *Invest Ophthalmol Vis Sci.* 2019;60:2248–2256.
17. Yamamoto T, Sakuma T, Kitazawa Y. An ultrasound biomicroscopic study of filtering blebs after mitomycin C trabeculectomy. *Ophthalmology.* 1995;102:1770–1776.
18. Singh M, Chew PT, Friedman DS, et al. Imaging of trabeculectomy blebs using anterior segment optical coherence tomography. *Ophthalmology.* 2007;114:47–53.
19. Shah M. Micro-invasive glaucoma surgery - an interventional glaucoma revolution. *Eye Vis.* 2019;6:29.
20. Grover DS, Godfrey DG, Smith O, Feuer WJ, Montes de Oca I, Fellman RL. Gonioscopy-assisted transluminal trabeculotomy, ab interno trabeculotomy: technique report and preliminary results. *Ophthalmology.* 2014;121:855–861.
21. Queen J, Shah M, Ayres MB. Ultrasound biomicroscopy of anterior chamber angle structures after gonioscopy-assisted transluminal trabeculotomy. *JAMA Ophthalmol.* 2017;135:e164931.
22. Carrillo MM, Trope GE, Pavlin C, Buys YM. Use of ultrasound biomicroscopy to diagnose Ahmed valve obstruction by iris. *Can J Ophthalmol.* 2005;40:499–501.
23. Lloyd MA, Minckler DS, Heuer DK, Baerveldt G, Green RL. Echographic evaluation of glaucoma shunts. *Ophthalmology.* 1993;100:919–927.
24. Baig NB, Lin AA, Freedman SF. Ultrasound evaluation of glaucoma drainage devices in children. *J AAPOS.* 2015;19(3):281–284.
25. Queiroz WS, Lucena Dda R, Ferreira Jde L, Rodrigues Mde L, Paula JS. Correlation between cup-to-disc ratio and cup/retrobulbar optic nerve diameter proportion assessed by high-resolution ultrasound in glaucomatous eyes. *Arq Bras Oftalmol.* 2013;76:274–277.

7

Anterior Segment Tumors

ANA MARISA PIRES CASTELLO BRANCO, MELINA CORREIA MORALES, AND NORMA ALLEMANN

Ultrasonography is the preferred imaging exam for assessing anterior segment tumors. Ultrasound biomicroscopy (UBM) uses higher-frequency transducers (35–60 MHz) with 12-mm penetration and axial resolution of 35 μm. This provides a better image of small lesions, especially in cases of opaque media.[1] Conventional contact B- and A-scan ultrasound is used for large lesions of the ciliary body and choroid, and if UBM is unavailable, an immersion technique can be adapted to allow imaging of anterior segment structures and to evaluate the anterior margins of the lesions. Standardized A-scan ultrasonography has lower resolution. For the reliable detection of anterior segment tumors, iris lesions must be at least 1.0 mm and cliliary body lesions at least 1.5 mm in thickness. The use of UBM is usually limited to larger than 2.0 mm.[2]

IRIS CYSTS

Iris cystic lesions are classified into primary and secondary:

- Primary cysts: Iris pigment epithelium and/or stromal cysts.[3]
- Secondary cysts: Epithelial (postsurgical, posttraumatic), drug-induced, parasitic.[4]

The most common primary cyst of the iris is iris pigment epithleium cyst and originates in the iris pigment epithelium.[2] On slit lamp examination, iris pigment cysts are usually observed as bulging of the peripheral iris. When the iris is dilated, iris pigment epithelium cyst can sometimes be observed with slit lamp examination.[2,3]

The pigmented epithelium originated cysts are usually identified at the iridociliary junction, and their echographic characteristics are a thin-walled, well-circumscribed, round or oval echolucent lesion[3] (Fig. 7.1). UBM exam is mandatory to differentiate between a solid mass and a cystic lesion.[3]

Acquired iris cysts commonly occur following trauma or surgery, close to the wound site, as a result of the implantation of epithelial cells from the eyelid, conjunctiva or cornea.[1,2] The epithelium cells find a favorable environment for their multiplication at the iris due to the local blood supply.[2] Acquired iris cysts usually present as a translucid mass with a smooth surface on or within the iris stroma, and they can be filled with fluid debris[5] (Fig. 7.2).

On UBM, acquired iris cysts can have large dimensions. They are well outlined, echolucent, and often have an irregular shape. When located at the anterior surface of the iris, they tend to grow toward the anterior chamber, causing sectorial angle closure or endothelium touch.[2,3]

IRIS NEVUS

Iris nevus is the most common iris lesion. In a review of 3680 iris tumors, iris nevus corresponds to 25% of all iris lesions in children, 36% in young adults, and 47% in middle-aged and senior adults.[5] Transformation of iris nevus into melanoma ranges from 5% at a mean follow-up of 5 years to 8% by 15 years.[6,7]

Iris nevus can be flat to dome shaped, large and diffuse, small and circumscribed, and usually has a deeper penetration in the iris stroma.[5] More than 80% are located in the inferior half of the iris.[8]

Predictive factors for evolution of iris nevus into melanoma include: younger age at presentation (≤ 40 years), episode of hyphema, inferior location from 3 o'clock to 9 o'clock, diffuse tumor involving entire iris surface, ectropion uveae, and feathering tumor margins. These characteristics correspond to the ABCDEF mnemonic.[6]

The ultrasonographic characteristic of iris nevus is a high reflective surface plaque on a thickened iris area.[9] UBM should be performed to monitor the nevus dimensions (radial, transverse, and thickness measurements) and echographic characteristics (Fig. 7.3).

IRIS MELANOMA

Iris melanomas are malignant melanocytic neoplasms which arise in the iris stroma.

They can be circumscribed or, less commonly, diffuse. They present as variably pigmented flat or elevated masses in the iris stroma with a predilection to the inferior iris. Secondary glaucoma can occur when the tumor infiltrates the trabecular meshwork. A variant form of iris melanoma is anterior chamber angle melanoma, when the tumor grows diffusely, confined to the anterior chamber angle without forming a mass, affecting around 10 o'clock position, usually causing ipsilateral glaucoma.[4]

Iris melanoma is less frequent, and was reported to comprise only 2% of uveal melanomas (285 eyes with iris melanoma) in a series of 8033 eyes with uveal melanoma. In

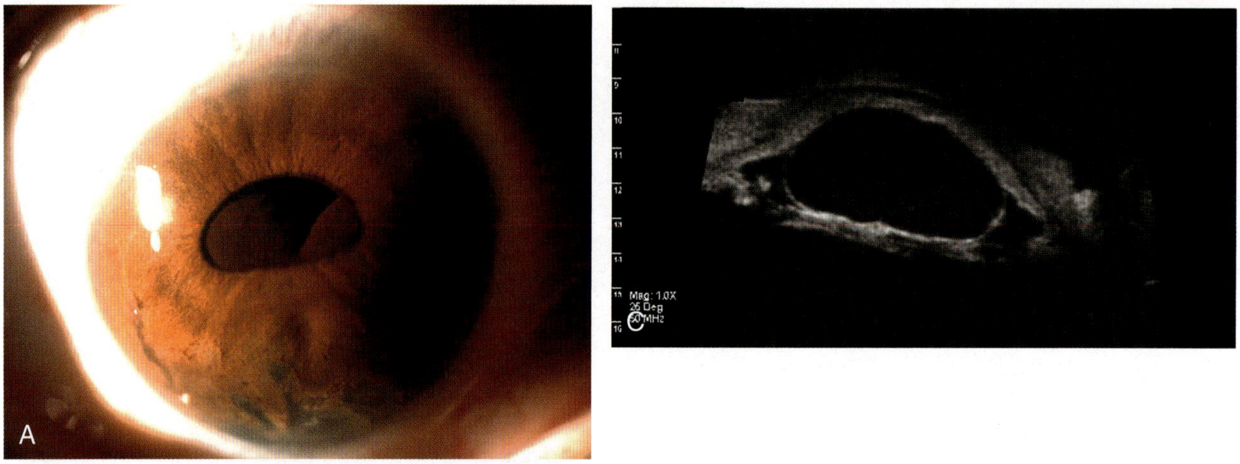

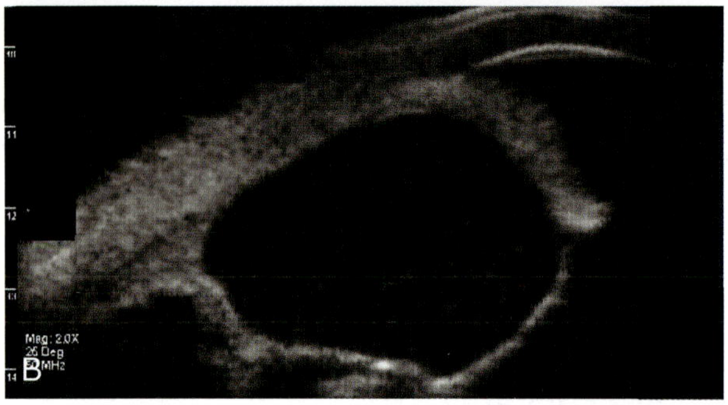

• **Fig. 7.1** A 57-year-old woman was referred for evaluation of a pigmented lesion observed in the pupillary area, posterior to the iris of the right eye. Best corrected visual acuity was 20/25. Diagnosis: Primary pigment epithelial cyst. **(A)** Slit lamp photography shows pigmented lesions protruding from the posterior chamber into the nasal pupillary area. A thinning of the peripheral iris can be seen inferiorly. **(B–C)** UBM evaluation, 50 MHz, immersion technique shows a well-delimited echolucent cystic lesion protruding from the posterior chamber into the pupillary area and determining the anterior displacement of the iris and local angle closure ([B] longitudinal scan; [C] transverse scan).

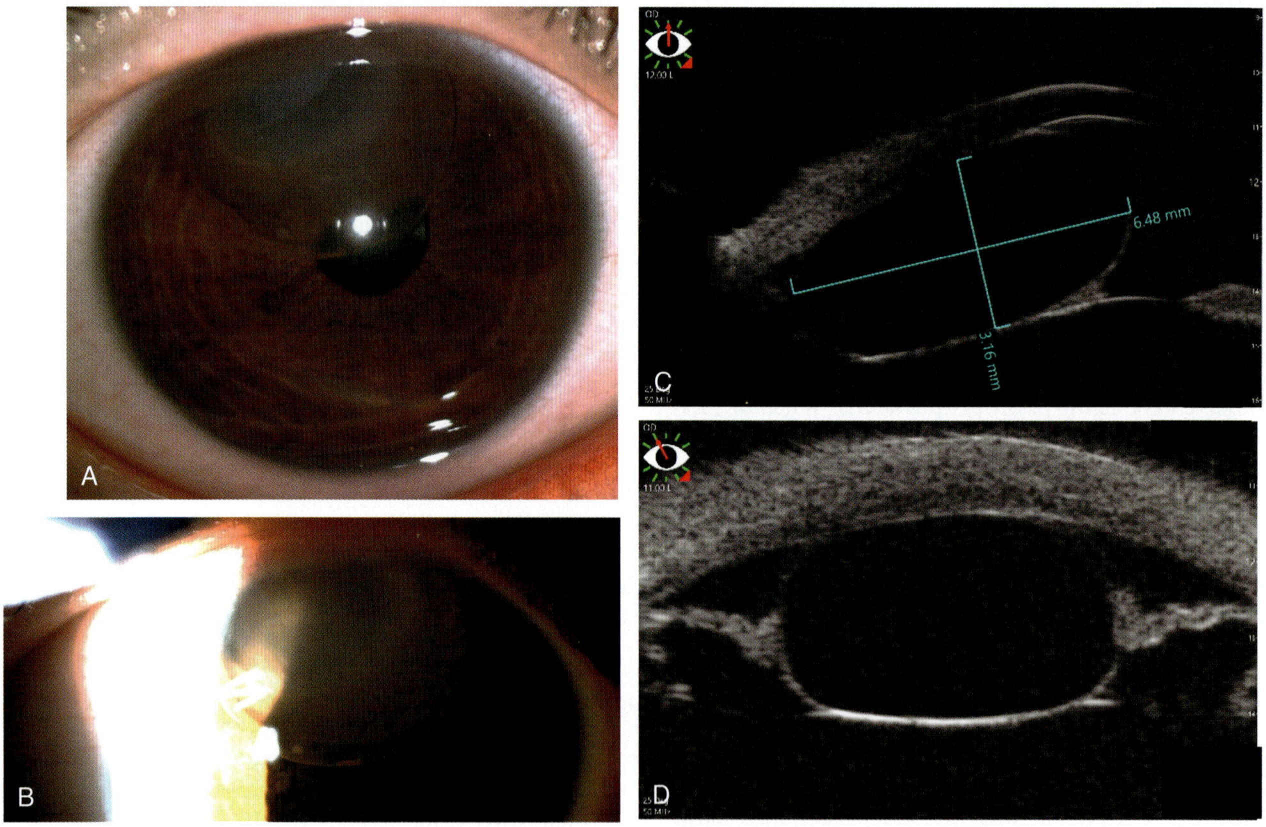

• **Fig. 7.2** A 10-year-old girl was referred for evaluation of a right eye anterior chamber lesion without complaints. Best corrected visual acuity was 20/40. Diagnosis: stromal iris cyst. **(A–B)** Slit lamp photography demonstrates a translucid cystic lesion occupying the anterior chamber superiorly and obstructing partially the pupillary area. **(C–D)** UBM, 50 MHz, immersion technique demonstrates longitudinal (C) and transverse (D) scans, a lesion that is well-delimited with a thin wall, echolucent content, anterior cyst wall in contact with the endothelium. In the transverse (D) scan, it is possible to determine that the cyst originates from the iris stroma. Measurements: longitudinal: 6.48 mm; height: 3.16 mm.

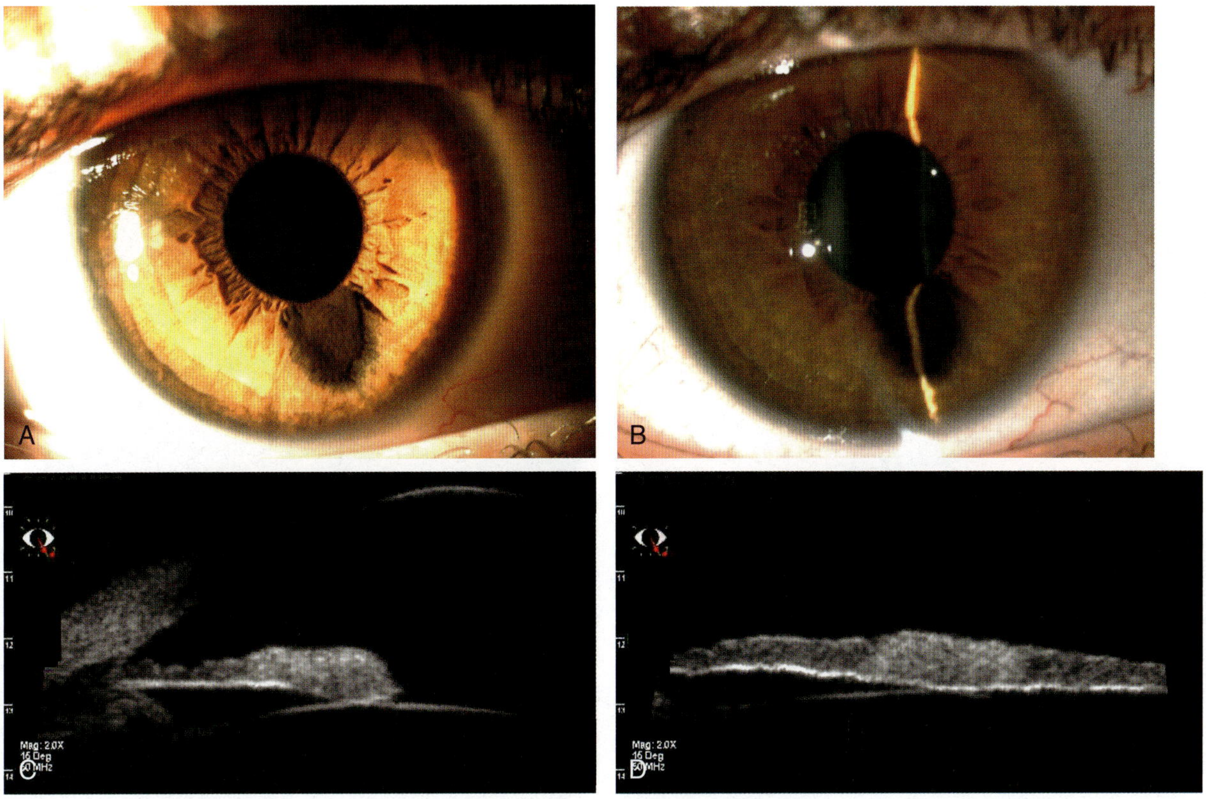

• **Fig. 7.3** 18-year-old woman was referred for evaluation of a pigmented iris lesion of the right eye. Best corrected visual acuity was 20/25. Diagnosis: Iris nevus. **(A–B)** Slit lamp photography instead of showed a pigmented slightly elevated iris lesion in the inferior quadrant, occupying medium and pupillary areas of the iris with no apparent pupil retraction. **(C–D)** UBM ultrasonography with a 50-MHz transducer shows longitudinal (B) and transverse (C) scans of a local thickening of the iris, stromal hyper-reflectivity with no interruption of the iris pigment epithelium.

this series of 285 eyes with uris melanoma the mean tumor thickness was 2.7mm, and metastasis occurred in 0.5%, 4%, and 7% at 3, 5, and 10 years, respectively.[10] This metastasis rate is much lower than the one in choroidal melanomas.

At UBM examination, iris melanoma appears as a solid lesion that varies in shape and usually presents with a medium internal reflectivity. Depending on thickness, it is possible to detect internal vascularity. UBM is important to evaluate if there is a possible extension into the ciliary body or image the iris pigment epithelium, since iris melanoma tend to invade and cause an interruption of retina pigment epithelium.

Iris melanomas are measured by UBM to monitor the tumor size and guide a possible treatment, usually brachytherapy or surgical excision. After treatment, UBM is still necessary to monitor the therapeutic response, analyze the tumor size and its internal reflectivity, and rule out any recurrence. If surgery was performed, it is recommended to evaluate the surrounding iris structure (Fig. 7.4).

IRIS HEMANGIOMA

Vascular iris lesions are rare and classified as capillary hemangioma, cavernous hemangioma, racemose hemangioma, and varix.[11]

Iris hemangiomas are usually sporadic, and rarely associated with vascular neuro-oculocutaneous syndromes.

Children with congenital periocular cutaneous capillary hemangioma may have associated iris capillary hemangioma. It presents as a circumscribed or diffuse red mass that usually regresses spontaneously with the cutaneous lesion.

Iris cavernous hemangioma is generally very small and located at the pupillary margin but can also occur in the iris stroma away from the pupil. It can bleed and cause hyphema, that can resolve and recur periodically.[4,12,13]

There are few reports in literature describing these vascular lesions and to our knowledge, no report of UBM alterations was found.

The authors present a case of a middle-aged female patient who presented a red iris mass on the mid-zonal iris at 6 o'clock (Fig. 7.5). She had bleeding episodes and raised intraocular pressure. UBM revealed an irregular multiloculated mass with medium internal reflectivity. The iris pigment epithelium was preserved. After an episode of bleeding, the mass presented an enlargement, internal structures became more heterogeneous, with a multilobulated aspect, and the pigmented epithelium were preserved.

CILIARY BODY MELANOMA

Ciliary body melanomas often reach large dimensions before they are clinically suspected because of its location.

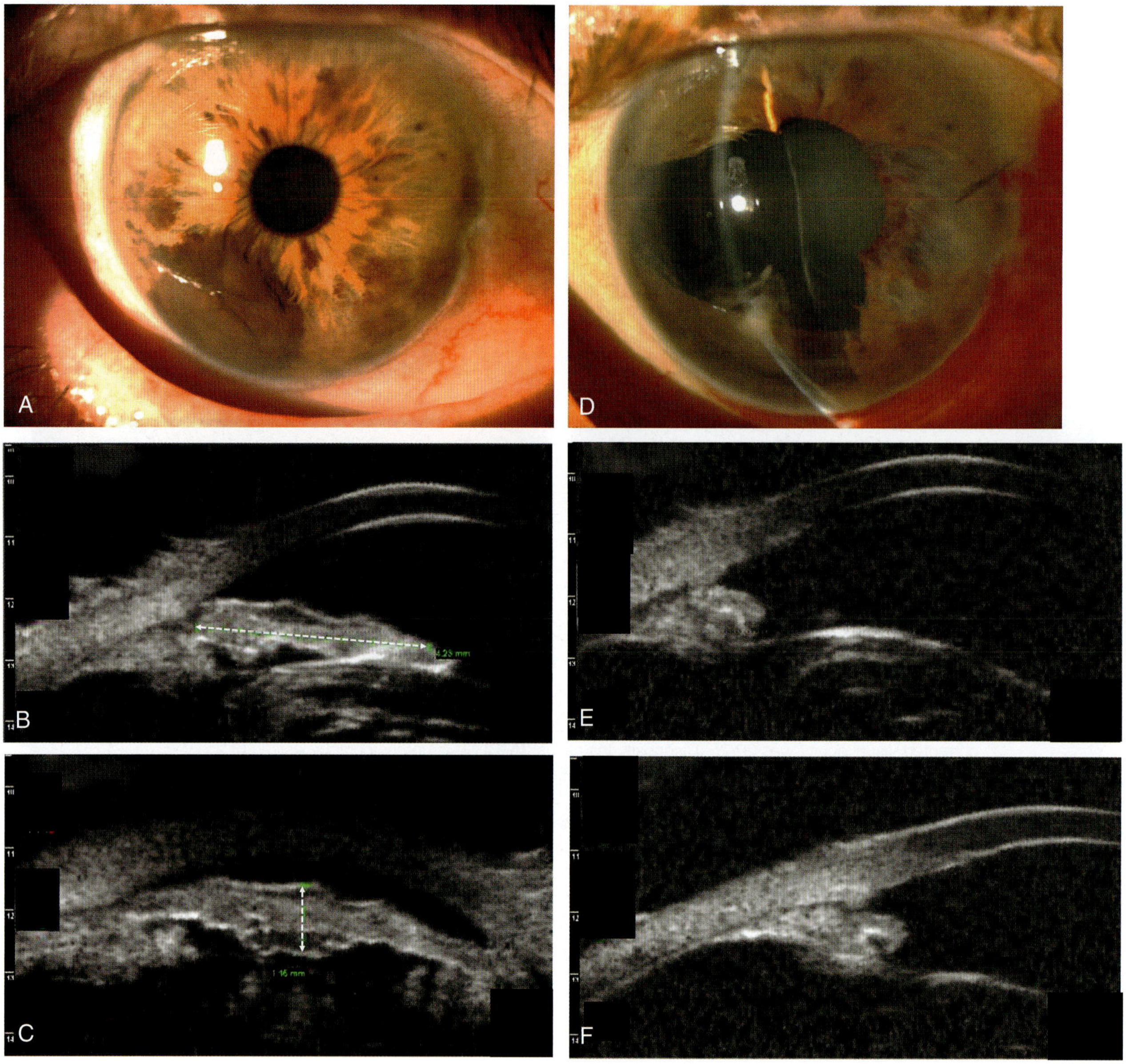

• **Fig. 7.4** A 80-year-old female presented with a pigmented iris lesion (A) that has been followed. **(A)** Slit lamp photography shows a temporal inferior pigmented iris lesion with irregular margins and endothelial touch. **(B–C)** UBM, 50 MHz, immersion technique. Serial UBM evaluation showed a discrete growth, associated with a break and an irregularity of the iris pigmented epithelium. **(B)** Longitudinal scan, radial extension: 4.23 mm. **(C)** Transverse scan, thickness: 1.16 mm. **(D)** Slit lamp photography after surgical excision of the iris lesion. Histopathology confirmed: iris melanoma. **(E–F)** UBM performed 1 month after surgery, showing no recurrence and iris discontinuity at 6 o'clock **(E)** and 9 o'clock **(F)** margins.

When the tumor is large, it is sometimes possible to visualize the pigmented ciliary body lesion through the dilated pupil.[4] They usually develop dilated feeder episcleral vessels that are visible on the ocular surface.

In a series of 8033 consecutive eyes with uveal melanoma, ciliary body comprised 6% of uveal melanomas. The mean tumor thickness was 6.6 mm and metastasis occurred in 12%, 19%, and 33% at 3, 5, and 10 years, respectively.[10]

There is a variant that shows a diffuse circumferential growth pattern (ring melanoma) that may be difficult to diagnose. This variant should be suspected when there is unilateral and refractory glaucoma.[4]

On UBM, ciliary body melanomas are usually dome shaped or collar button shaped, and show low-to-medium internal reflectivity, possible posterior extension to the peripheral choroid, and one or more internal cystic cavities (cavitary melanoma) (Fig. 7.6). Small lesions and ring melanoma are difficult to identify on conventional B-scan ultrasonography and UBM is recommended.

UBM is also useful to investigate adjacent angle and iris involvement.

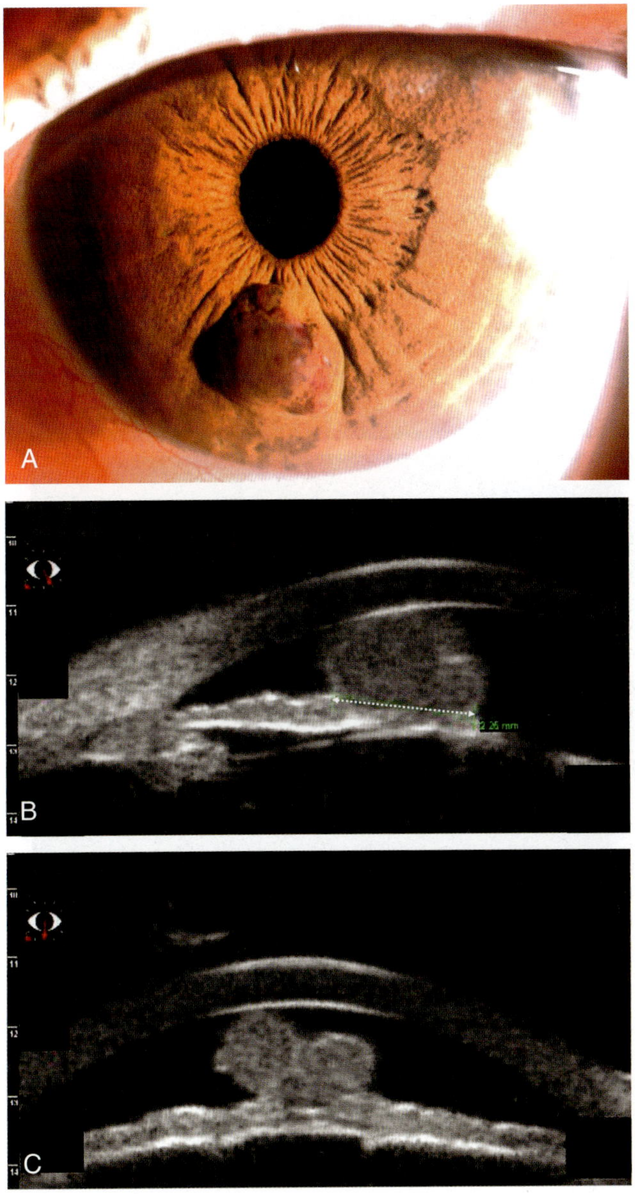

• **Fig. 7.5** A 46-year-old female presented with local pain and an iris lesion in the left eye. **(A)** Slit lamp photography shows a reddish brown multilobulated mass in the lower mid-zonal iris. **(B–C)** UBM, 50 MHz transducer, immersion technique shows longitudinal (5B) and transverse **(C)** scans of a lobulated iris lesion with normal deep stroma. Due to recurrent intralesional bleeding, surgical excision was performed, and histopathology confirmed the diagnosis of iris hemangioma.

MEDULLOEPITHELIOMA

Medulloepithelioma is a tumor originating from the primitive medullary epithelium, and usually diagnosed in childhood. It involves the ciliary body, but the retina and optic disc can be affected in rare cases. Occasionally, the tumor can remain undiagnosed until adulthood.[14]

The clinical findings can include a pink to tan ciliary body mass with cysts, lens "coloboma" (secondary to congenital absence of zonule on the quadrant of the tumor), glaucoma, cataract, neoplastic cyclitic membrane, and iris neovascularization. Intralesional cysts are common and can be found in 60% of cases. Some patients may also have an associated persistent fetal vasculature (PFV).[14]

The histopathologic classification divides these tumors into teratoid and nonteratoid, and either benign or malignant. More than 80% of medulloepitheliomas are malignant. The teratoid type comprises neuroepithelium and heteroplastic tissues such as cartilage, rhabdomyoblasts, and brain tissue. Therefore, echographic features reflect these different tissues.[4]

Echographic characteristics of medulloepithelioma usually include highly reflective dome-shaped mass with moderate intrinsic vascularity, irregular internal structure, and multiple cystic spaces (Fig. 7.7). When cartilage is present in medulloepithelioma, there are echoes of extremely high internal reflectivity.

RETINOBLASTOMA

The most common ocular malignant neoplasia in childhood is retinoblastoma and better described in the posterior intraocular tumors chapter.

UBM can display heterogeneous mass with medium internal reflective areas corresponding to the tumor, and some highly reflective areas corresponding to intratumoral calcification. Vitreous seeds appear as irregular and moderately echogenic punctiform or granular structures.[2]

UBM can evaluate the anterior chamber, anterior chamber angle, and ciliary body involvement (Fig. 7.8).

OTHER LESS FREQUENT TUMORS OF THE ANTERIOR SEGMENT

IRIS AND CILIARY BODY METASTASIS

Metastasis can appear in any part of the eye or orbit, but the uvea is the main affected part of the eye due to its vascular characteristics and a typical hematogenous spread.

Iris and ciliary body metastasis correspond to 10% of ocular metastasis and usually present with a iris or ciliary body mass and anterior segment involvement, like anterior uveitis, episcleritis, and raised intraocular pressure. The most common primary tumors that metastasize to the eye are breast (47%), lung (21%), and gastrointestinal tract (4%).[15]

Iris metastasis presents as amelanotic stromal nodules or ill-defined iris thickening (Fig. 7.9).

UBM is used to help diagnose and monitor these tumors, but it does not have a classic characteristic or pathognomonic findings since metastatic lesions depend on the primary tumor and have variable presentations.[16]

CILIARY BODY LYMPHOMA

Lymphoid proliferations of the uvea can be a primary uveal tumor or a secondary intraocular manifestation of systemic lymphoma. Primary uveal lymphoma is rare and usually indolent in nature. The ciliary body involvement is exceptionally rare.[17] The ciliary body lymphoma can be localized,

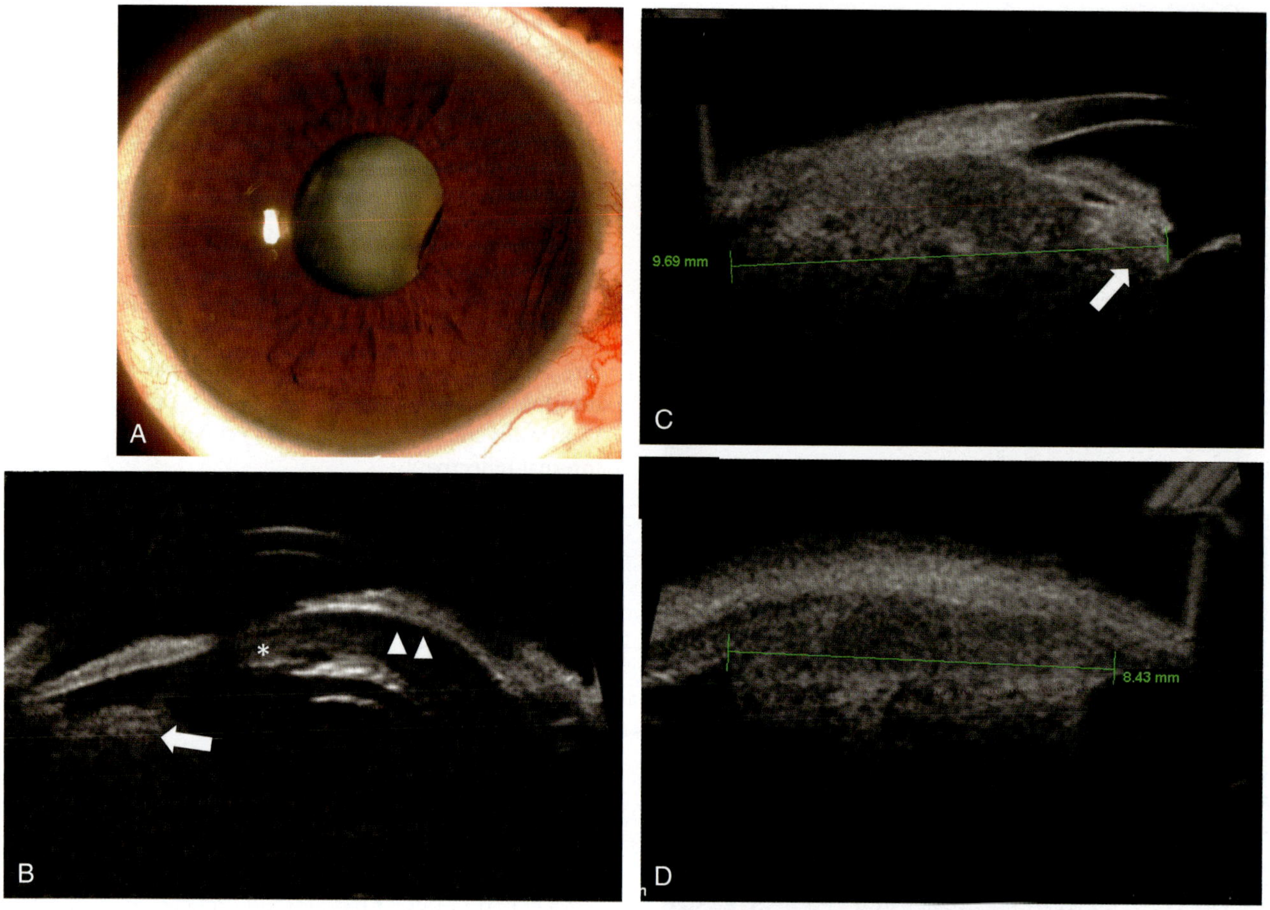

• **Fig. 7.6** A 58-year-old female presented with recent development of a dense cataract. No history of ocular trauma. Diagnosis: ciliary body melanoma. **(A)** Pigmented ciliary body mass protruding from the posterior chamber was observed nasally at the pupil. It causes the anterior displacement of the iris. **(B–D)** UBM, 50 MHz transducer, immersion technique. **(B)** Horizontal axial scan showing a hyperreflective lens (*), displaced in relation to the pupil, determined by a ciliary body mass (*arrow*). Anterior displacement of iris induced by the subluxated lens can be observed (*arrowheads*). **(C)** Longitudinal scan, radial diameter: 9.69 mm. Observe the anterior margin of the lesion occupying the posterior chamber, touching the iris and in contact with the lens arrow). **(D)** Transverse scan, diameter: 8.43 mm. UBM allows the observation of the internal architecture with a limited depth of focus and sound attenuation, showing a homogenous medium-reflective lesion with homogeneous architecture.

solitary mass or grow in a ring-like pattern, with 360° ciliary body involvement and low acoustic reflectivity.[18]

Pei et al. reported a case of bilateral mantle cell lymphoma in a 59-year-old male who presented with redness, pain, and blurred vision in the left eye. Ocular examination revealed elevated intraocular pressure, anterior chamber reaction, pseudohypopyon, and anterior placement of the peripheral iris. On UBM examination, there were confluent ciliary body masses with almost 360° involvement in both eyes. They were dome-shaped and had homogeneous internal structure, and medium to low internal reflectivity. B-scan ultrasonography demonstrated no anomalies in the vitreous and choroid. After treatment, UBM was performed to confirm treatment response with complete regression of the ciliary tumor in the right eye and reduction of tumor size in the left eye.[19]

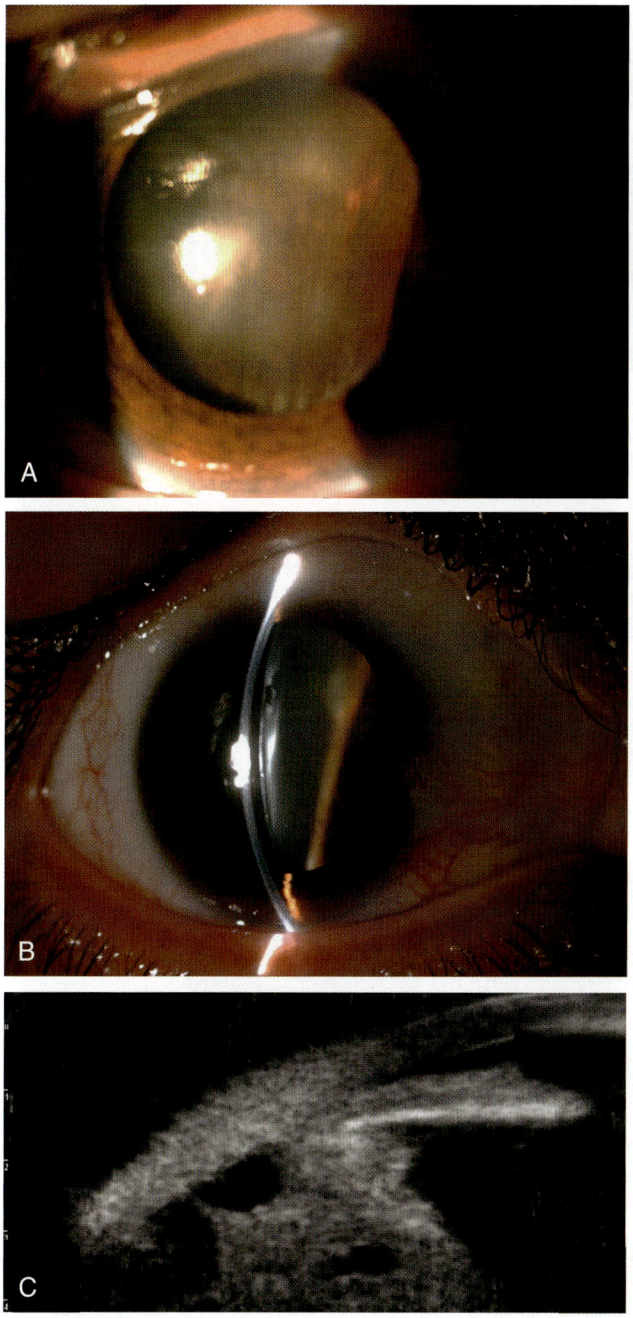

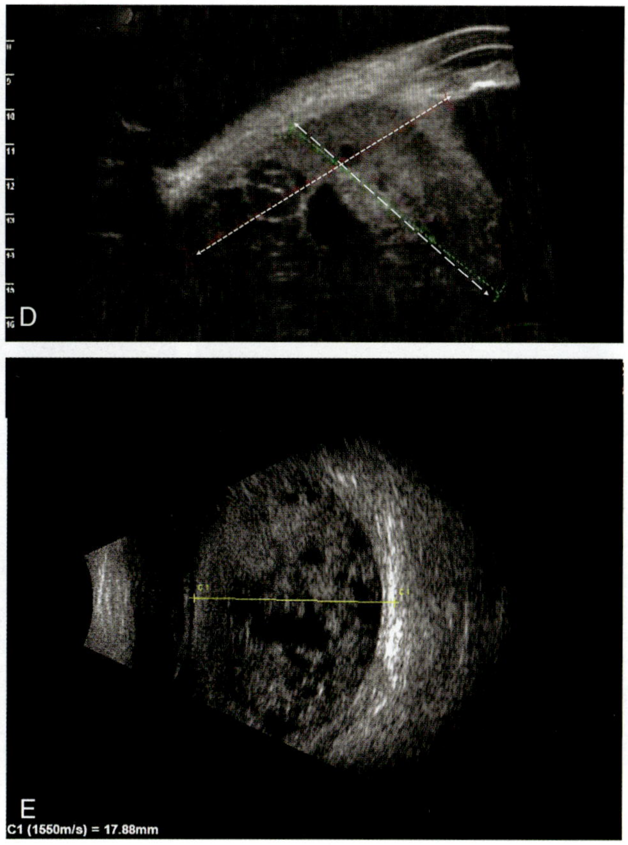

• **Fig. 7.7** A 50-year-old male presented with visual impairment in the right eye. **(A–B)** Clinical exam showed a brown mass located posterior to the lens. **(C–D)** UBM, 50 MHz transducer, immersion technique showed a large lesion with multiple intralesional hypoechogenic spaces. Lesions approximate dimensions: radial, 9.80 mm (*dotted line*); height measured at the anterior portion, 9.12 mm (*hatched line*). **(E)** Due to its large size, 10-MHz B-scan evaluation was conducted to evaluate its posterior margins. Height measured at the posterior portion: 11.88 mm. Enucleation was performed and histopathology confirmed a medulloepithelioma.

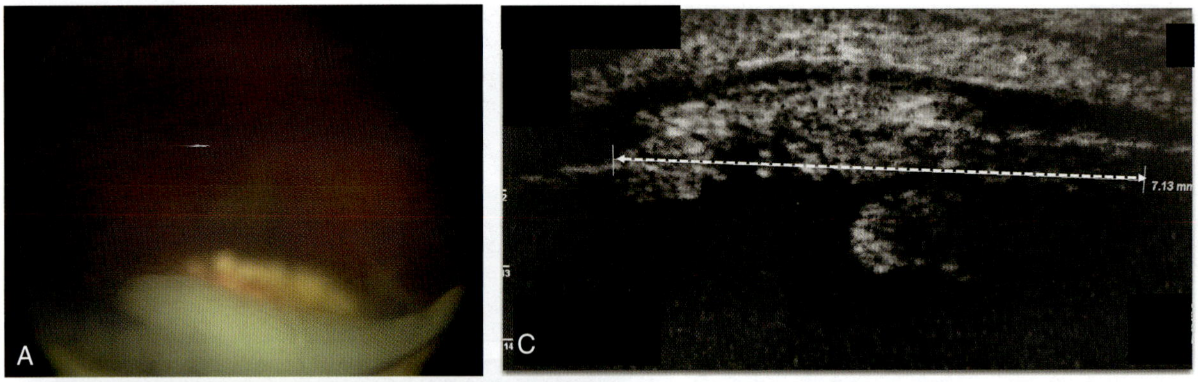

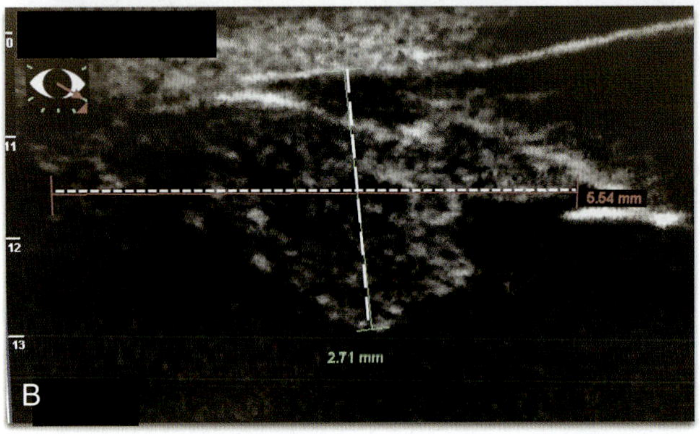

• **Fig. 7.8** A 7-year-old female under chemotherapy for retinoblastoma in the right eye. **(A)** RetCam photography demonstrates a white lesion in the ciliary body. **(B–C)** UBM, 50 MHz transducer, transpalpebral technique because of poor cooperation, demonstrated an enlarged ciliary body, with irregular contour and scarce highly reflective particles, in radial **(B)** and transverse scans **(C)** compatible with retinoblastoma in the ciliary body. Dimensions: radial: 5.54 mm; thickness: 2.71 mm; transverse: 7.13 mm.

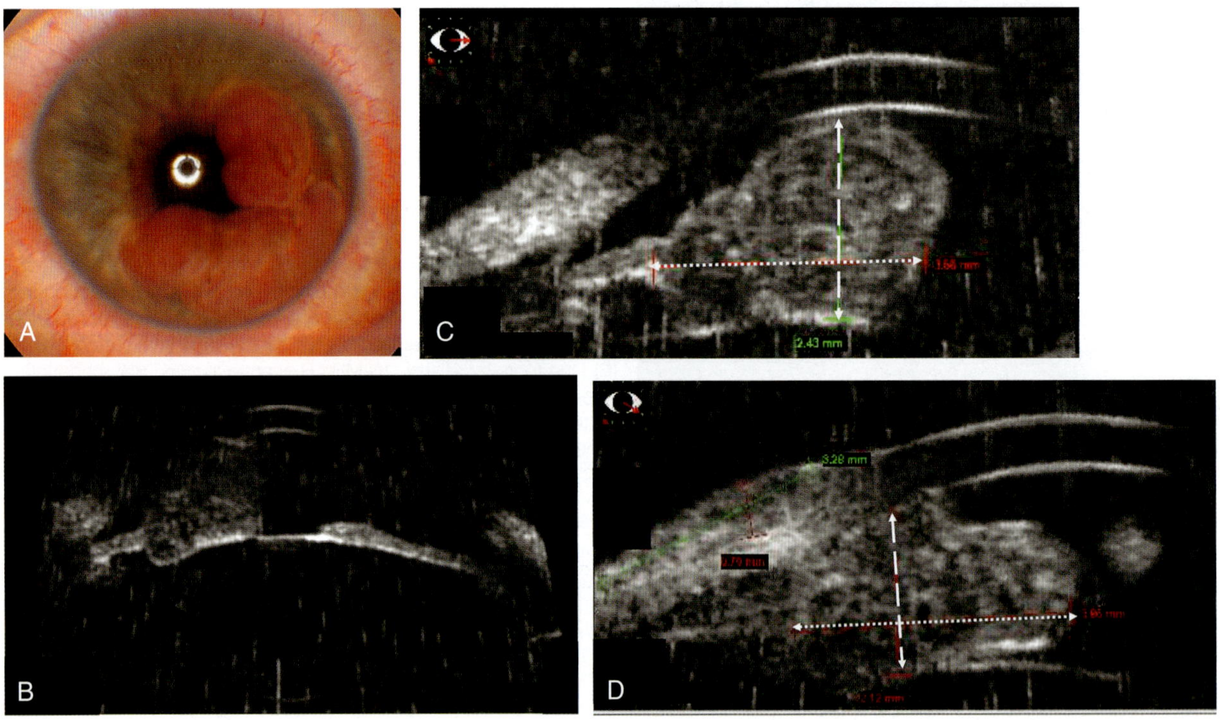

• **Fig. 7.9** A 60-year-old male developed a reddish-colored iris lesion on the left iris for 45 days. He was treated with systemic chemotherapy and chest external beam radiotherapy for small cell lung cancer about 1 year ago. He was receiving external beam radiotherapy for intracranial metastasis. **(A)** Slit lamp photography shows a nodular reddish lesion of the temporal and inferior iris partially obstructing the pupil. **(B–D)** UBM, 50 MHz, immersion technique. **(9B)** Horizontal axial scan demonstrates the iris multilobulated solid lesion occupying the anterior chamber and touching endothelium and the anterior capsule of the lens. **(C)** 3 o'clock radial scan showing a solid multilobulated lesion of the mid and distal zones of the iris, sparing the proximal iris and angle. Measurements obtained: radial: 3.66 mm; thickness: 2.43 mm. **(D)** 4 o'clock radial scan demonstrates the involvement of the entire extension of the iris and ciliary body, occupying the angle. Measurements obtained: radial: 3.95 mm; thickness: 2.12 mm.

REFERENCES

1. Silverman RH. High-resolution ultrasound imaging of the eye—a review. *Clin Exp Ophthalmol.* 2009;37(1):54–67.
2. Bianciotto C, Shields CL, Guzman JM, et al. Assessment of anterior segment tumors with ultrasound biomicroscopy versus anterior segment optical coherence tomography in 200 cases. *Ophthalmology.* 2011;118(7):1297–1302.
3. Marigo FA, Esaki K, Finger PT, et al. Differential diagnosis of anterior segment cysts by ultrasound biomicroscopy. *Ophthalmology.* 1999;106(11):2131–2135.
4. Ayres B, Allemann N, Nakanami C, Adan CBD. Primary cysts of the iris and ciliary body pigment epithelium: ultrasound biomicroscope features. *Arq Bras Oftalmol.* 2000;63(5):337–343.
5. Shields CL, Shields PW, Manalac J, Jumroendararasame C, Shields JA. Review of cystic and solid tumors of the iris. *Oman J Ophthalmol.* 2013;6(3):159–164.
6. Shields CL, Kaliki S, Hutchinson A, et al. Iris nevus growth into melanoma: analysis of 1611 consecutive eyes: the ABCDEF guide. *Ophthalmology.* 2013;120(4):766–772.
7. Territo C, Shields CL, Shields JA, Augsburger JJ, Schroeder RP. Natural course of melanocytic tumors of the iris. *Ophthalmology.* 1988;95(9):1251–1255.
8. van Klink F, de Keizer RJ, Jager MJ, Kakebeeke-Kemme HM. Iris nevi and melanomas: a clinical follow-up study. *Doc Ophthalmol.* 1992;82(1–2):49–55.
9. Pavlin CJ, Foster FS. *Ultrasound Biomicroscopy of the Eye.* Springer; 1995.
10. Shields CL, Furuta M, Thangappan A, et al. Metastasis of uveal melanoma millimeter-by-millimeter in 8033 consecutive eyes. *Arch Ophthalmol.* 2009;127(8):989–998.
11. Shields JA. Vascular tumors of the Iris in 45 patients. *Arch Ophthalmol.* 2010;128(9):1107.
12. Woo SJ, Kim CJ, Yu YS. Cavernous hemangioma of the iris in an infant. *J AAPOS.* 2004;8(5):499–501.
13. Strauss EC, Aldave AJ, Spencer WH, et al. Management of prominent iris vascular tufts causing recurrent spontaneous hyphema. *Cornea.* 2005;24(2):224–226.
14. Shields JA, Eagle Jr RC, Shields CL, Singh AD, Robitaille J. Pigmented medulloepithelioma of the ciliary body. *Arch Ophthalmol.* 2002;120(2):207–210.
15. Cohen VM. *Ocular metastases. Eye (Lond).* 2013;27(2):137–141.
16. Shields CL, Kaliki S, Crabtree GS, et al. Iris metastasis from systemic cancer in 104 patients: the 2014 Jerry A. Shields Lecture. *Cornea.* 2015;34(1):42–48.
17. Coupland SE, Damato B. Understanding intraocular lymphomas. *Clin Exp Ophthalmol.* 2008;36(6):564–578.
18. Konstantinidis L, Angi M, Coupland SE, Damato B. Primary B-cell lymphoma of the ciliary body with 360° (ring-like) growth pattern. *Eye (Lond).* 2014;28(3):355–356.
19. Pei M, Zhao C, Gao F, Zhang M. Bilateral mantle cell lymphoma of the ciliary body that responded to a combined local radiotherapy and chemotherapy regimen: a case report. *BMC Cancer.* 2019;19(1):355.

8

Tumors of the Posterior Segment

BERNADETE AYRES, ZELIA M. CORREA, AND HAKAN DEMIRCI

Ultrasonography is an ideal imaging modality for detecting and assessing an intraocular tumor. It is widely available and does not involve ionizing radiation. It evaluates specific acoustic features that assist in the differential diagnosis of intraocular tumors and establishes an accurate diagnosis when combined with indirect ophthalmoscopy. Furthermore, ultrasonography provides accurate measurements of intraocular tumors, which is essential in treatment decision and planning. It can detect extraocular extension of an intraocular tumor, which is often hidden from clinical visualization. Ultrasonography is particularly useful for following the response to the treatment, providing a safe tool for disease surveillance by monitoring tumor regression or recurrence.

A detailed ultrasonographic examination of an eye with suspected intraocular tumor should be performed with B-scan mode and standardized A-scan. The B-scan mode, using transverse and longitudinal approaches can assess the morphology, location, internal structure, intrinsic vascularity, and margins of lesions and surrounding tissues. The A-scan mode is used to estimate the tissue reflectivity of the lesion.

Choroidal Tumors

Choroidal Nevus

Choroidal nevus is the most common benign intraocular tumor. Although choroidal nevus is benign. It may still cause vision loss especially if located in the macula or posterior pole. It may grow, and undergo malignant transformation into a choroidal melanoma.

Clinically, a choroidal nevus can be flat or minimally elevated, melanotic or amelanotic. It usually measures between 1.5 to 58.0 mm in basal diameter and usually less than 2.0 mm in thickness.[1] Most nevi are diagnosed early due to their location in the posterior pole, between the macula and the equator. Risk factors of transformation of choroidal nevus into choroidal melanoma include thickness >2.0 mm, subretinal fluid, symptoms of vision loss, orange pigment on the surface, low reflectivity, and diameter >5.0 mm.[2]

On ultrasonographic examination, elevated choroidal nevi are typically dome shaped and highly reflective. They can have mild intrinsic vascularity that is detectable with B-scan and A-scan.[3]

CASE

A 55-year-old male patient was found to have a melanocytic lesion in the macula of his right eye, just temporal to the fovea (Fig. 8.1 and Video 8.1). A complete multimodal imaging examination showed a choroidal lesion of about 1.5 mm in thickness with drusens and some subretinal fluid overlying the lesion. A diagnosis of choroidal nevus was made, and a follow-up was planned.

CASE

A 58-year-old female was referred for an evaluation of a melanotic choroidal lesion in the left eye. Best-corrected visual acuity was 20/20 in both eyes. Anterior segment examination was unremarkable. Funduscopic examination was significant for a melanotic choroidal lesion along superior vascular arcade with overlying orange pigment and subretinal fluid (Fig. 8.2 and Video 8.2). Ultrasound exam revealed a dome-shaped, highly reflective lesion measuring 2.0 mm in thickness, and 7.3 mm in the greatest basal diameter. At this time, observation was elected. Upon follow-up 10 months later, the choroidal lesion demonstrated growth with an increase of 1.0 mm in thickness.

Melanocytoma of the Optic Disc

Melanocytoma is also known as magnocellular nevus, it is an intensely melanotic variant of uveal nevus that classically occurs on the optic disc but can involve any site of the uveal tract. The mean age at diagnosis is 50 years and appears to have a slight predilection for females and an equal incidence in all races. The lesion is usually unilateral. Although most melanocytomas do not cause significant visual impairment; visual loss can occur due to either mild exudation or choroidal neovascular membrane involving the fovea or secondary to central retinal vein obstruction or spontaneous tumor necrosis. Some tumors can grow slowly and may rarely

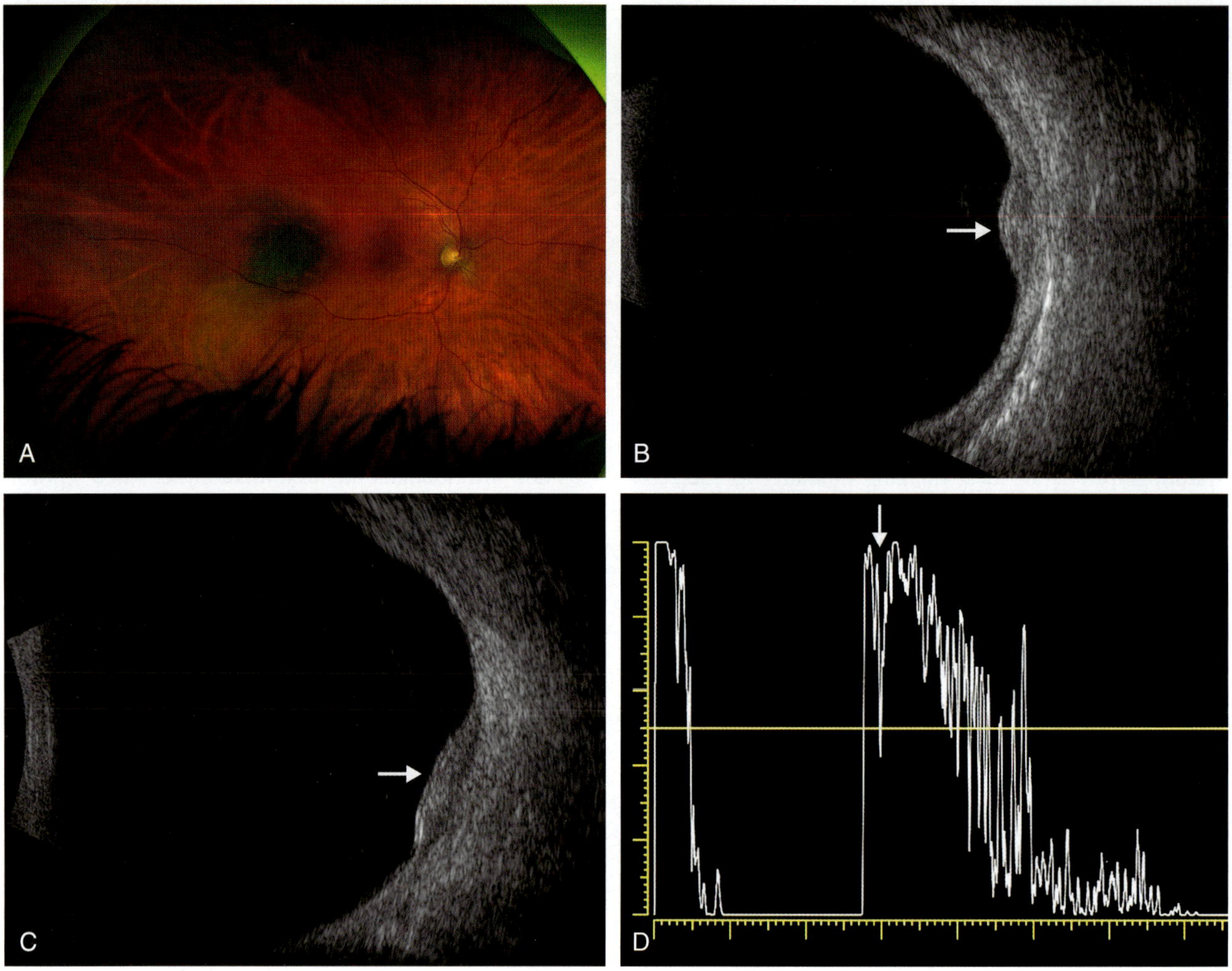

• **Fig. 8.1** Choroidal nevus. **(A)** Wide-angle fundus photography shows a melanotic choroidal nevus just temporal to the fovea. **(B)** Transverse and **(C)** longitudinal B-scans show a slightly elevated, dome-shaped choroidal lesion (*arrow*) with a minimal overlying subretinal fluid. **(D)** A-scan demonstrates high internal reflectivity (*arrow*).

exhibit malignant transformation; therefore, patients with melanocytoma should be monitored periodically.[4]

On ultrasound, melanocytomas are typically mildly elevated, dome-shaped, regularly structured, and highly reflective.

CASE

A 25-year-old female was referred for a melanocytic fundus lesion in the left eye detected on a routine ophthalmic exam. The fundus examination revealed an intensely melanotic mass overlying the optic disc and involving the surrounding choroid (Fig. 8.3). Ultrasound exam revealed a highly reflective lesion overlying the optic disc measuring 2.4 mm in thickness and 6.2 mm in the largest basal diameter.

Choroidal Melanoma

Choroidal melanoma is the most common primary intraocular malignancy in the adult population.[5] It is more common in adults with Caucasian ancestry. The diagnosis is generally prompted during a routine eye exam as few patients have vision symptoms usually associated with posterior tumor location and/or exudative retinal detachment.

Choroidal melanoma exhibits various growth patterns and degrees of melanotic pigmentation. The choroidal melanoma presents as a dome-shaped or mushroom-shaped solid mass when the tumor growth ruptures through Bruch's membrane. Other less frequent configurations include lobulated, diffuse (large diameter and thickness less than 20% of tumor largest diameter), and ring melanoma (circular involvement of the uvea). In some cases, the tumor can be amelanotic or partially melanotic.

Echographic features characteristic of choroidal melanoma include low to medium internal reflectivity (5%–60% spike height), regular internal structure, sound attenuation, and intrinsic vascularity.[6,7] Although a mushroom shape is highly suggestive of melanoma, other fundus lesions like metastasis and retinal capillary hemangioblastomas can present the similar configuration. The presence of an overlying or adjacent subretinal fluid or a more extensive exudative retinal detachment is common.

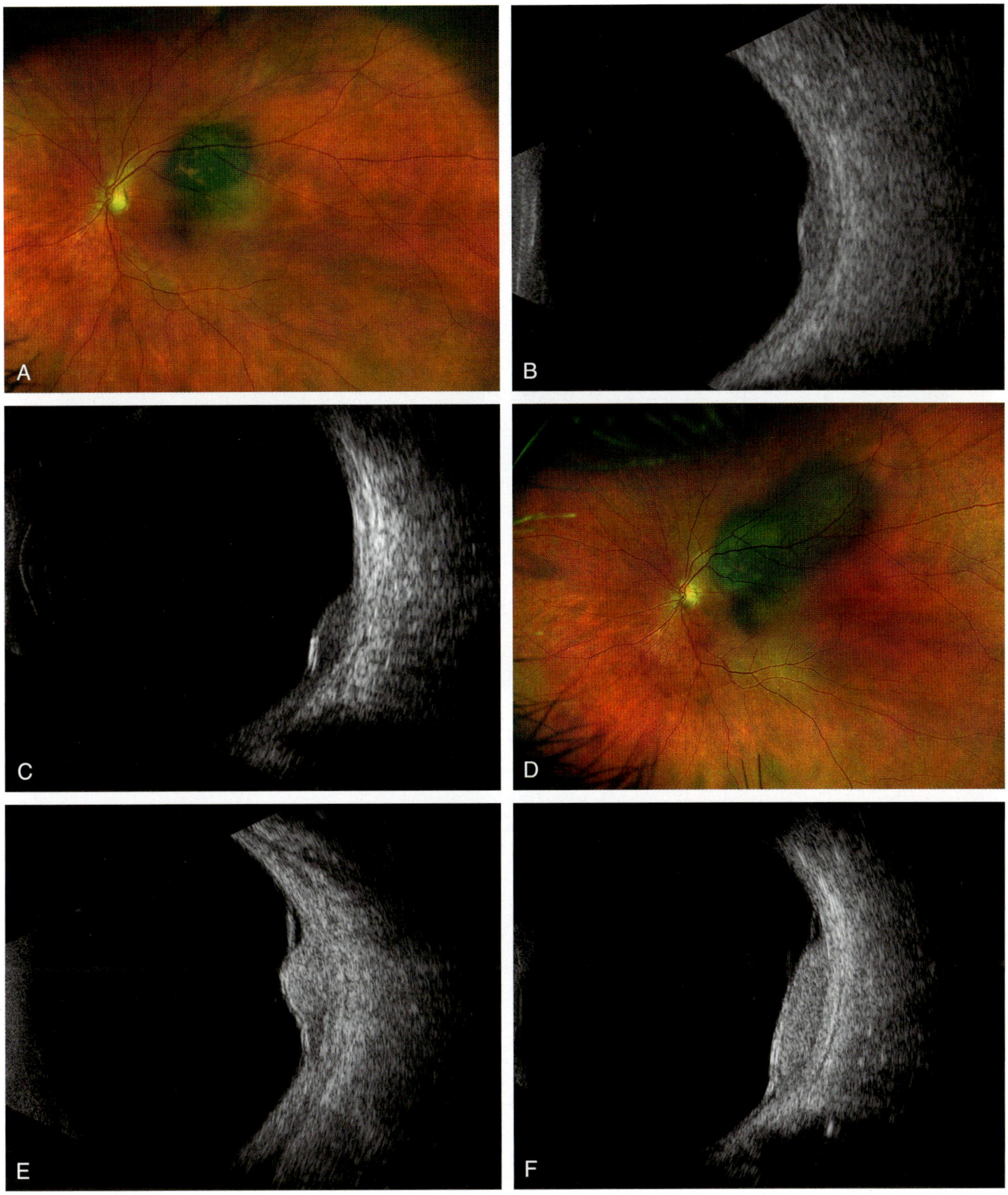

• **Fig. 8.2** Growth of suspicious choroidal nevus. **(A–C)** Fundus photography and ultrasonography of suspicious choroidal nevus on the initial visit. **(B)** Transverse and **(C)** longitudinal B-scans show a dome-shaped choroidal lesion. **(D–F)** Ten months later, fundus photography and ultrasonography revealed the growth of the lesion. **(E)** Transverse and **(F)** longitudinal B-scans show the choroidal lesion with increased dimensions—height and basal diameter—and surrounding subretinal fluid.

CASE

A 67-year-old female, presented with a history of melanotic fundus lesion in the left eye. Anterior segment examination was unremarkable. The fundoscopic examination was significant for a partially melanotic choroidal mass with associated subretinal fluid along its margins (Fig. 8.4 and Video 8.3). Ultrasound revealed a dome-shaped choroidal lesion with medium reflectivity and intrinsic vascularity, measuring 3.7 mm in thickness and 12.9 mm in largest basal diameter.

CASE

A 59-year-old male, presented with recently decreased vision in his left eye. A fundoscopic exam revealed a partially melanotic choroidal lesion with an overlying retinal hemorrhage (Fig. 8.5 and Video 8.4). Ultrasonography disclosed a large, mushroom-shaped choroidal lesion with low to medium internal reflectivity, and associated exudative retinal detachment.

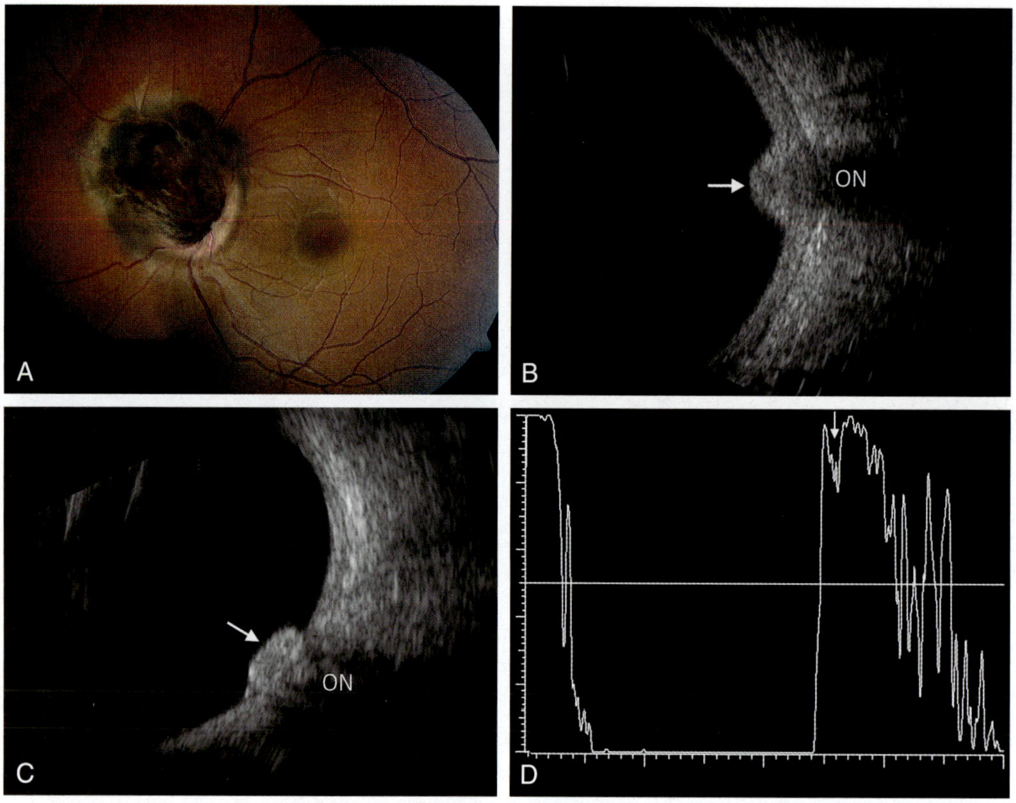

• **Fig. 8.3** Melanocytoma of the optic disc. **(A)** Fundus photography shows a melanocytoma overlying the optic disc with a surrounding choroidal component. **(B)** Transverse and **(C)** longitudinal B-scans show a dome-shaped mass lesion overlying the optic disc (*arrow*). **(D)** A-scan demonstrates regular internal structure and high reflectivity (*arrow*). ON, Optic nerve.

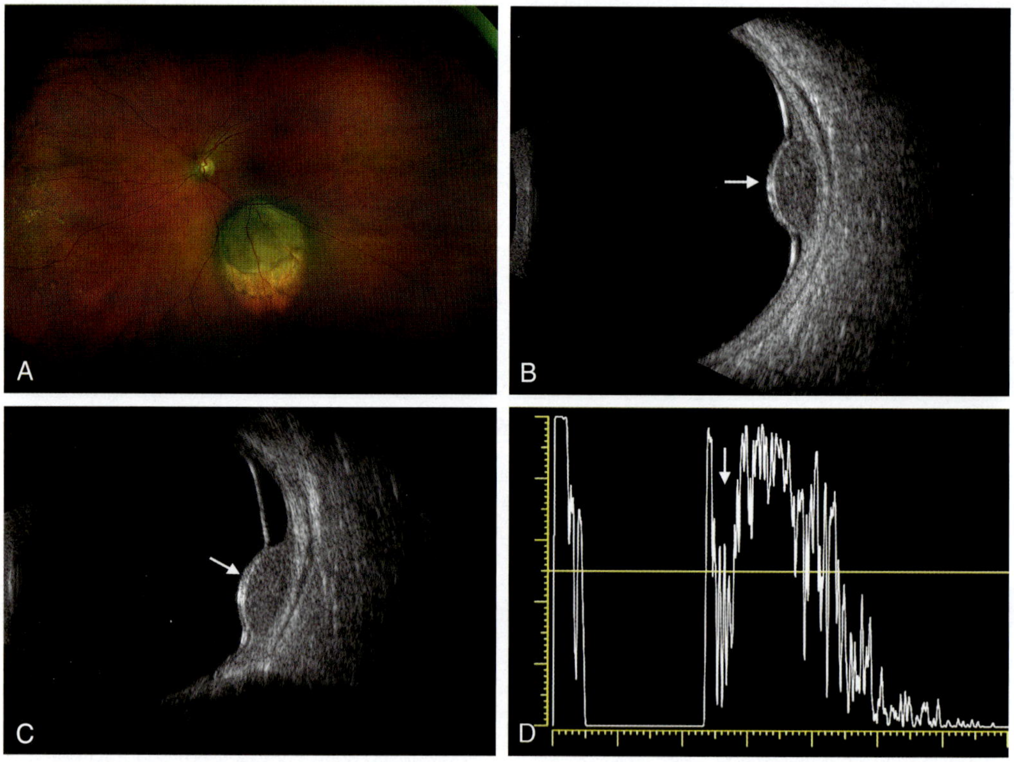

• **Fig. 8.4** Choroidal melanoma. **(A)** Fundus photography of a partially melanotic choroidal melanoma. **(B)** Transverse and **(C)** longitudinal B-scans show a dome-shaped, regularly structured choroidal lesion (*arrow*) with subretinal fluid along the margins. **(D)** The corresponding A-scan shows medium internal reflectivity (*arrow*).

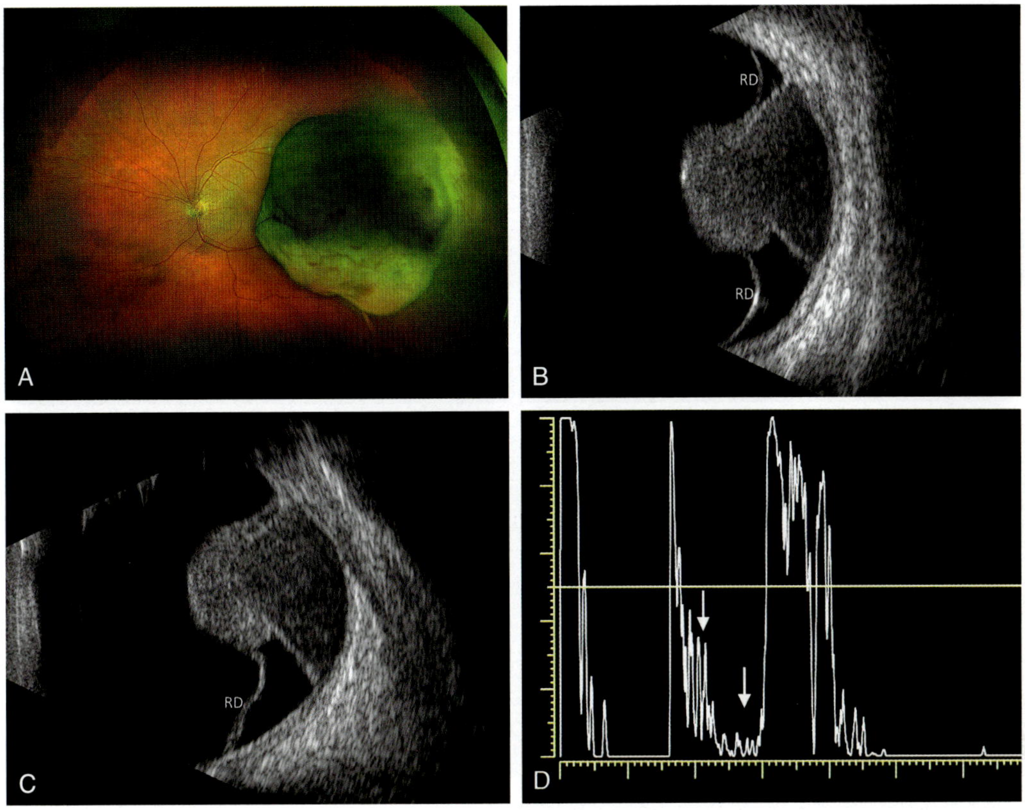

• **Fig. 8.5** Mushroom-shaped choroidal melanoma. **(A)** Fundus photography shows a partially melanotic choroidal melanoma just temporal to the macula, with overlying retinal hemorrhage. **(B)** A transverse B-scan shows a mushroom-shaped choroidal melanoma with a nearly echolucent base due to moderate sound attenuation. There is an associated exudative retinal detachment (*RD*). **(C)** A longitudinal view of the lesion shows a choroidal excavation. **(D)** A-scan shows low to medium internal reflectivity with a decay slope of the spikes (angle Kappa) typical of sound attenuation (*arrows*).

CASE

An 80-year-old male was referred for a melanotic fundus lesion in the right eye. Ultrasonographic exam revealed a dome-shaped, low-reflective choroidal lesion with an extrascleral extension (Fig. 8.6).

CASE

A 42-year-old male was referred for a choroidal melanoma. Ultrasonography revealed a dome-shaped, low-reflective lesion with intrinsic vascularity, and associated subretinal fluid, measuring 2.3 mm in thickness. Systemic workup was negative. The patient underwent Iodine-125 brachytherapy. Five years later, the patient presented with decreased vision. Ultrasonography revealed a regressed choroidal melanoma measuring 1.0 mm in thickness and a massive extrascleral lesion with low internal reflectivity adjacent to the treated melanoma measuring 12.8 mm in diameter (Fig. 8.7).

Choroidal Melanoma Associated With Ocular Melanocytosis

Oculodermal melanocytosis is an uncommon congenital condition that represents an important predisposing factor for uveal melanoma. Overall, patients with ocular melanocytosis have a 35–50% higher risk of developing uveal melanoma compared to general population, and the life time prevelance of uveal melanoma in a patient with ocular melanocytosis is estimated to be 1 in 400. Additionally, patients with uveal melanoma and ocular melanocytosis have a relative risk for metastasis of 1.6 times greater compared with those without melanocytosis.[8]

CASE

A 15-year-old female with congenital ocular melanocytosis was referred for evaluation of a choroidal mass in the left eye. External and slit lamp examinations revealed scleral hyperpigmentation (Fig. 8.8). Fundus examination of the left eye disclosed multiple choroidal patches involving all quadrants and an elevated, bilobed, melanocytic juxtapapillary mass. An A- and B-ultrasound showed lobulated, regularly structured, low-reflective choroidal mass with positive intralesional vascularity. The lesion dimensions were 5.6 mm in height and 13.1 in the largest basal diameter. After a diagnosis of choroidal melanoma was made, the patient was treated with enucleation. A histopathology exam revealed mixed-cell choroidal melanoma.

Intraoperative Ultrasonographic Evaluation of Localization of the Radioactive Episcleral Plaque for Choroidal Melanoma

Radioactive episcleral plaque therapy is the most common form of radiotherapy for uveal melanoma (Fig. 8.9 and Video 8.5). B-scan ultrasonography has been used for intraoperative

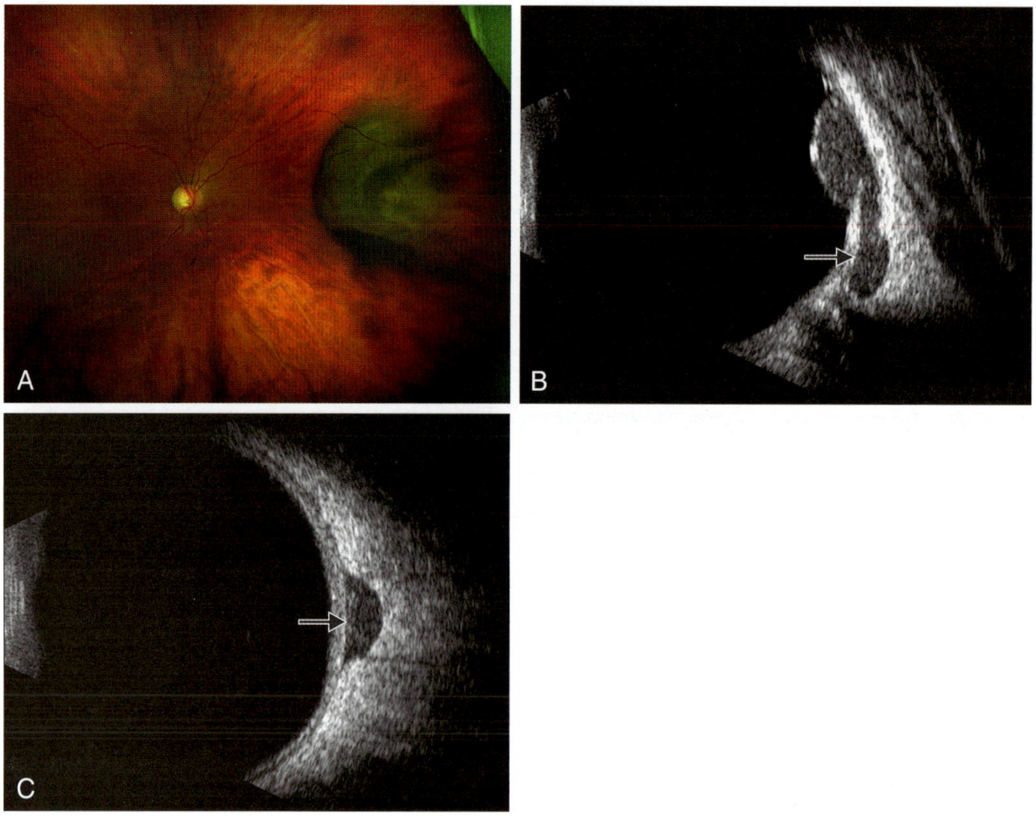

• **Fig. 8.6** Extrascleral extension of choroidal melanoma. **(A)** Fundus photography shows a melanotic choroidal melanoma nasal to the optic disc. **(B)** Ultrasound longitudinal view demonstrates a dome-shaped, regularly structured, low-reflective fundus lesion with an extrascleral extension (*arrow*). **(C)** A transverse view just posterior to the lesion shows an extrascleral low-reflective nodular lesion (*arrow*).

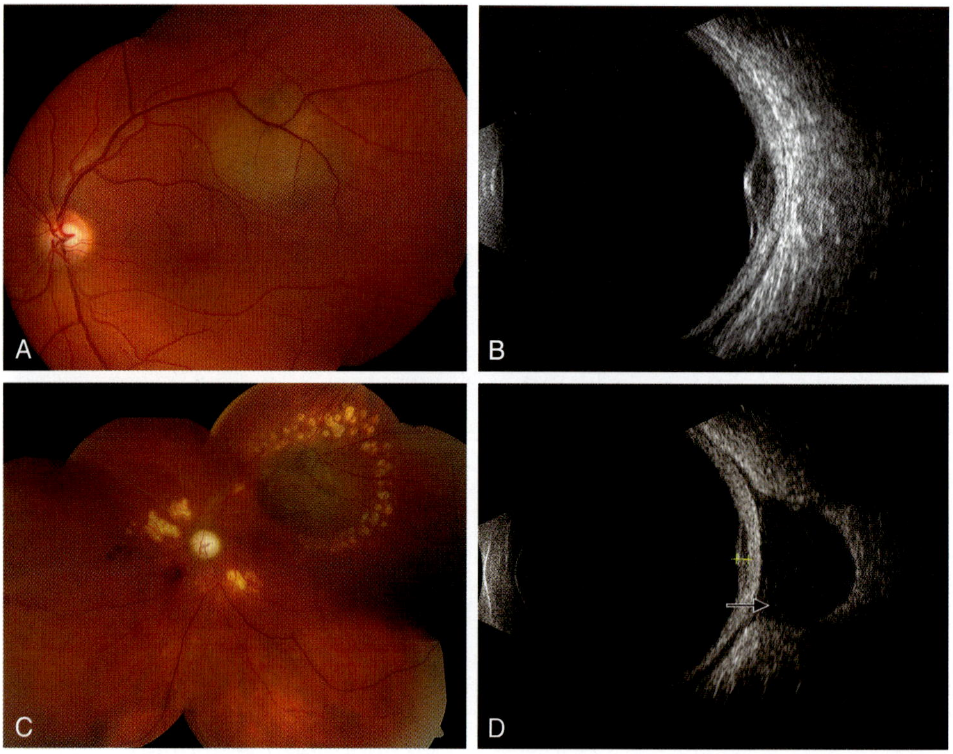

• **Fig. 8.7** Choroidal melanoma with an extrascleral extension after brachytherapy. **(A)** Fundus photography and, **(B)** transverse B-scan show choroidal melanoma on the initial visit **(C–D)**. Follow-up ultrasonography image 5 years after brachytherapy demonstrates a massive extrascleral extension (*arrow*) of a regressed choroidal melanoma. Notice the decreased thickness of the primary intraocular tumor.

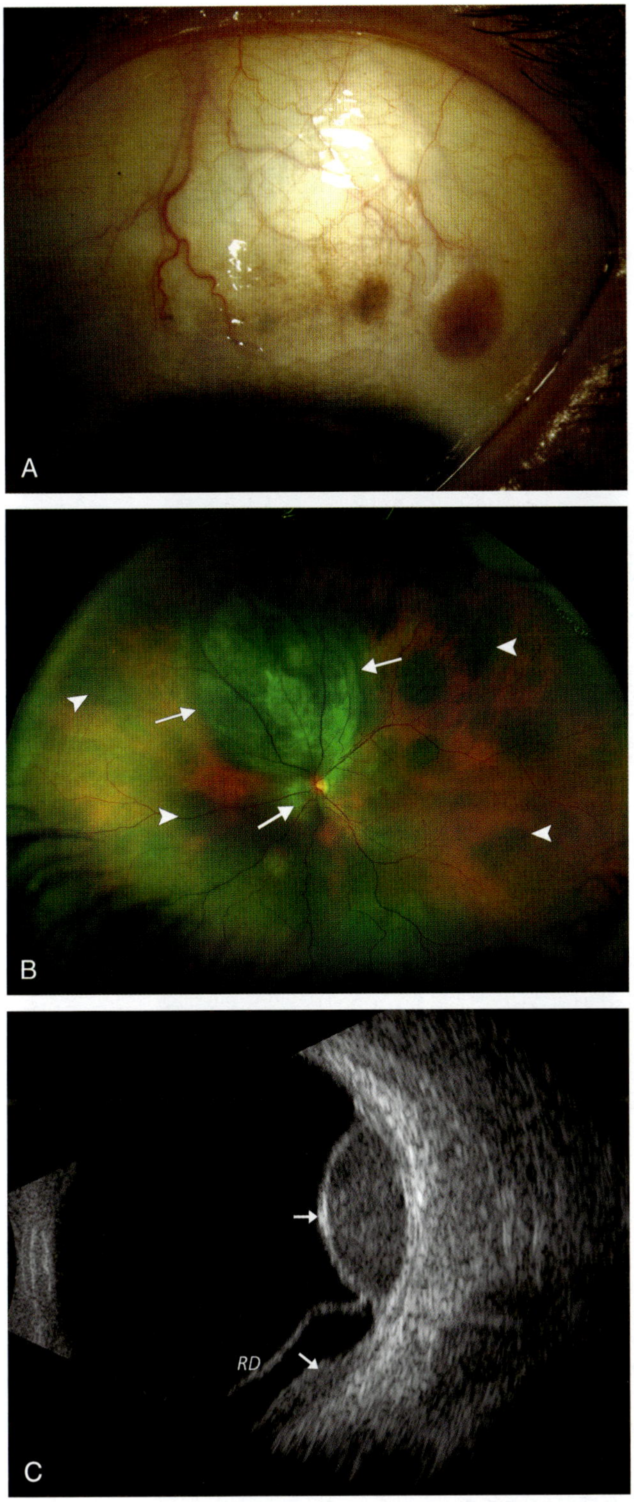

• **Fig. 8.8** Choroidal melanoma associated with ocular melanocytosis. **(A)** Slit lamp photography shows alternating areas of dispersed and densely patched scleral melanotic pigmentation. **(B)** Fundus photography exhibits dispersed melanocytosis involving all quadrants (*arrowheads*), and an elevated pigmented choroidal mass (*arrows*). **(C)** Ultrasound B-scan shows a lobulated, regularly structured, low reflective choroidal mass (*arrows*), with associated retinal detachment (*RD*).

confirmation of the optimal plaque placement. Under sterile conditions, a dynamic transverse, and longitudinal transocular scans of B-scan ultrasound are obtained using a coupling agent at an optimized gain. After the radioactive episcleral plaque has been fixated to the episcleral surface B-scan ultrasound is performed to confirm that the radioactive plaque was centered on the tumor episcenter and/or all tumor margins were covered. Radioactive plaques that were not correctly placed were repositioned, and echographic confirmation was repeated to evaluate the revised localization.[9,10]

Choroidal Metastasis

The choroid is the most common ocular site for metastasis. Choroidal metastases most often arise from primary cancer of the breast, and lung. Less common primary tumors include carcinoma of the gastrointestinal tract, prostate, kidney, and cutaneous melanoma. In some cases, a choroidal metastasis precedes the diagnosis of primary systemic cancer. Patients typically present with a complaint of blurred vision. Most metastatic choroidal tumors present as a creamy-yellow solid choroidal mass associated with a serous retinal detachment, and frequently located posterior to the equator. These metastatic lesions can be focal or multifocal, unilateral, or bilateral.[11,12]

On B-scan ultrasonography, most tumors are observed as a moderately elevated, relatively flat or dome-shaped choroidal lesion with an undulating surface and a central excavation. They usually present an irregular internal structure, and the internal reflectivity can vary from medium to high on an A-scan ultrasonography. These lesions are often associated with exudative retinal detachment that is often more extensive than those seen in choroidal melanoma of an equivalent size. Atypical presentation features include mushroom shape, internal cavitation, and low internal reflectivity on A-scan ultrasonography.

CASE

A 58-year-old male, presented with blurred vision in the right eye for one week. He had no history of cancer. A fundus examination revealed a yellowish, multilobulated, flat choroidal mass just temporal to the macula with associated exudative retinal detachment inferiorly (Fig. 8.10). A B-scan and A-scan ultrasonography examination disclosed a multilobulated, flat choroidal mass with medium-high internal reflectivity, measuring 2.6 mm in thickness and 17.0 mm in the largest basal diameter, and confirmed the exuadative retinal detachment inferiorly. The patient had systemic imaging workup with chest, abdomen, and pelvis CT scans, which revealed a mass in the upper lobe of the right lung and numerous nodules in both lungs. A diagnosis of choroidal metastatic disease secondary to lung cancer was made.

CASE

A 49-year-old male with a history of squamous cell carcinoma of the tongue was referred with blurred vision complaint in both eyes. The anterior segment was unremarkable. A dilated fundoscopic exam revealed an amelanotic choroidal lesion along the superotemporal temporal arcade in both eyes (Fig. 8.11 and Video 8.6). Ultrasound exam disclosed slightly heterogeneous choroidal mass with medium-high internal reflectivity at the posterior pole, temporally, and associated exudative shallow retinal detachment. Based on clinical and imaging features, a diagnosis of bilateral choroidal metastasis was made.

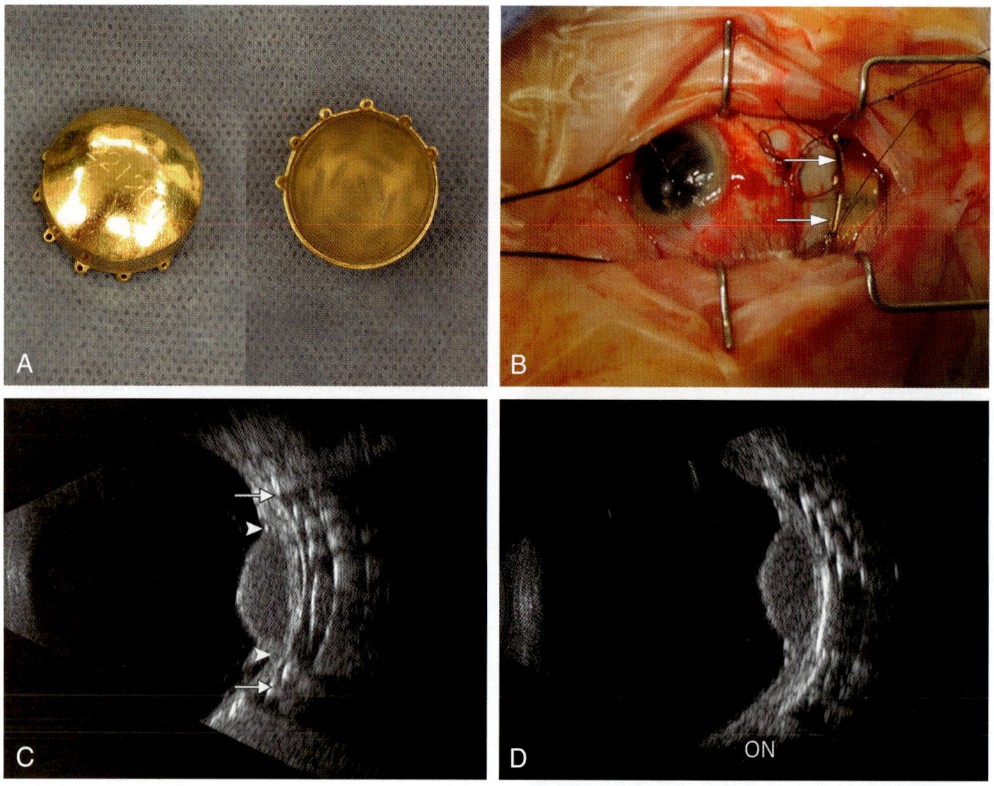

• **Fig. 8.9** Intraoperative echographic evaluation of localization of the for radioactive episcleral plaque for choroidal melanoma. **(A)** Gold-shielded round episcleral plaque with iodine-125 radioactive seeds. **(B)** Radioactive episcleral plaque sutured to the sclera (*arrows*). **(C)** A transverse B-scan aimed at the tumor's center shows optimally positioned plaque (*arrows*) covering the tumor margins (*arrowheads*). **(D)** Longitudinal B-scan shows adequate plaque position covering the anterior and posterior tumor margins. *ON*, Optic nerve.

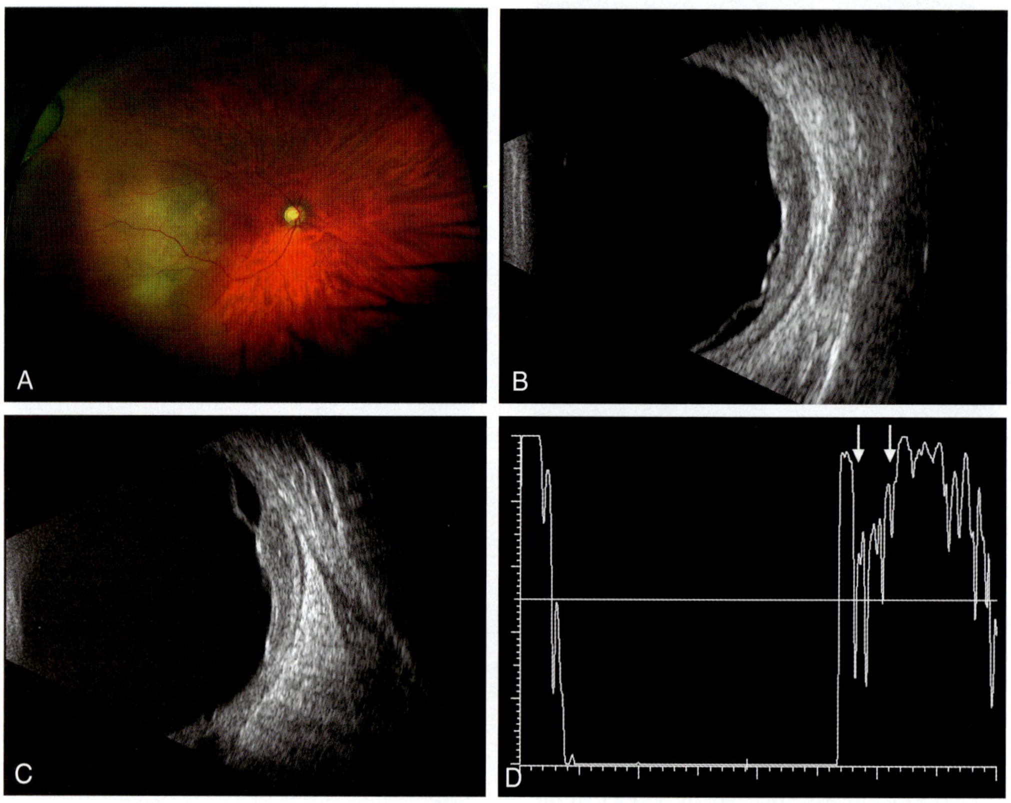

• **Fig. 8.10** Choroidal metastasis as an initial presentation of lung cancer. **(A)** Fundus photography shows a creamy-yellowish choroidal mass just temporal to the macula. **(B)** Transverse and **(C)** longitudinal ultrasound B-scans show a moderately elevated, flat, lobulated choroidal mass with associated exudative retinal detachment along the margin. **(D)** A-scan ultrasound at tissue sensitivity displays medium-high internal reflectivity (*arrows*).

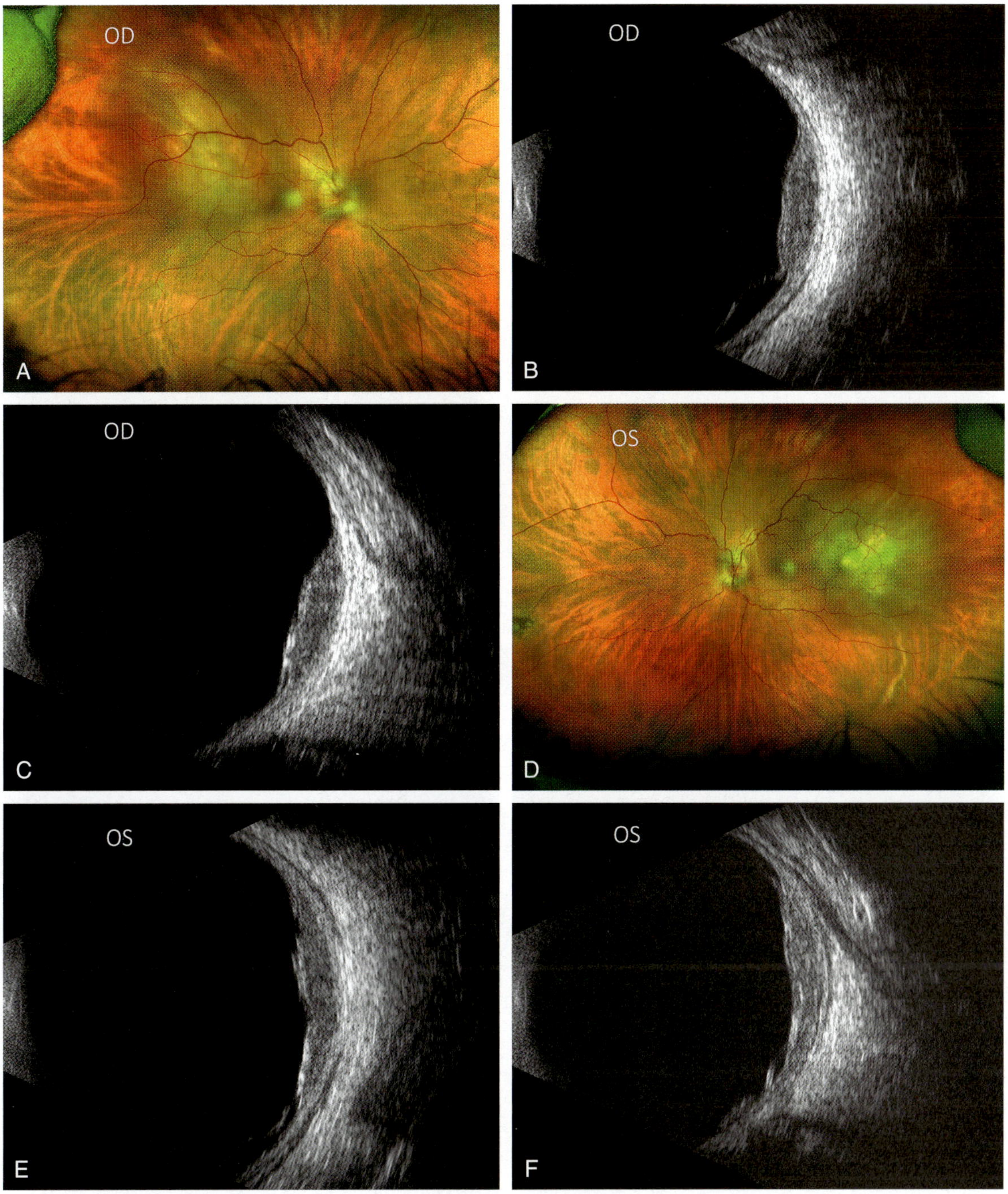

• **Fig. 8.11** Bilateral choroidal metastasis. **(A–C)** Right eye and **(D–F)** left eye images of bilateral choroidal metastasis showing yellow choirdal lesions superotemporal to the macula on fundus photography and elevated, flat choroidal masses with lobulated surface and medium highly internal reflectivity on transverse and longitudinal B-scans.

TEACHING POINTS

Although some imaging variances can occur, low to medium internal reflectivity and moderate to marked intrinsic vascularity are the typical acoustic features of choroidal melanoma.

Ultrasonography is essential to assess the extraocular tissue adjacent to a choroidal melanoma to detect extrascleral extension and accurately measure the tumor before any treatment and after the episcaleral plaque radiotherapy.

Circumscribed Choroidal Hemangioma

Circumscribed choroidal hemangioma typically presents as a solitary, unilateral tumor, at the posterior pole without any other ocular or systemic anomalies. Furthermore, this tumor is often misdiagnosed as a malignant lesion such as choroidal melanoma or metastasis.

Ophthalmoscopically, circumscribed choroidal hemangioma is seen as a round or oval, orange-red choroidal mass located posterior to the equator and most frequently temporal to the optic disc. Over time, secondary changes such as subretinal fluid or even extensive retinal detachment may occur, leading to visual loss.[13,14]

On B-scan ultrasonography, circumscribed choroidal hemangioma is characterized as a dome-shaped, regularly structured, hyperreflective choroidal lesion with shallow borders and a lack of choroidal excavation.[15] Mild intrinsic vascularity may be detected.

CASE

A 44-year-old female was referred for a choroidal lesion in the right eye. Ocular history, medical history, and anterior segment were unremarkable. Dilated fundus examination revealed an amelanotic choroidal lesion superotemporal to the fovea (Fig. 8.12 and Video 8.7). There was no orange pigment on the lesion surface. B-scan ultrasonography examination disclosed a solid, dome-shaped, highly reflective choroidal lesion measuring 2.5 mm in thickness, and 8.4 mm in the largest basal diameter. Based on clinical and imaging studies, a diagnosis of choroidal hemangioma was made.

Diffuse Choroidal Hemangioma

Diffuse choroidal hemangioma is usually part of neuro-oculo-cutaneous hemangiomatosis (Sturge-Weber syndrome). The lesion is typically ipsilateral to the facial cutaneous vascular malformation and causes choroidal thickening. A diffuse choroidal hemangioma can cause exudative retinal detachment and neovascular glaucoma.

On ultrasonography exam, the B-scan ultrasonography demonstrates a diffuse, shallowly elevated, highly reflective choroidal thickening more prominent or restricted to the temporal quadrants. In some cases, an exudative retinal detachment can be associated.

CASE

A 6-year-old girl, presented with left-sided facial hemangioma, diffuse choroidal hemangioma, and secondary glaucoma in the left eye in Sturge-Weber Syndrome. The best corrected visual acuity was 20/20 in the right eye, and no light perception in the left eye. Dilated indirect ophthalmoscopy showed a total retinal detachment in the left eye. Ultrasound imaging revealed features of diffuse choroidal hemangioma (Fig. 8.13 and Video 8.8).

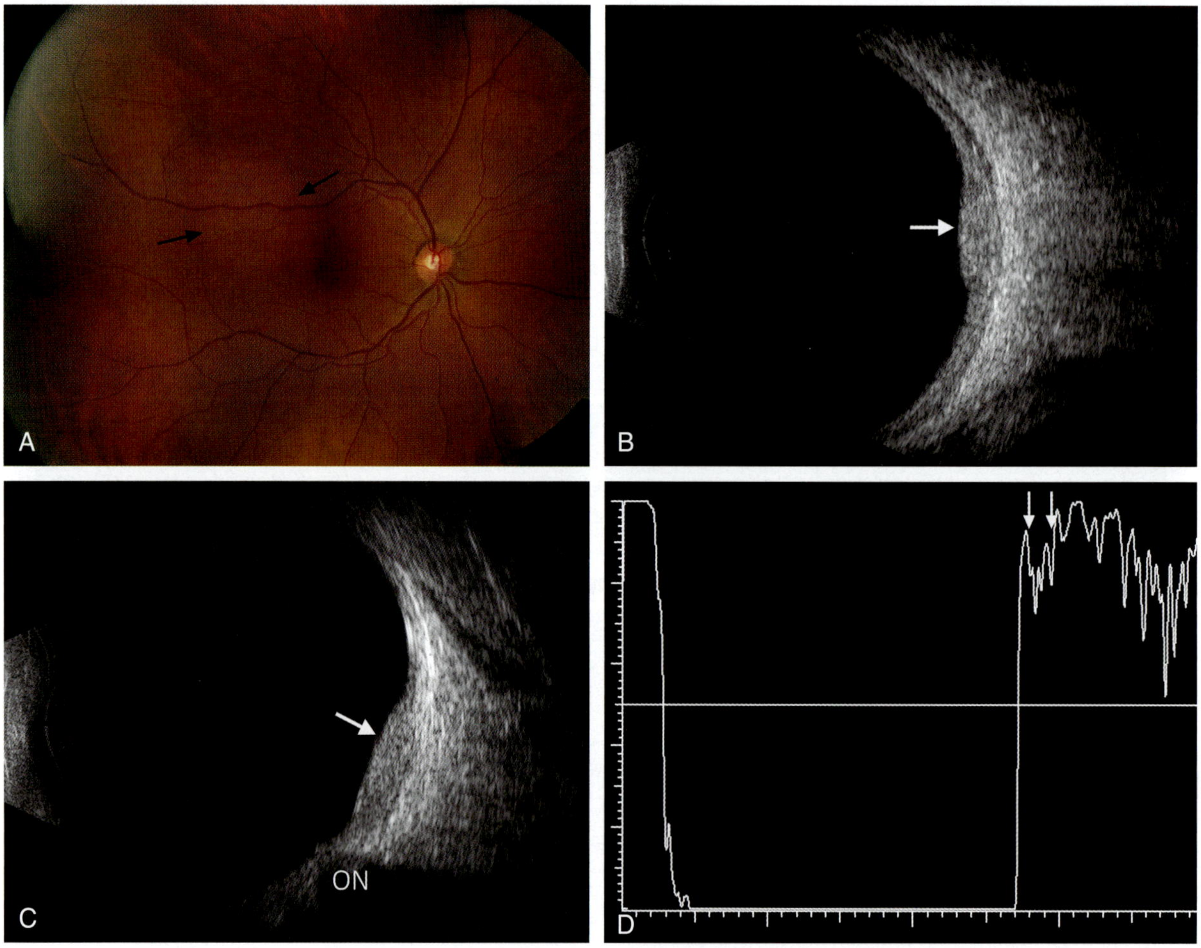

• **Fig. 8.12** Circumscribed choroidal hemangioma. **(A)** Fundus photography shows an orange choroidal lesion along the superior temporal arcade (*arrows*). **(B)** Transverse B-scan exhibits a regularly structured, highly reflective dome-shaped lesion, with shallow borders (*arrow*). **(C)** Longitudinal B-scan exhibits a choroidal melanoma close to the optic disc. *ON*, Optic nerve. **(D)** A-scan shows high internal reflectivity (*arrows*).

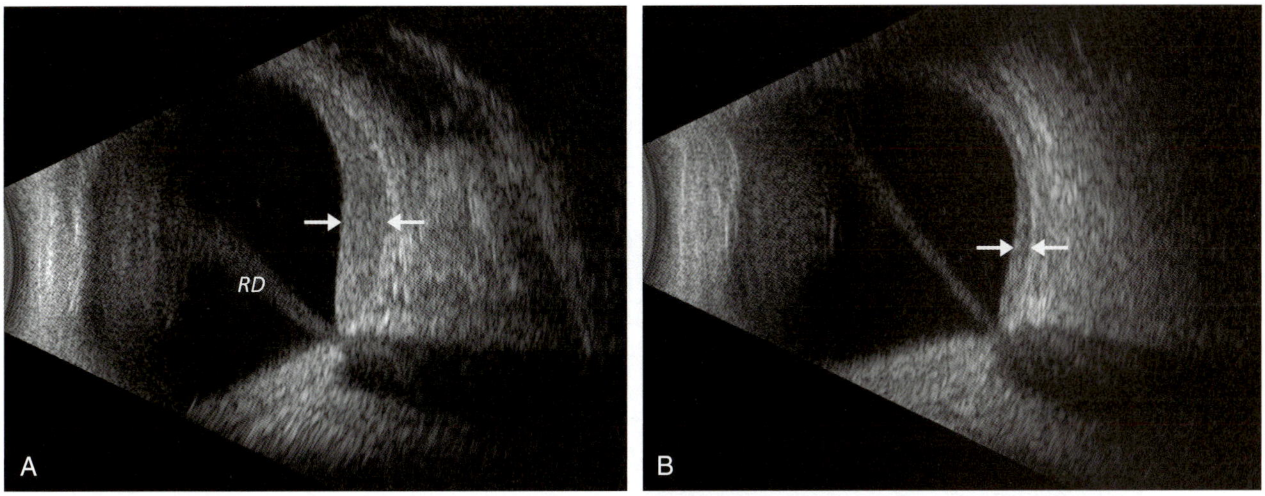

• **Fig. 8.13** Diffuse choroidal hemangioma. **(A)** Longitudinal B-scan aimed temporally shows diffuse, homogeneous, highly reflective choroidal thickening (*arrows*) extending from the optic disc to the periphery, and total closed funnel retinal detachment (RD). **(B)** A longitudinal scan through the nasal fundus shows average choroidal thickness (*arrows*).

Osseous Tumor of the Uvea – Choroidal Osteoma

Choroidal osteomas are rare benign ossifying tumors typically found in healthy young females in the second or third decade of life. They appear irregular, slightly elevated, yellow-white choroidal masses with well-defined geographic borders. The tumor is unilateral in most cases and tends to be in the juxtapapillary area. The major complication of choroidal osteoma is the development of choroidal neovascularization or decalcification of choroidal osteoma leading to visual loss.[16,17]

On B-scan ultrasonography, choroidal osteomas are minimally elevated with a broad base. Due to the presence of calcified components, they are highly reflective with a marked acoustic shadow of the orbital tissue. They remain highly reflective at lower gain settings.[18]

CASE

A 24-year-old female was referred for a fundus lesion in the left eye. The patient had no systemic disease. The best corrected visual acuity was 20/20 in the right eye and 20/70 in the left eye. Dilated fundus examination revealed a chalky-white juxtapapillary lesion superotemporally with macular involvement (Fig. 8.14). Ultrasonography exam revealed a plaque-like hyperreflective fundus lesion causing distinct orbital shadowing. Lesion dimensions were 1.2 mm in thickness and 10.5 mm in largest basal diameter.

CASE

A 23-year-old female, presented with a history of bilateral choroidal osteoma complicated by choroidal neovascularization treated with anti-VEGF injection. The best corrected visual acuity was 20/400 in the right eye and 20/20 in the left eye. Fundus examination showed a juxtapapillary yellow choroidal tumor with well-defined margins in both eyes (Fig. 8.15 and Video 8.9).

See Table 8.1 for clinical and acoustic characteristics of choroidal tumors summary.

TEACHING POINTS

Choroidal metastasis is the most common intraocular cancer in adults.

The most common primary tumors are breast cancer in women and lung cancer in men. These lesions usually display higher internal reflectivity and present a disproportional amount of associated serous retinal detachment.

Tumors of the Retina

Retinoblastoma

Retinoblastoma is the most common intraocular malignancy of childhood, with an estimated 300 cases annually in the United States, or approximately 1 in 18,000 live births. Retinoblastoma primarily affects children of very young age, and most patients are diagnosed before the age of 2 years. It is rare after 7 years of age. Early detection and treatment by a multidisciplinary specialty team maximize the chance for survival and ocular/vision salvage while minimizing treatment-related toxicity. The tumor can be unilateral or bilateral, sporadic or familial, intraocular (confined to the globe), or extraocular (extension of the tumor beyond the globe).[19,20]

Leukocoria, or a white pupillary reflex, is the most frequent presenting sign of retinoblastoma. The second most common presenting sign of retinoblastoma is strabismus. In its earliest clinical stage, a small retinoblastoma appears ophthalmoscopically transparent lesion in the sensory retina. Slightly larger tumors lead to dilated retinal blood vessels on the surface. Some larger tumors show foci of chalk-like calcification that resemble cottage cheese.

Retinoblastoma growth patterns are subdivided into intraretinal, endophytic, and exophytic. Intraretinal tumors are limited to the substance of the retina. Endophytic

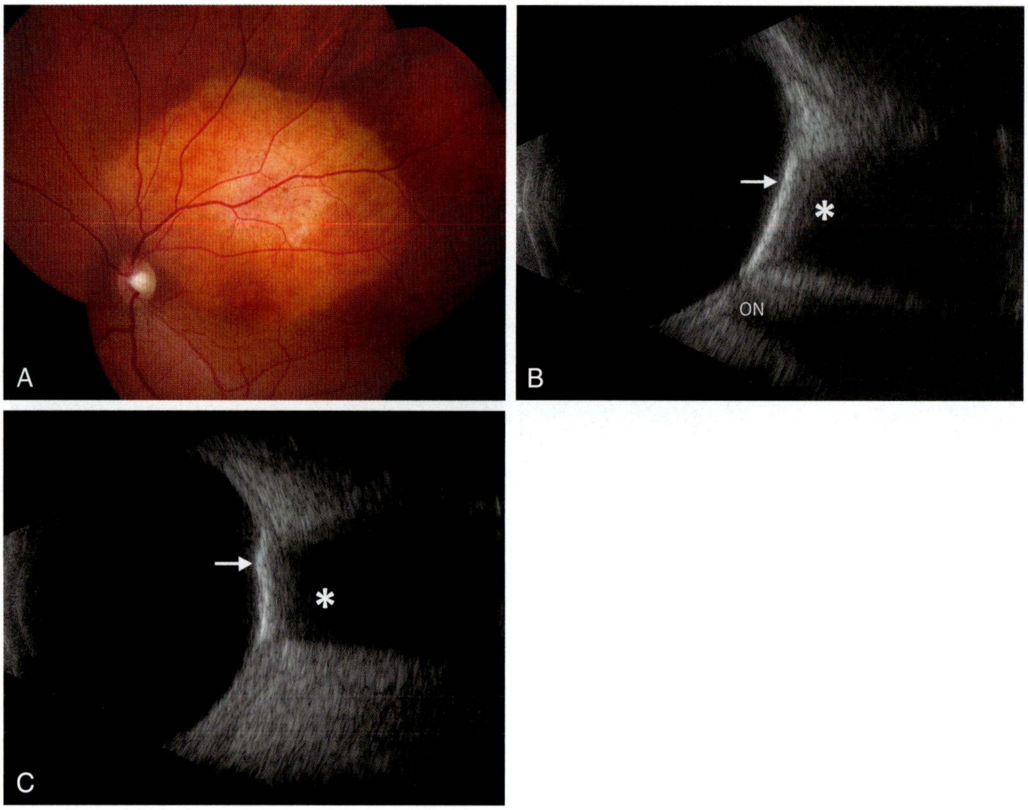

• **Fig. 8.14** Choroidal osteoma. **(A)** Fundus photo montage shows a choroidal osteoma adjacent to the optic disc. **(B)** Transverse and, **(C)** longitudinal B-scans reveal a plaque-like hyperreflective choroidal lesion (*arrow*) causing distinct orbital shadowing (asterisk). *ON*, Optic nerve.

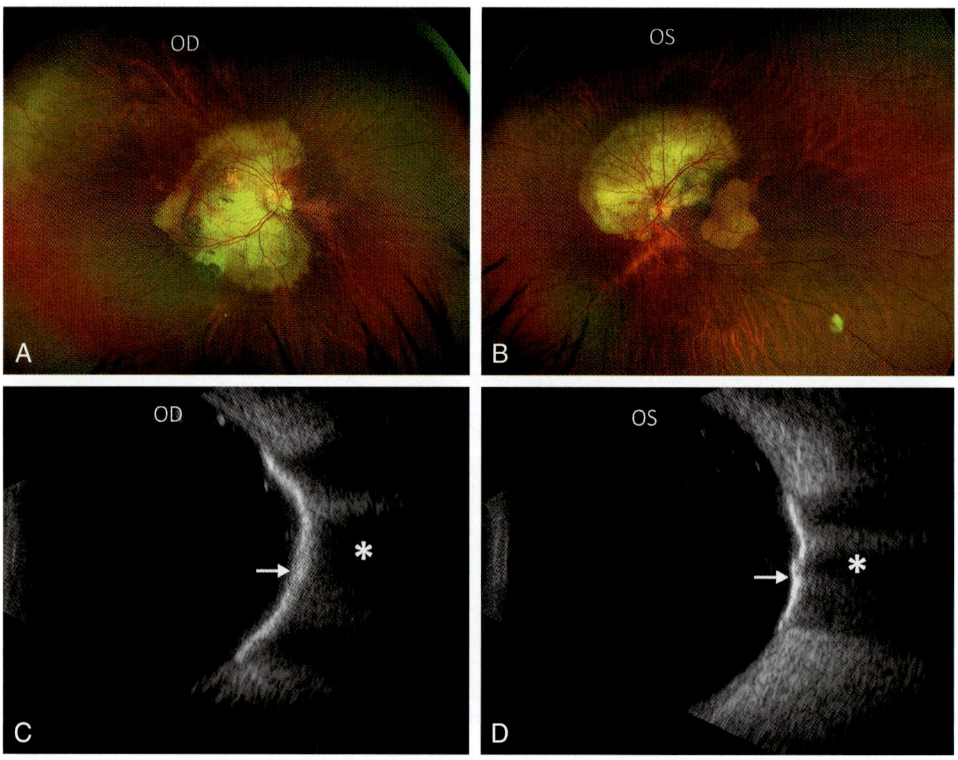

• **Fig. 8.15** Bilateral choroidal osteoma. Fundus photography shows a juxtapapillary, partially decalcified choroidal osteoma temporally on the macula of the right eye **(A)**, and superiorly in the left eye **(B)**. Transverse B-scans of the right eye **(C)**, and left eye **(D)** show flat, highly reflective choroidal lesions (*arrow*), causing a strong sound attenuation of the orbital tissue (*asterisk*).

TABLE 8.1 Clinical and Acoustic Characteristics of Choroidal Tumors

Tumor	Clinical Features	Shape/Height	Internal Reflectivity	Intrinsic Vascularity
Melanoma	Melanotic or partially melanotic or amelanotic Associated orange pigment (lipofuscin) Associated subretinal fluid (SRF)	Dome or mushroom >2.0 mm	Low to medium	Mild to intense
Nevus	Melanotic or amelanotic Overlying drusen Atrophic separation of the retina instead of SRF	Flat or dome <2.0 mm	High	None to mild
Melanocytoma	Dark brown to black Usually over the optic disc margin Can present in the ciliary body, and iris root	Flat or dome <2.0 mm	High	None to mild
Metastasis	Creamy yellow and mostly amelanotic Solitary/multifocal Disproportional associated SRF	Irregular or lobulated Shallowly elevated	Medium to high	None to mild
Circumscribed Hemangioma	Orange-red color with associated retinal pigment epithelium changes Usually in the macula or around the optic disc Variable subretinal fluid	Dome with shallow borders Mean = 2.4 mm	High	None to mild
Osteoma	Whitish-yellow Well-defined geographic borders Usually, juxtapapillary	Plaque or ridge-like Mean = 1.5 mm	Extremely high causing x acoustic shadowing	None

retinoblastoma grows from the retina inward toward the vitreous cavity. An exophytic retinoblastoma is one that grows from the retina outward into the subretinal space producing a progressive retinal detachment and subretinal seeding.[19]

The gold standard diagnostic approach for a child with retinoblastoma is direct visualization of the tumor under anesthesia. Ophthalmic ultrasonography is very valuable in providing additional diagnosis evidence for retinoblastoma. Magnetic resonance imaging should be performed to assess for orbital, optic nerve, and intracranial involvement.[20]

On the B-scan ultrasonography, the tumor is usually dome-shaped or round with a smooth or slightly lobulated surface. Less frequently, a diffuse form with irregular thickening of the retina can occur.

Intratumoral calcification is a frequent and essential diagnostic feature. The amount and distribution of calcium within the tumor will determine the internal reflectivity of the lesion; therefore, the lesion can vary from non-calcified with a medium internal reflectivity, to highly calcified with high reflectivity. The distribution of calcium can have a multiple punctate pattern or a totaly calcified appearance.

CASE

A 5-week-old infant, presented with bilateral leukocoria. The family history was negative for intraocular tumor. The ophthalmoscopic exam under anesthesia revealed a bilateral, white retinal lesion with overlying dilated retinal vessels (Fig. 8.16 and Video 8.10).

CASE

A 13-month-old girl was referred for an intraocular mass in the right eye. The patient has had torticollis since she was born. There is no history of eye cancer in the family. The fundus exam under anesthesia revealed three, amelanotic retinal lesions at the posterior pole, temporally in the right eye, and a small opaque white retinal lesion in the inferonasal periphery in the left eye (Fig. 8.17).

CASE

A 4-month-old girl with a positive family history of retinoblastoma presented with a bilateral retinal mass. The infant had been screened for intraocular tumors since birth. The ophthalmoscopic exam under anesthesia revealed multiple retinoblastomas in the left eye (Fig. 8.18 and Video 8.11).

CASE

A 6-year-old girl was referred for evaluation of an intraocular mass in the left eye. The ophthalmoscopic exam under anesthesia revealed a normal fundus in the right eye. Indirect ophthalmoscopy of the left eye revealed an extensive retinal detachment and a subretinal solitary retinal tumor with tortuous, dilated intrinsic vessels located inferonasally anterior to the equator and extending to the posterior pole. The ultrasonography examination disclosed intratumoral calcification (Fig. 8.19).

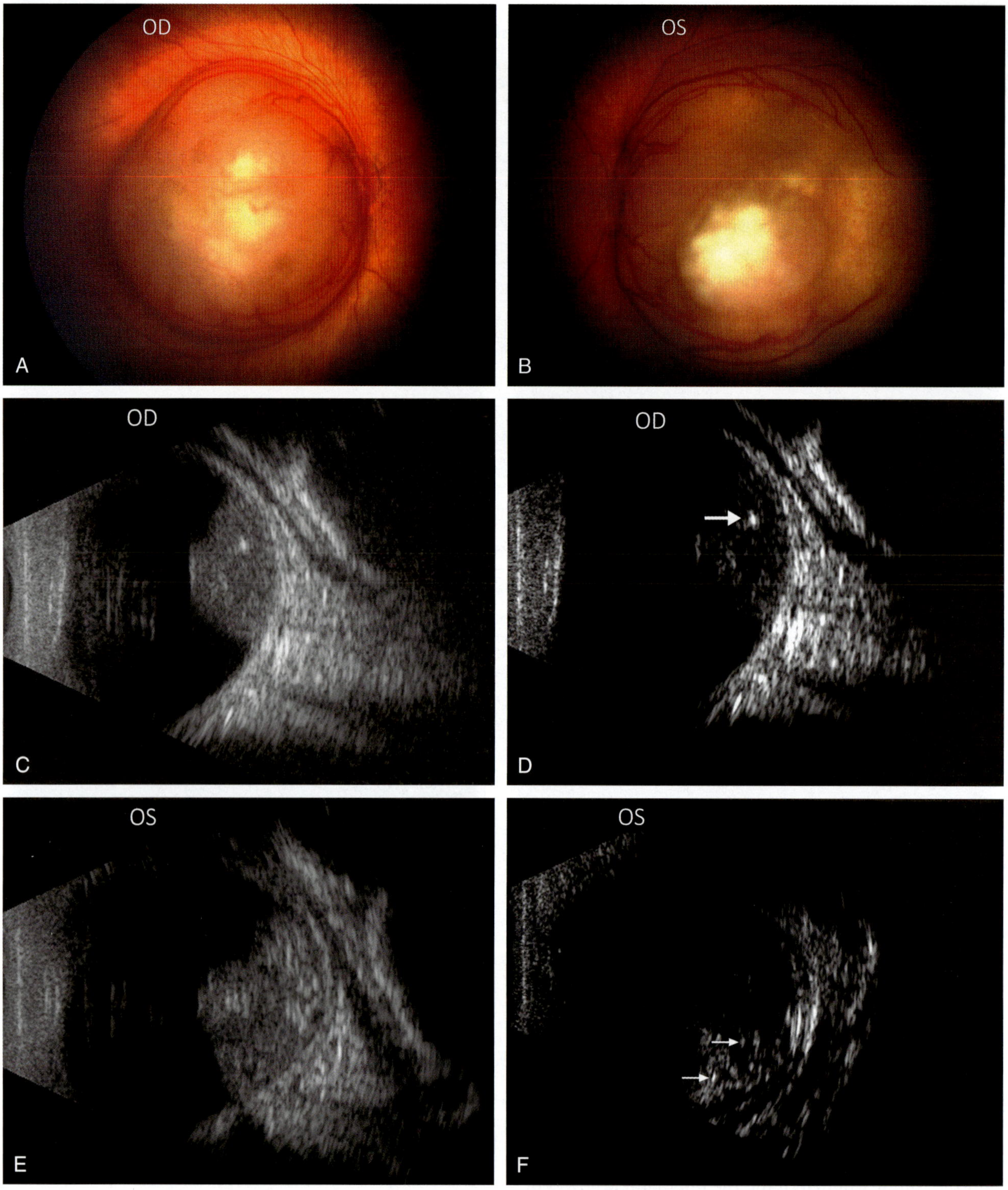

• **Fig. 8.16** Bilateral retinoblastoma. **(A–B)** Fundus photographs of retinoblastoma centered in the macula in both eyes. **(C)** A longitudinal B-scan of the right eye shows a solid retinal lesion with an irregular surface. **(D)** The same view as C at lower gain displays a solitary focus of calcium within the lesion (*arrow*). **(E)** Longitudinal B-scan left eye shows a retinoblastoma with multiple punctate calcium sources. **(F)** The same view as image E, at lower gain shows bright punctate calcium (*arrows*).

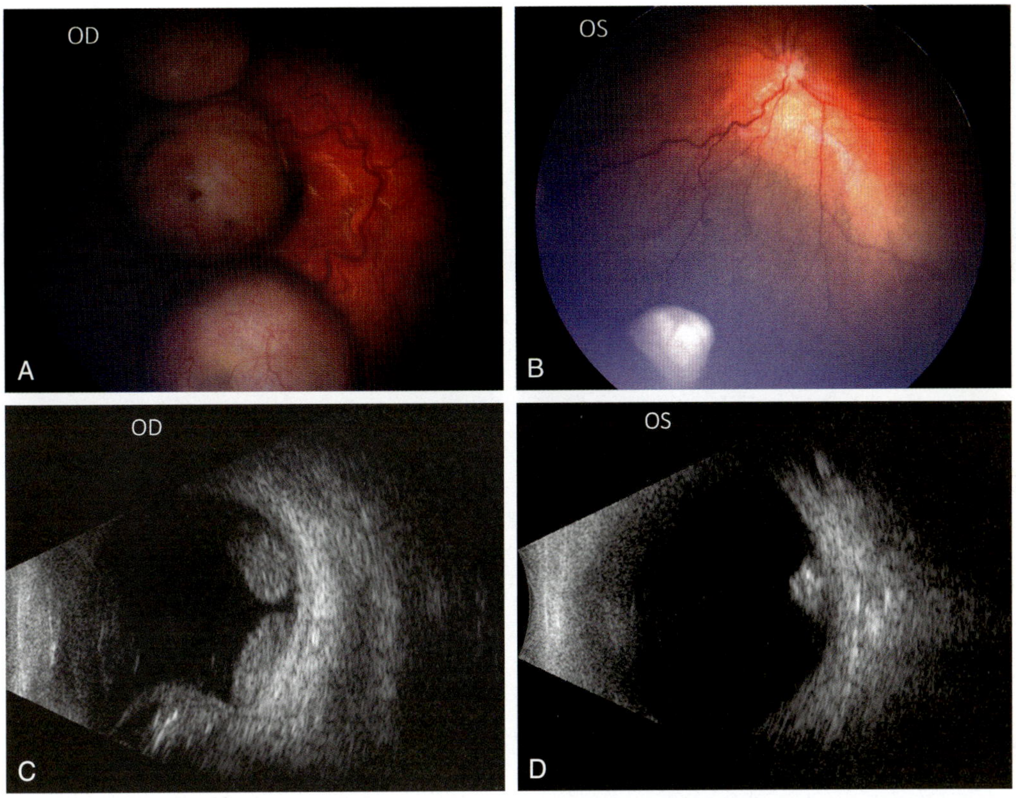

• **Fig. 8.17** Multiple retinoblastomas. **(A)** Fundus photographs show multiple retinal masses occupying the macular area in the right eye and, **(B)** a solitary, small, peripheral retinal lesion in the left eye. **(C)** Traverse view of B-scan ultrasonography shows a solid, trilobed retinal lesion in the right eye and, **(D)** a peripheral, minimally calcified retinal lesion in the left eye.

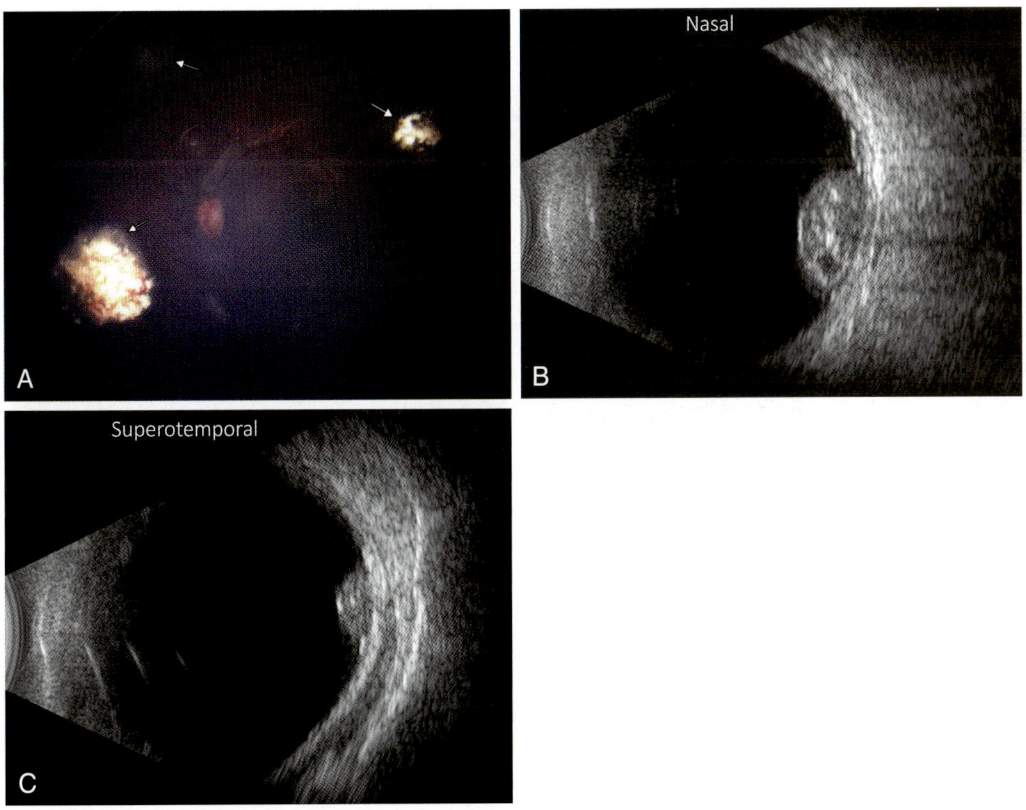

• **Fig. 8.18** Familial multiple retinoblastomas. **(A)** Wide-angle fundus photography displays three retinoblastomas (*arrows*) at midperiphery. **(B)** Transverse B-scan aimed nasally shows a medium-sized, dome-shaped retinal lesion with intrinsic calcium foci causing acoustic shadowing. **(C)** Transverse B-scan of another slightly elevated retinoblastoma located superotemporally.

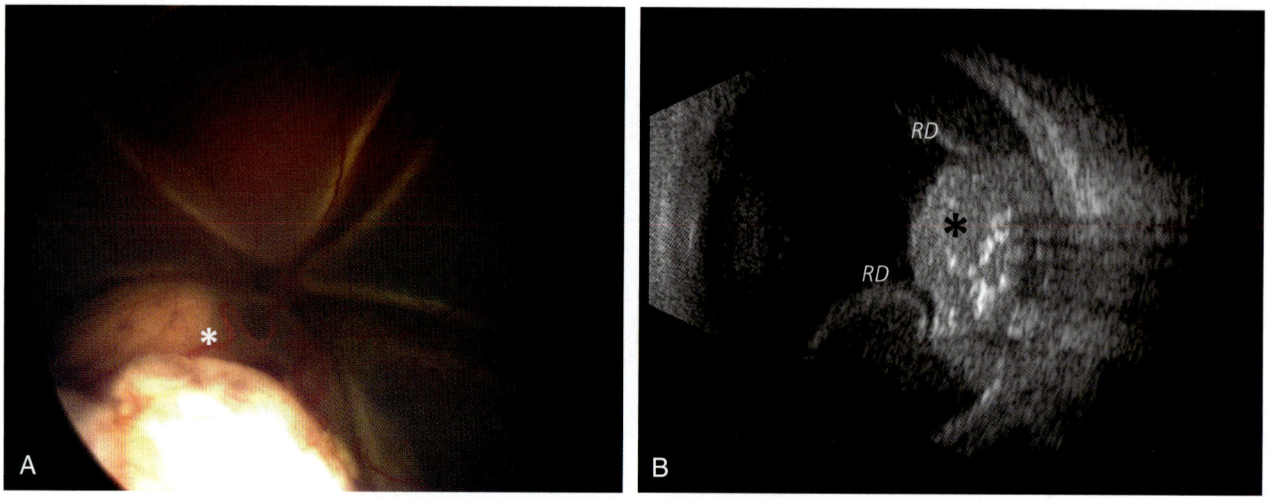

• **Fig. 8.19** Exophytic retinoblastoma. **(A)** Fundus photography shows an extensive retinal detachment and, subretinal retinoblastoma (*asterisk*). **(B)** Ultrasound B-scan shows a dome-shaped, highly reflective retinal tumor (*asterisk*), with internal calcification causing acoustic shadowing. A retinal detachment (RD) is noted at the tumor's margins.

Cavitary retinoblastoma is a variant of retinoblastoma characterized by the presence of ophthalmoscopically visible translucent cavities within the solid tumor.

CASE

A 2-year-old girl presented with leukocoria of the right eye. The ophthalmoscopic exam under anesthesia revealed a white cream retinal lesion with distinct cavitations (Fig. 8.20).

TEACHING POINTS

Intratumoral calcification presenting as an acoustic shadow is the hallmark of retinoblastoma.

The most common differential diagnoses include persistent fetal vasculature, Coat's disease, and ocular toxocariasis, all of which may mimic diffuse retinoblastoma.

Retinocytoma or Retinoma

Retinocytoma or retinoma is a benign variant of retinoblastoma. The typical ophthalmoscopic appearance of a retinocytoma is a translucent retinal mass; other frequent features are calcification, retinal pigment epithelial changes, and chorioretinal atrophy. Malignant transformation of retinocytoma into retinoblastoma rarely occurs. Despite the rarity of malignant transformation, patients with retinocytoma should be observed regularly.[21]

The median patient age at presentation is 5 years, and the mean thickness of the tumor is 2.3 mm. The tumor can be sited at the macula or have an extramacular location.[22]

Echographically, retinocytomas are slightly elevated, highly reflective retinal lesions without the involvement of the underlying choroid.[23,24]

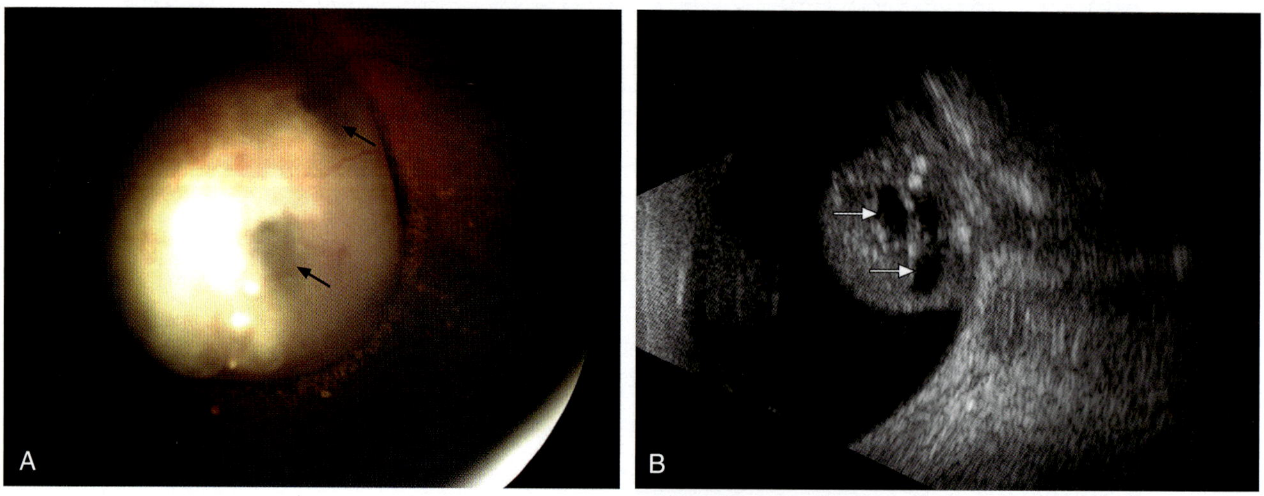

• **Fig. 8.20** Cavitary retinoblastoma. **(A)** Fundus photography shows a retinoblastoma with gray translucent cavities (*arrows*). Notice subretinal tumor seeds at the base of the lesion. **(B)** Ultrasound B-scan shows a solid dome-shaped, mainly highly reflective retinal tumor with multiple echolucent cavitated areas (*arrows*), and scattered intrinsic calcification.

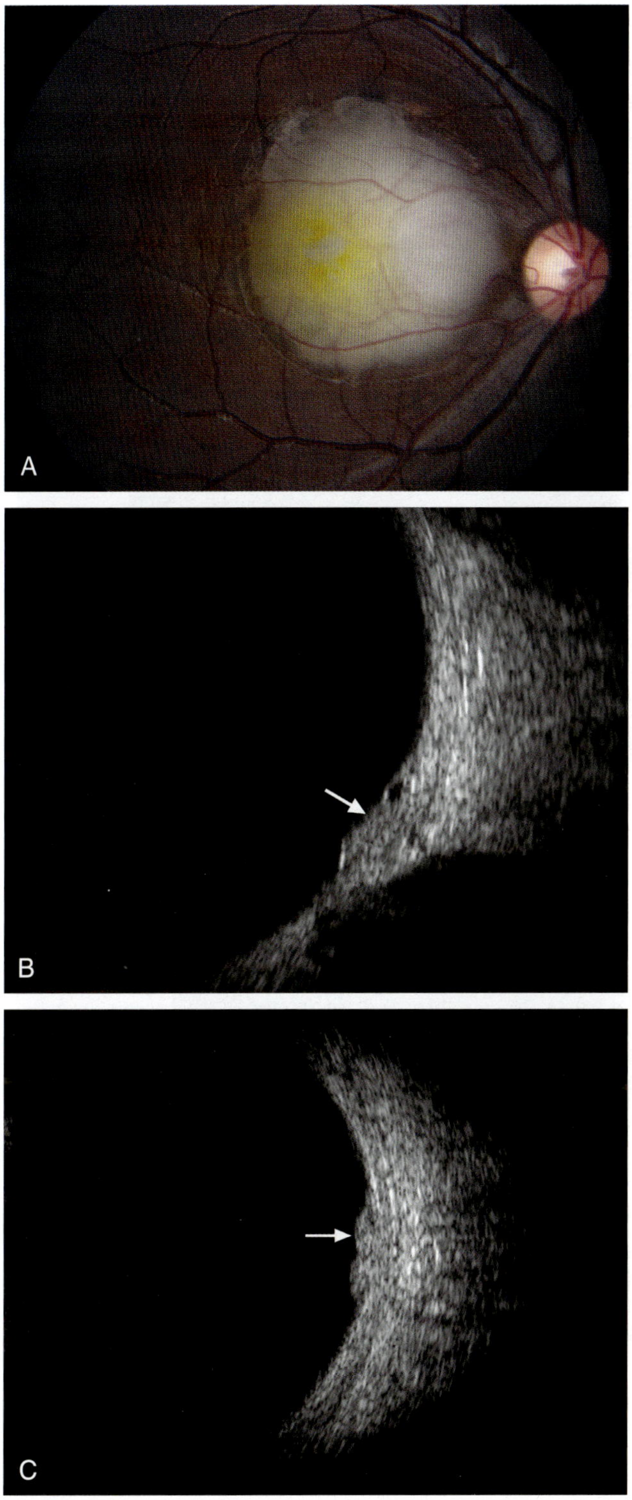

• **Fig. 8.21** Retinocytoma. **(A)** Fundus photography of a retinocytoma. **(B)** Longitudinal and **(C)** transverse B-scans show a plateau-like, highly reflective retinal lesion (*arrow*) at the macula.

CASE

A 4-year-old boy was referred for exotropia, and intraocular mass in the right eye. Ophthalmoscopy revealed a grayish, semitranslucent mass at the macula, surrounded by retinal pigment epithelial changes (Fig. 8.21). B-scan ultrasonography demonstrated a highly reflective retinal lesion measuring 1.5 mm in thickness, and 4.3 mm in largest basal diameter.

Retinal Hemangioblastoma

Retinal hemangioblastoma is a benign vascular tumor that presents as a round, orange-red mass with a dilated retinal feeding artery, and tortuous draining vein located in the juxtapapillary or peripheral retina. This tumor can present as a sporadic unifocal mass or as a manifestation of von Hippel-Lindau (VHL) disease, often with multifocal or bilateral tumors, or both.[25]

Retinal hemangioblastoma can lead to decreased visual acuity, often resulting due to tumor location on the macula and macular extension of intraretinal or subretinal fluid. Additionally, vitreous hemorrhage and tractional retinal detachment can develop.

On B-scan ultrasound, retinal hemangioblastomas are characterized as dome-shaped, mildly elevated retinal lesions with reflectivity predominately medium-high and mild intrinsic vascularity.[26]

CASE

A 34-year-old male with unremarkable ocular and systemic history presented with decreased visual acuity in the right eye for two months. Fundus examination of the right eye revealed a retinal hemangioblastoma along the superior temporal arcade with a prominent feeding artery and draining vein, and lipid exudation (Fig. 8.22 and Video 8.12).

CASE

A 32-year-old male with unremarkable ocular and medical history presented with blurry vision in the left eye. A dilated fundus exam disclosed retinal hemangioblastoma over the optic disc (Fig. 8.23 and Video 8.13).

Retinal Astrocytic Hamartoma

Retinal astrocytic hamartoma is a benign hamartomatous proliferation originating from retina glial cells (predominantly, astrocytes). The tumor is located in the retinal nerve fiber layer and appears as a sessile or slightly elevated yellow-grey mass, that may or may not be calcified. It can be present as an isolated entity or as a part of the tuberous sclerosis complex.[27]

Retinal astrocytic hamartoma can have a plaque-like or dome-shaped appearance on ultrasonography. The lesion is extremely high-reflective and causes an acoustic shadowing that varies from minimal to marked, depending on the level of calcification.[28]

CASE

An 18-year-old male has been followed for an asymptomatic, stable-in-size retinal astrocytic hamartoma for eight years. Multimodal imaging of the lesion is illustrated in Fig. 8.24 and Video 8.14. Systemic history was negative for tuberous sclerosis.

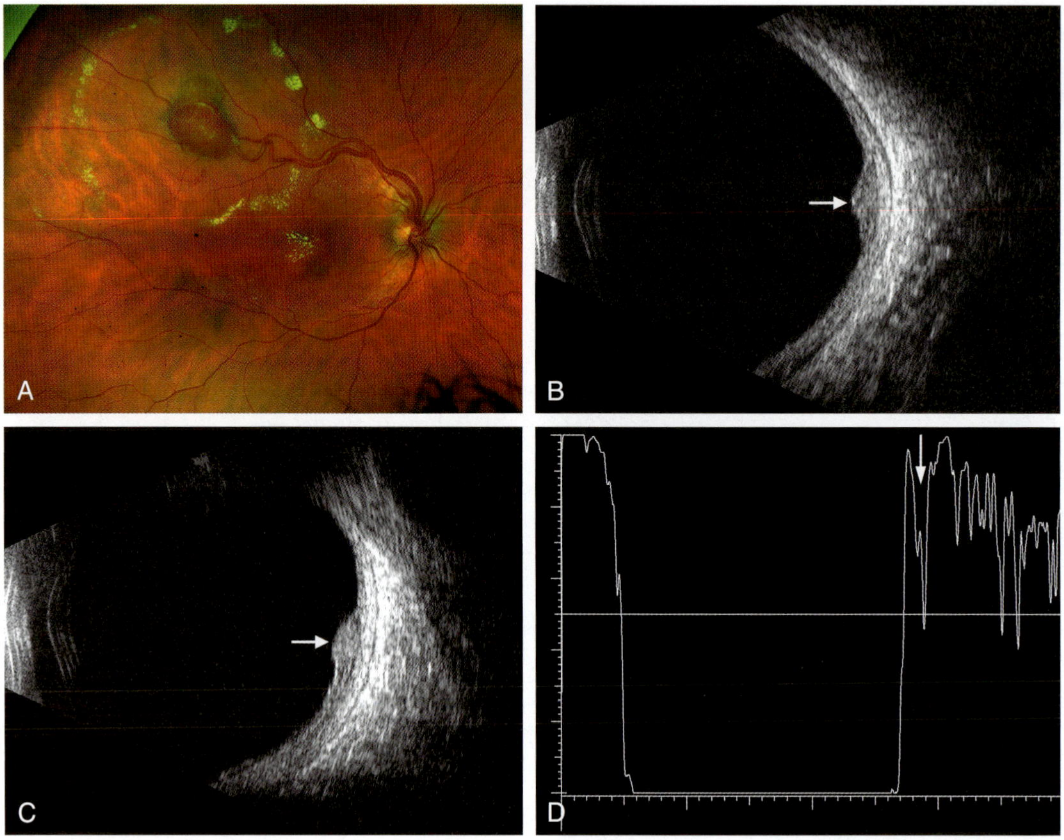

• **Fig. 8.22** Retinal Hemangioblastoma. **(A)** Fundus photography shows a retinal hemangioblastoma located superotemporal to the macula. **(B)** Transverse and **(C)** longitudinal B-scans show a mildly elevated, dome-shaped retinal lesion (*arrow*). **(D)** Corresponding A-scan shows medium-highly internal reflectivity (*arrow*).

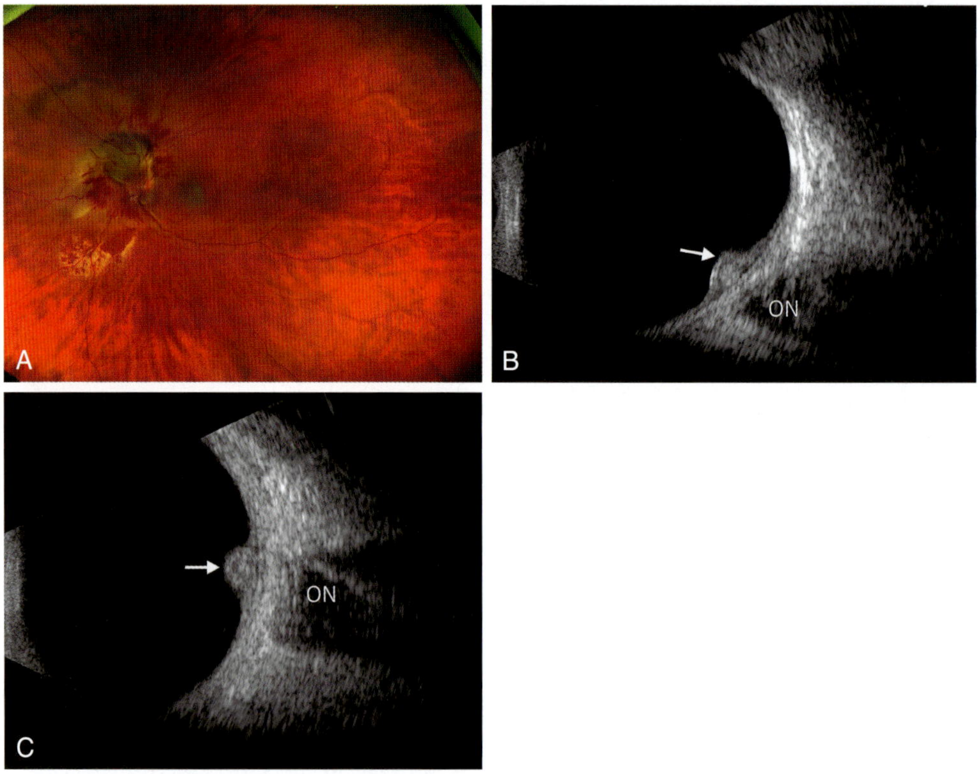

• **Fig. 8.23** Juxtapapillary Retinal Hemangioblastoma. **(A)** Fundus photography shows a hemangioblastoma surrounded by retinal hemorrhage, hard exudates, and subretinal fluid. **(B)** Longitudinal and **(C)** transverse ultrasound B-scans show a dome-shaped, hyperechoic juxtapapillary lesion (*arrow*). *ON*, Optic nerve.

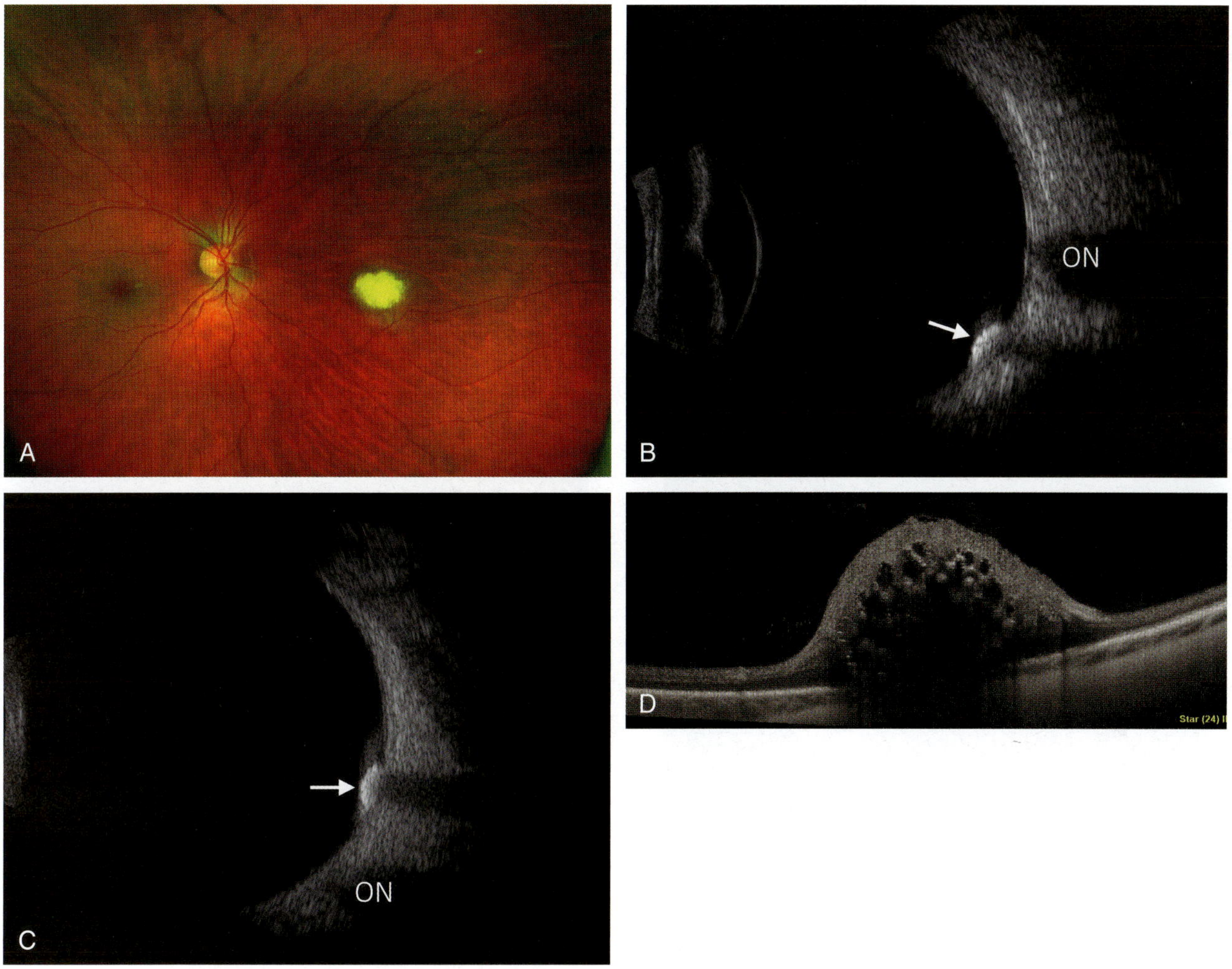

• **Fig. 8.24** Acquired retinal astrocytic hamartoma. **(A)** Fundus photography of a calcified, mulberry-type retinal astrocytic hamartoma nasal to the optic disc. **(B)** Axial horizontal and **(C)** longitudinal scans show a slightly elevated, dome-shaped, hyperreflective retinal lesion (*arrow*) causing acoustic shadowing of posterior tissues. *ON*, Optic nerve. **(D)** Optical coherence tomography shows a gradual transition from a normal retina to a hyperreflective intraretinal mass. Note the moth-eaten optically empty spaces representing intralesional calcification, and prominent optical shadowing posteriorly.

Intraocular Lymphoid Tumors

Lymphoma

Most intraocular lymphomas are of the non-Hodgkin type, most of which are B cell in origin. Based on their site of involvement and whether the disease is primary or secondary, intraocular lymphomas can be divided into primary vitreoretinal lymphoma, primary uveal lymphoma, secondary vitreoretinal lymphoma secondary to central nervous system lymphom or systemic lymphoma, and secondary to uveal lymphoma secondary to systemic lymphoma.[29]

Primary Vitreoretinal Lymphoma is a subtype of primary central nervous system lymphoma that can occur preceding, concurrent, or after central nervous system lymphoma. It is usually bilateral, and the most common presenting features are blurred vision and floaters. The typical clinical findings are vitreous cells and multifocal yellowish retinal and subretinal infiltrates.[30,31]

B-scan ultrasonography can demonstrate moderately dense vitreous opacities. These cells tend to be larger, but less dense than those seen in vitritis. Posterior vitreous detachment and sub-hyaloid opacities are common findings.

CASE

A 68-year-old female with a history of central nervous system lymphoma was referred with a complaint of blurred vision in both eyes. The best visual acuity was 20/60 in the right eye and 20/30 in the left eye. The anterior segment was unremarkable. A dilated fundus exam revealed moderate vitreous cells without retinal or choroidal infiltration (Fig. 8.25). B-scan ultrasonography showed bilateral, moderately dense vitreous haze secondary to cellularity, and no uveal thickening.

Primary uveal lymphoma is predominantly unilateral and seen in the elderly population, commonly in the fifth

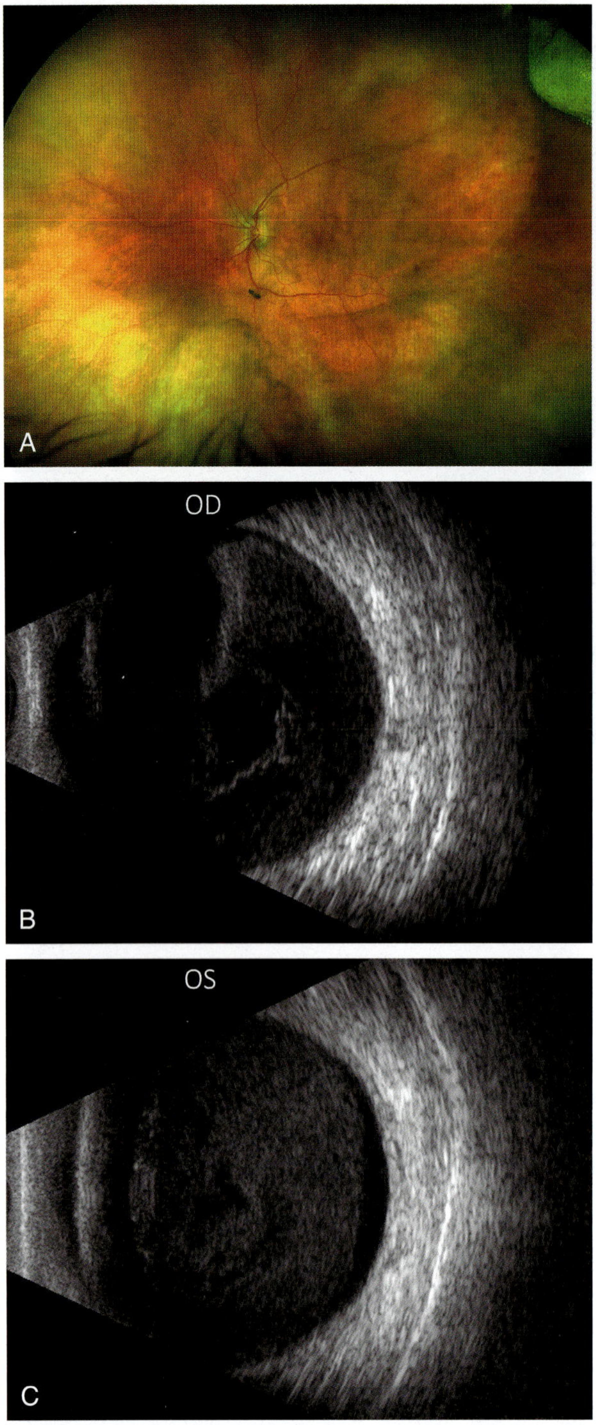

• **Fig. 8.25** Vitreoretinal lymphoma. **(A)** Wide-angle fundus photography of the left eye exhibits vitreous haze. **(B)** B-scan ultrasound of the right eye and, **(C)** left eye exhibits moderately dense vitreous haze secondary to cellularity.

to seventh decades. It is generally a low-grade B-cell lymphoma with an indolent clinical course. Primary uveal lymphoma mainly involves the choroid and, less frequently, the iris and ciliary body. Patients with uveal lymphoma typically present episodes of painless, blurred vision, and metamorphopsia secondary to exudative retinal detachment. In advanced disease, patients may develop secondary angle-closure glaucoma. Dilated fundus examination usually shows multiple yellow, creamy choroidal infiltrates. Ultimately, diffuse thickening of the uveal develops and is often associated with exudative retinal detachment. In some cases, there may be subconjunctival extension appearing as a nonmobile "salmon" patch.[29]

B-scan ultrasonography typically reveals low reflective, diffuse, or nodular choroidal thickening. Overlying subretinal fluid can be detected. Extrascleral extension, usually around the optic nerve, is a common finding. Rarely, anterior extension with infiltration of the ciliary body and iris can occur.

CASE

A 68-year-old male, presented with blurry vision and metamorphopsia in the left eye. Systemic history was negative for any neoplasm. The anterior segment was unremarkable. Ophthalmoscopy disclosed irregularly depigmented choroidal thickening with multifocal yellow infiltrates in all quadrants (Fig. 8.26). The patient had a systemic workup that revealed marginal zone lymphoma.

CASE

A 69-year-old male was referred with an initial diagnosis of posterior uveitis in the left eye, unresponsive to clinical treatment. The best corrected visual acuity was 20/25 in the right eye and hand motion in the left eye. A dilated fundus exam of the left eye revealed a yellowish diffuse choroidal lesion with retinal pigment epithelium changes and shallow retinal detachment (Fig. 8.27). B-scan ultrasonography detected a low reflective, diffuse choroidal thickening, inferior serous retinal detachment and an extrascleral extension. The patient underwent an ultrasound-guided biopsy of the extraocular lesion, and pathology revealed marginal zone lymphoma of mucosa-associated lymphoid tissue (MALT lymphoma).

TEACHING POINTS

Intraocular lymphomas frequently masquerade as inflammatory and infectious processes, resulting in the delay of accurate diagnosis.

Non-Neoplastic Disorders Simulating Intraocular Tumors

There are many lesions that may be mistaken for an intraocular tumor. Ophthalmic ultrasound combined with a detailed clinical examination can assist in the differentiation and accurate diagnosis.

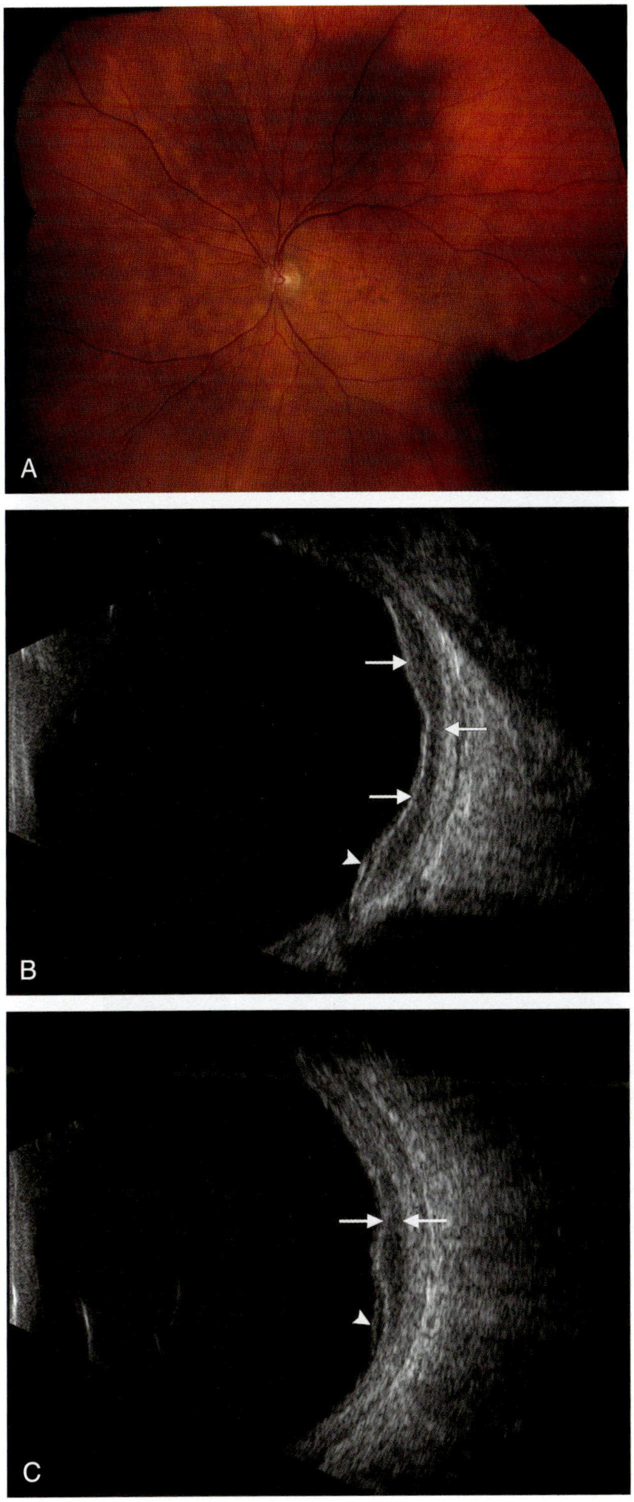

• **Fig. 8.26** Uveal lymphoma. **(A)** Fundus photo shows multiple yellow choroidal infiltrates dispersed in all quadrants. **(B)** Longitudinal and, **(C)** transverse B-scan shows a diffuse, low-reflective choroidal thickening (*arrows*) and focal subretinal fluid (*arrowhead*). There was no extrascleral extension detected.

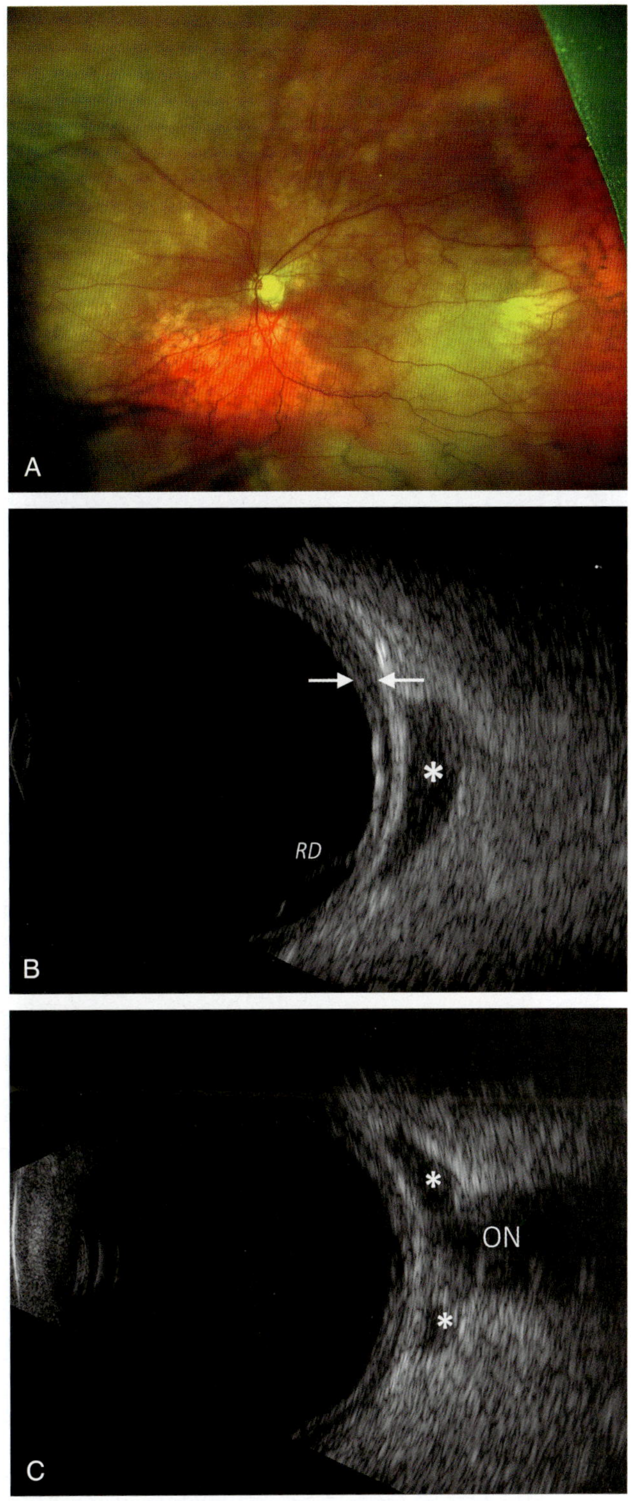

• **Fig. 8.27** Uveal lymphoma with extraocular extension. **(A)** Fundus photography exhibits diffuse choroidal infiltration with retinal pigment changes. **(B)** Transverse B-scan demonstrates a shallowly elevated, diffuse, low-reflective choroidal thickening (*arrows*) with a focal retinal elevation (*arrowhead*) and a crescent-like, low-reflective extraocular extension (*asterisk*). **(C)** Transverse B-scan through the optic disc area demonstrates a perineural location of the extraocular extension (*asterisks*). *ON*, Optic nerve.

Peripheral Exudative Hemorrhagic Chorioretinopathy

Peripheral exudative hemorrhagic chorioretinopathy (PEHCR) is an age-related, bilateral, asymmetric disorder of the peripheral ocular fundus. It typically presents in the temporal quadrants, between the equator and ora serrata. PEHCR is often misinterpreted as an intraocular tumor, particularly choroidal melanoma.

On B-scan ultrasonography, PEHCR is characterized by a dome or irregularly shaped peripheral fundus lesion. The internal structure is irregular, varying from a low reflective, exudative area to a highly reflective fibrotic area. There is no observed choroidal excavation.

CASE

An 85-year-old man was referred for evaluation of a pigmented peripheral lesion in the left eye. The best corrected visual acuity was 20/60 in the right eye, and 20/80 in the left eye. The anterior segment findings were unremarkable. Based on ophthalmoscopic and ultrasonographic exams (Fig. 8.28), a diagnosis of PEHCR was made.

Sclerochoroidal Calcification

Sclerochoroidal calcification usually manifests as asymptomatic, multiple discrete yellow placoid lesions in the midperipheral fundus of older Caucasian patients. Although most cases may be idiopathic, some patients may have underlying systemic calcium disorders. Sclerochoroidal calcification is often misdiagnosed as choroidal metastasis.

B-scan ultrasonography typically shows multifocal, plaque-like, or minimally elevated hyperreflective lesions at the sclerochoroidal interface with marked shadowing of the orbital tissues. Ultrasound can detect subtle lesions that are clinically not apparent.

CASE

A 73-year-old male was referred for possible metastatic disease after multiple, yellow-white elevated choroidal lesions were found in both eyes. He has had a history of prostate cancer treated with prostatectomy 3 years ago. Fundus examination revealed bilateral, multifocal whitish-yellow lesions at the posterior pole (Fig. 8.29 and Video 8.15). Ultrasonography demonstrated features typical of sclerochoroidal calcification.

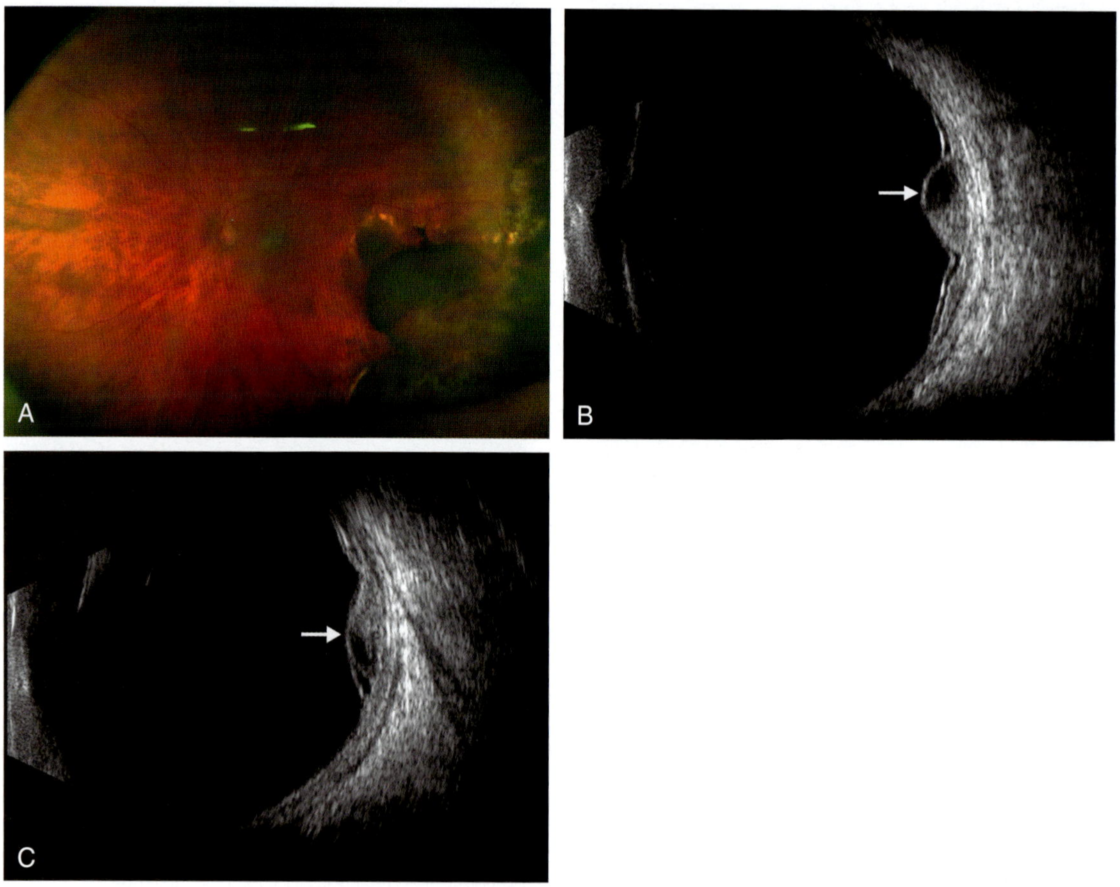

• **Fig. 8.28** Peripheral exudative hemorrhagic chorioretinopathy. **(A)** Wide-angle fundus photography demonstrates an inferotemporal peripheral fundus lesion with sub-retinal pigment epithelial hemorrhage, subretinal fluid, and lipid exudation. **(B)** Transverse and **(C)** Longitudinal B-scans show an irregularly shaped, irregularly structured chorioretinal lesion with echodense and echolucent areas. Note an area of pigmented epithelial detachment (*arrow*), with typical dome configuration and sharp insertions.

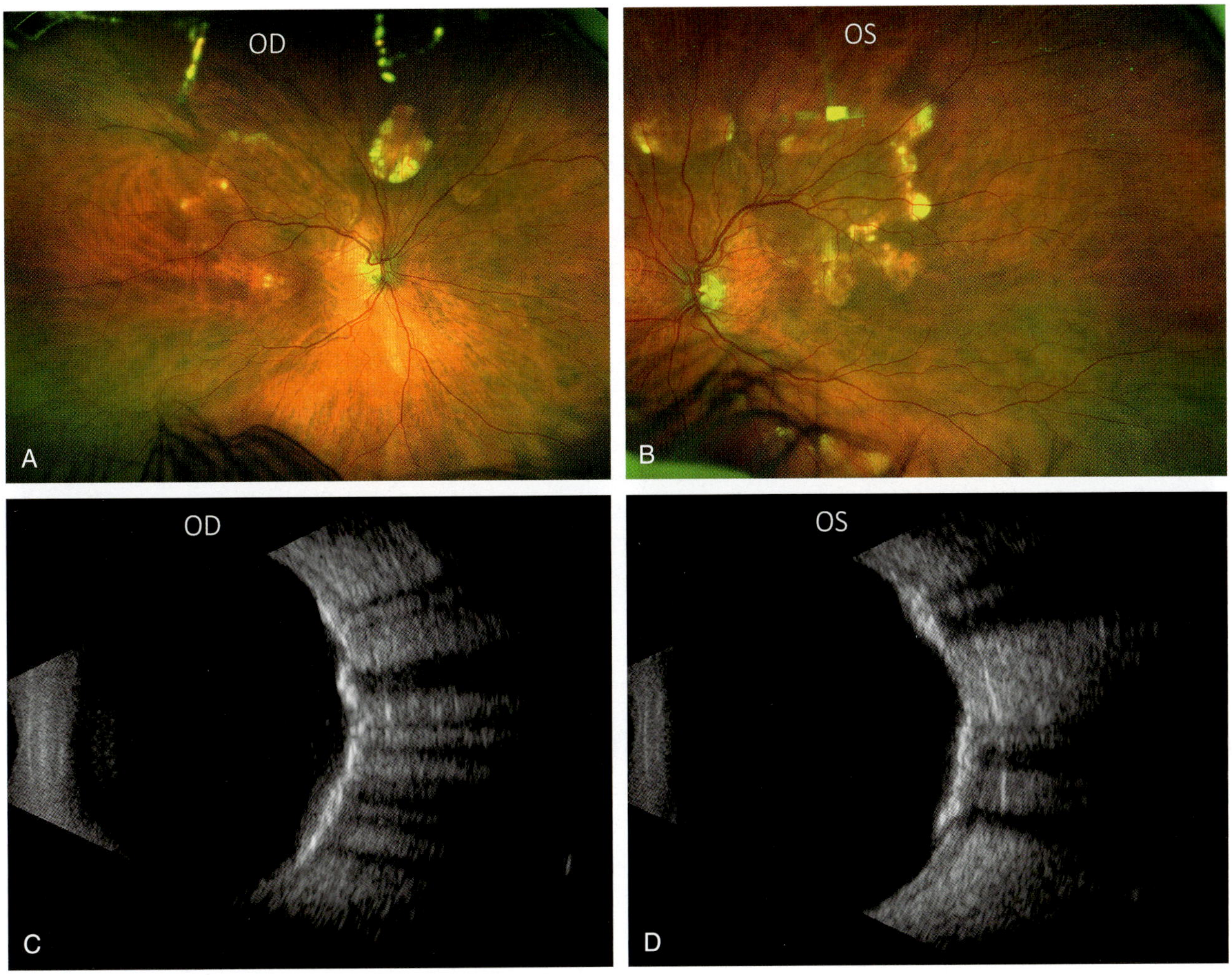

• **Fig. 8.29** Sclerochoroidal calcification. **(A–B)** Fundus photographs show multifocal, placoid, yellow lesions, located at the vascular arcades in both eyes. Transverse B-scan of the right eye **(C),** and the left eye **(D)** show plaque-like hyperreflective, mildly elevated fundus lesions with posterior acoustic shadowing.

References

1. Augsburger JJ, Corrêa ZM, Trichopoulos N, Shaikh A. Size overlap between benign melanocytic choroidal nevi and choroidal malignant melanomas. *Invest Ophthalmol Vis Sci*. 2008;49:2823–2828.
2. Shields CL, Dalvin LA, Ancona-Lezama D, et al. Choroidal nevus imaging features in 3,806 cases and risk factors for transformation into melanoma in 2,355 Cases. *Retina*. 2019;39(10):1840–1851.
3. Ayres MB, Provenzano G, Demirci H. Ultrasound Assessment of Vascularity in Choroidal Nevus. 2019 [Poster Presentation]. International Society of Ocular Oncology Biennial Conference, Los Angeles, USA.
4. Shields JA, Demirci H, Mashayekhi A, Shields CL. Melanocytoma of the optic disc in 115 cases: the 2004 Samuel Johnson Memorial Lecture, part 1. *Ophthalmology*. 2004;111:1739–1746.
5. Singh AD, Turell ME, Topham AK. Uveal melanoma: trends in incidence, treatment, and survival. *Ophthalmology*. 2011;118:1881–1885.
6. Ossoinig KC, Blodi FC. Preoperative differential diagnosis of tumors with echography. III. Diagnosis of intraocular tumors. In: Blodi FC, ed. St. Louis: Mosby; 1974. *Current Concepts in Ophthalmology*. IV:296–312.
7. Collaborative Ocular Melanoma Study Group, Boldt HC, Byrne SF, et al. Baseline echographic characteristics of tumors in eyes of patients enrolled in the Collaborative Ocular Melanoma Study: COMS report no. 29. *Ophthalmology*. 2008;115(8):1390–1397.
8. Shields CL, Kaliki S, Livesey M, et al. Association of ocular and oculodermal melanocytosis with the rate of uveal melanoma metastasis: analysis of 7872 consecutive eyes. *JAMA Ophthalmol*. 2013;131:993–1003.
9. Harbour JW, Murray TG, Byrne SF, et al. Intraoperative echographic localization of iodine 125 episcleral radioactive plaques for posterior uveal melanoma. *Retina*. 1996;16:129–134.
10. Aziz HA, Al Zahrani YA, Bena J, et al. Episcleral brachytherapy of uveal melanoma: role of intraoperative echographic confirmation. *Br J Ophthalmol*. 2017;101:747–751.
11. Demirci H, Shields CL, Chao AN, Shields JA. Uveal metastasis from breast cancer in 264 patients. *Am J Ophthalmol*. 2003;136:264–271.
12. Arepalli S, Kaliki S, Shields CL. Choroidal metastases: origin, features, and therapy. *Indian J Ophthalmol*. 2015;63:122–127.
13. Shields JA, Shields CL, Materin MA, Marr BP, Demirci H, Mashayekhi A. Changing concepts in management of circumscribed

choroidal hemangioma: the 2003 J. Howard Stokes Lecture, Part 1. *Ophthalmic Surg Lasers Imaging.* 2004;35:383–394.
14. Krohn J, Rishi P, Froystein T, Singh AD. Circumscribed choroidal haemangioma: clinical and topographical features. *Br J Ophthalmol.* 2019;103:1448–1452.
15. Verbeek AM, Koutentakis P, Deutman AF. Circumscribed choroidal hemangioma diagnosed by ultrasonography. A retrospective analysis of 40 cases. *Int Ophthalmol.* 1995;19:185–189.
16. Aylward GW, Chang TS, Pautler SE, Gass JD. A long-term follow-up of choroidal osteoma. *Arch Ophthalmol.* 1998;116(10):1337–1341.
17. Shields CL, Shields JA, Augsburger JJ. Choroidal osteoma. *Surv Ophthalmol.* 1988;33(1):17–27.
18. Gass JD, Guerry RK, Jack RL, Harris G. Choroidal osteoma. *Arch Ophthalmol.* 1978;96(3):423–428.
19. Shields CL, Shields JA. Diagnosis and management of retinoblastoma. *Cancer Control.* 2004;11:317–327.
20. Lin FY, Chintagumpala MM. Neonatal retinoblastoma. *Clin Perinatol.* 2021;48:53–70.
21. Singh AD, Santos CM, Shields CL, Shields JA, Eagle Jr RC. Observations on 17 patients with retinocytoma. *Arch Ophthalmol.* 2000;118:199–205.
22. Shields CL, Srinivasan A, Lucio-Alvarez JA, Shields JA. Retinocytoma/retinoma: comparative analysis of clinical features in 78 tumors and rate of transformation into retinoblastoma over 20 years. *J AAPOS.* 2021;25:147.e1–147.e8.
23. Rb Garoon, Medina CA, Scelfo C, Harbour JW. Retinocytoma with vitreous seeding: new insights from enhanced depth imaging optical coherence tomography and high-resolution posterior segment ultrasonography. *Retin Cases Brief Rep.* 2021;15:68–70.
24. Temkar S, Pujari A, Chawla R, Kumar A. Multimodal imaging in a case of retinocytoma. *Indian J Ophthalmol.* 2018;66:444–447.
25. Di Nicola M, Williams Jr BK, Hua J, et al. Photodynamic therapy for retinal hemangioblastoma: treatment outcomes of 17 consecutive patients. *Ophthalmol Retina.* 2022;6:80–88.
26. Russell JF, Villegas VM, Schwartz SG, et al. Multimodal imaging in the diagnosis of exophytic juxtapapillary retinal capillary hemangioblastoma. *Am J Ophthalmol.* 2021;225:128–136.
27. Shields CL, Benevides R, Materin MA, Shields JA. Optical coherence tomography of retinal astrocytic hamartoma in 15 cases. *Ophthalmology.* 2006;113:1553–1557.
28. Stacey AW, Pefkianaki M, Ilginis T, et al. Clinical features and multi-modality imaging of isolated retinal astrocytic hamartoma. *Ophthalmic Surg Lasers Imaging Retina.* 2019;50:e1–e9.
29. Aronow ME, Singh AD. The use of imaging in the diagnosis and management of intraocular lymphoma. *Int Ophthalmol Clin.* 2012;52:199–208.
30. Dalvin LA, Lim LS, Ancona-Lezama D, et al. Clinical features predictive of survival in patients with vitreoretinal lymphoma: analysis of 70 patients at a single ocular oncology center. *Asia Pac J Ophthalmol.* 2020;9(2):110–116.
31. Cani AK, Hovelson DH, Demirci H, Johnson MW, Tomlins SA, Rao RC. Next generation sequencing of vitreoretinal lymphomas from small-volume intraocular liquid biopsies: new routes to targeted therapies. *Oncotarget.* 2017;8:7989–7998.

9

Orbit Tumors and Tumor-Like Lesions

BERNADETE AYRES, CHRISTINE C. NELSON, AND HAKAN DEMIRCI

Introduction

The orbit is a small anatomic space with a wide range of distinct anatomical and histological structures. The orbit and ocular adnexa include a broad spectrum of tissues, including skin, bone, ocular globe, muscles, nerves, meninges, fat, vessels, lacrimal gland, and others. This diversity of tissues can be the site of origin for the various tumor and tumor-like lesions, both in adults and children.

A compressive history-taking, systemic, and ophthalmic examinations are essential in assessing a patient with orbital pathology. Multimodality imaging with computed tomography (CT), magnetic resonance imaging (MRI), and ultrasonography (US) can provide crucial information for diagnosing and managing orbital lesions. Of course, the histopathological exam, either by fine-needle aspiration or incisional/excisional biopsy, is still the gold standard in the definitive diagnosis of orbital lesions.

Cystic Lesions

Dermoid Cyst

Dermoid cyst is the most frequent orbital tumor in children, accounting for nearly 14% of all orbital lesions,[1] and it is generated from epithelial sequestration.[2]

It is typically located extraconally and in superolateral quadrant along the frontozygomatic suture. Dermoid cysts usually contain skin appendages, including hair, also bone, and teeth.

Clinically, it presents as a painless mass in the periocular or periorbital region; this may be soft, or firm, moveable, or fixed to the bone. Dermoid cysts are slow-growing benign lesions; however, they may occasionally rupture and cause acute inflammation.

On B-scan ultrasonography, dermoid cysts are cystic lesions with well-circumscribed, oval or rounded shape, and a smooth margin. The internal reflectivity is usually low; however, cysts rich in epidermal appendages have a more heterogeneous structure and higher internal reflectivity.

CASE

A 6-month-old infant presented with a visible mass in the superolateral area of the left upper lid that was noticed at 2 months of age. The mass was palpable, firm, nontender, and located along the superotemporal orbital rim (Fig. 9.1).

CASE

A 25-year-old male presented for evaluation of a recurrent enlarging mass in the left brow region. On examination, the lesion was mobile, soft, superficial, and non-tethered. The patient underwent surgical excision. During the surgery, the cyst ruptured with gentle manipulation, releasing contents that included keratin debris and hair follicles, consistent with a dermoid cyst (Fig. 9.2 and Video 9.1). The lesion was firmly attached to the zygomaticofrontal suture line of the lateral orbital rim.

Microphthalmos With Orbital Cyst

Microphthalmos with orbital cyst is a rare congenital anomaly of the embryonic eye caused by improper fusion of the margins of the fetal fissure. The neuroectodermal tissue of retina and optic nerve protrudes through the congenital defect (coloboma) in the wall of a microphthalmic eye and form a cyst lined by a neuroectoderm. The resulting globe remains stable, leading to microphthalmia. Most cases are unilateral and may appear either as an isolated finding or in association with other systemic abnormalities.[3,4]

These lesions are often visible at birth. At presentation, a large, compressible mass occupying the orbit and stretching the lid is noted. The cyst may be large enough to obscure the microphthalmic eye.

On B-scan ultrasonography, the cyst appears as a well-outlined, smooth, echolucent cavity displacing the microphthalmic globe. A-scan ultrasonography demonstrates low internal reflectivity.

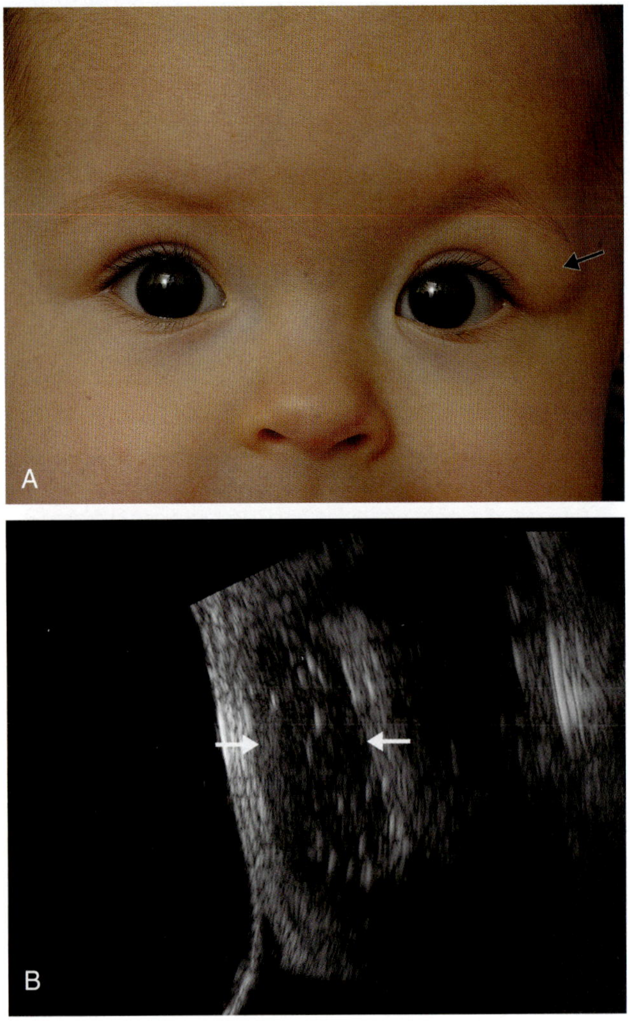

• **Fig. 9.1** Dermoid cyst. **(A)** External photography shows a left superotemporal superficial dermoid cyst (*arrow*). **(B)** Paraocular immersion B-scan showing well-circumscribed, oval, and mainly low-reflective lesion (*arrows*) with heterogeneous contents.

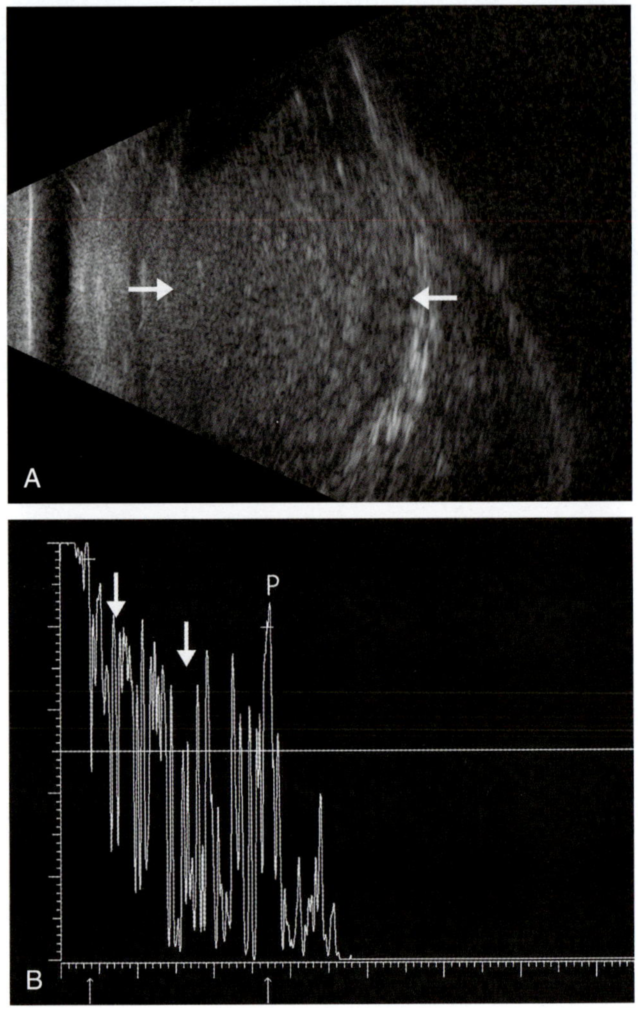

• **Fig. 9.2** Dermoid cyst. **(A)** B-scan ultrasonography exhibits a homogeneous oval lesion (*arrows*). **(B)** Corresponding A-scan ultrasonography exhibits medium-high reflective lesion (*arrows*) with moderate sound attenuation. *P*, posterior margin spike.

CASE

A 2-week-old boy presented with a large orbital lesion, bulging eyelids, and a microphthalmic eye. Systemic evaluation disclosed agenesis of the corpus callosum and cerebral ventriculomegaly. The patient underwent surgical excision of the orbital cyst and enucleation of the microphthalmic eye (Fig. 9.3).

Respiratory Epithelial Orbital Cysts

Cysts lined by respiratory epithelium in the orbit are most commonly mucoceles, secondary to chronic paranasal sinus disease and sometimes due to previous sinus trauma many years earlier. Rarely, they may occur following orbital trauma or as a choristoma.

Post-traumatic respiratory epithelial cysts are formed by the proliferation of respiratory epithelium deposited into the orbit through a fracture from previous orbital trauma or following orbital surgery.[5,6]

Patients usually present with unilateral proptosis and globe displacement. Most of the post-traumatic cysts are located inferiorly in the orbit cavity, while congenital cysts usually are located inferomedially.

On B-scan ultrasonography, respiratory epithelial orbital cysts are typically well-circumscribed, smooth, round, or oval-shaped, compressible lesions. The internal structure can vary from homogeneous and low reflectivity to more heterogeneous images with increased reflectivity, depending on the amount of mucoid contents.

CASE

A 32-year-old man presented with progressive left upper lid swelling and a palpable mass. His past history included congenital anophthalmia and orbital floor surgery. The patient underwent surgical excision of the orbital cyst, and the histopathological exam revealed a respiratory epithelial-lined inclusion cyst (Fig. 9.4 and Video 9.2).

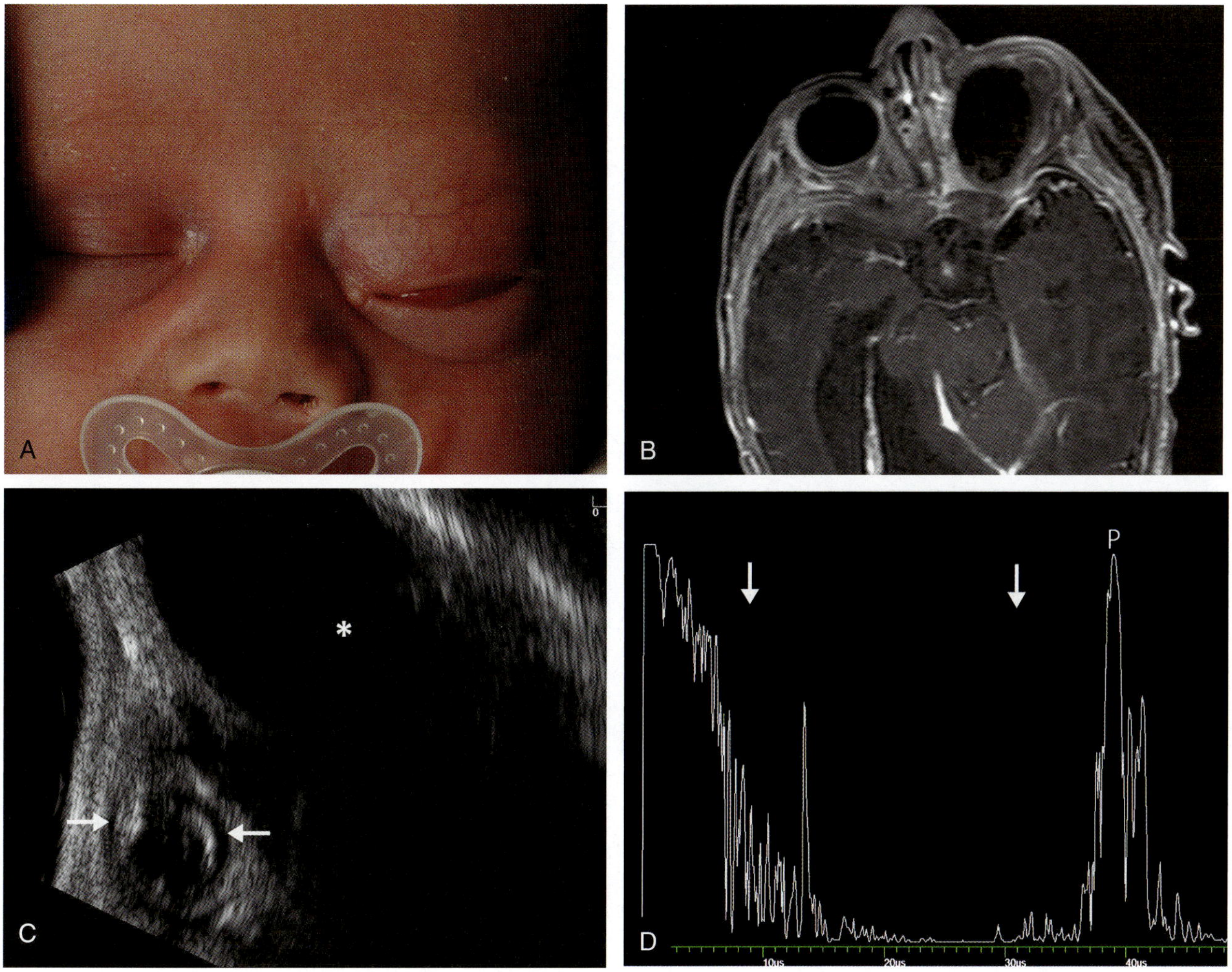

• **Fig. 9.3** Microphthalmos with orbital cyst. **(A)** External photography of a 2-week-old boy with a large orbital mass that is bulging eyellids. **(B)** T1-weighted axial MR image of the orbit shows a large left orbital cyst and a microphtalmic eye. **(C)** Immersion B-scan ultrasonography shows a large orbital cystic lesion (*asterisk*) and a microphthalmic eye (*arrows*). **(D)** The corresponding A-scan shows a low-reflective lesion (*arrow*). *P*, Posterior margin spike.

Orbital Mucocele

Mucoceles are cystic lesions that arise from obstruction of the paranasal sinus and can erode through the orbit. The lesion occurs in all decades of life but is mostly seen in the fifth to seventh decades. The frontal and frontoethmoidal sinus are the most frequent sources of mucoceles.[3]

Patients often have a history of sinusitis. The history is usually of gradual onset over weeks to months. The initial presentation usually shows proptosis displacement of the globe, upper eyelid swelling, a palpable mass, and orbital pain.

Mucoceles are identified on the B-scan ultrasonography as a large, well-outlined, extraconal, round or oval, hypoechoic mass that extends from the adjacent sinus. The lesions are usually cystic and located superonasally. A bone defect can be detected. A-scan ultrasonography displays a low internal reflective, regular internal structure.

CASE

A 64-year-old female presented with left-sided proptosis and pain around the eye. She had a history of frontal sinus surgery. She had swelling of the left upper lid, displacement of the eye inferiorly, and a palpable mass at the superior orbital rim. Orbital ultrasound and CT scan showed a left orbital mucocele originating from the frontal sinus. The patient underwent an excision of the mass, and the histopathological exam was consistent with a mucocele (Fig. 9.5).

CASE

A 45-year-old male presented with a 6-month history of right-sided proptosis and upper lid swelling. CT scan and ultrasound showed a mass extending from the frontal sinus to the orbital cavity through a bone defect in the orbital roof. The mass was compressing and displacing the eyeball downward (Fig. 9.6 and Video 9.3).

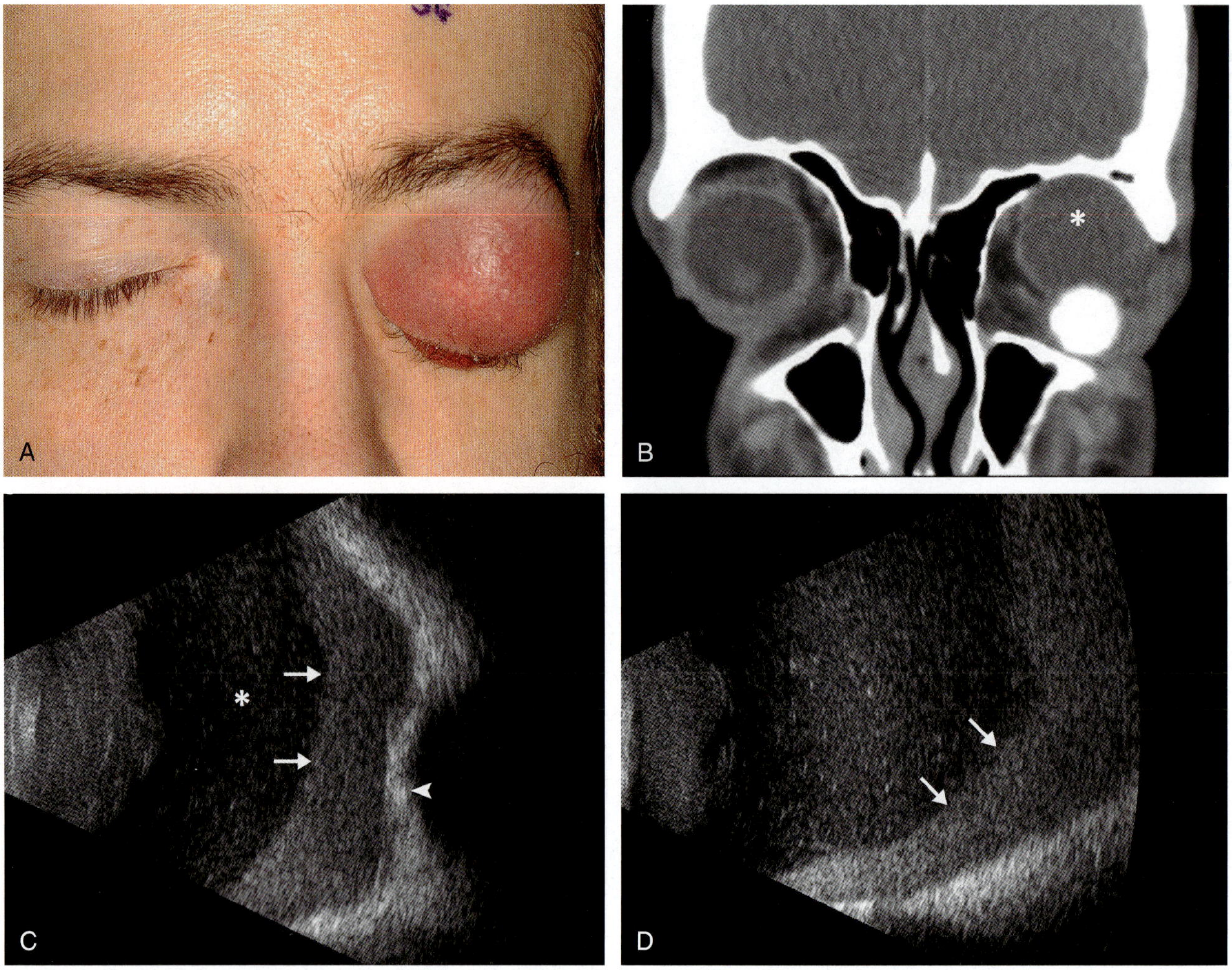

• **Fig. 9.4** Respiratory epithelial orbital cyst. **(A)** External photography shows a significant left proptosis and swelling of the upper eyelid. **(B)** A coronal CT scan shows a large orbital cystic lesion (*asterisk*) and spherical hyperattenuating orbital implant inferiorly. **(C)** B-scan ultrasonography shows a large orbital lesion (*asterisk*) with moderately dense mucoid content with a fluid level (*arrows*). Note the edge of an echodense orbital implant inferior to the cyst (*arrowhead*). **(D)** On a dynamic exam, with changing head position, the mucoid contents were shifted (*arrows*).

Vascular Tumors

Infantile Hemangioma

Infantile hemangiomas are congenital hamartomas of blood vessels, predominately of capillary. Infantile hemangioma is the most common tumor of the orbit and periorbital areas in childhood.

The lesions can be superficial in the eyelid or extend deeper into the orbit. The tumor may be present at birth, but in most cases, it becomes apparent within the first few weeks to months of life. They undergo a proliferative phase during the first year of life, followed by an involution phase over several years.[7]

Orbital infantile hemangioma appears as a red or bluish eyelid mass. Deep orbital tumors can cause proptosis and displacement of the eye. The lesion becomes more prominent when the child cries, as observed by the parents.[3]

On B-scan ultrasound, infantile hemangiomas are usually poor-outlined, irregularly shaped lesions with heterogeneous internal structures. On kinetic study, the masses are compressible, and exhibit marked spontaneous internal motion, consistent with vascularity.

On the A-scan ulreasound exam, infantile hemangiomas exhibit irregular structures and mainly medium-high to high amplitude spikes.[8]

CASE

An eight-week-old male infant presented with a four-week history of left upper left swelling. The external exam showed a redhued mass causing mechanical ptosis and obstruction of the visual axis. Imaging studies were consistent with infantile hemangioma (Fig. 9.7 and Video 9.4). The patient had oral propranolol therapy, with significant improvement.

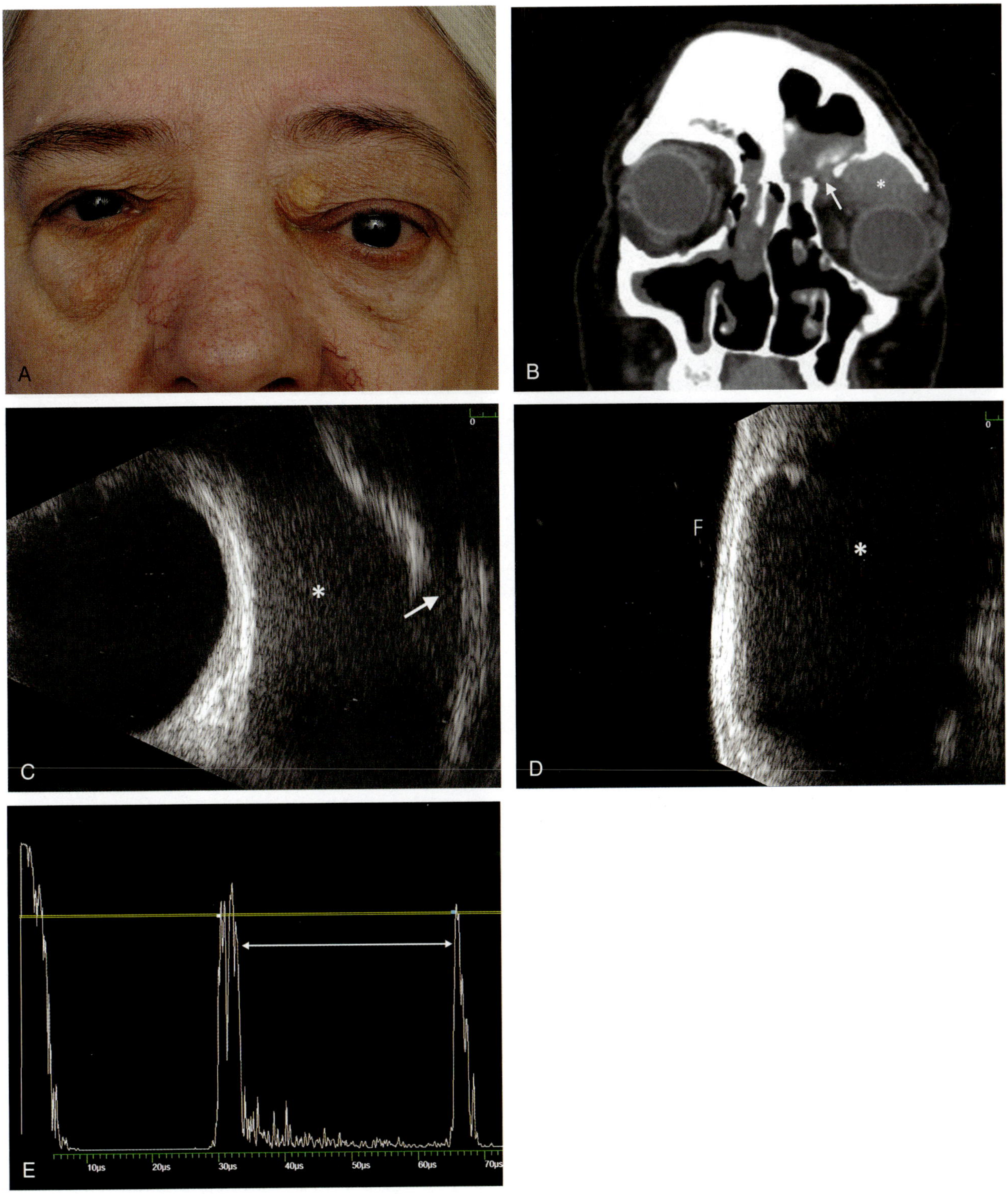

• **Fig. 9.5** Orbital mucocele. **(A)** External photography shows left-upper lid swelling, proptosis, and inferior eye displacement in a patient presenting orbital mucocele. **(B)** A coronal CT scan shows a large expansile left fronto-orbital mucocele (*asterisk*) and hypoglobus. There was a focal area of bony defect (*arrow*). **(C)** Longitudinal B-scan ultrasound aimed superiorly, through a mucocele, showing a large, well-outlined, low-reflective lesion (*asterisk*) with associated bone defect (*arrow*). **(D)** Modified immersion B-scan ultrasound showing low-reflective lesion (*asterisk*); *F*, Fluid **(E)** A-scan ultrasound showing extremely low internal reflectivity (*arrow*).

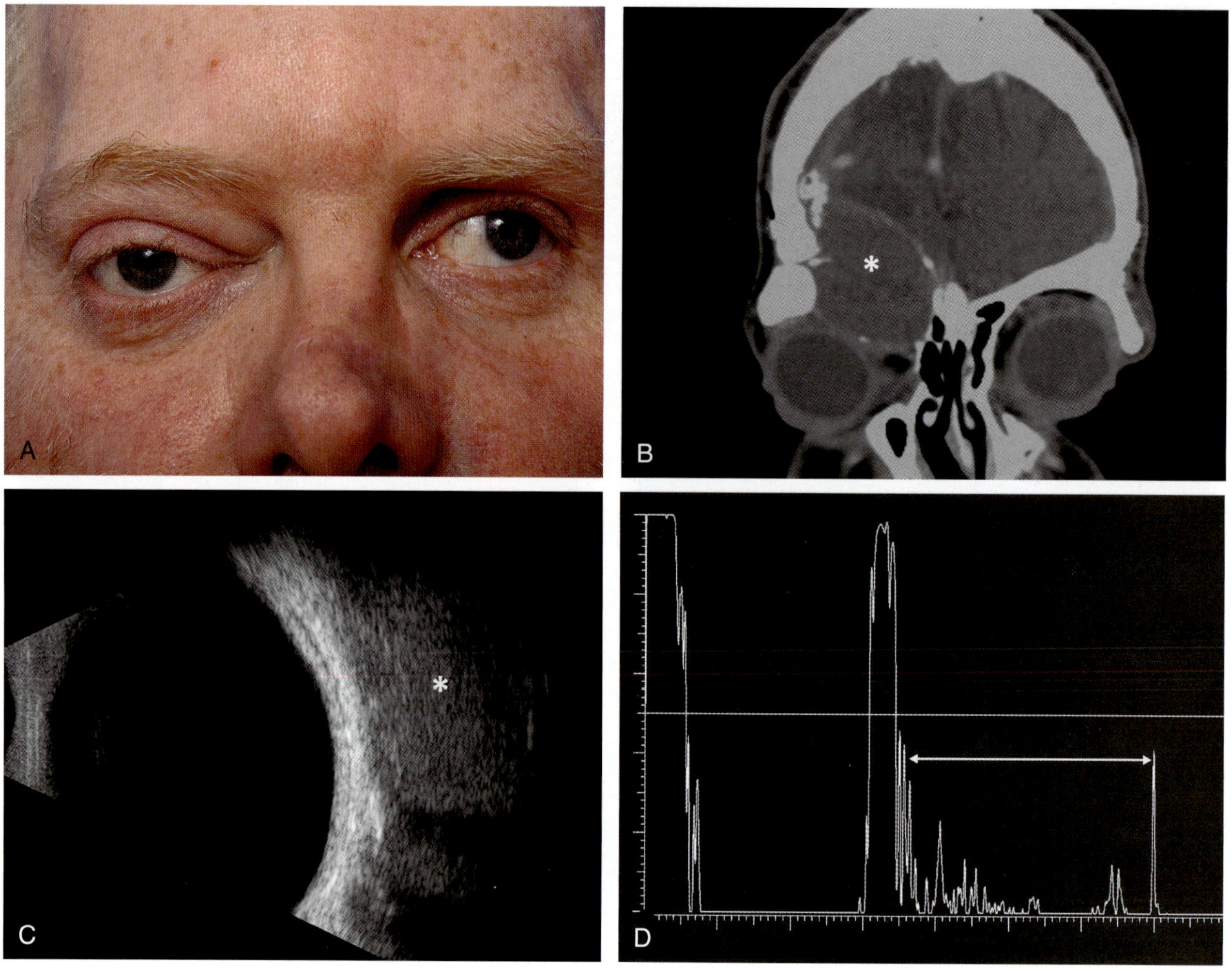

• **Fig. 9.6** Orbital mucocele. **(A)** External photography shows right-sided proptosis and upper lid swelling. The right globe was inferiorly displaced. **(B)** Coronal CT scan shows a large frontal and orbital mucocele (*asterisk*) with extensive bone erosion of the orbital roof. **(C)** Transverse B-scan ultrasound aimed superiorly shows a large low-reflective lesion (*asterisk*). **(D)** A-scan ultrasound shows low-reflective internal echoes (*arrow*).

CASE

A 3-month-old male infant born at 34 weeks gestational age, presented to the clinic with a two-week history of rapidly progressive left proptosis. The pregnancy was uneventful. Imaging studies were consistent with infantile hemangioma (Fig. 9.8 and Video 9.5). The patient underwent oral propranolol treatment with excellent response and decreased lesion size.

Cavernous Venous Malformation

Cavernous venous malformation of the orbit, previously called cavernous hemangioma, is a common primary orbital lesion of adults. It occurs more often in women, with a peak incidence in the fifth decade.[9]

The most common sign of cavernous venous malformation is a painless, unilateral, slow progressive proptosis from the preferential involvement of the intraconal orbital space. Decreased vision can be related to the hyperopic shift caused by a posterior globe indentation. Edema, pallor, or atrophy of the optic disc can be present.

A significant number of cavernous venous malformations present as incidental, asymptomatic lesions discovered on CT or MRI performed for unrelated reasons.[10]

On B-scan ultrasound, cavernous venous malformation appears as a well-circumscribed, round, or oval lesion with a smooth surface. The lesion is homogeneous and has a firm consistency. Mild intrinsic vascular flow can be detected. Flattening of the globe, optic nerve, or muscle deviation can be observed in the case of large masses. The A-scan ultrasound typically shows a regular internal structure with medium-high to high reflectivity and moderate to strong acoustic attenuation.

CASE

A 46-year-old female presented with a four-year history of macular change in the left eye and hyperopic shift. The external examination showed left-sided proptosis. A fundoscopic examination revealed choroidal folds on the macula. The imaging study was consistent with a cavernous venous malformation (Fig. 9.9 and Video 9.6). The patient underwent an excision of the leison, and pathology confirmed cavernous venous malformation.

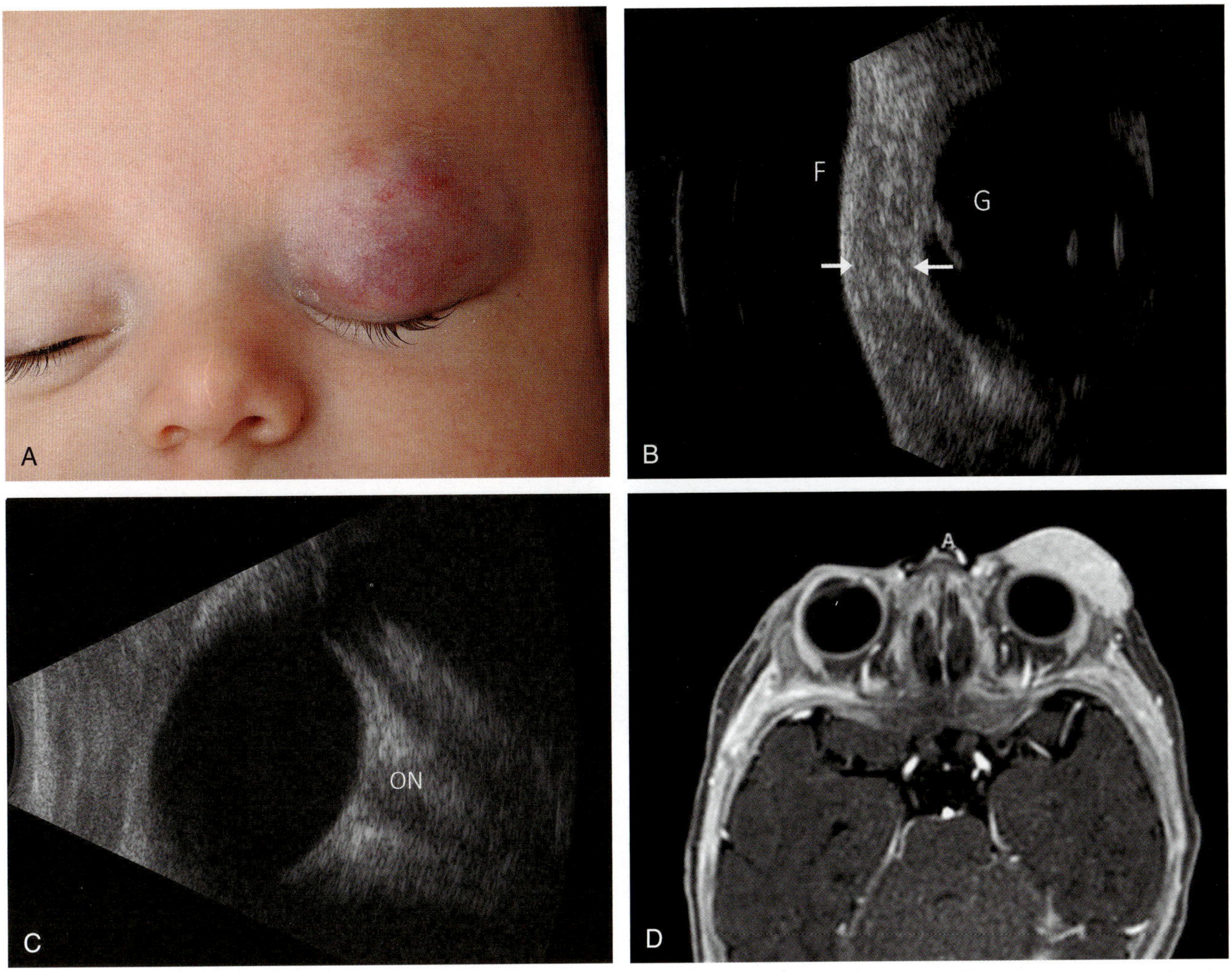

• **Fig. 9.7** Infantile hemangioma. **(A)** External photography shows a reddish left-upper lid mass. **(B)** Modified immersion B-scan through the lids displays a large, irregularly structured, hyperechoic, anterior orbital mass (*arrows*) adjacent to the globe (G). *F*, Fluid. **(C)** Longitudinal B-scan shows no extension of the lesion to the retrobulbar space; *ON*, optic nerve. (D) Axial post-contrast T1-weighted MRI shows periorbital lobulated mass.

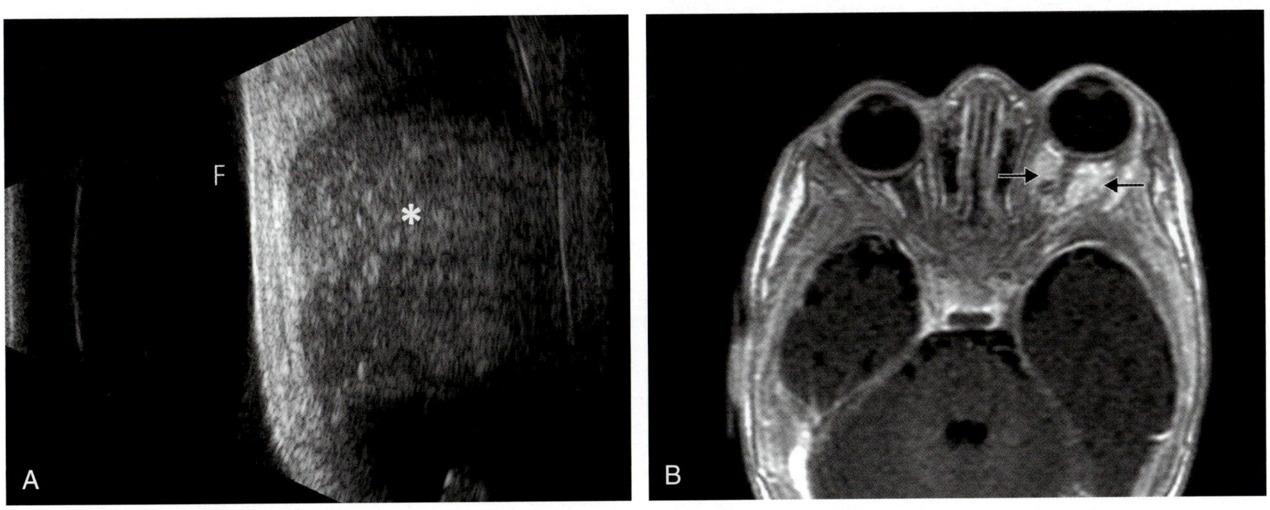

• **Fig. 9.8** Infantile Hemangioma. **(A)** Modified immersion B-scan demonstrates lid lesion (*asterisk*) with a heterogeneous internal structure. *F*, Fluid. **(B)** Axial T1-weighted MRI of infantile hemangioma extending to the retrobulbar space (*arrows*).

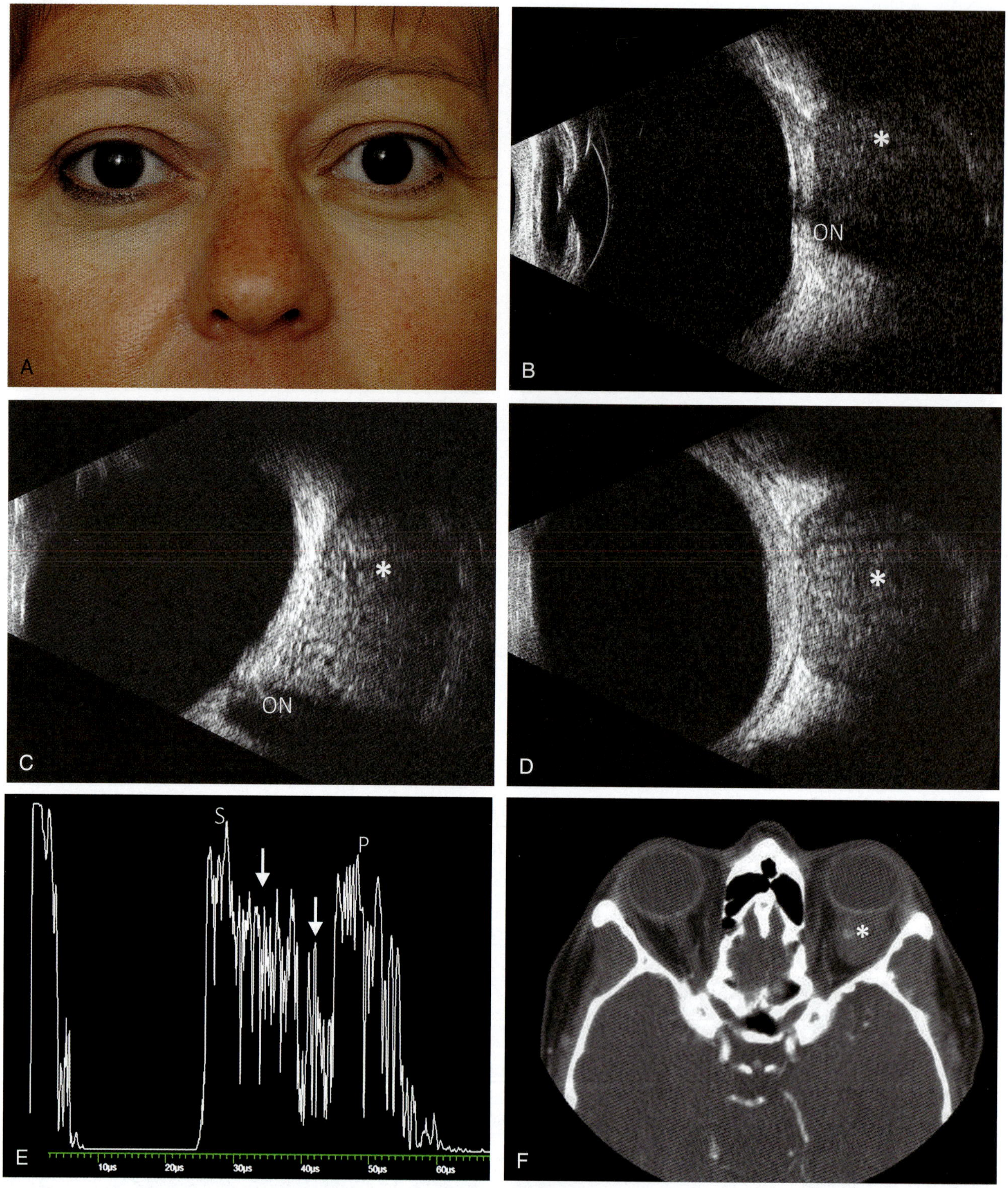

• **Fig. 9.9** Cavernous Venous Malformation. **(A)** External photography shows a slight left-sided proptosis. **(B)** Axial B-scan ultrasound shows a large cavernous venous malformation (*asterisk*) abutting the optic nerve (ON). **(C)** Longitudinal B-scan ultrasound shows a well-outlined, oval-shaped, homogeneous orbital lesion (*asterisk*). *ON*, Optic nerve. **(D)** Transverse B-scan ultrasound shows a smooth, well-outlined orbital lesion indenting the globe. **(E)** A-scan ultrasound shows high reflectivity and moderate sound attenuation (*arrows*); *S*, Sclera; *P*, Posterior lesion margin spike. **(F)** Axial CT scan shows a large intraconal mass (*asterisk*).

Venous-Lymphatic Malformation

Venous-lymphatic malformation is a benign congenital tumor composed of venous and lymphatic channels. Lymphatic malformations account for 4% of all orbital masses and 25% of orbital vascular masses. Most patients develop symptoms in the first or second decade.[11]

At presentation, patients can have progressive periocular swelling, proptosis, resricted eye mobility or an eyelid mass. A sudden increase in proptosis indicates hemorrhage within the lesion, leading to periocular pain and compressive neuropathy. Episcleral and conjunctival involvement can be present.[12]

B-scan ultrasonography shows a poorly outlined, irregularly shaped orbital lesion infiltrating the adjacent orbital tissues. The lesion is heterogeneous, with low reflective lymph-filled channels separated by septa and vessel walls. On compressibility maneuver, lymphangiomas are soft. In case of intralesional hemorrhage, the loculated spaces become dilated, and fluid-air or fluid-fluid level can occasionaly be noticed. A-scan ultrasound exam displays irregularly structured lesions with multiple low reflective spaces intercalated by high amplitude spikes, corresponding to septations and vascular walls.

CASE

A 9-year-old girl presented with progressive right-sided proptosis and a bluish subcutaneous mass involving the upper and lower eyelid. Eye motility was within normal limits. The patient underwent MRI and ultrasound exams (Fig 9.10 and Video 9.7).

Vascular Malformation

Orbital Varix

The varix is a slow-flow, distensible venous malformation. These lesions can be located superficially in the epibulbar or lid region, or deep in the orbital area.[13] It usually manifests in infancy or early childhood, but its appearance may be delayed until the first or second decade. Most cases occur unilaterally as intermittent, painless, positional proptosis, with a head-down position. Occasionally, varix can present acutely with the onset of painful proptosis resulting from thrombosis or hemorrhage of the affected vein. Long-standing lesions can be associated with enophthalmos, attributed to atrophy of the orbital fat.[14]

Ultrasonography shows a well-outlined, low reflective mass-like or tubular image that exhibits enlargement during the Valsalva maneuver. In some cases, varix can have poorly defined borders due to the tangle of malformed vessels. Their reflectivity can be irregular because of alternating areas of low reflective blood-filled spaces and high reflective vessel walls.[12]

CASE

A 70-year-old man presented with a 10-year history of occasional left retrobulbar pressure sensation and proptosis when bending over. The patient was worked up and found to have a left orbit varix (Fig. 9.11 and Video 9.8), which underwent a successful sclerosant agent injection.

Neoplasms of Lacrimal Gland

Pleomorphic Adenoma of the Lacrimal Gland

Pleomorphic adenoma is the most common benign lacrimal gland tumor, representing 20% of all lacrimal gland tumors.[15]

The initial presenting sign is a painless, unilateral growing mass superotemporally, causing downward displacement of the eyeball and ptosis. The duration of the symptoms at the time of presentation is typically 1–2 years.

B-scan ultrasonography demonstrates a round or oval, smooth, well-outlined mass. The tumor is firm and can cause indentation of the adjacent eye wall and bone remodeling.

On A-scan ultrasonography, pleomorphic adenoma shows a regular internal structure, mainly medium reflectivity, with moderate sound attenuation.[16]

CASE

A 36-year-old female presented with left upper eyelid swelling for 12 months. There was a downward displacement of the eye. Choroidal folds were detected in the fundoscopic exam. MRI revealed a heterogeneously enhanced well-circumscribed mass in the lacrimal fossa (Fig. 9.12 and Video 9.9).

Adenoid Cystic Carcinoma of the Lacrimal Gland

Adenoid cystic carcinoma is the most common malignant epithelial tumor of the lacrimal gland, comprising 20%–30% of all malignant lacrimal gland tumors.[15]

Most patients are in the fifth decade of life. They typically have a 6-month history of symptoms. The clinical signs are similar to those of other lacrimal gland masses, like upper eyelid swelling, ptosis, proptosis, and downward displacement of the eye. Pain is a cardinal symptom and may be secondary to perineural invasion.

On B-scan ultrasound, adenoid cystic carcinoma can be well-outlined in the early process. In more advanced cases, the lesion turns into an infiltrative appearance. The lesion is firm to hard in consistency. The finding of bone erosion in patients with more advanced diseases suggests the presence of malignancy. The A-scan ultrasound exhibits medium to medium-high internal reflectivity with marked sound attenuation.

CASE

A 38-year-old patient presented with a six-month history of right-sided proptosis with orbital pain. MRI of the orbit revealed a solid, enhancing right orbital mass with both intra- and extraconal components. Incisional biopsy disclosed adenoid cystic carcinoma (Fig. 9.13 and Video 9.10).

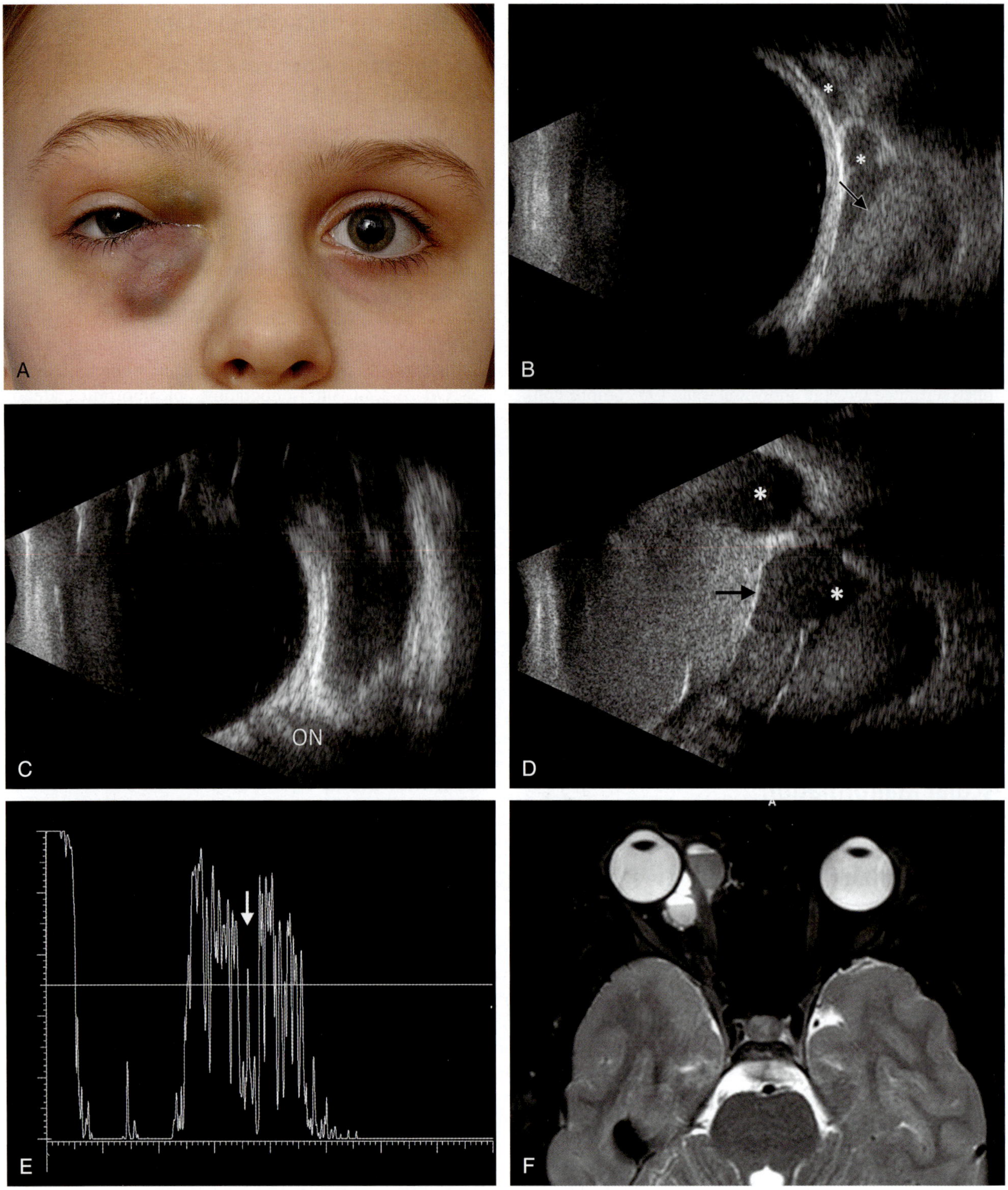

• **Fig. 9.10** Orbital venous-lymphatic malformation with intrinsic hemorrhage. **(A)** External photography of a 9-year-old girl with bluish subcutaneous upper and lower lid lesions. **(B)** Transverse B-scan ultrasound showing infiltrative, multiloculated mass with multiple distended channels (*asterisks*) with blood-fluid level (*arrow*). Firm consistency was detected in the compressibility right aneuver. **(C)** Longitudinal B-scan ultrasound showing the posterior extension of the mass in proximity to the optic nerve (ON). **(D)** B-scan ultrasound with the probe positioned on the lower eyelid displays a large loculated mass with dilated channels (*asterisks*) and thin walls (*arrow*). **(E)** A-scan ultrasound shows irregularly structured, low-reflective area (*arrow*), and high-amplitude spikes. **(F)** Axial MRI shows an enhancing multiloculated extraconal and intraconal mass with blood-fluid level, abutting the medial aspect of the optic nerve.

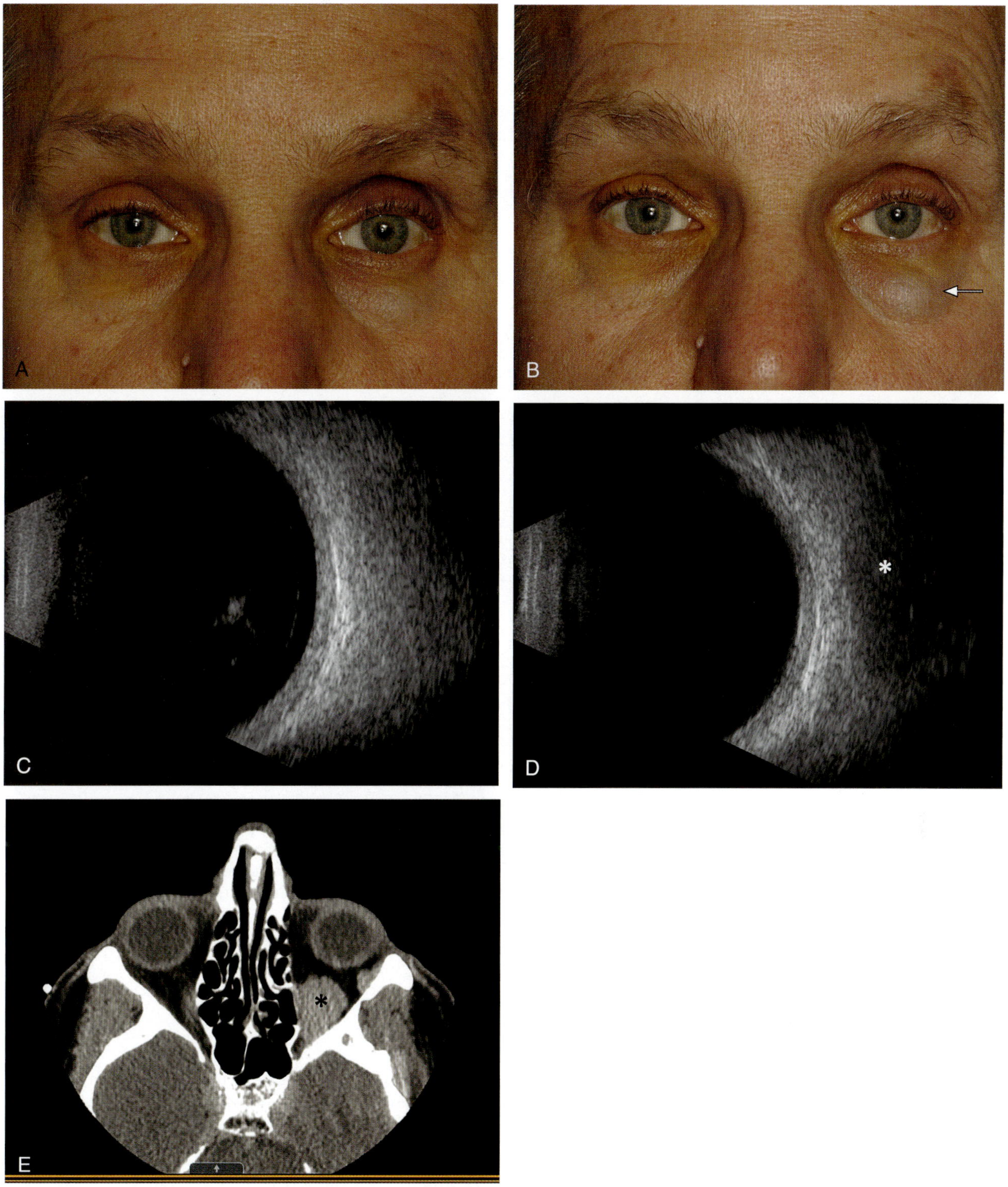

• **Fig. 9.11** Orbital varix. **(A)** External photography before the Valsalva maneuver shows minimal fullness of the left lower lid. **(B)** External photography during the Valsalva maneuver demonstrates increased fullness of the left lower lid (*arrow*). **(C)** Transverse B-scan ultrasound through the lower eyelid shows a normal pattern of orbital soft tissue. **(D)** Transverse B-scan ultrasound through the lower eyelid, while the patient sustained a bending over position, demonstrates a well-outlined, round, low-reflective orbital lesion (*asterisk*). **(E)** Axial CT scan shows retrobulbar lesion (*asterisk*).

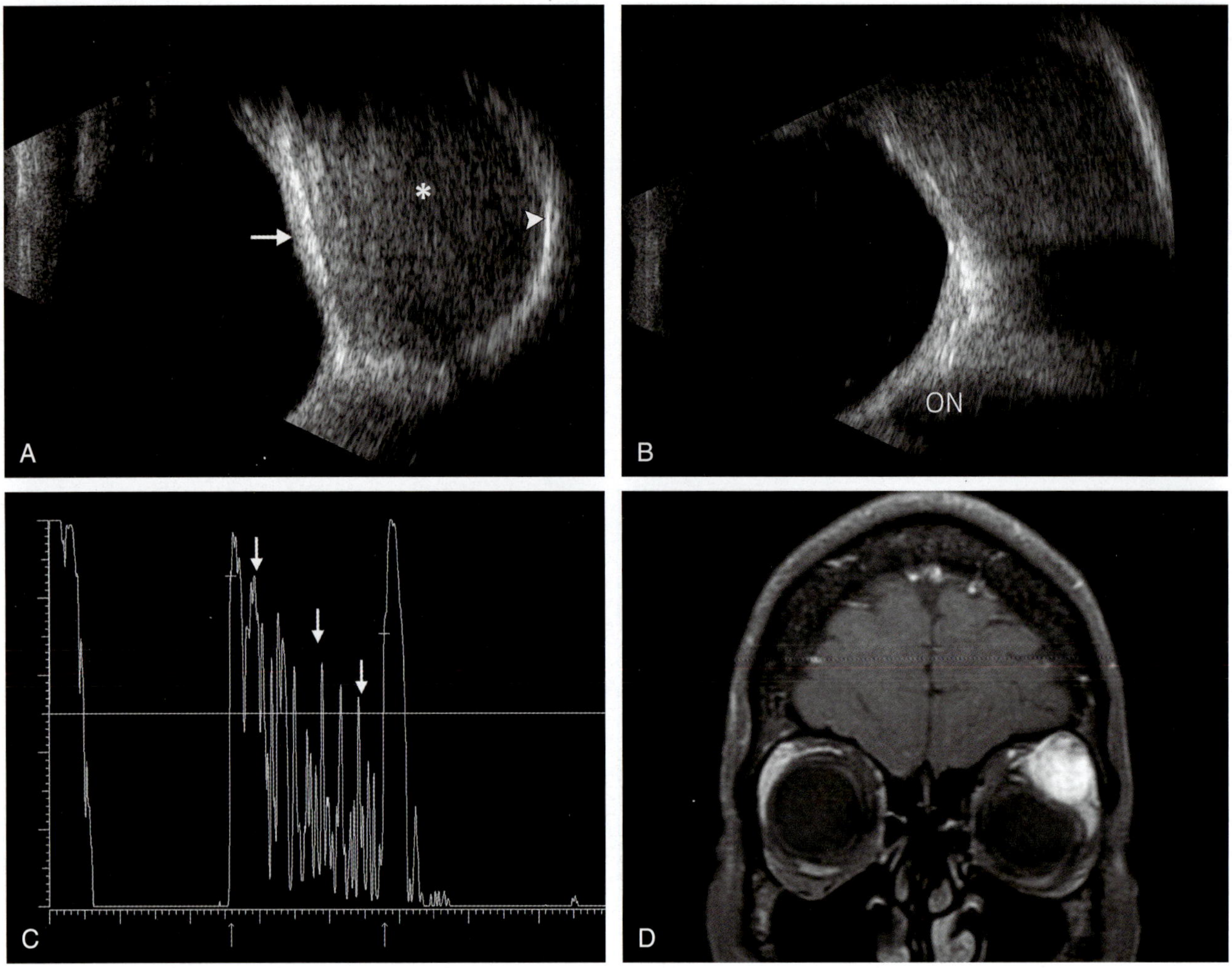

• **Fig. 9.12** Pleomorphic adenoma of the lacrimal gland. **(A)** Transverse B-scan ultrasound aimed superotemporally shows a large, well-circumscribed, medium reflective orbital lesion (*asterisk*) indenting the eye (*arrow*) and causing orbital bone excavation (*arrowhead*). **(B)** Longitudinal B-scan ultrasounds shows the anteroposterior extension of the lesion. *ON*, Optic nerve. **(C)** The corresponding A-scan ultrasound shows mostly medium internal reflectivity and moderate sound attenuation (*arrows*). **(D)** Coronal post-contrast T1-weighted MRI revealed a heterogeneously enhanced mass in the lacrimal fossa.

Tumors of Hematopoietic and Lymphoid Tissues

Orbital Lymphoma

Ocular adnexal lymphoma can arise in the conjunctiva, eyelids, and orbit, including the lacrimal gland. Lymphoma is the most frequent malignancy of the ocular adnexa and comprises 5%–10% of all extranodal lymphomas. Orbital lymphomas (OL) constitute 50%–60% of ocular adnexal lymphomas.

Most OL is of B-cell origin and affects patients older than 50 years, with a slight male predominance. The majority of B-cell lymphomas arise as a primary orbital disease and less frequently occur secondarily, either as a metastatic spread or as a local invasion from adjacent periorbital structures.[17,18]

The onset of the disease is insidious, with a mean duration of symptoms of 10 months.[14]

The principal sign at presentation is a painless lid swelling. Proptosis and a palpable mass are also common signs. A smooth, red-salmon color mass can be present on the conjunctiva, especially along the fornix. The majority of the tumors are unilateral.[17]

On B-scan ultrasound, OL can present as smooth, circumscribed, or diffuse, usually an extraconal mass with molding to the globe. The lesion is homogeneous and contains connective tissue septa. The tumor is soft in consistency. On the A-scan ultrasound, OL shows a regular internal structure with low to medium internal reflectivity, weak sound attenuation, and mild internal vascularity.

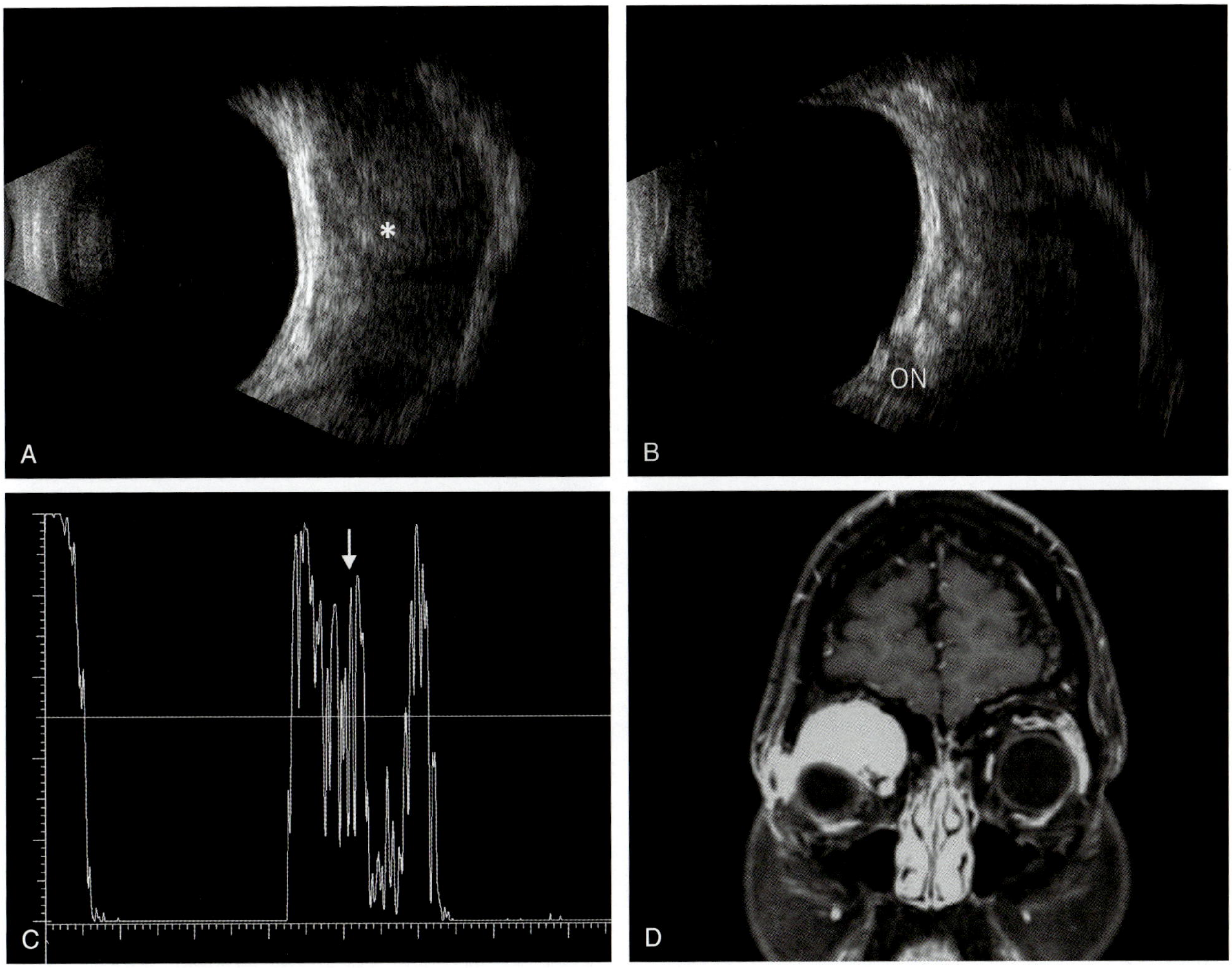

• **Fig. 9.13** Adenoid cystic carcinoma of the lacrimal gland. **(A)** Transverse B-scan ultrasound aimed superotemporally shows a well-outlined large lesion (*asterisk*) causing mild indentation of the globe wall. **(B)** Longitudinal B-scan through the superior orbit showing a large mass extending posteriorly. *ON*, Optic nerve. **(C)** A-scan ultrasound displaying mainly medium-high internal reflectivity with sound attenuation (*arrow*). **(D)** Coronal post-contrast T1-weighted MRI scan revealed a large orbital mass superiorly with marked enhancement, displacing the right eye inferiorly.

CASE

A 66-year-old male presented with bilateral upper and lower lid swelling for one year. On external exam, there was bilateral upper and lower lid swelling and left-sided proptosis. There were multiple moveable nodules around both eyes. CT scan showed lobulated extraconal masses (Fig. 9.14 and Video 9.11). The patient underwent an incisional biopsy, and pathology demonstrated B-cell lymphoma.

Orbital Plasmacytoma

Plasmacytoma is a monoclonal proliferation of plasma cells or plasmacytoid lymphocytes. It can occur as a primary or secondary tumor. Solitary orbital extramedullary plasmacytoma (primary plasmacytoma), without evidence of systemic disease, is extremely rare. Orbital plasmacytoma is usually associated with multiple myeloma, diagnosed before or immediately after the initial orbital presentation.[14,19]

The median age of patients at diagnosis is 57 years, with an equal gender distribution. The mean duration of symptoms is 1.9 months.[20] Patients present with a unilateral, droopy, swollen eyelid associated with eye displacement.

On B-scan ultrasound, plasmacytomas are well-outlined, firm in consistency, and internal vascularity can be visible within the mass. On A-scan ultrasound, plasmacytomas exhibit low internal reflectivity. Bone erosion can be demonstrated Histologically, the plasmacytoma comprises a dense, monotonous population of plasma cells producing a regular structured lesion.

CASE

A 65-year-old male presented with left upper and lower lid swelling for 10 weeks. A left-sided proptosis was seen on examination, and a palpable, firm, non-tender mass was detected in the superior quadrant of the orbit. CT scan revealed orbital soft tissue eroding through the roof. He underwent left orbitotomy with biopsy, and histopathology revealed a plasmacytoma (Fig. 9.15).

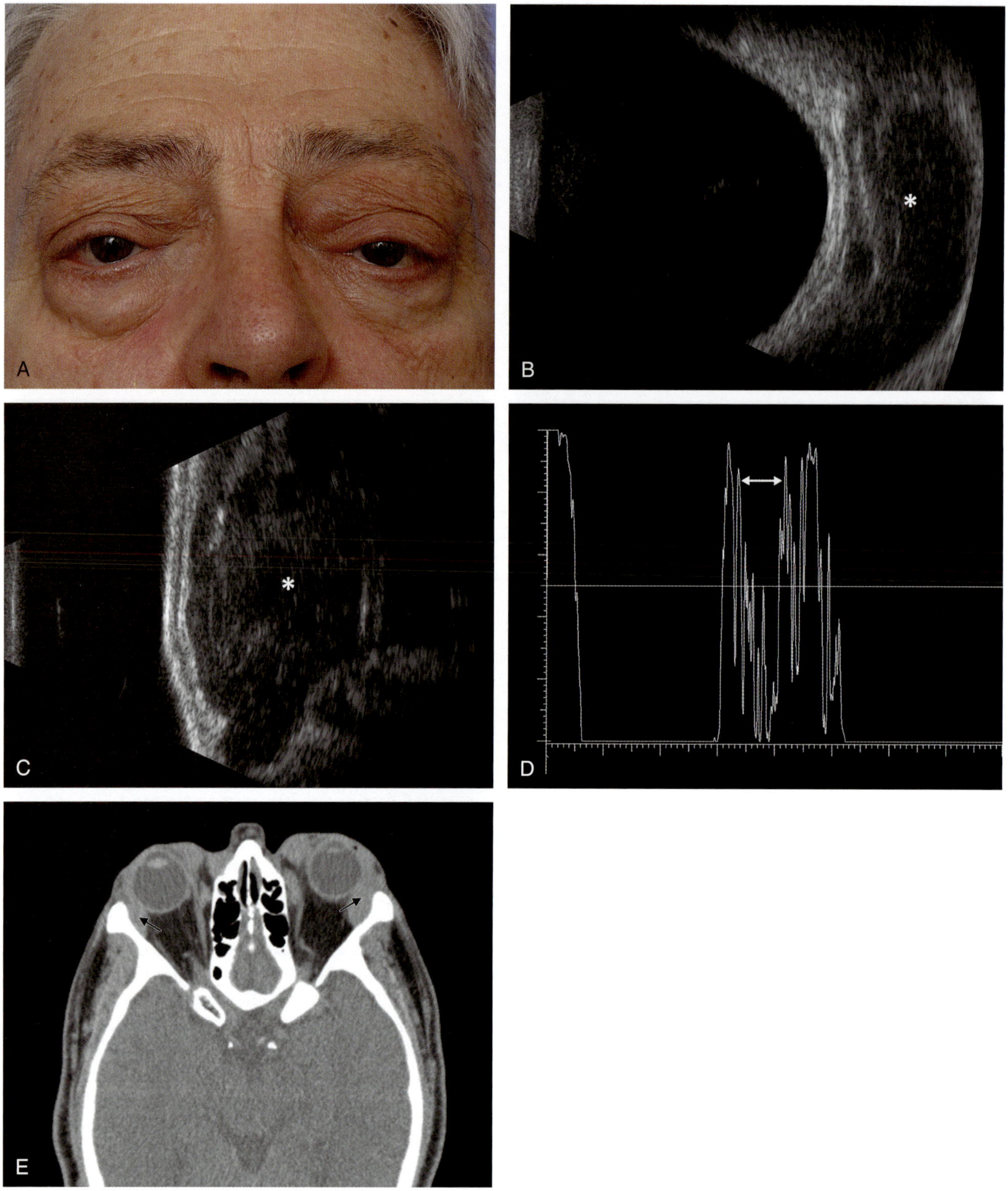

• **Fig. 9.14** Orbital lymphoma. **(A)** External photography shows bilateral lid swelling. **(B)** Transverse B-scan shows a well-outlined, low-reflective orbital mass (*asterisk*) molding the globe. **(C)** Modified immersion technique B-scan ultrasound through closed eyelids showing the anterior margin of a large, homogeneous, low-reflective lesion (*asterisk*) in the lid. **(D)** A-scan ultrasound showing low-medium internal reflectivity (*arrows*). **(E)** Axial CT scan shows bilateral, multiple orbital soft tissue lesions molding the globe and orbital walls.

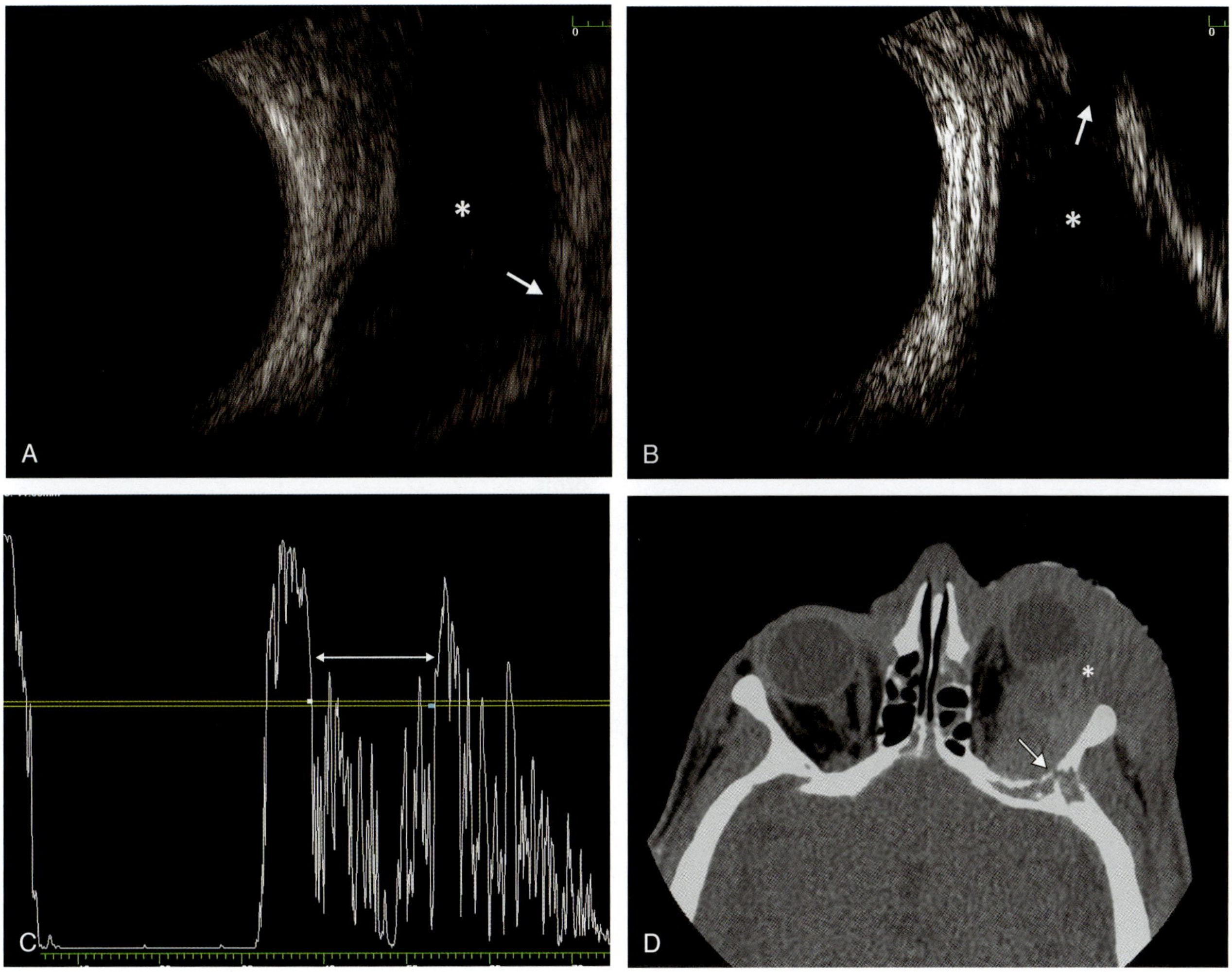

• **Fig. 9.15** Orbital plasmacytoma. B-scan ultrasound in **(A)** transverse and **(B)** longitudinal views, aimed superotemporally, exhibits a well-outlined, homogeneous orbital lesion (*asterisks*) with adjacent bone defect (*arrow*). **(C)** A-scan ultrasound showing low internal reflectivity (*arrow*). **(D)** Axial CT scan demonstrates a large soft tissue mass (*asterisks*) with aggressive bone erosion (*arrow*).

Orbital Leukemic Tumor

All types of leukemia may involve the orbit; however, orbital involvement is more common in acute leukemia than in chronic. Orbital leukemic tumors are mostly seen in the myelogenous forms, also denominated as granulocytic sarcoma, and occur most commonly in the first decade of life. These tumors may present before, concurrently, or appear during a remission stage of leukemia. The presenting features include proptosis, extraocular motility restriction, displacement of the eye, a palpable mass, and pain. The involvement is usually unilateral.[21–23]

On B-scan ultrasound, orbital leukemic tumors are well-outlined, homogeneous, and low to medium reflective lesions. On kinetic exam, the tumor is slightly compressible. The mass is typically located in the extraconal space, adjacent to an area of bone remodeling.

CASE

A 5-year-old boy presented with a five-week history of left upper and lower lid swelling, complaints of fatigue, and left leg and foot pain. An ocular adnexal exam disclosed left upper lid edema and a rubbery mass in the left lower lid (Fig. 9.16 and Video 9.12). The slit lamp and fundoscopy were unremarkable. Blood count was significant for normocytic anemia and neutropenia. MRI revealed an extraconal mass in the inferolateral portion of the left orbit with extraorbital extension into the zygoma. The patient underwent an incisional biopsy of the orbital mass, and the pathology was consistent with B-cell lymphoblastic leukemia. Bone narrow examination was consistent with the diagnosis of leukemia.

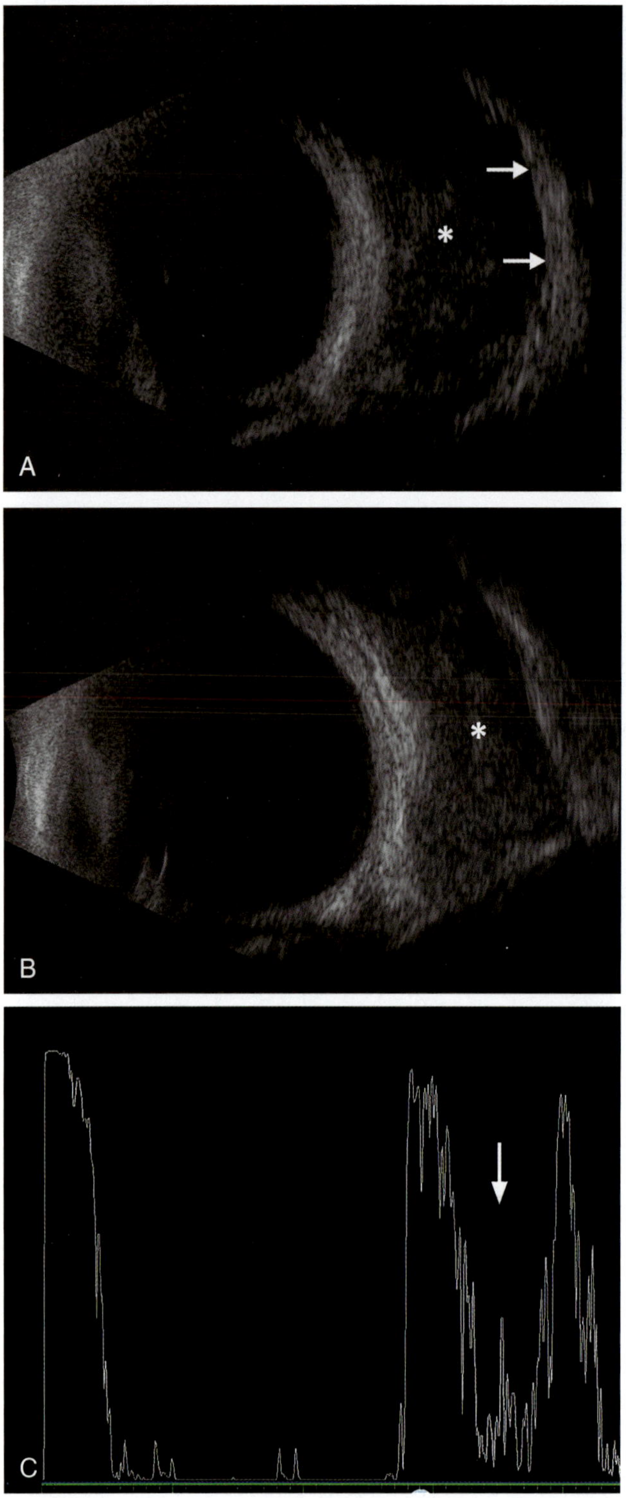

• **Fig. 9.16** Orbital leukemic tumor. **(A)** Transverse B-scan shows a well-outlined, homogeneous, low-reflective lesion (*asterisk*) with associated bone remodeling (*arrows*). **(B)** Longitudinal B-scan shows the posterior extension of the lesion (*asterisk*). **(C)** A-scan shows a low-reflective orbital lesion (*arrow*). The patient underwent an incisional biopsy of the orbital mass, and the pathology was consistent with B-cell lymphoblastic leukemia. Bone marrow examination was consistent with the diagnosis of leukemia.

Mesenchimal Tumors

Rhabdomyosarcoma

Rhabdomyosarcoma is the most common primary orbital malignancy of childhood. Orbital rhabdomyosarcoma probably arises from primitive pluripotent mesenchymal cells that possess the capacity to differentiate into striated muscle. It most commonly occurs in the first decade of life, with a mean age at diagnosis at 8 years.[24]

Patients typically develop a rapidly progressive proptosis and displacement of the eye. Other common signs and symptoms include ptosis, conjunctival and eyelid swelling, and pain. The tumor is invariably unilateral and is usually located superiorly or superonasal in the anterior orbit.

On B-scan ultrasound, rhabdomyosarcoma appears as an extraconal, well-circumscribed, oval-shaped, homogeneous mass of low to medium echogenicity. The lesion is firm in consistency and can cause globe indentation. Larger tumors have less well-defined margins and can be associated with bone erosion. A-scan ultrasonography demonstrates a regular internal structure with low to medium internal reflectivity.

CASE

A 9-year-old boy was referred with a four-week history of a right-sided orbital lesion. At presentation, the patient had lower lid swelling, chemosis, and an anterior orbital palpable mass inferotemporally. The patient underwent a biopsy. Histopathology was consistent with embryonal rhabdomyosarcoma (Fig. 9.17 and Video 9.13).

Solitary Fibrous Tumor

Solitary fibrous tumor is a rare tumor of mesenchymal origin that most often involves the pleura; rarely, the orbit is involved. Although usually benign, it can recur locally and rarely metastasizes.

The tumor typically presents with painless proptosis of fewer than six months' duration. The age at presentation is usually during mid-adulthood but can occur in all age groups.[25]

On B-scan ultrasonography, solitary fibrous tumors are smooth-walled, well-outlined, oblong, firm lesions. The lesion is typically in the superior quadrants of the intraconal or extraconal spaces in the orbit. On A-scan ultrasonography, it typically has a regular internal structure with low to medium internal reflectivity.[25,26]

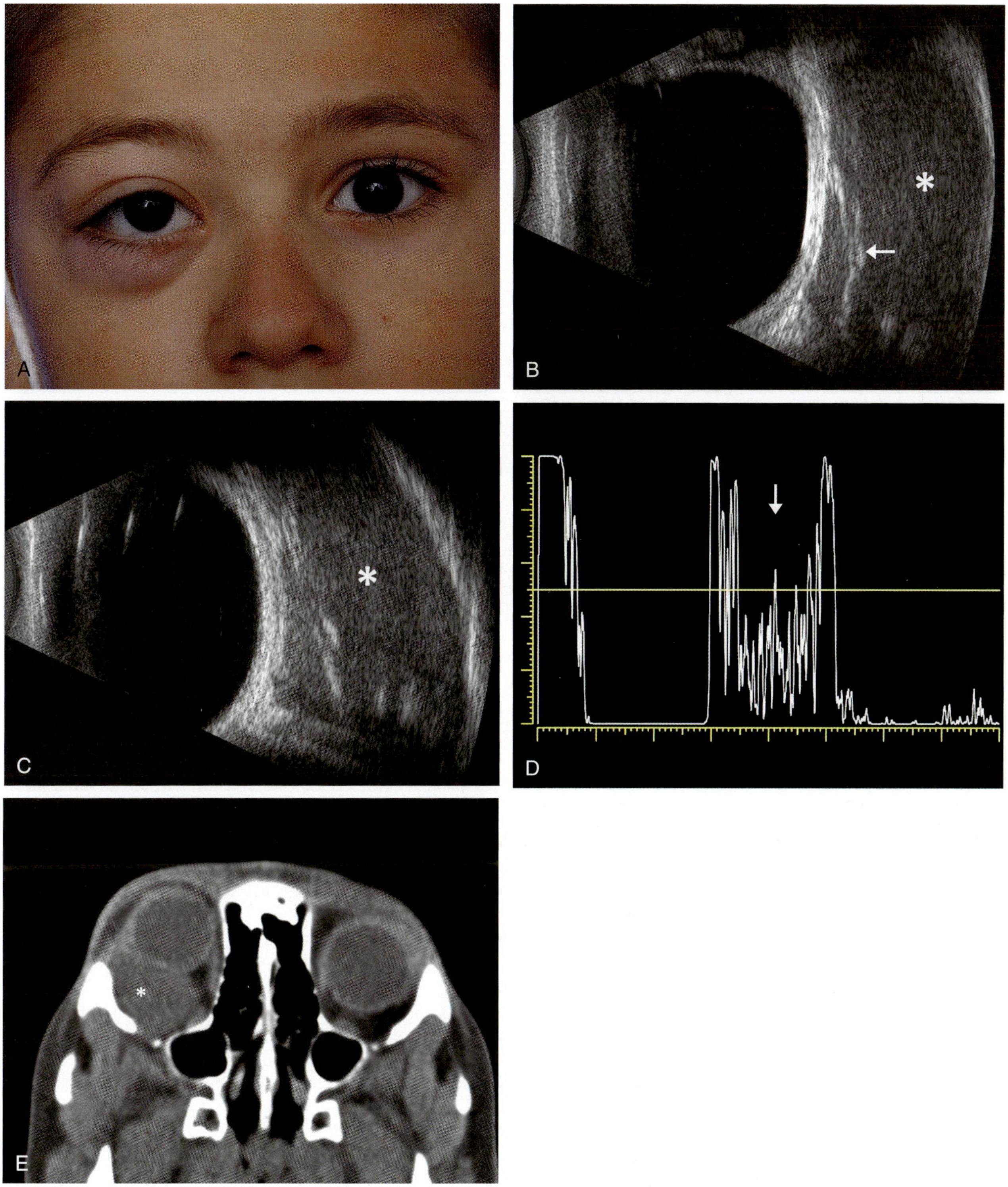

• **Fig. 9.17** Orbital rhabdomyosarcoma. **(A)** External photography shows a right-sided proptosis with upward eye displacement and a lower lid mass. **(B)** Transverse B-scan ultrasound shows a large, homogeneous orbital rhabdomyosarcoma (*asterisk*) with an intrinsic septae (*arrow*). **(C)** Longitudinal B-scan ultrasound demonstrates the mass extending deep in the orbit. **(D)** The corresponding A-scan ultrasound shows predominantly low to medium internal reflectivity (*arrow*). **(E)** CT scan shows a well-circumscribed, homogeneous soft tissue mass (*asterisk*) temporally.

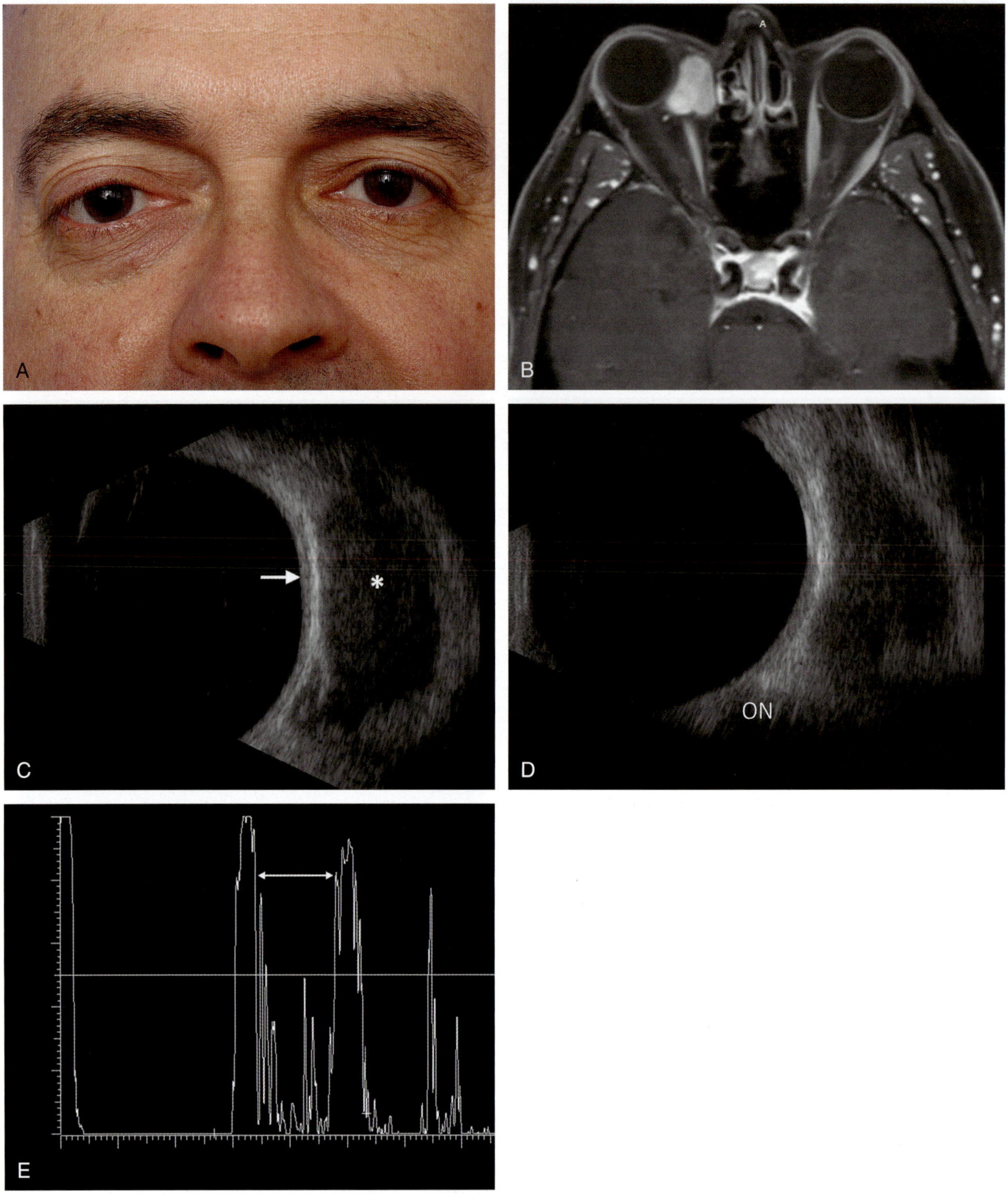

• **Fig. 9.18** Orbital solitary fibrous tumor. **(A)** External photo showing proptosis and inferior displacement of the right eye. **(B)** Post-contrast axial MR imaging showing a well-circumscribed, extraconal, enhanced mass. **(C)** Transverse B-scan ultrasound showing a well-outlined, oval orbital lesion (*asterisk*) and mild indentation of the globe (*arrow*). **(D)** Longitudinal B-scan ultrasound showing a large orbital lesion with no bone erosion; *ON*, Optic nerve. **(E)** A-scan ultrasound demonstrating a regularly structured, low-internal reflective lesion (*arrow*).

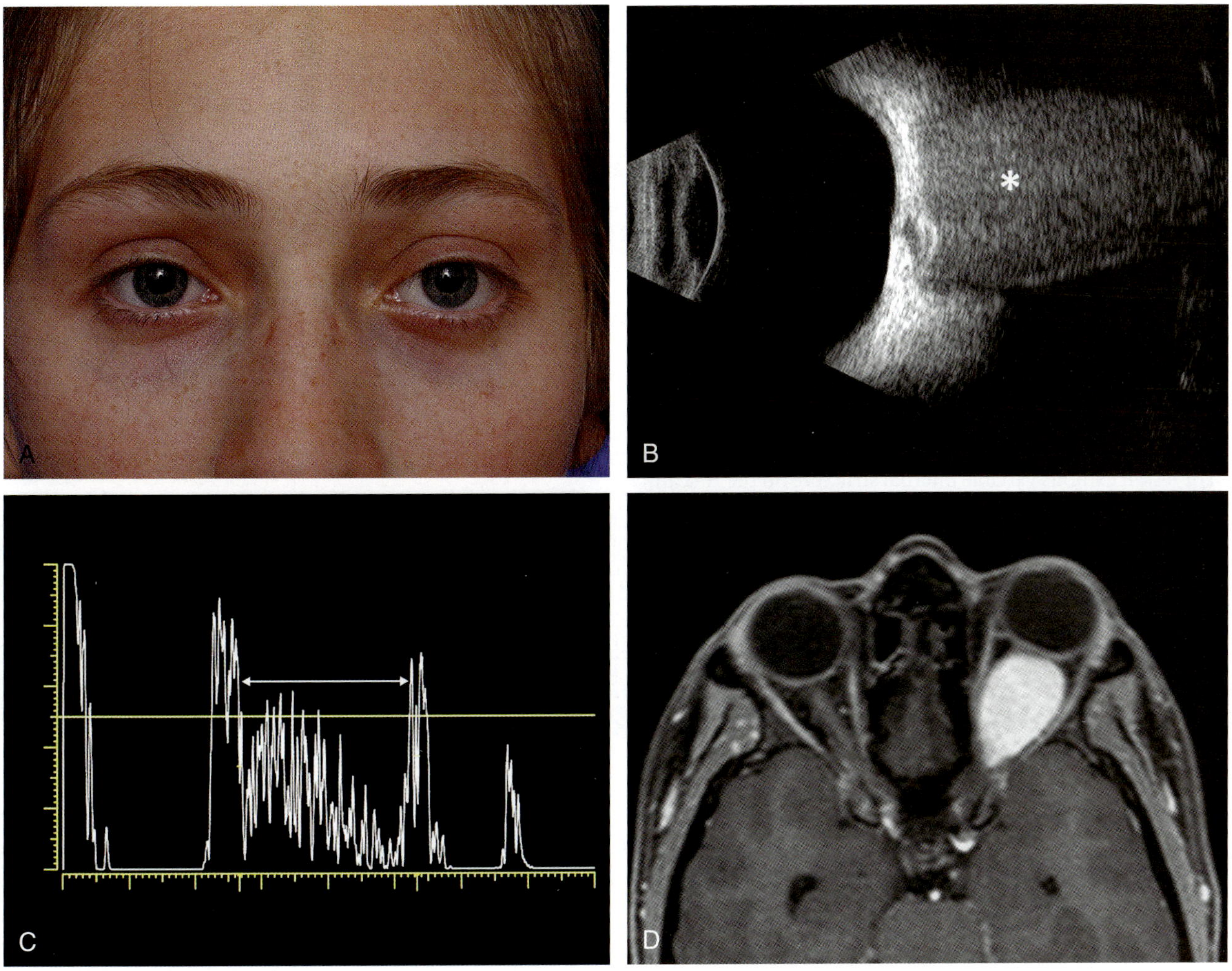

• **Fig. 9.19** Optic nerve glioma. **(A)** External photography shows left-sided axial proptosis. **(B)** Axial B-scan ultrasound shows a large, well-circumscribed, medium reflective enlargement of the optic nerve (*asterisk*), causing globe indentation. **(C)** The corresponding A-scan ultrasound shows a typical medium reflective (*arrow*) mass with moderate sound attenuation. **(D)** Post-contrast axial MRI exhibits an enhanced, large fusiform mass affecting the optic nerve.

CASE

A 55-year-old male presented with right proptosis and diplopia. The patient had an eight-year history of right-sided orbital tumor excision, and histopathology was consistent with a solitary fibrous tumor (Fig. 9.18). The patient underwent to an orbital biopsy, and a histopathology exam revealed a recurrent solitary fibrous tumor.

Neural Tumors

Optic Nerve Glioma

Optic nerve glioma is a slow-growing, unilateral tumor that may occur at any age, but most become symptomatic in childhood and are also commonly seen in patients with neurofibromatosis type 1.

The symptoms and signs in patients with optic nerve gliomas include decreased visual function, proptosis (often associated with infradisplacement of the globe), optic disc swelling or pallor, and strabismus. However, not all optic nerve gliomas are symptomatic; some are found during general screening of children with neurofibromatosis type 1 or other neuroimaging studies.[27]

On B-scan ultrasonography, optic nerve glioma appears as a smooth fusiform or tubular enlargement of the optic nerve with firm consistency. A-scan ultrasonography shows a regular internal structure with low to medium internal reflectivity.

CASE

A healthy 18-year-old female presented with a history of visual loss and left-sided axial proptosis for two years. The best-corrected visual acuity was 20/20 in the right eye and hand motion in the left eye. There was a positive relative afferent pupillary defect in the left eye. Given the clinical manifestations, ultrasonography and MRI were ordered, revealing an optic nerve glioma (Fig. 9.19 and Video 9.14).

Schwannoma

Schwannomas are benign tumors of the peripheral nerve sheath that originate from Schwann cells. Orbital schwannomas are rare, accounting for 1%–2% of all orbital neoplasms. They are usually solitary and occur in adults in the third to sixth decade.[28] Orbital schwannomas tend to arise from trigeminal nerve branches and commonly involve the superior orbit.[29]

The main symptom of orbital schwannoma is slowly progressive, painless proptosis. Late manifestations include diplopia, extraocular motility restriction, and mild worsening of visual acuity.

On the gross pathological exam, these tumors are well-circumscribed, encapsulated, and well-vascularized.[30]

On B-scan ultrasound, orbital schwannoma is typically extraconal, located at the superior orbit, and appears as a well-outlined, round, or elliptical mass with a smooth boundary. The tumor can be slightly compressible or firm. Bone remodeling can be observed in longstanding cases.

The lesion exhibits variable internal structure on the A-scan, ranging from a homogeneous low internal reflective pattern to a heterogeneous appearance with internal cystic spaces.

CASE

A 25-year-old female patient presented with painless, slowly progressive right-sided proptosis for two years. On ocular exam, a palpable firm mass was detected superotemporally, extending deep into orbit. The patient underwent orbitotomy with lesion excision. A histopathological exam revealed a schwannoma (Fig. 9.20).

CASE

A 31-year-old male presented with the main complaint of right-sided proptosis and decreased vision. The patient had a previous history of biopsy-proven right optic nerve schwannoma. MRI showed recurrence of the orbital lesion. The patient underwent orbitozygomatic craniotomy and resection of the orbital lesion; histopathology revealed schwannoma with degenerative changes (Fig. 9.21).

Neuroblastoma

Neuroblastoma derives from neural crest cells and can arise anywhere along the sympathetic chain, most commonly affecting the adrenal glands. It is predominantly a tumor of early childhood. Orbital metastasis is the most common ocular manifestation.

Rapid unilateral proptosis, periorbital swelling, and periorbital ecchymosis (raccoon eyes) are the common presenting signs.[31]

B-scan ultrasound demonstrates an extraconal, well-circumscribed, irregularly shaped, homogeneous mass. Associated bone defect can be observed. A-scan ultrasonography shows medium internal reflectivity.

CASE

An 8-month-old girl presented with left-sided proptosis for one week. A systemic workup revealed a retroperitoneal abdominal primary neuroblastoma (Fig. 9.22).

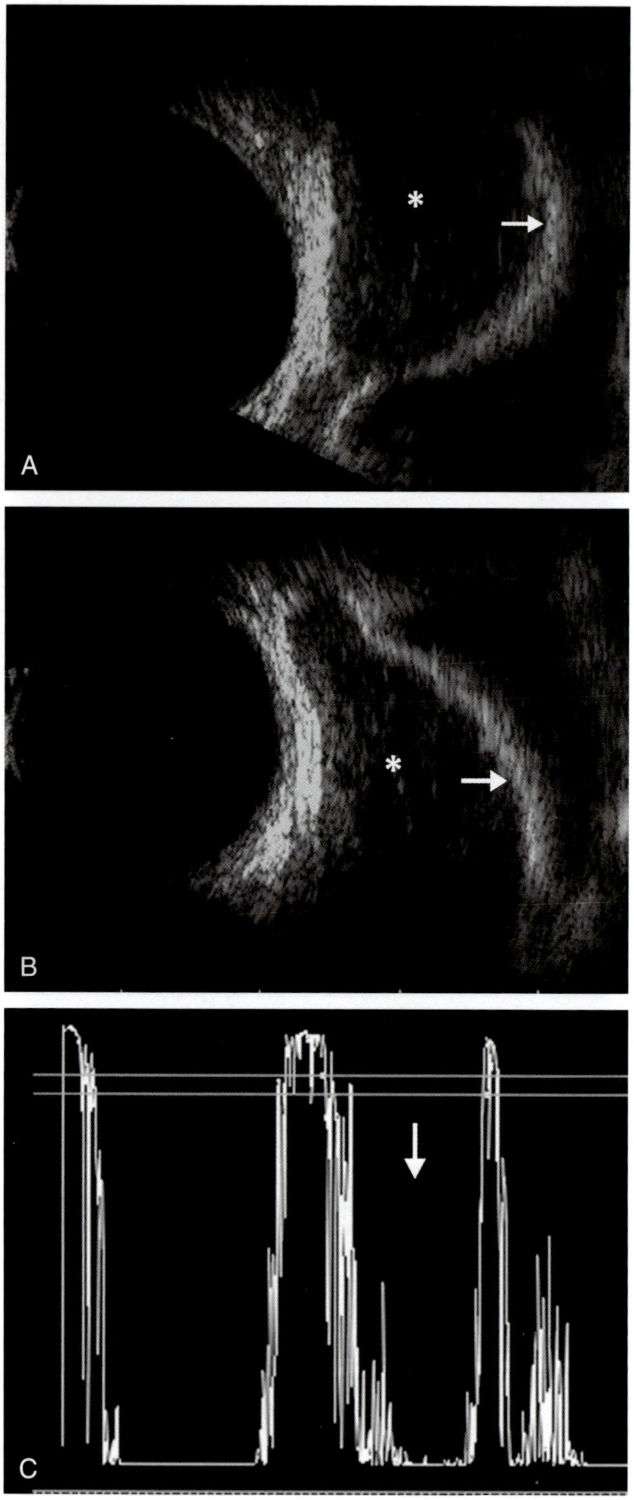

• **Fig. 9.20** Orbital schwannoma. **(A)** Transverse B-scan ultrasound through the upper eyelid shows a well-outlined, low-reflective lesion (*asterisk*) with associated bone excavation (*arrow*). **(B)** Longitudinal B-scan ultrasound shows a well-defined large orbital lesion (*asterisk*) with a smooth contour causing bone excavation (*arrow*). **(C)** Corresponding A-scan ultrasound displays a low-internal reflective lesion.

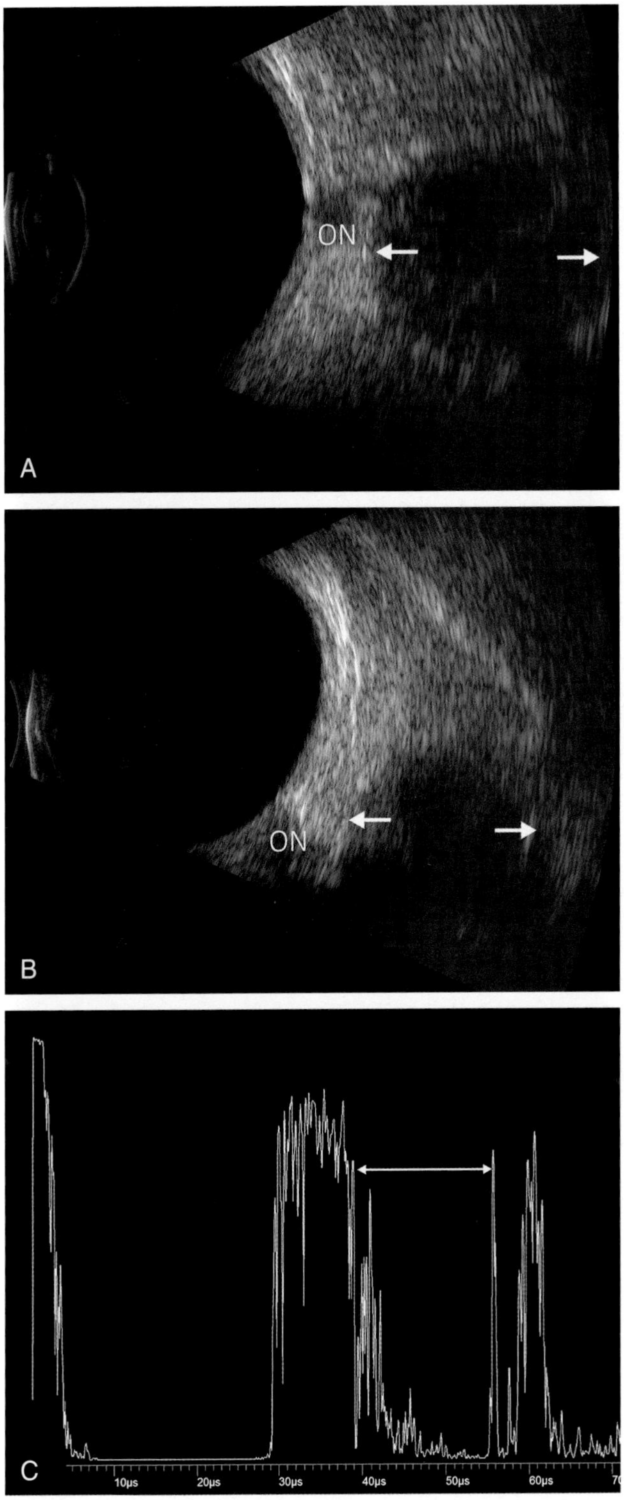

• **Fig. 9.21** Orbital schwannoma. **(A)** Vertical axial B-scan ultrasound showing an intraconal, round, low-reflective lesion (*arrows*) adjacent to the optic nerve (ON). **(B)** Longitudinal B-scan ultrasound showing the lesion (*arrows*) located deep in the orbit. **(C)** The corresponding A-scan ultrasound shows the low internal reflectivity of the lesion (*arrow*).

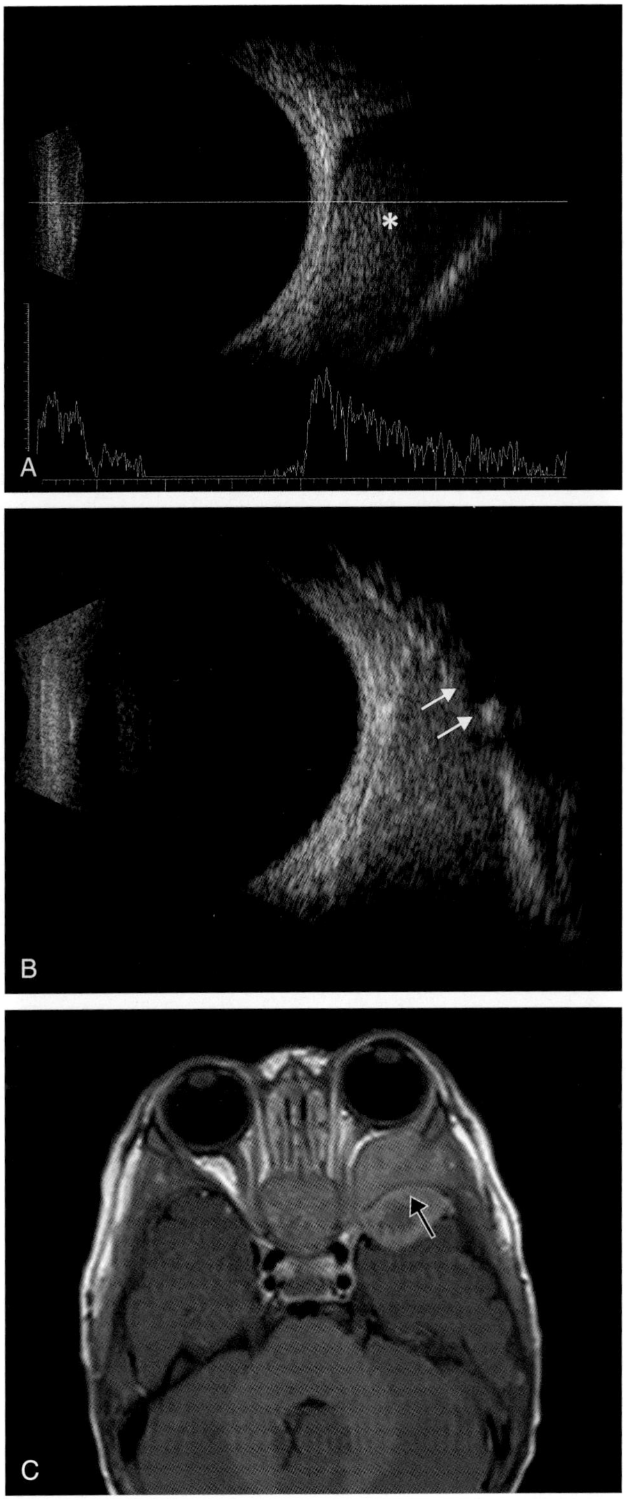

• **Fig. 9.22** Orbital neuroblastoma. **(A)** Transverse B-scan ultrasound shows a well-outlined, extraconal, homogeneous medium reflective mass (*asterisk*). **(B)** Longitudinal B-scan ultrasound shows the posterior extension of the orbital mass and a defect in the bone wall (*arrows*). **(C)** Axial T1-weighted post-contrast MRI shows a mass lesion centered in the greater wing of the left sphenoid bone with orbital extension (*arrow*).

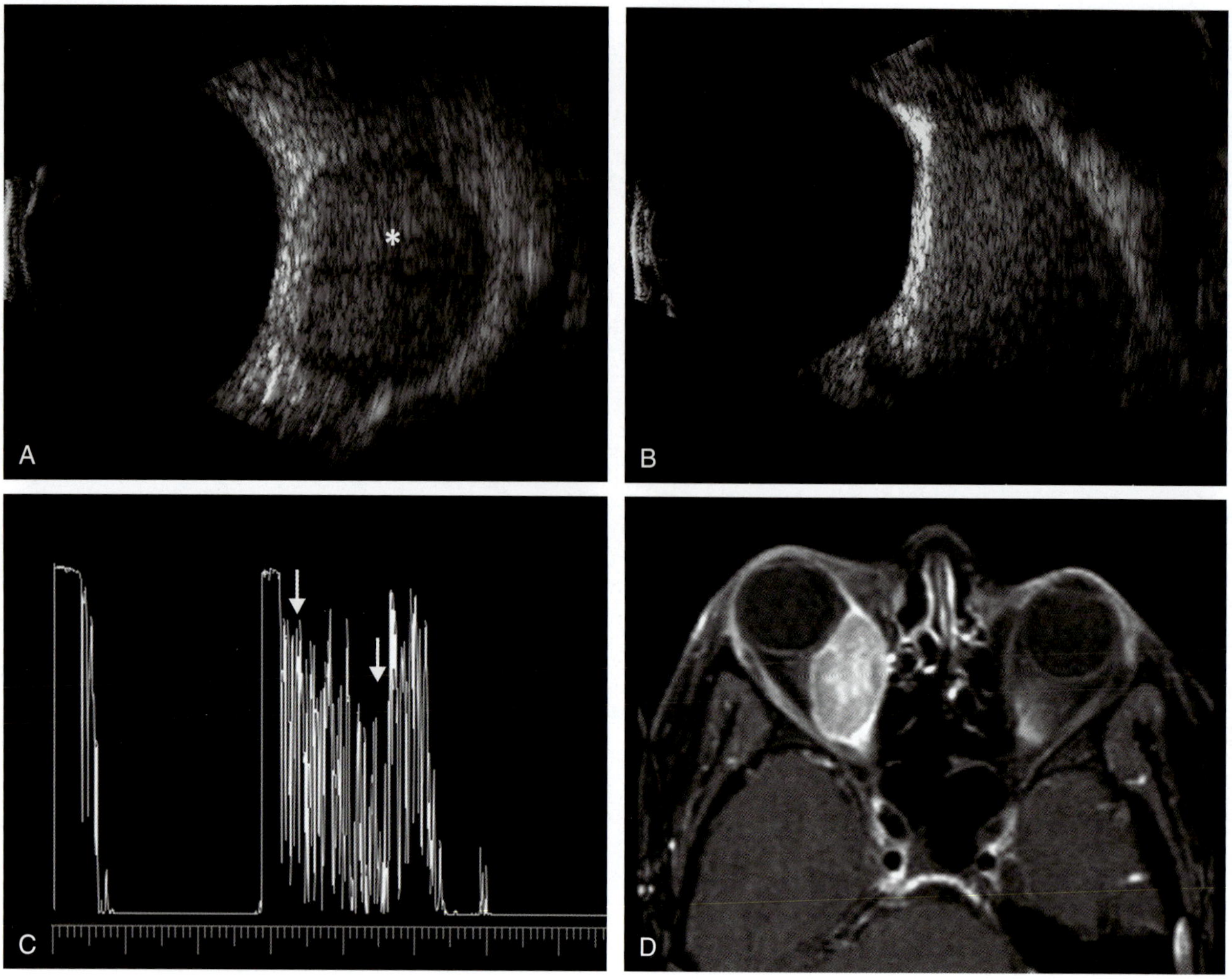

• **Fig. 9.23** Orbital granular cell tumor. **(A)** Transverse and **(B)** longitudinal B-scans ultrasound aimed medially shows a large, oval-shaped, well-outlined, intraconal lesion (*asterisk*) indenting the globe. During the dynamic examination, infiltration of the medial rectus muscle was noted. **(C)** The corresponding A-scan ultrasound shows regularly structured, medium-high reflective lesion with moderate sound attenuation (*arrows*). **(D)** Fat-suppressed T1-weighted axial MR image demonstrates a well-outlined, ovoid intraconal enhanced mass that can't be separable from the medial rectus muscle.

Granular Cell Tumor

Granular cell tumor (GCT) is a benign neoplasm, probably of Schwann cell origin, occurring in various sites in the body, including the breast, skin, subcutaneous tissue, digestive, respiratory, urogenital tracts, and pituitary stalk.[32] The occurrence of GCT in the orbit and ocular adnexal structures is rare,[33] and extraocular involvement is noticeable.[34,35]

The clinical presentation is typical of a slow-growing painless mass with proptosis and diplopia.

On B-scan ultrasound examination, granular cell tumors appear as round to oval, well-outlined, intraconal lesions. The internal structure is regular, and the reflectivity is medium to high. These tumors are firm in consistency and produce moderate sound attenuation. Bone remodeling can be associated, and muscular attachment can be demonstrated.

CASE

A 31-year-old woman was referred with a history of right-sided proptosis, diplopia, and mild pain around the right eye. On the external exam, there was a mild conjunctival injection over the medial rectus muscle insertion. Ultrasound and MRI exams were performed (Fig. 9.23). The patient underwent an orbitotomy with complete excision of the tumor. Intraoperatively, the tumor was noted to have a well-developed capsule and to be adherent to the medial rectus muscle. Pathology was consistent with granular cell tumor.

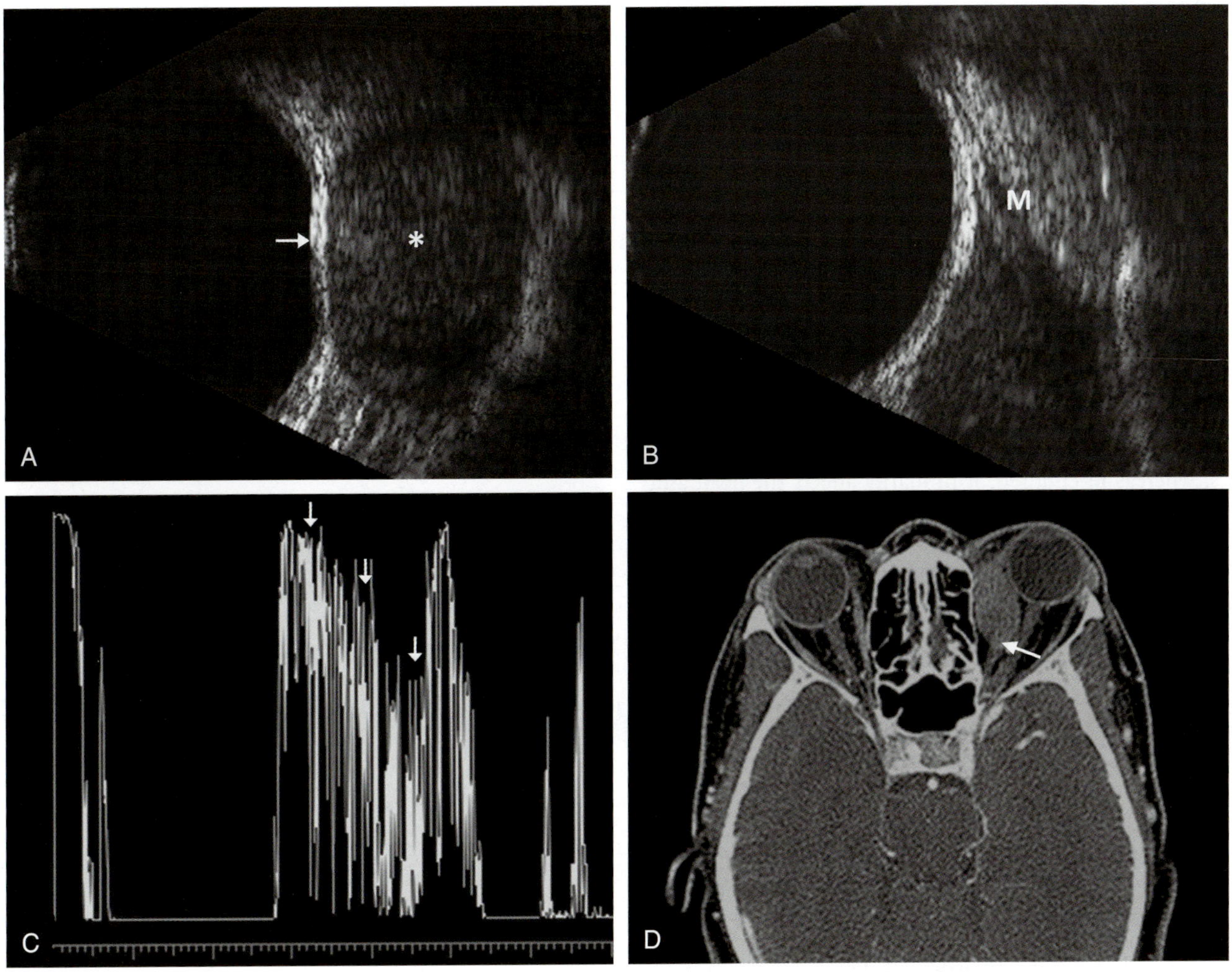

• **Fig. 9.24** Orbital granular cell tumor. **(A)** Transverse B-scan ultrasound shows a well-circumscribed, oval, homogeneous lesion (*asterisk*) causing mild indentation of the globe (*arrow*). **(B)** Longitudinal B-scan ultrasound shows the anteroposterior extension of a lesion adherent to the extraocular muscle (M). **(C)** The corresponding A-scan ultrasound shows a medium-high reflective lesion with moderate sound attenuation. **(D)** CT scan shows a large enhancing left orbital mass involving the medial rectus (*arrow*).

CASE

A 54-year-old woman was referred with a history of an enlarging left orbital mass. On examination, there were proptosis and motility restriction on abduction of the left eye. Anterior segment and dilated fundus examinations of both eyes were unremarkable. Ultrasound and CT scan exams were performed (Fig. 9.24). Systemic workup was negative. The patient underwent orbitotomy with complete excision of the tumor. The histological and immunohistochemical findings were consistent with granular cell tumor.

Miscellaneous

Orbital Metastasis

Orbital metastasis accounts for 7% of all orbital lesions. The most frequent primary tumors are breast carcinoma, prostatic cancer, and melanoma.[36] In one series, cutaneous melanoma was the second most common cause of orbital metastasis.[37] Most of the orbital metastasis presents in patients with known primary disease; however, in 15% of the cases, the orbital tumor can be the initial presentation.[38]

The mean age of patients at presentation is 60 years. Proptosis, diplopia, restriction of extraocular motility, and mass effect with ocular displacement are common signs and symptoms. Enophthalmos may be present with scirrhous tumors such as breast carcinoma.[38,39]

The presentation varies depending on the underlying primary tumor. Melanoma and breast carcinoma tend to localize in the orbital fat and muscle, whereas prostatic cancer tends to metastasize to bone. The infiltrative pattern is more commonly seen in breast carcinoma. Muscle thickening is highly associated with metastatic melanoma.

CASE

A 64-year-old female presented with right-sided ptosis and inferior displacement of the globe. The patient had a history of cutaneous melanoma. An ultrasonography exam revealed a mass lesion attached to the right superior rectus muscle (Fig. 9.25 and Video 9.15). Systemic workup with positron emission tomography showed lung, liver, bones, and orbit lesions. A liver biopsy showed metastatic melanoma.

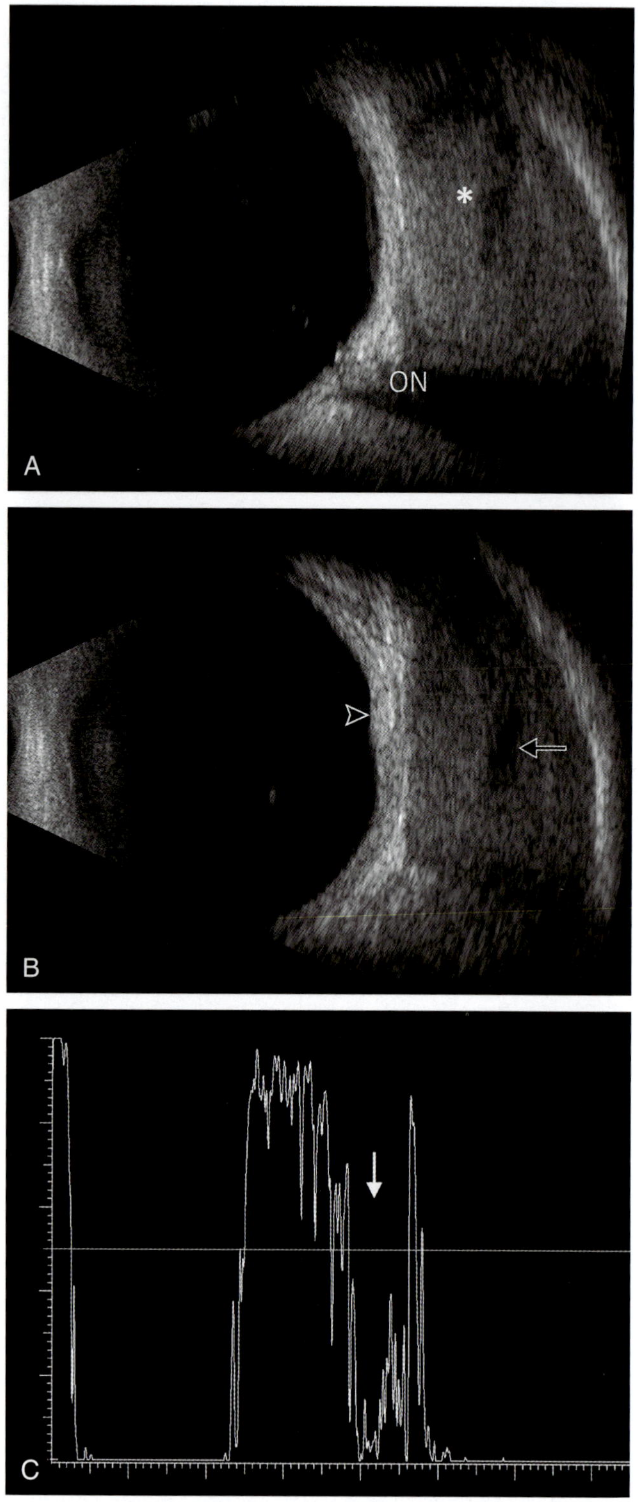

• **Fig. 9.25** Orbital metastasis. **(A)** Longitudinal B-scan ultrasound oriented superiorly exhibits a circumscribed, elliptical orbital massive lesion (*asterisk*) surrounding the superior rectus. **(B)** Transverse B-scan ultrasound shows a large orbital mass with a low-reflective space (*arrow*), causing a globe wall indentation (*arrowhead*). **(C)** Corresponding A-scan ultrasound exhibits low internal reflectivity (*arrow*).

Alveolar Soft-Part Sarcoma

Alveolar soft-part sarcoma may occur at any age but mainly affects young patients, with a slight female preponderance. In adults, the tumor typically manifests in the lower extremities, whereas in children, it primarily affects the head and neck, particularly the orbit and tongue.[40]

The course of the disease is usually short, with patients presenting painless proptosis, abnormal position of the eye, and eyelid swelling. When the mass is located more anteriorly, conjunctival congestion with dilated and tortuous vessels can be detected.[40,41]

On B-scan ultrasound, alveolar soft-part sarcoma appears well-outlined with a smooth surface mass with heterogeneous internal echoes. Marked intrinsic vascular flow is observed. The tumor is firm in consistency and can be indistinguishable or abutting an adjacent extraocular muscle.

A-scan ultrasound shows an irregular internal structure, with reflectivity varying from low to medium and intense internal vascularity.[42]

CASE

A 34-year-old female presented with a two-month history of a painless mass in the left nasal canthal area, displacing the globe temporally (Fig. 9.26 and Video 9.16). Extraocular motility restriction, conjunctival swelling, engorged episcleral vessels, and optic disc elevation were detected. The patient underwent an incisional biopsy, and the histopathology was consistent with alveolar soft-part sarcoma.

Summary

Evaluation of orbital masses requires a multimodality approach combining ultrasonography, computed tomography, and magnetic resonance imaging. Ultrasonographic evaluation of the orbit provides unique dynamic and readily available information. Differential diagnosis of orbital tumors and tumor-like lesions is accomplished by a combination of an accurate medical history, precise clinical examination, and knowledge of the distinct sonographic features of the orbital masses (Table 9.1).

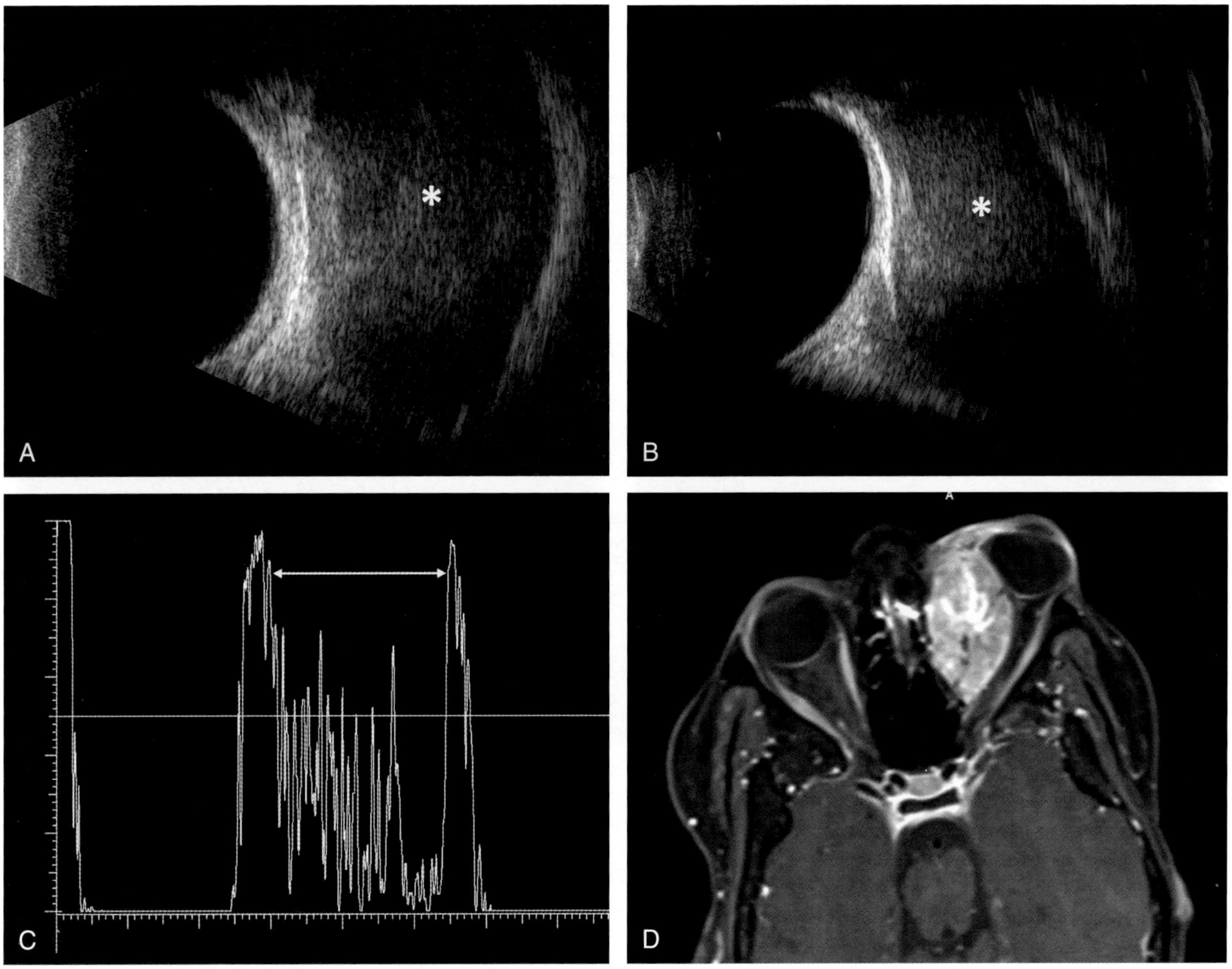

• **Fig. 9.26** Orbital alveolar soft-part sarcoma. **(A)** Transverse B-scan ultrasound shows a well-outlined, with smooth borders orbital mass (*asterisk*). **(B)** Longitudinal B-scan ultrasound shows a large lesion (*asterisk*) extending back into the orbit. **(C)** Transocular A-scan ultrasound shows an irregular internal structure with low- and medium-intensity spikes (*arrow*). **(D)** Axial T1-weighted contrast-enhanced MRI shows a large orbital mass indistinguishable from the medial rectus muscle.

TABLE 9.1 Clinical and Acoustic Features of Common Orbital Tumors and Tumor-Like Lesions

Lesion	Age	Onset	Shape/Borders	Structure	Reflectivity	Consistency	Specific
Dermoid cyst	Infants/middle-aged adults	Slow growth	Oval/round Well-outlined	Variable	Low to high	Firm	Often superotemporal
Microphthalmos with cyst	Newborns & infants	Acute at birth	Round Well-outlined	Regular	Extremely low	Soft	Bluish mass bulging in the lower lid
Respiratory epithelial cyst	Children/young adults	Slow growth	Round/oval Well-outlined	Regular	Low	Soft	Possible history of trauma
Mucocele	Adults & older adults	Slow growth	Round/oval Well-outlined	Regular	Low	Firm	Bone defect
Infantile hemangioma	Newborn and infants	Fast growth	Irregular Poorly outlined	Irregular	Medium-high to high	Soft	Locations: cutaneous/ subcutaneous and deep in the orbit
Cavernous venous malformation	Adults	Slow growth	Round/oval Well-outlined	Regular	Medium-high to high	Firm	Intraconal in most cases
Venous-lymphatic malformation	Children/young adults	Slow growth	Irregular Poorly outlined	Irregular (multilocular)	Low	Soft	A sudden increase in proptosis indicates hemorrhage
Varix	Children/young adults	Slow progressive	Variable Well-outlined	Regular	Low	Soft	Intermittent proptosis on straining
Pleomorphic adenoma	Adults	Slow growth	Round/oval Well-outlined	Regular	Medium-high	Firm	Palpable mass superotemporally
Adenoid cystic carcinoma	Adults	Fast growth	Oval/irregular Well-outlined	Variable	Medium to medium-high	Firm	Painful, palpable mass Bone defect
Lymphoma	Adults & older adults	Slow growth	Variable Well-outlined, molding eye and wall	Regular	Low to medium	Slightly soft	Intrinsic septae
Plasmacytoma	Adults & older adults	Fast growth	Variable Well-outlined	Regular	Low to medium	Firm	Bone defect Can be multiple myeloma associated
Leukemic tumor	Children	Fast growth	Variable Well-outlined, molding eye and wall	Regular	Low to medium	Slightly soft	History of systemic leukemia
Rhabdomyosarcoma	Children	Fast growth	Variable Well-outlined	Regular	Low to medium	Firm	Typical rapidly progressive proptosis
Solitary fibrous tumor	Adults	Variable – few months to years	Oval Well-outlined	Regular	Low to medium	Firm	
Optic nerve glioma	Children	Slow growth	Fusiform or tubular Well-outlined	Regular	Low to medium	Firm	Progressive visual loss and proptosis Can be neurofibromatosis associated
Schwannoma	Adults	Slow growth	Round/oval Well-outlined	Regular	Low-medium	Firm	Occasionally intrinsic cysts are found
Granular cell tumor	Adults	Slow growth	Oval Well-outlined	Regular	Medium to high	Firm	Muscle associated
Alveolar soft-part sarcoma	Children & adolescents	Fast growth	Oval Well-outlined	Regular	Medium	Firm	Muscle associated

REFERENCES

1. Bonavolontà G, Strianese D, Grassi P, et al. An analysis of 2,480 space-occupying lesions of the orbit from 1976 to 2011. *Ophthalmic Plast Reconstr Surg.* 2013;29:79–86.
2. Purohit BS, Vargas MI, Ailianou A, et al. Orbital tumours and tumour-like lesions: exploring the armamentarium of multiparametric imaging. *Insights Imaging.* 2016;7:43–68.
3. Garrity JA. *Henderson's Orbital Tumors.* 4th ed. Lippincott Williams & Wilkin; 2007.
4. Pahwa S, Sharma S, Das CJ, Dhamija E, Agrawal S. Intraorbital cystic lesions: an imaging spectrum. *Curr Probl Diagn Radiol.* 2015;44:437–448.
5. Thanos A, Jakobiec FA, Mendoza PR, Hatton MP. Ectopic (choristomatous) orbital respiratory cyst: histopathology and immunohistochemistry. *Surv Ophthalmol.* 2014;59:328–333.
6. Goh RL, Hardy TG, Williams RA, McNab AA. Respiratory epithelial cysts of the orbit. *Orbit.* 2016;35:245–249.
7. Reem RE, Golden RP. Periocular hemangiomas and lymphangiomas. *Pediatr Clin North Am.* 2014;61:541–553.
8. Byrne S, Green R. *Ultrasound of the Eye and Orbit.* 2nd ed. Mosby; 2002.
9. Calandriello L, Grimaldi G, Petrone G, et al. Cavernous venous malformation (cavernous hemangioma) of the orbit: current concepts and a review of the literature. *Surv Ophthalmol.* 2017;62:393–403.
10. McNab AA, Tan JS, Xie J, et al. The natural history of orbital cavernous hemangiomas. *Ophthalmic Plast Reconstr Surg.* 2015;31:89–93.
11. Tunç M, Sadri E, Char DH. Orbital lymphangioma: an analysis of 26 patients. *Br J Ophthalmol.* 1999;83:76–80.
12. Ko F, DiBernardo CW, Oak J, Miller NR, Subramanian PS. Confirmation of and differentiation among primary vascular lesions using ultrasonography. *Ophthalmic Plast Reconstr Surg.* 2011;27:431–435.
13. Rootman J. Vascular malformations of the orbit: hemodynamic concepts. *Orbit.* 2003;22(2):103–120.
14. Garrity J, Henderson J. *Orbital Tumors.* 4th ed. Lippincott Williams & Wilkins; 2007.
15. Andreasen S, Esmaeli B, Holstein SL, Mikkelsen LH, Rasmussen PK, Heegaard S. An update on tumors of the lacrimal gland. *Asia Pac J Ophthalmol.* 2017;6:159–172.
16. DiBernardo CW, Greenberg EF. *Ophthalmic Ultrasound a Diagnostic Atlas.* 2nd ed. Thieme; 2007:127.
17. Olsen TG, Heegaard S. Orbital lymphoma. *Surv Ophthalmol.* 2019;64:45–66.
18. Demirci H, Shields CL, Karatza EC, Shields JA. Orbital lymphoproliferative tumors: analysis of clinical features and systemic involvement in 160 cases. *Ophthalmology.* 2008;115:1626–1631.
19. Adkins JW, Shields JA, Shields CL, Eagle Jr RC, Flanagan JC, Campanella PC. Plasmacytoma of the eye and orbit. *Int Ophthalmol.* 1996-1997;20:339–343.
20. Thuro BA, Sagiv O, Shinder R, et al. Clinical presentation and anatomical location of orbital plasmacytomas. *Ophthalmic Plast Reconstr Surg.* 2018;34:258–261.
21. Kincaid MC, Green WR. Ocular and orbital involvement in leukemia. *Surv Ophthalmol.* 1983;27:211–232.
22. Reddy SC, Jackson N, Menon BS. Ocular involvement in leukemia: a study of 288 cases. *Ophthalmological.* 2003;217:441–445.
23. Bidar M, Wilson MW, Laquis SJ, et al. Clinical and imaging characteristics of orbital leukemic tumors. *Ophthalmic Plast Reconstr Surg.* 2007;23:87–93.
24. Shields JA, Shields CL. Rhabdomyosarcoma: review for the ophthalmologist. *Surv Ophthalmol.* 2003;48:39–57.
25. Blessing NW, Bermudez-Magner JA, Fernandez MP, Rosenberg AE, Dubovy SR, Johnson TE. Solitary fibrous tumor of the orbit: a case series with clinicopathologic correlation and evaluation of STAT6 as a diagnostic marker. *Ophthalmic Plast Reconstr Surg.* 2020;36:164–171.
26. Johnson TE, Onofrey CB, Ehlies FJ. Echography as a useful adjunct in the diagnosis of orbital solitary fibrous tumor. *Ophthalmic Plast Reconstr Surg.* 2003;19:68–74.
27. Miller NR. Primary tumours of the optic nerve and its sheath. *Eye.* 2004;18:1026–1037.
28. Rootman J. *Diseases of the Orbit.* 2nd ed. Lippincott Williams & Wilkins; 2003:250–254.
29. Pointdujour-Lim R, Lally SE, Shields JA, Eagle Jr RC, Shields CL. Orbital schwannoma: radiographic and histopathologic correlation in 15 cases. *Ophthalmic Plast Reconstr Surg.* 2018;34:162–167.
30. Ghassibi MP, Ulloa-Padilla JP, Dubovy SR. Neural tumors of the orbit—what is new? *Asia Pac J Ophthalmol (Phila).* 2017;6:273–282.
31. Graef S, Irwin MS, Wan MJ. Incidence and prognostic role of the ocular manifestations of neuroblastoma in children. *Am J Ophthalmol.* 2020;213:145–152.
32. Ordóñez NG, Mackay B. Granular cell tumor: a review of the pathology and histogenesis. *Ultrastruct Pathol.* 1999;23:207–222.
33. Jaeger MJ, Green WR, Miller NR, Harris GJ. Granular cell tumor of the orbit and ocular adnexa. *Surv Ophthalmol.* 1987;31:417–423.
34. Ribeiro SF, Chahud F, Cruz AA. Oculomotor disturbances due to granular cell tumor. *Ophthal Plast Reconstr Surg.* 2012;28:23–27.
35. Yanoff M, Sassani J. *Ocular Pathology.* 6th ed. Mosby; 2009:562.
36. Shields JA, Shields CL, Scartozzi R. Survey of 1264 patients with orbital tumors and simulating lesions: the 2002 Montgomery Lecture, part 1. *Ophthalmology.* 2004;111:997–1008.
37. El-Hadad C, Koka K, Dong W, et al. Multidisciplinary management of orbital metastasis and survival outcomes. *Ophthalmic Plast Reconstr Surg.* 2021;37:541–545.
38. Valenzuela AA, Archibald CW, Fleming B, et al. Orbital metastasis: clinical features, management and outcome. *Orbit.* 2009;28:153–159.
39. Goldberg RA, Rootman J. Clinical characteristics of metastatic orbital tumors. *Ophthalmology.* 1990;97:620–624.
40. Hei Y, Kang L, Yang X, et al. Orbital alveolar soft part sarcoma: a report of 8 cases and review of the literature. *Oncol Lett.* 2018;15:304–314.
41. Kim HJ, Wojno T, Grossniklaus HE, Shehata BM. Alveolar soft-part sarcoma of the orbit: report of 2 cases with review of the literature. *Ophthalmic Plast Reconstr Surg.* 2013;29:138–142.
42. Grant GD, Shields JA, Flanagan JC, Horowitz P. The ultrasonographic and radiologic features of a histologically proven case of alveolar soft-part sarcoma of the orbit. *Am J Ophthalmol.* 1979;87:773–777.

10

Orbital Inflammatory Diseases

BERNADETE AYRES, VICTOR ELNER, AND HAKAN DEMIRCI

Introduction

Orbital inflammatory disease encompasses a spectrum of specific and nonspecific entities. Specific causes include infection and systemic inflammatory diseases such as immunoglobin G4-related disease (IgG4) orbital inflammation, sarcoidosis, and granulomatosis with polyangiitis. Meanwhile, nonspecific orbital inflammation, also known as idiopathic orbital inflammation (IOI), is a noninfectious inflammatory condition, probably immunopathologic dysfunction with no identifiable local or systemic etiology.

Idiopathic Orbital Inflammation (Orbital Pseudotumor)

Idiopathic orbital inflammation is a noninfection inflammatory process of unknown etiology.

It accounts for 5–10% of orbital lesions and mostly involves middle-aged patients without gender predilection. Mixed inflammatory infiltration can be seen in any area of the orbit and takes a form of a mass.[1] IOI can be classified, according to the site or tissue involved, including anterior, diffuse, apical or posterior, myositis, and dacryoadenitis. The disease can have an acute, subacute, or chronic presentation based on the onset and duration of symptoms. The patients typically present with lid swelling, proptosis, orbital pain, and restricted motility.[2,3] Unilateral presentation is typical, but a bilateral presentation can occur.

On ultrasound imaging, the lesion is usually unilateral, multifocal, irregularly shaped, and regularly structured with internal low to medium reflectivity. Internal vascularity sometimes is positive. The lesion has firm consistency under the probe pressure test.

TEACHING POINTS

Idiopathic Orbital Inflammation may mimic lymphoproliferative diseases as well as thyroid ophthalmopathy. The presence of pain is an important clue to the diagnosis of idiopathic orbital inflammation.

CASE

A 60-year-old female patient presented with right upper lid swelling, ptosis, and palpable orbital mass superiorly for 2 months. The patient underwent an excisional biopsy, and the exam revealed chronic inflammation with mild fibrosis (Fig. 10.1).

Idiopathic sclerosing orbital inflammation

Is a rare pathological subgroup of orbital inflammation characterized as an insidious, chronic, and progressive sclerosing process. It exhibits fewer inflammatory signs than nonspecific orbital inflammation.

CASE

A 57-year-old woman presented with a 1-month history of left upper lid swelling and diplopia. Upon examination, a palpable firm orbital mass was detected superiorly. Imaging studies revealed an infiltrative orbital mass (Fig. 10.2). The patient underwent an orbitotomy with excisional biopsy. Histopathology exam revealed sclerosing orbital inflammation.

Idiopathic Myositis

Is an acute, usually unilateral inflammatory condition involving single or multiple extraocular muscles, including the tendinous insertion. There is orbital pain, exacerbated by eye movement, with diplopia, often some eyelid swelling, ptosis, and conjunctival chemosis. There may be an injection over the insertion of the affected muscle.

CASE

A 36-year-old female presented to the emergency room with a 2-day history of left eye pain exacerbated by eye movement and diplopia. There was no history of trauma or systemic disease. Ultrasound revealed enlargement of the inferior rectus in the left orbit (Fig. 10.3).

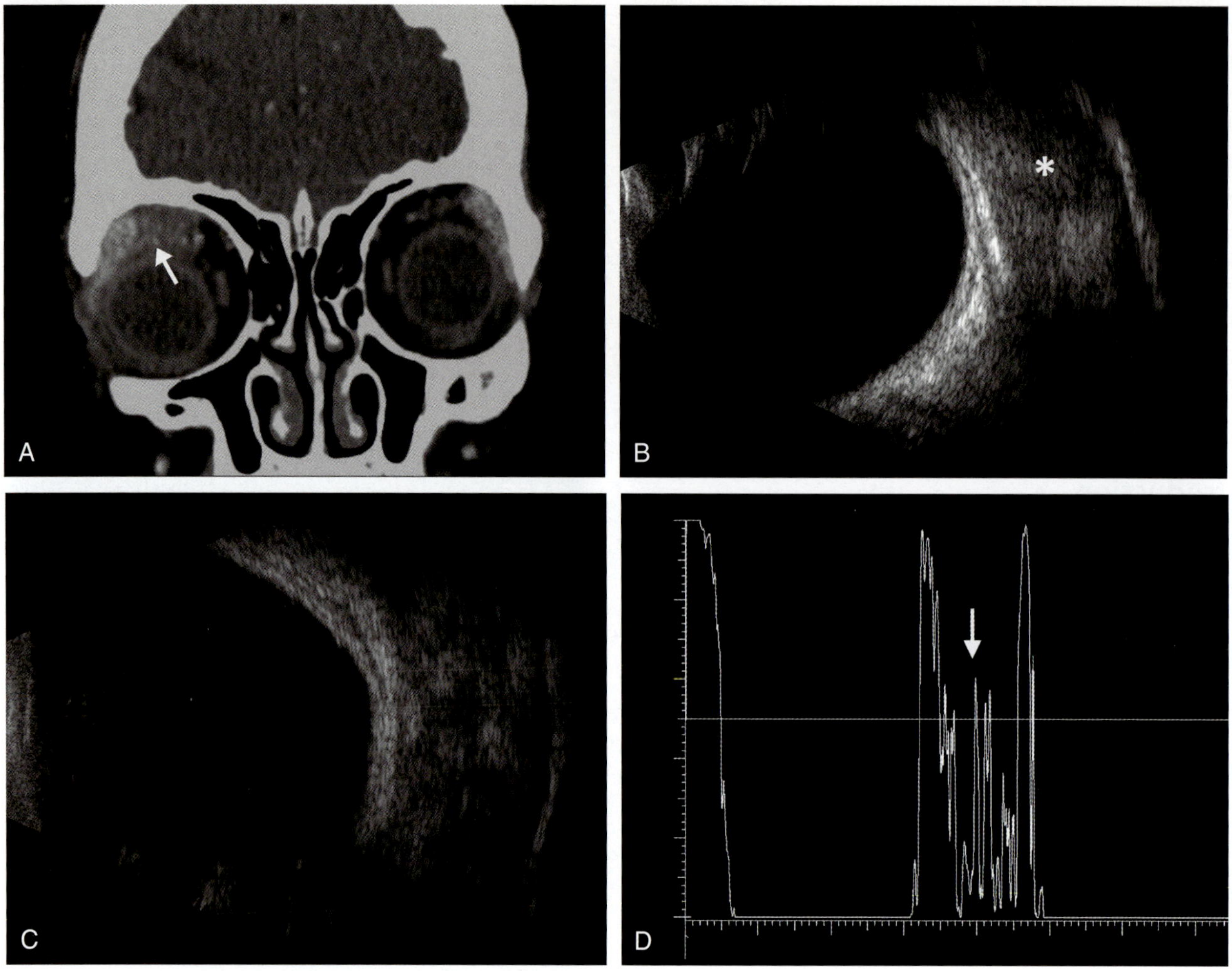

• **Fig. 10.1** Idiopathic Orbital Inflammation. **(A)** A coronal CT scan demonstrates a mass in the superior extraconal compartment of the right orbit (*arrow*). **(B)** Longitudinal B-scan through superior orbit demonstrates well-outlined, extraconal, low-reflective lesion (*asterisk*). **(C)** Transverse B-scan through the superior orbit region displays large low-reflective mass lesion. **(D)** The corresponding A-scan demonstrates a low-reflective orbital lesion (*arrow*).

IgG4-Related Dacryoadenitis

IgG4-related disease, recognized only recently, is a multi-organ fibro-inflammatory disease with characteristic histopathology showing lymphoplasmacytic infiltration, increased IgG4+ plasma cells, and elevated IgG4/IgG ratios (>40%). The lacrimal gland is the most common ocular site of involvement,[4,5] and characteristically presents as an indolent, painless bilateral gland enlargement. Less involved tissues are extraocular muscles, orbital fat, and nerves.

Ultrasound can demonstrate a well-outlined, oval, medium-reflective, with honeycomb pattern enlargement of the lacrimal gland. The mass is slightly compressible.

CASE

A 50-year-old female presented with a 2-year history of painful, bilateral asymmetric upper eyelid swelling. On ophthalmic exam, a palpable lacrimal gland was detected bilaterally (Fig. 10.4 and Video 10.1). The patient had a lacrimal gland biopsy, and the pathology demonstrated IgG4-rich reactive lymphoid hyperplasia.

Sarcoidosis

Sarcoidosis is an idiopathic, multisystem disorder characterized histopathologically by noncaseating granulomas.[6]

Ocular involvement in sarcoidosis is common, with anterior uveitis the most frequent manifestation. Orbital and adnexal involvement can occur in 8–10% of patients.[7,8] Within the orbit, sarcoidosis can affect the lacrimal gland, soft tissue, extraocular muscles, and optic nerve. The lacrimal gland is the most common site affected by extraocular sarcoidosis.

The most signs and symptoms at the initial presentation of orbital and adnexal sarcoidosis are eyelid swelling, painless palpable eyelid mass, proptosis, ptosis, discomfort, restricted ocular motility, dry eye, diplopia, and decreased vision. The patient may have been previously diagnosed with systemic disease, or orbital and adnexal sarcoidosis can be the initial manifestation.[9]

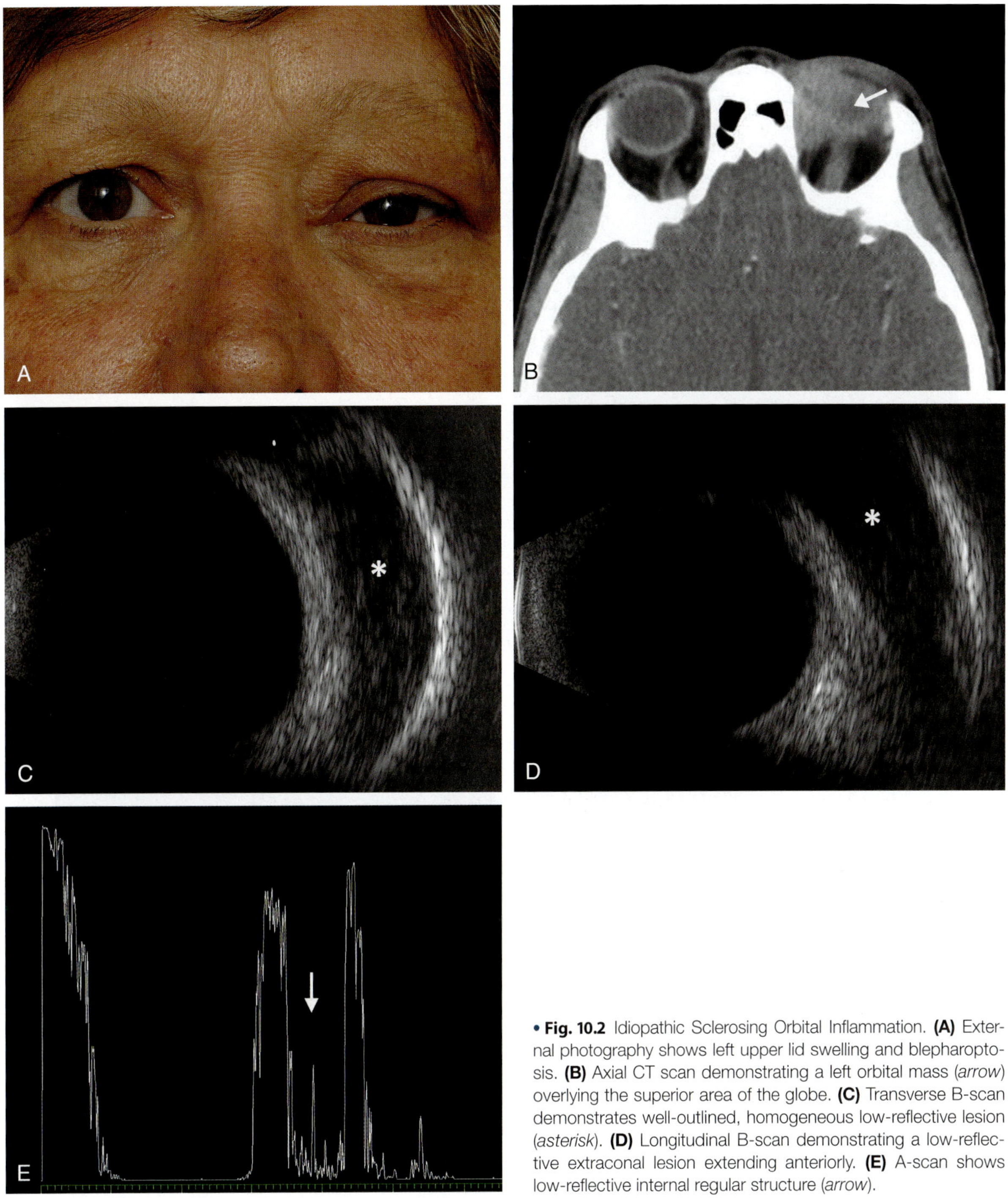

• **Fig. 10.2** Idiopathic Sclerosing Orbital Inflammation. **(A)** External photography shows left upper lid swelling and blepharoptosis. **(B)** Axial CT scan demonstrating a left orbital mass (*arrow*) overlying the superior area of the globe. **(C)** Transverse B-scan demonstrates well-outlined, homogeneous low-reflective lesion (*asterisk*). **(D)** Longitudinal B-scan demonstrating a low-reflective extraconal lesion extending anteriorly. **(E)** A-scan shows low-reflective internal regular structure (*arrow*).

On B-scan, patients with lacrimal involvement show well-outlined, somewhat homogeneous enlargement. The cases with soft orbital tissue involvement tend to be diffuse but can be focal. On A-scan, the lesion shows a regular internal structure with low to medium reflectivity.

CASE

A 46-year-old male presented with a 4-week history of bilateral upper eyelid swelling and dry eye sensation. A physical exam demonstrated bilateral ptosis and palpable, enlarged parotid and lacrimal glands. Imaging studies demonstrated bilateral enlarged lacrimal glands on CT scan (Fig. 10.5) and hilar lymphadenopathy on chest x-ray. The patient underwent a lacrimal gland biopsy for a definitive diagnosis. The pathology revealed noncaseating granuloma consistent with sarcoidosis.

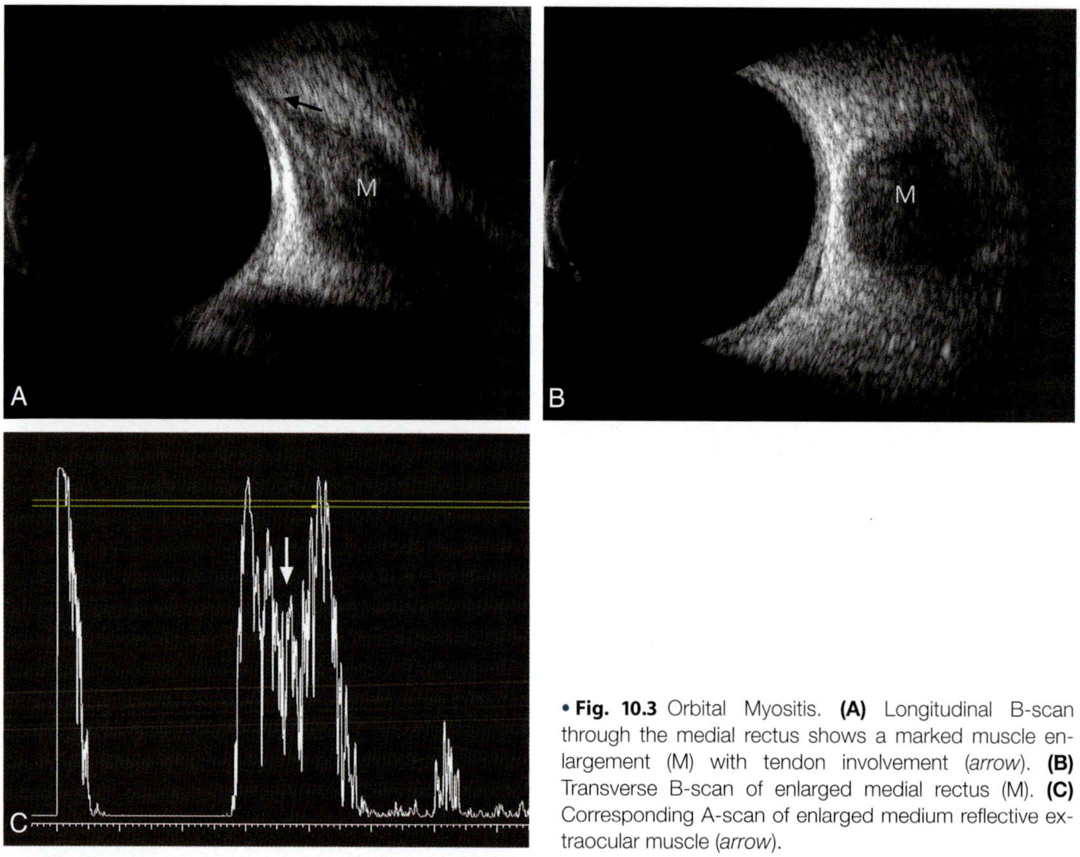

• **Fig. 10.3** Orbital Myositis. **(A)** Longitudinal B-scan through the medial rectus shows a marked muscle enlargement (M) with tendon involvement (*arrow*). **(B)** Transverse B-scan of enlarged medial rectus (M). **(C)** Corresponding A-scan of enlarged medium reflective extraocular muscle (*arrow*).

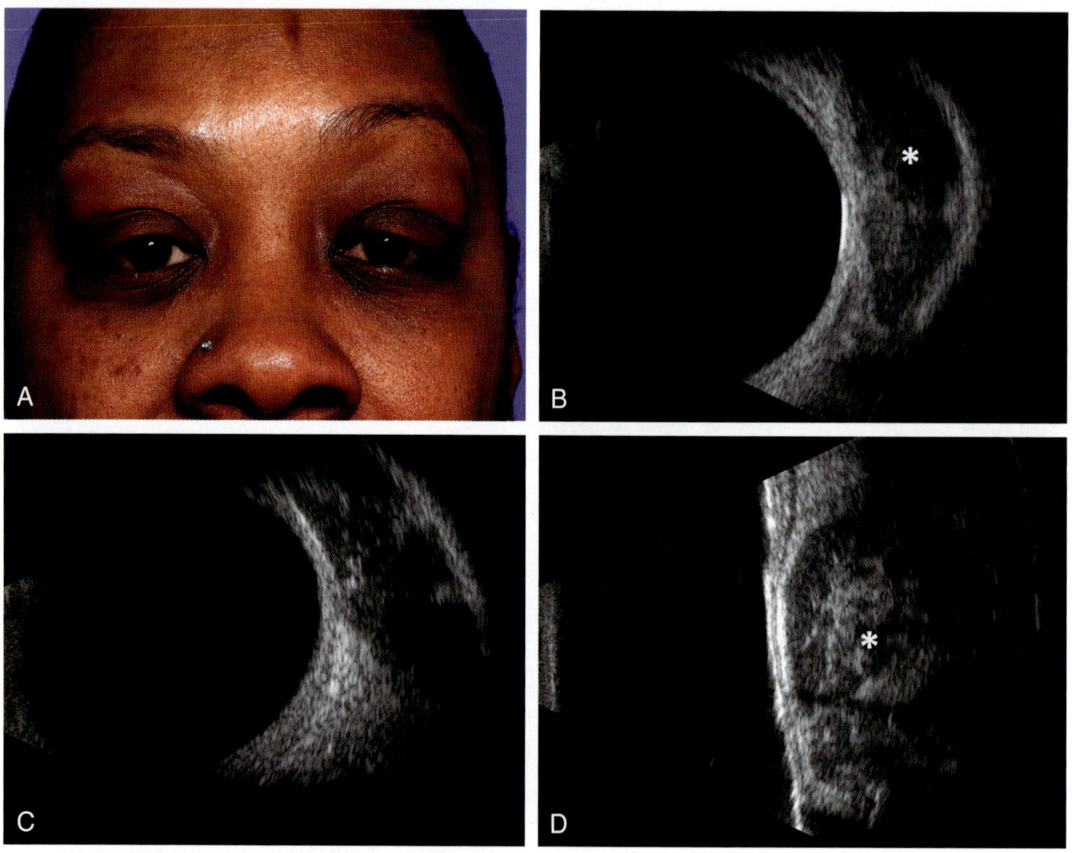

• **Fig. 10.4** IgG4 Related Dacryoadenitis. **(A)** External photography shows bilateral upper eyelid fulness and blepharoptosis. **(B)** Transverse B-scan aimed superotemporally, left eye, shows a well-outlined, medium reflective orbital lesion (*asterisk*) molded to the globe. There is no bone defect. **(C)** Longitudinal B-scan view of an enlarged left lacrimal gland. **(D)** Paraocular modified immersion over the left lacrimal gland shows a superficial, medium reflective lesion (*asterisk*).

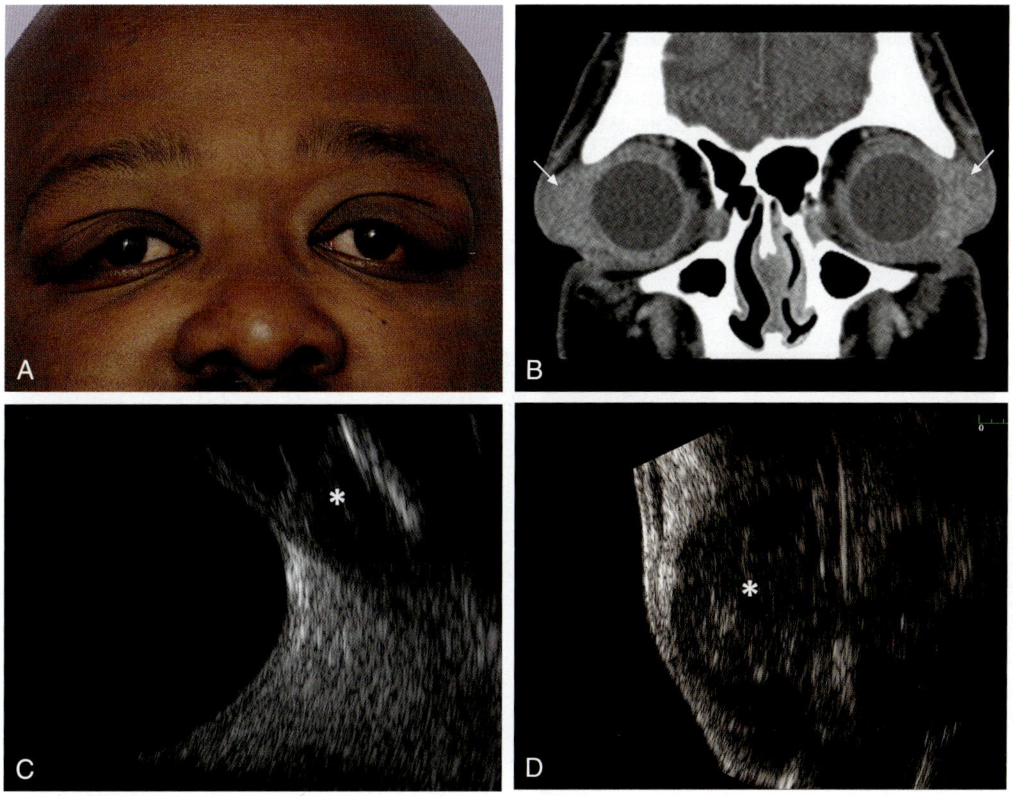

• **Fig. 10.5** Lacrimal Gland Involvement in Sarcoidosis. **(A)** External photography shows bilateral upper eyelid swelling and s-shaped ptosis. **(B)** A coronal CT scan shows a bilateral enhanced enlargement of the lacrimal glands (*arrows*). **(C)** Longitudinal B-scan with the probe aimed superotemporally, right eye, shows a well-outlined hyporreflective anterior orbital lesion (*asterisk*). **(D)** Paraocular modified Immersion B-scan through closed lids of the enlarged left lacrimal gland (*asterisk*) in case of sarcoidosis.

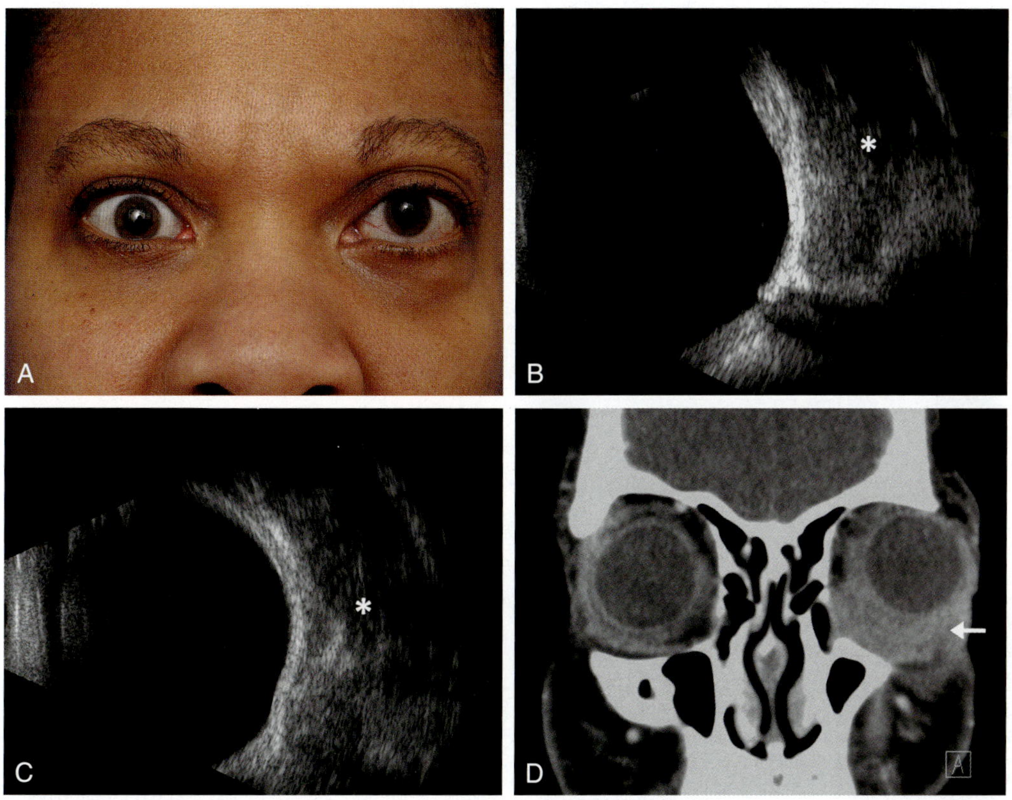

• **Fig. 10.6** Orbital Sarcoidosis. **(A)** External photography showing fullness of the left lower lid and upward eye displacement. **(B)** Longitudinal B-scan of a hypo-reflective orbital lesion extending posteriorly in her left orbit (*asterisk*). **(C)** Transverse B-scan displays orbital lesion causing mild indentation of the globe in the left orbit. **(D)** The post-contrast coronal CT scan shows a large, enhanced mass within the left inferior orbit (*arrow*).

CASE

A 53-year-old female was referred for evaluation of orbital mass of the left orbit for 2 months. External exam revealed left-side proptosis, upward eye displacement, and palpable mass in the lower eyelid (Fig. 10.6 and Video 10.2). Chest x-ray showed bilateral hilar adenopathy. The patient underwent an incisional biopsy, and pathology demonstrated noncaseating granuloma.

TEACHING POINTS

Chest x-ray usually reveals hilar lymphadenopathy in cases of systemic sarcoidosis. Definitive diagnosis relies on histopathologic analysis with the presence of characteristic noncaseating granuloma.

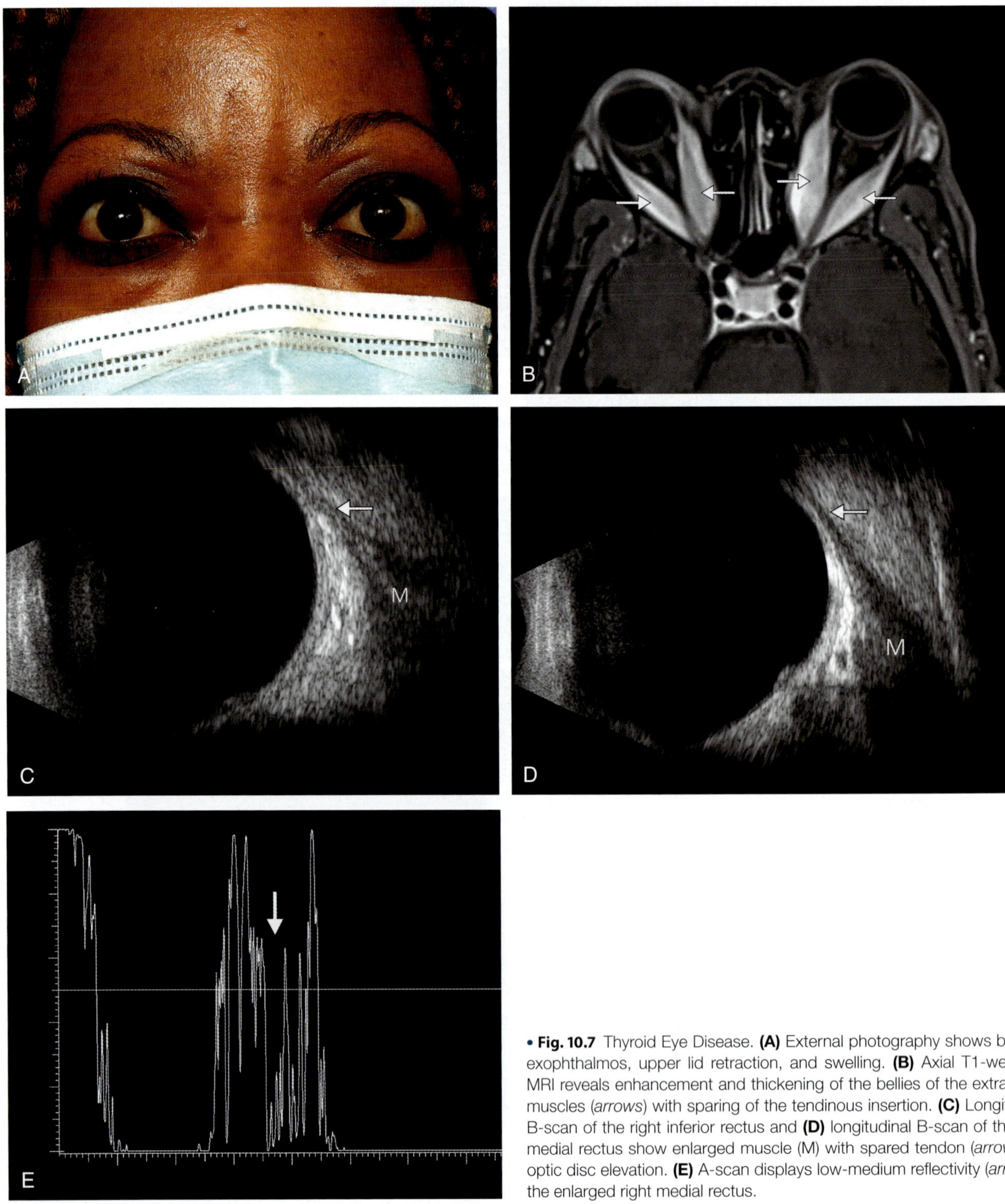

• **Fig. 10.7** Thyroid Eye Disease. **(A)** External photography shows bilateral exophthalmos, upper lid retraction, and swelling. **(B)** Axial T1-weighted MRI reveals enhancement and thickening of the bellies of the extraocular muscles (*arrows*) with sparing of the tendinous insertion. **(C)** Longitudinal B-scan of the right inferior rectus and **(D)** longitudinal B-scan of the right medial rectus show enlarged muscle (M) with spared tendon (*arrow*) and optic disc elevation. **(E)** A-scan displays low-medium reflectivity (*arrow*) of the enlarged right medial rectus.

Thyroid Eye Disease

Thyroid eye disease results from an autoimmune process closely associated with Graves' disease. Nearly 90% of cases occur in hyperthyroidism, with the remaining 10% associated with euthyroidism or hypothyroidism.

Swelling of the orbital soft tissues is the fundamental process underlying most of the clinical manifestations.

Based on the level of disease activity, thyroid eye disease can be classified into two phases: an active phase characterized by soft tissue inflammation, and an inactive phase associated with orbital fibrosis.[10]

Typical clinical findings of thyroid eye disease include bilateral eyelid erythema and edema, chemosis, exophthalmos, upper lid retraction, and restricted ocular motility. The disease may be insidious with only subtle clinical signs. Compressive optic neuropathy is a serious complication affecting about 5% of patients.

On ultrasound, thyroid eye disease presents bilateral, symmetric, and multiple muscle enlargement. Usually, the muscle bellies are enlarged, whereas the tendons are spared.[11] The internal reflectivity of an enlarged muscle can be low in the active phase and then become more reflective in the fibrotic phase. Other manifestations include swelling of the orbital fat, low reflective thickening of the periorbita, and lacrimal gland enlargement.[12]

CASE

A 36-year-old female presented with a history of Grave's disease and total thyroidectomy for hyperthyroidism. On examination, there were bilateral proptosis, eyelid swelling, and lid retraction (Fig. 10.7 and Video 10.3). Imaging studies revealed enlargement of the extraocular muscles and proptosis.

TEACHING POINTS

Thyroid eye disease characteristically affects the belly of the extraocular muscles and spares the tendinous insertions.

Orbital involvement may precede endocrine abnormalities in a small group of patients.

References

1. Aygun N, Shah G, Gandhi D (eds.). Idiopathic orbital pseudotumor. In: *Pearls and Pitfalls in Head and Neck and Neuroimaging: Variants and Other Difficult Diagnoses*. Cambridge University Press; 2013:331.
2. Garrity JA. *Henderson's Orbital Tumors*. 4th ed. Lippincott Williams & Wilkin; 2007:343.
3. Pemberton JD, Fay A. Idiopathic sclerosing orbital inflammation: a review of demographics, clinical presentation, imaging, pathology, treatment, and outcome. *Ophthalmic Plast Reconstr Surg*. 2012;28:79–83.
4. Kamisawa T, Zen Y, Pillai S, Stone JH. IgG4-related disease. *Lancet*. 2015;385:1460–1471.
5. Maehara T, Pillai S, Stone JH, Nakamura S. Clinical features and mechanistic insights regarding IgG4-related dacryoadenitis and sialoadenitis: a review. *Int J Oral Maxillofac Surg*. 2019;48:908–916.
6. Statement on sarcoidosis. Joint Statement of the American Thoracic Society (ATS), the European Respiratory Society (ERS) and the World Association of Sarcoidosis and Other Granulomatous Disorders (WASOG) adopted by the ATS Board of Directors and by the ERS Executive Committee, February 1999. *Am J Respir Crit Care Med*. 1999;160:736–755.
7. Smith JA, Foster CS. Sarcoidosis and its ocular manifestations. *Int Ophthalmol Clin*. 1996;36:109–125.
8. Demirci H, Christianson MD. Orbital and adnexal involvement in sarcoidosis: analysis of clinical features and systemic disease in 30 cases. *Am J Ophthalmol*. 2011;151:1074–1080.
9. Demirci H. *Orbital inflammatory diseases and their differential diagnosis*. Springer; 2015:35.
10. Joseph S, Douglas R. Thyroid eye disease: a comprehensive review. In: Demirci H, ed. *Orbital Inflammatory Diseases and their Differential Diagnosis*. Springer; 2015:73.
11. Byrne S, Green R. *Ultrasound of the Eye and Orbit*. 2nd ed. Mosby; 1992:396.
12. Gerding MN, Prummel MF, Wiersinga WM. Assessment of disease activity in Graves' ophthalmopathy by orbital ultrasonography and clinical parameters. *Clin Endocrinol*. 2000;52:641–646.

11

Conjuctival, Eyelids, and Lacrimal System Diseases

NORMA ALLEMANN AND RENATO LANDRE FILETI

The evaluation of ocular structures is well established with ultrasonography (10–60 MHz probes). However, extraocular structures and ocular adnexa are not well explored. Limited number of study shows the correlation between ultrasound biomicroscopy (UBM) and conjunctival diseases, eyelid cancers, or lacrimal system.

This chapter will evalute the use of ultrasonography for the diseases of the conjunctiva, eyelids, and lacrimal system.

Conjunctiva

Even though most of cases with conjunctival diseases are diagnosed clinically, the use of ultrasound can be complementary in the evaluations of conjunctival tumors; the UBM can provide information such as size, depth, internal reflectivity, and their relationship with adjacent structures.[1]

Benign Lesions

Conjunctival Cyst

UBM of a conjunctival cyst shows a well-delineated cystic lesion, with a continuous hyperreflective wall and hypoechoic internal content (Fig. 11.1). Surrounding conjunctiva shows no change in reflectivity.[2]

Pterygium

Pterygium is a fibrovascular overgrowth of the conjunctival and subconjunctival tissue over the cornea. It is usually triangular and invades the cornea more frequently medially and laterally.[3]

Risk factors for pterygium are immune mechanisms, genetic predisposition, and exposure to environmental factors such as ultraviolet rays, hot and dry weather, and wind.[3]

On UBM ultrasonography, it is a homogeneous conunctival thickening with blurred edges and high reflectivity compared to the surrounding conjunctiva (Fig. 11.2). Compared to the cornea, the tissue is more reflective and clearly demarcated.[2]

Pyogenic Granuloma

Pyogenic granuloma is a common acquired benign vascular tumor arising in tissues such as the skin and mucous membranes. The lesion grossly appears as a solitary, red, pedunculated, and very friable papule. In rare situations, they present as a sessile plaque. Often related to postoperative periods, it has a rapid exophytic growth, often with an ulcerated surface.[4]

They usually present as a homogeneous lesion with medium-to-high internal reflectivity and borders that are not so well defined in comparison to the surrounding tissue.[2]

Malignant Lesions

Ocular Surface Squamous Neoplasia

Ocular surface squamous neoplasia (OSSN) are tumors that are more commonly seen in adults, mainly males, and associated with exposure to ultraviolet radiation, human papilloma virus, and immunodeficiency such as human immunodeficiency virus infection.

The lesions are usually located on the perilimbal bulbar conjunctiva and may or may not involve the cornea, or can be located only on the cornea.[1]

The term OSSN encompasses the histopathological variations including dysplasia, carcinoma *in situ*, and squamous cell carcinoma (SCC) of the conjunctiva.

The differentiation of the three types of OSSN is possible using impression cytology and histopathological examination. Epithelial atypia associated with disruption of the epithelial basement membrane, and keratin pearls and dyskeratosis are histopathologic features of SCC.

For SCC, UBM examination is useful for evaluating of structures adjacent to the tumor and the deep margins over the cornea and the sclera.

In general, on the UBM exam, conjunctival SCC has a highly reflective epithelial surface with medium/low-reflective stroma. In some cases, their internal reflectivity may be heterogeneous. The image of the tumor can vary from a focal thickening of the conjunctiva to an elevated lesion with a nodular shape and a generally irregular surface (Fig. 11.3A–C).[5]

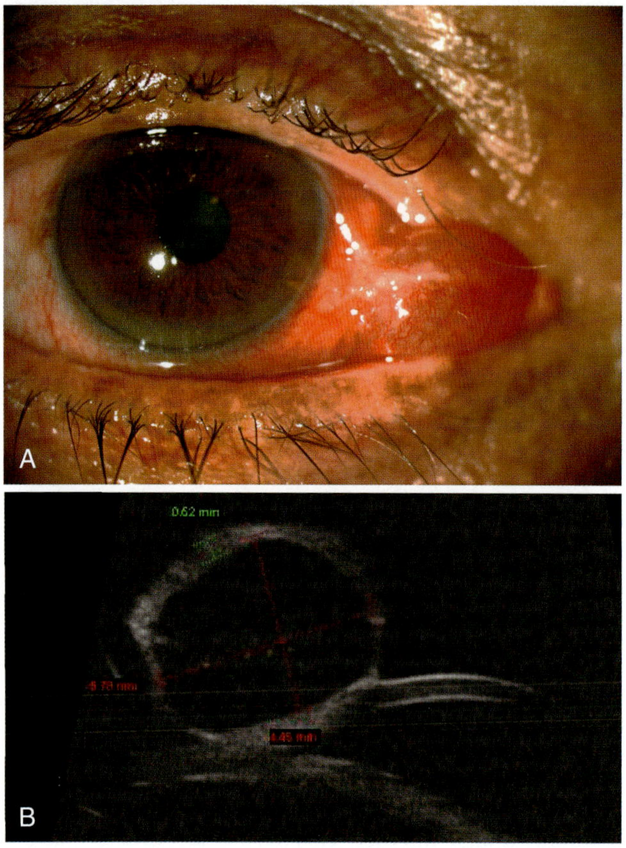

• **Fig. 11.1** **(A)** Conjunctival inclusion cystover the medial bulbar conjunctiva in a patient with a previous history of trauma. **(B)** UBM demonstrates a thin-walled benign cystic lesion lined with a non-keratinizing epithelium containing serous fluid, well delimited from the sclera. Dimensions measured radial: 5.78 mm; height: 4.45 mm, wall thickness: 0.52 mm.

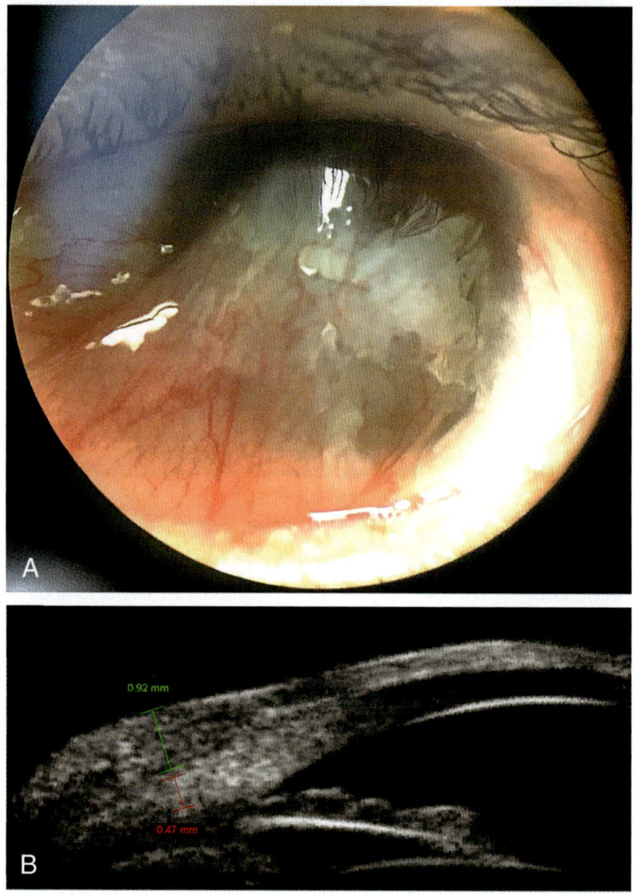

• **Fig. 11.2** **(A)** Recurrent pterygium, inferomedial lesion with extension over the cornea impairing the visual axis. **(B)** UBM with 50-MHz probe and immersion technique shows heterogeneous, highly reflective thickening of the perilimbal conjunctiva (thickness: 0.92 mm) and extension to the cornea, no invasion of the sclera or the cornea. The underlying sclera is normal: high reflectivity and thickness: 0.47 mm.

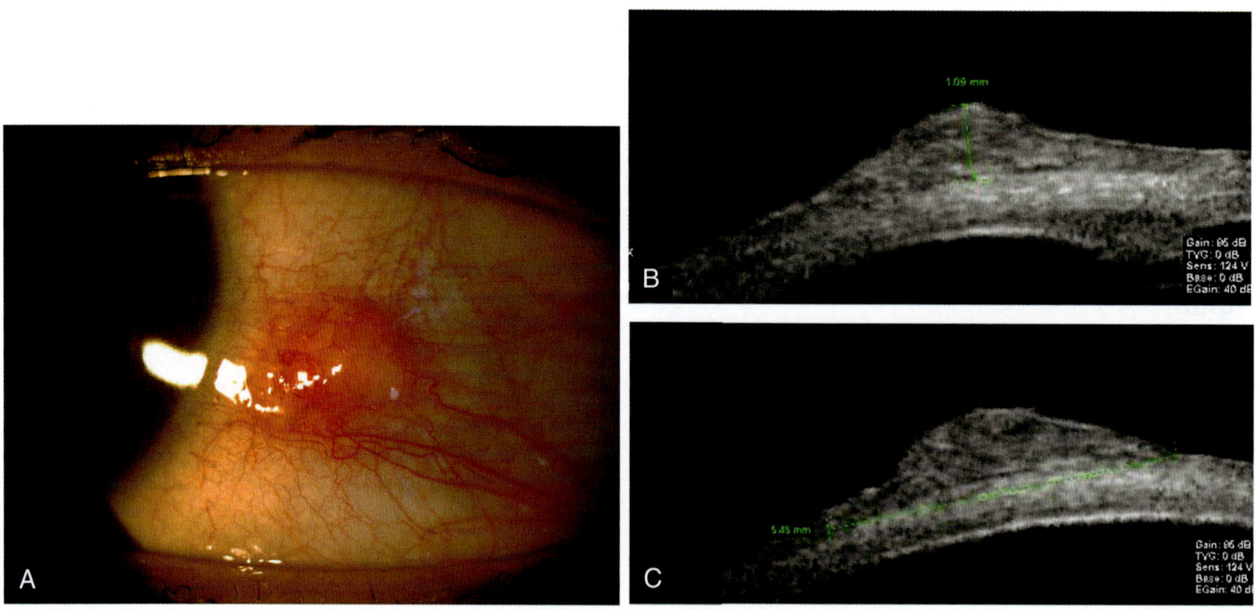

• **Fig. 11.3** **(A)** Slit-lamp photography of conjunctiva *in situ* shows elevated, focal thickening of the conjunctiva, with a nodular shape. **(B and C)** UBM in longitudinal and transverse scans demonstrate a focal thickening of the conjunctiva, with a heterogeneous structure with medium reflectivity and normal scleral bed. Measurements obtained: height: 1.09 mm; transverse extension: 5.45 mm. **(D)** Slit-lamp photography of a squamous cell carcinoma of the conjunctiva with nodular shape and irregular surface. **(E)** UBM in longitudinal scan demonstrates an elevated lesion of the perilimbal conjunctiva that extends over the cornea with heterogeneous structure and medium-to-high internal reflectivity. Scleral margin is intact.

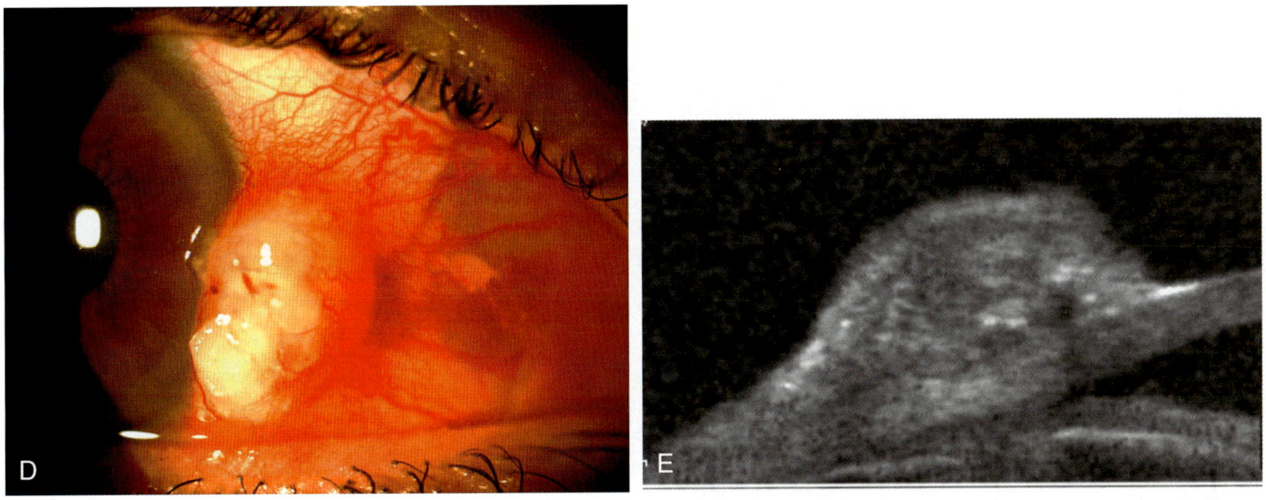

• **Fig. 11.3** cont'd

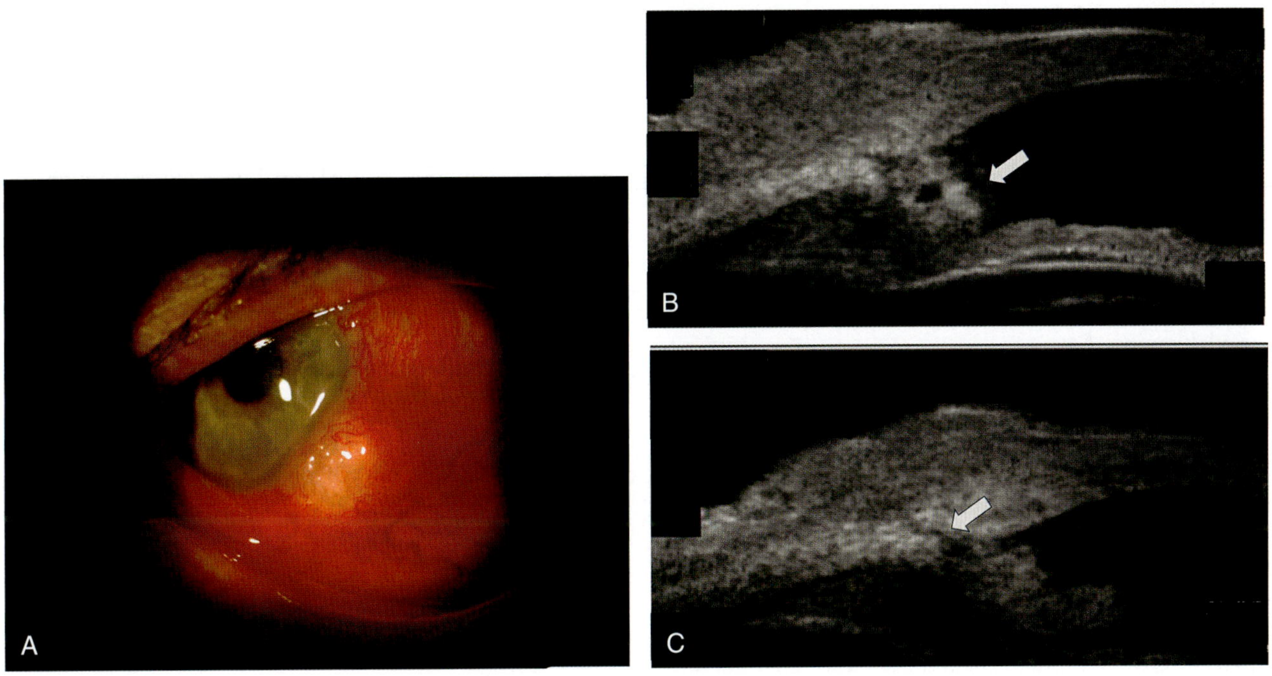

• **Fig. 11.4** Squamous cell carcinoma of the conjunctiva. **(A)** Slit-lamp photo demonstrates a nodular lesion in the inferomedial perilimbal area with pronounced hyperemia. In the same photo, a whitish and irregular tissue is observed in the anterior chamber angle, obstructing the observation of the iris and angle details. **(B–C)** UBM demonstrates thickening of the conjunctiva with a heterogeneous structure and suspected invasion of the sclera, anterior chamber angle, iris, and anterior chamber. **(B)** Nodular lesion in the anterior chamber occupying the anterior chamber angle and hindering details of the iris (*arrow*). **(C)** At the base of the conjunctival lesion, there is a scleral hypoechogenic path communicating the conjunctival lesion to the intraocular extension (*arrow*).

It is important to identify the limits of the lesion and to measure its dimensions using a caliper tool to assess the thickness as well as radial (antero-posterior) and transverse dimensions (Fig. 11.3D–E). The distance of the tumor margin in relation to a reference point such as cornea or sclera is very important both for surgical planning and follow-up after treatment.[1]

If the deep posterior margin is disrupted or compromised, hyperreflectivity and thickening of the cornea can be noticed, showing invasion to the cornea. If there is a disruption of the scleral base of the conjunctival tumor, scleral invasion even possible intraocular invasion is possible (Fig. 11.4).

Conjunctival Melanoma

Conjunctival melanoma is a rare, pigmented or non-pigmented lesion of the conjunctiva, which may correspond to 2% of all ocular tumors and 5% of ocular melanomas. It is aggressive and can cause local invasion and systemic disease due to its possible dissemination through the lymphatic or hematogenous system. Local recurrence can occur after treatments.[6]

On UBM exams, the internal reflectivity is homogeneously low due to the regular arrangement of their small cells. Tumor thickness measurement must be performed

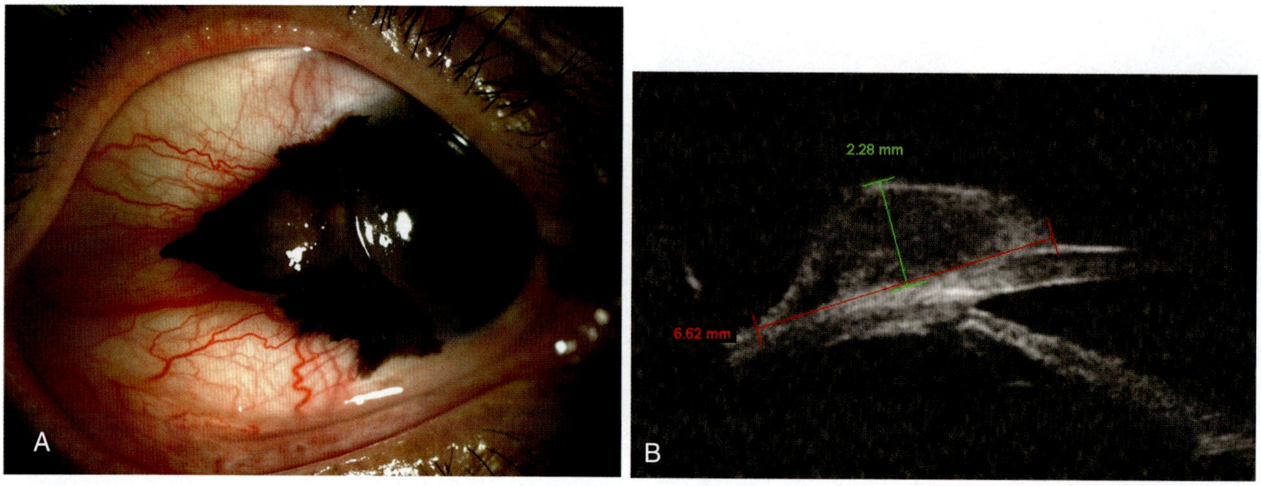

• **Fig. 11.5** **(A)** Slit-lamp biomicroscopy photo shows a conjunctival melanoma as a highly pigmented and elevated conjunctival lesions on the perilimbal area. **(B)** UBM demonstrates a homogeneous low internal reflectivity; measurements obtained: radial extension: 6.62 mm; height: 2.28 mm. The lesion is well delimited, with intact underlying sclera and cornea.

during UBM exam (Fig. 11.5). The tumor measurements and the evaluation of the tumor invasion to adjacent structures (cornea, sclera, iridocorneal angle, and uveal tissue) are important in the follow-up of patients.[7] Some authors have identified a significant correlation between tumor thickness on UBM exams and histopathologic results.[1]

The differential diagnoses of conjunctival melanoma should include previous staphylomas (scleral thinning) or cases with extrascleral extension of primary ciliary body or choroidal lesions.

Conjunctival Lymphoma

Lymphomas of the conjunctiva may appear as a primary lesion or associated with systemic lymphoma.

Clinically, the conjunctival lymphoid lesion appears as an orange–pink lesion, classically described as a salmon patch and a localized thickening of the conjunctiva.

The clinical differentiation between lymphoma and benign reactive lymphoid hyperplasia can be difficult, and histopathology plays an important role in the differential diagnosis. Conjunctival lymphoma is usually seen in elderly patients, while benign reactive lymphoid hyperplasia is observed in children. Upon UBM examination, we observe an area of conjunctival thickening with low internal reflectivity, generally without underlying scleral involvement.[1]

Eyelids

History and clinical examination are important for the diagnosis of eyelid lesions. In some cases, it is necessary to perform a incisional or excisional biopsy.

Noninvasive imaging exams become a great ally for evaluating the lesions, determining internal structure, depth, and correlation with adjacent tissues.[8] Serial evaluation provides information about the growth and possible extension to adjacent structures.

Capillary Hemangioma

Capillary hemangioma of the eyelid is known to be the most common benign tumor in childhood, with rapid proliferation and slow and gradual involution. Even though most hemangiomas remain asymptomatic, in some cases the morbidity can be significant, causing visual impairment.[9]

Capillary hemangioma has an internal composition of capillaries, endothelial cells, and endothelium-lined free spaces. Due to this internal composition, it appears poorly delimited at ultrasonography as an irregular lesion with low-to-medium internal reflectivity (density of blood vessels). The detection of internal vascularization by Color Doppler contributes to the diagnosis (Fig. 11.6). It presents as a soft, compressible lesion with detectable internal blood flow.[10]

Treatment with systemic drugs or surgical excision may be necessary. In case of treatment with systemic drugs, a gradual involution may be followed using ultrasonography.

Immersion technique using B-scan ultrasound may allow better evaluation of eyelid tumors that are superficial.

Lacrimal System

Lacrimal Gland

Ultrasonography can make an important contribution to the diagnosis of lacrimal gland diseases, in addition to magnetic resonance imaging and computed tomography.

In ultrasonography, the normal lacrimal gland and the adjacent orbital fat cannot be differentiated from adjacent tissues and present a high reflectivity.[10]

The incidence of lacrimal gland lesions is estimated at 1–1,000,000 people per year and can be divided into epithelial and non-epithelial lesions.

- Non-epithelial tumors account for 55–80% of lacrimal gland masses. Among the no-nepithelial ones, there are dacryoadenitis (non-granulomatous and granulomatous inflammation), and lymphoproliferative tumors.[11]

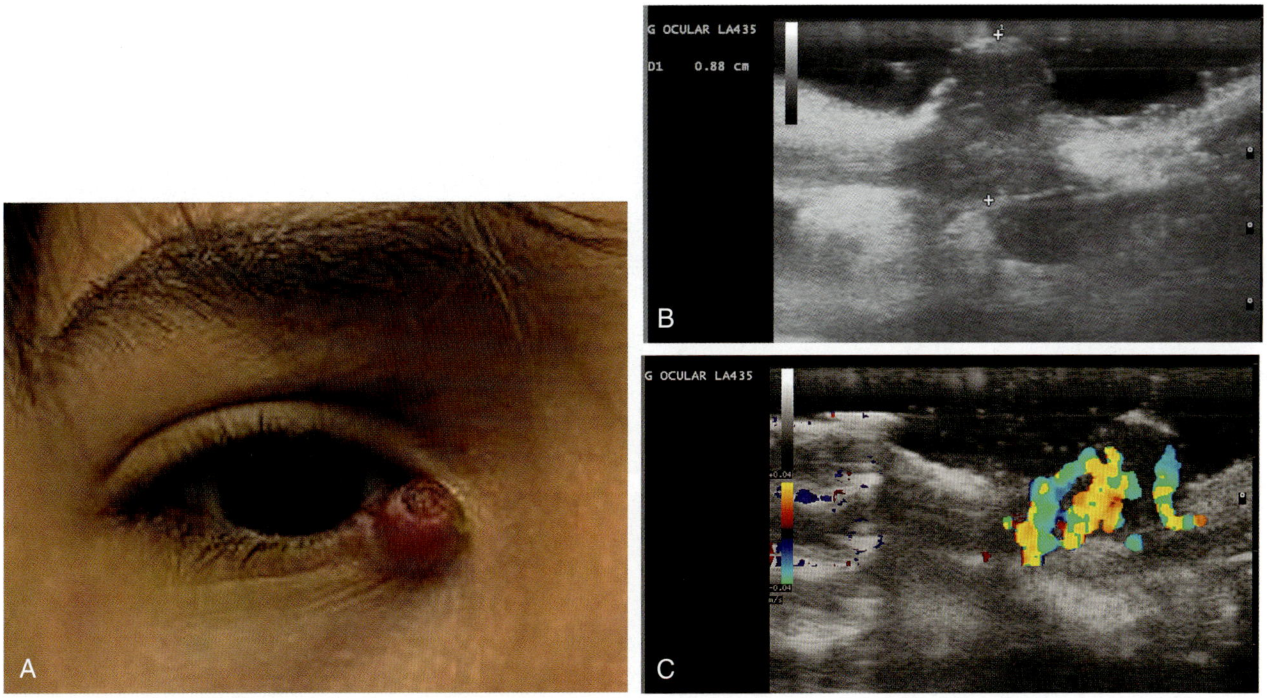

• **Fig. 11.6** **(A)** External view of a 10-year-old male presenting a solid, elevated, nodular, purplish, with central ulceration lesion on the medial portion of the lower eyelid. **(B–C)** B-scan and color Doppler, 7.5–15-MHz linear transducer. **(B)** B-mode ultrasound with immersion technique shows a superficial hypoechoic and superficial lesion with poor margins. Thickness: 8.8 mm. **(C)** Color Doppler ultrasound demonstrates high internal vascularity compatible with capillary hemangioma.

Dacryoadenitis

The inflammatory process of the lacrimal gland can be difficult to differentiate from an inflammatory pseudotumor when using ultrasonography. Some characteristics that appear on ultrasonographic examination are diffuse thickening of the lacrimal gland, with high internal reflectivity, and absence of internal vascularization. Adjacent orbital fat also presents changes in reflectivity due to the inflammatory process.

Lymphoproliferative Disorders

Lymphoproliferative disorders of the lacrimal gland can be unilateral or bilateral and are very common in the lacrimal gland fossa.

It includes a spectrum of conditions such as reactive lymphoid hyperplasia, atypical lymphoid hyperplasia, and malignant lymphoma. In B-scan ultrasonography they have an irregular spindle-shaped shape with a regular or slightly irregular internal structure and medium-to-low internal reflectivity and small degree of sound attenuation. Color Doppler exam shows internal vascularization.[10]

- Epithelial tumors represent about 20–45% of lacrimal gland tumors, divided into benign and malignant. Benign epithelial tumors include lacrimal ductal cysts and pleomorphic adenoma (benign mixed tumor). Malignant epithelial tumors include adenoid cystic carcinoma (ACC) and malignant adenocarcinoma (see Chapter 9).

Pleomorphic Adenoma (Benign Mixed Tumor)

Pleomorphic adenoma is the most common benign epithelial tumor of the lacrimal gland. It affects the orbital lobe of the lacrimal gland more commonly than the palpebral lobe. It presents a medium-to-high internal reflectivity with moderate attenuation. They are well delineated with their surrounding capsule, have a firm consistency and lack intrinsic vascularization. Internally, they may have small cysts. As a differential diagnosis, cavernous hemangioma may be considered; however, the latter has a softer consistency and rarely presents itself in the lacrimal gland fossa.[10]

Adenoid Cystic Carcinoma

Adenoid cystic carcinoma is the second most common epithelial tumor and most common primary malignant tumor of the lacrimal gland.

On B-scan ultrasonography, it usually has a medium-to-high internal reflectivity with irregular internal structures. It lacks vascularization and has firm consistency. A well-circumscribed carcinoma can be difficult to differentiate from a pleomorphic adenoma or even a dermoid cyst based on its ultrasonographic features.[10]

Lacrimal Drainage System

The lacrimal sac is a structure covered by columnar epithelium located between the anterior and posterior lacrimal crests. It comprises the widest portion of the lacrimal

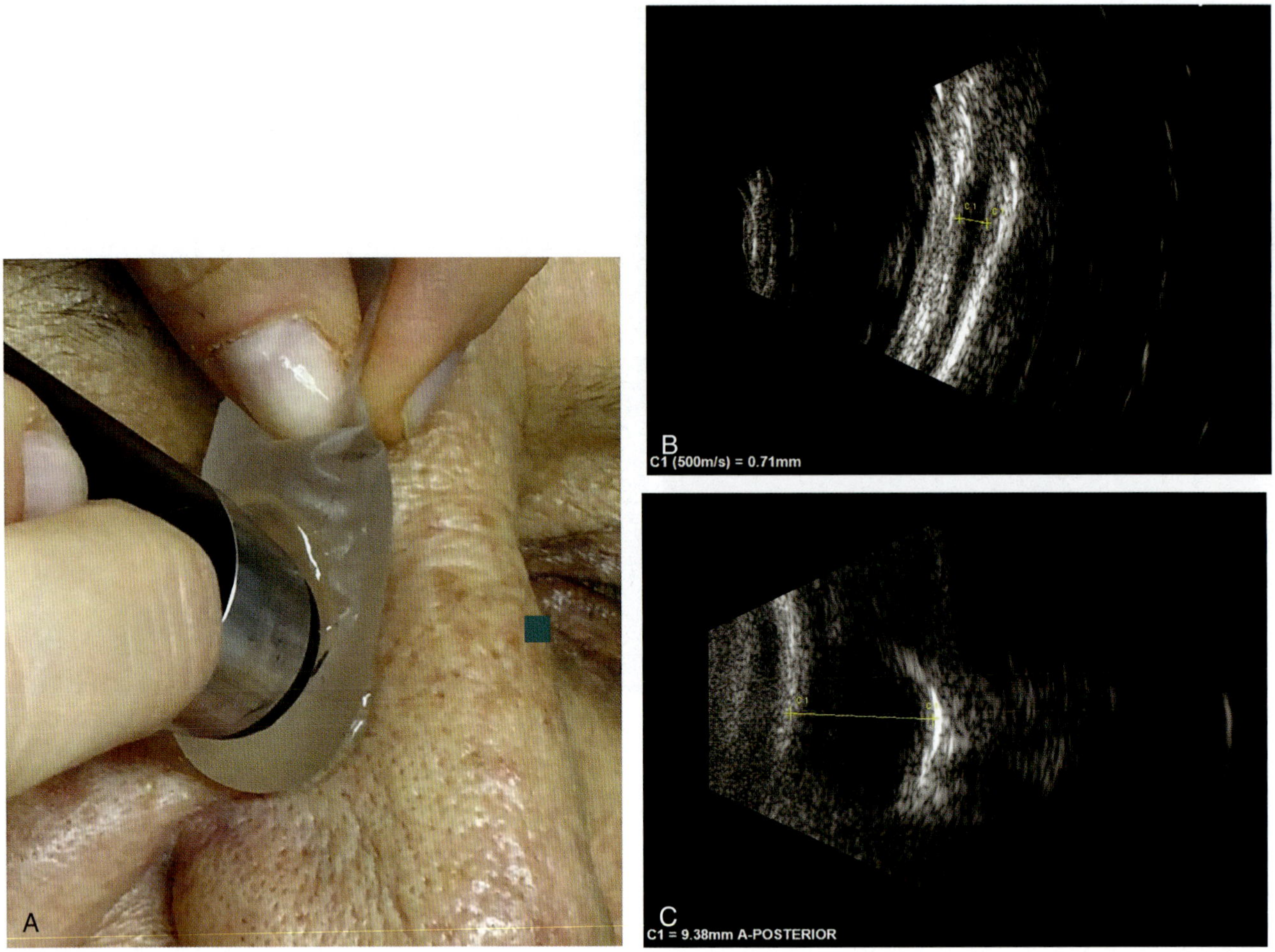

• **Fig. 11.7** **(A)** Technique of immersion on the lacrimal fossa, distancing the transducer from the skin surface to better evaluate superficially placed lesions. **(B)** Normal lacrimal sac; small and elongated shaped structure with low internal reflectivity, anteroposterior extension: 0.71 mm. **(C)** Enlarged lacrimal sac due to chronic dacryocystitis; dilated structure with a rounded shape and low internal reflectivity. Anteroposterior extension: 9.38 mm.

duct measuring 4–8 mm anteroposteriorly and 10–12 mm vertically.[12]

Ultrasonography can be useful to detect changes in the lacrimal sac as a painless and noninvasive method. In the preoperative evaluation, it can be used to determine the size and evaluate the characteristics of the lacrimal sac, including abnormal dilations, presence of diverticula, or exudative inflammatory processes.[13]

Dacryocystitis

Dacryocystitis is an inflammation or infection of the lacrimal sac.

Under normal conditions, the lacrimal sac appears as a small structure, with low and homogeneous internal reflectivity.[10,12,13]

When dilated secondary to an inflammation or infection, ultrasound shows an enlarged lacrimal sac with low internal reflectivity (Fig. 11.7).

In chronic dacryocystitis, the lacrimal sac may be completely or partially filled by low reflectivity and show punctate echoes associated with the inflammatory process.[12]

References

1. Branco AMPC, Fileti RL, Allemann N. Ultrassonografia biomicroscópica na avaliação de tumores oculares de segmento anterior. In: Conselho Brasileiro de Oftalmologia; Lavinsky D, Lavinsky F, Rocha JCP, organizadores. PRO-OFTALMO Programa de Atualização em Oftalmologia: Ciclo 5. Artmed Panamericana; 2021:9–58.
2. Buchwald HJ, Müller A, Spraul CW, Lang GK. Ultraschallbiomikroskopie bei Bindehauttumoren [Ultrasound biomicroscopy of conjunctival lesions]. *Klin Monbl Augenheilkd*. 2003;220(1-2):29–34. https://doi.org/10.1055/s-2003-37576.
3. Sarkar P, Tripathy K. *Pterygium*. StatPearls Publishing; 2023. https://www.ncbi.nlm.nih.gov/books/NBK558907/.
4. Sarwal P, Lapumnuaypol K. *Pyogenic Granuloma*. StatPearls Publishing; 2023. https://www.ncbi.nlm.nih.gov/books/NBK556077/.
5. Nanji AA, Mercado C, Galor A, Dubovy S, Karp CL. Updates in ocular surface tumor diagnostics. *Int Ophthalmol Clin*. 2017;57(3):47–62.
6. Wong JR, Nanji AA, Galor A, Karp CL. Management of conjunctival malignant melanoma: a review and update. *Expert Rev Ophthalmol*. 2014;9(3):185–204.
7. Conway RM, Chew T, Golchet P, Desai K, Lin S, O'Brien J. Ultrasound biomicroscopy: role in diagnosis and management in

130 consecutive patients evaluated for anterior segment tumours. *Br J Ophthalmol.* 2005;89(8):950–955. https://doi.org/10.1136/bjo.2004.059535.

8. Kikkawa DO, Ochabski R, Weinreb RN. Ultrasound biomicroscopy of eyelid lesions. *Ophthalmologica.* 2003;217(1):20–23. https://doi.org/10.1159/000068253.
9. Ceisler E, Blei F. Ophthalmic issues in hemangiomas of infancy. *Lymphat Res Biol.* 2003;1(4):321–330. https://doi.org/10.1089/153968503322758148.
10. Byrne SF, Green RL. Vascular lesions. In: Byrne SF, Green RL. Ultrasound of the Eye and Orbit. Mosby Year Book; 1992:347–366.
11. Gündüz AK, Yeşiltaş YS. Shields CL. Overview of benign and malignant lacrimal gland tumors. *Curr Opin Ophthalmol.* 2018;29(5):458–468. https://doi.org/10.1097/ICU.0000000000000515.
12. Milder B, Demorest BH. Dacryocystography. The pathologic lacrimal apparatus. *Arch Ophthalmol.* 1955;54(3):410–421.
13. Machado MAC, Silva JAF, Garcia EA, Allemann N. Ultrasound parameters of normal lacrimal sac and chronic dacryocystitis. *Arq Bras Oftalmol.* 2017;80(3):172–175. https://doi.org/10.5935/0004-2749.20170042.

12

Pediatric Ophthalmic Ultrasound

CARLA MOREIRA ALBHY AND NORMA ALLEMANN

Introduction

Pediatric eye examination can often be challenging, so B-scan ultrasonography is especially helpful, as it does not require any sedation or additional anesthesia. It can be easily performed by an experienced physician or certified ultrasonographer, even in uncooperative patients.

B-scan ultrasonography is especially important in evaluation of leukocoria or eye with opaque media. In this chapter, ultrasonographic features of some common pediatric ocular conditions are presented and exemplified.

Retinoblastoma

Retinoblastoma is the most common primary malignant intraocular tumor of childhood[1] and often presents as leukocoria in children. Further explanation and clinical presentation can be found in chapter about tumors of the posterior segment.

Coats Disease

Coats disease is a telangiectatic neovascular disease of the retina of unknown etiology. It usually affects one eyes and is more frequently seen in young males.[2]

On fundus examination, aneurysms and telangiectatic vessels, usually located on the temporal retina, are observed. These abnormal vessels are leaky, and there is exudation in various degrees that can lead to the serous retinal detachment, which is easily detected by the B-scan ultrasonography examination. The most typical ultrasonographic features are the presence of dispersed opacities corresponding to exudative lipid material in the subretinal space of serous retinal detachment[3] (Fig. 12.1). Areas of choroidal thickening can sometimes be demonstrated, but there is usually an absence of solid mass lesion and calcification.

Severe cases can evolve to atrophic stages (Fig. 12.2).

Retinopathy of Prematurity

Retinopathy of prematurity (ROP) is typically a bilateral condition that affects infants who are born early (premature birth), particularly before 31 weeks or who weight less than 3 pounds at birth.[4] The manifestation and timing of ROP differ greatly throughout the world, depending on the technology and resources of infant care. High unregulated oxygen at birth is one of the main risk factors for ROP, in addition to the prematurity itself. Other risk factors associated to ROP are low birth weight and poor postnatal growth.

In the intrauterine environment, the fetus is in a hypoxic state. After birth, the sudden increase in the oxygen level can damage retinal capillaries. ROP is caused by a mismatch between normal retinal vascularization and oxygen need by a premature developing retina.

Each eye should be classified using the following parameters: zone, plus disease, stage, and extent.[4] The acute disease has five stages: thin and flat line separating vascular retina from and avascular retina in stage 1; ridge arises from the demarcation line and vessels arise from the ridge to enter the posterior retina in stage 2; extraretinal neovascular proliferation or intravascular vascularization in stage 3; partial retinal detachment with fovea attached in stage 4A and fovea detached in stage 4B; and total retinal detachment with visible optic disc, suggesting open-funnel detachment in stage 5A, without visble optic dics due to retrolental fibrovascular tissue or closed-funnel detachment in stage 5B, and associated anterior segment changes in stage B disease in stage 5C.

B-scan ultrasonography can detect all stages of ROP,[5] although the sensitivity to detect stage 1 ROP is significantly low, and stage 1 disease should be diagnosed based on the fundus examination performed by an experienced physician. This is because the demarcation line in stage 1 ROP that represents hyperplasia of the spindle cells is too thin to be detected by the ultrasound, even in the most modern devices. A good correlation was demonstrated between the fundoscopic examination and ultrasonographic features in stage 2 ROP and above. Ultrasonography can demonstrate the presence of ridges and peripheral loops in earlier stages as well as the size and configuration of the tractional retinal detachment in advanced cases. When measuring the axial ocular length, the adjusted age of the premature patient should be considered (Figs. 12.3 and 12.4).

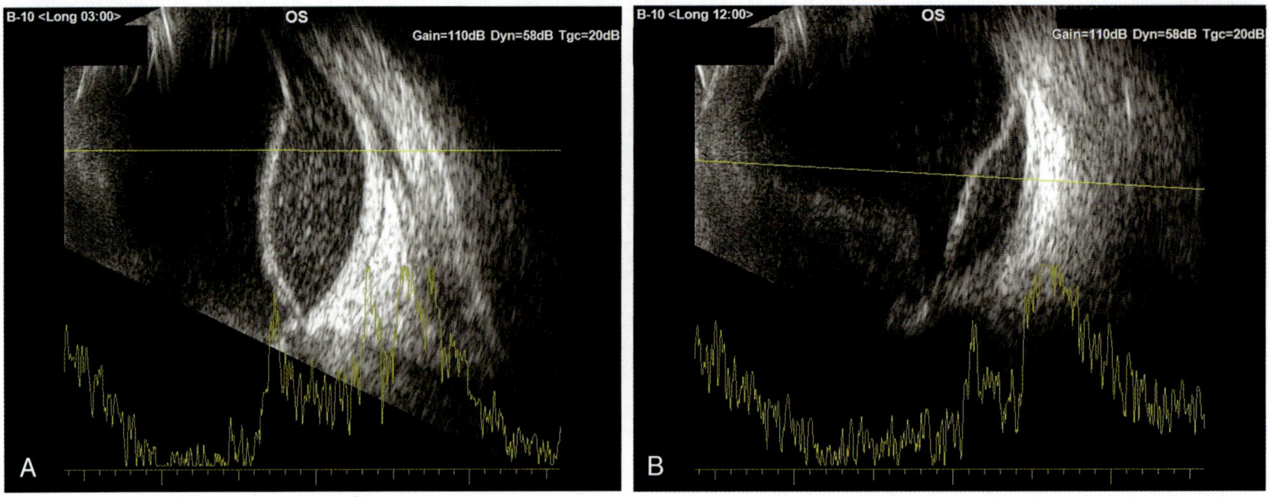

• **Fig. 12.1** B-scan ultrasound in a 3-year-old male demonstrating bullous retinal detachment with dispersed subretinal opacities (exudative lipid material) and more subretinal material in the inferior meridians **(A)**, sparing the superior periphery **(B)**.

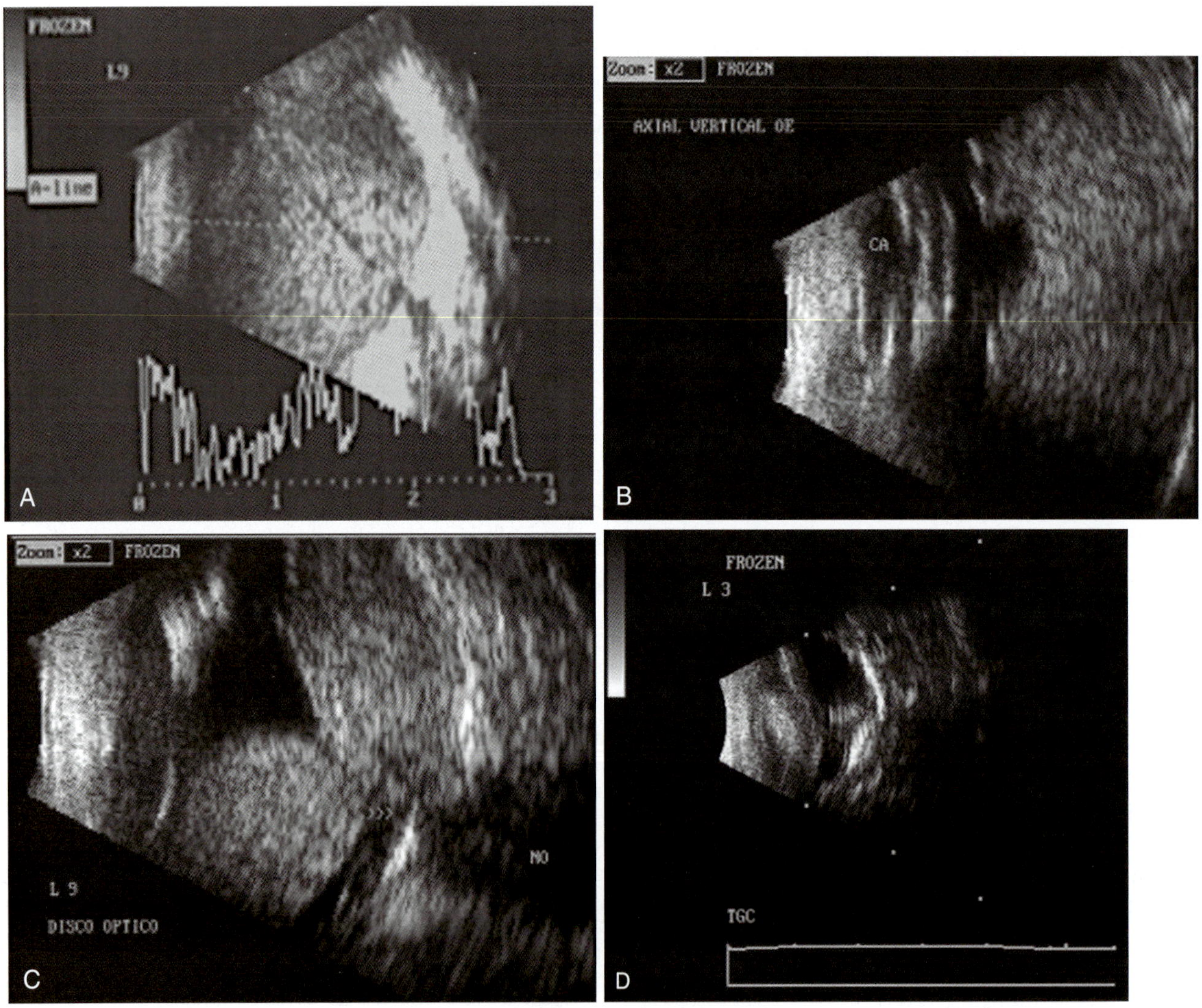

• **Fig. 12.2** **(A)** A 2-year-old female presents with strabismus of the left eye and total retinal detachment. Ultrasound exam demonstrates a dense collection of dispersed opacities in the subretinal space along with serous retinal detachment. Note that the detached retina appears echolucent when surrounded by dense opacities. **(B–C)** At 1-year follow-up, there is lens opacification (B), and B-scan ultrasonography shows total retinal detachment with dense subretinal debris and a peripapillary hyperreflective deposit or calcification (*arrows*). **(D)** At 6-year follow-up, the evolution to phthisis bulbi is observed. B-scan ultrasound demonstrates reduced axial length, multiple sites of calcification, disorganization of internal ocular structures, and orbital fat attenuation.

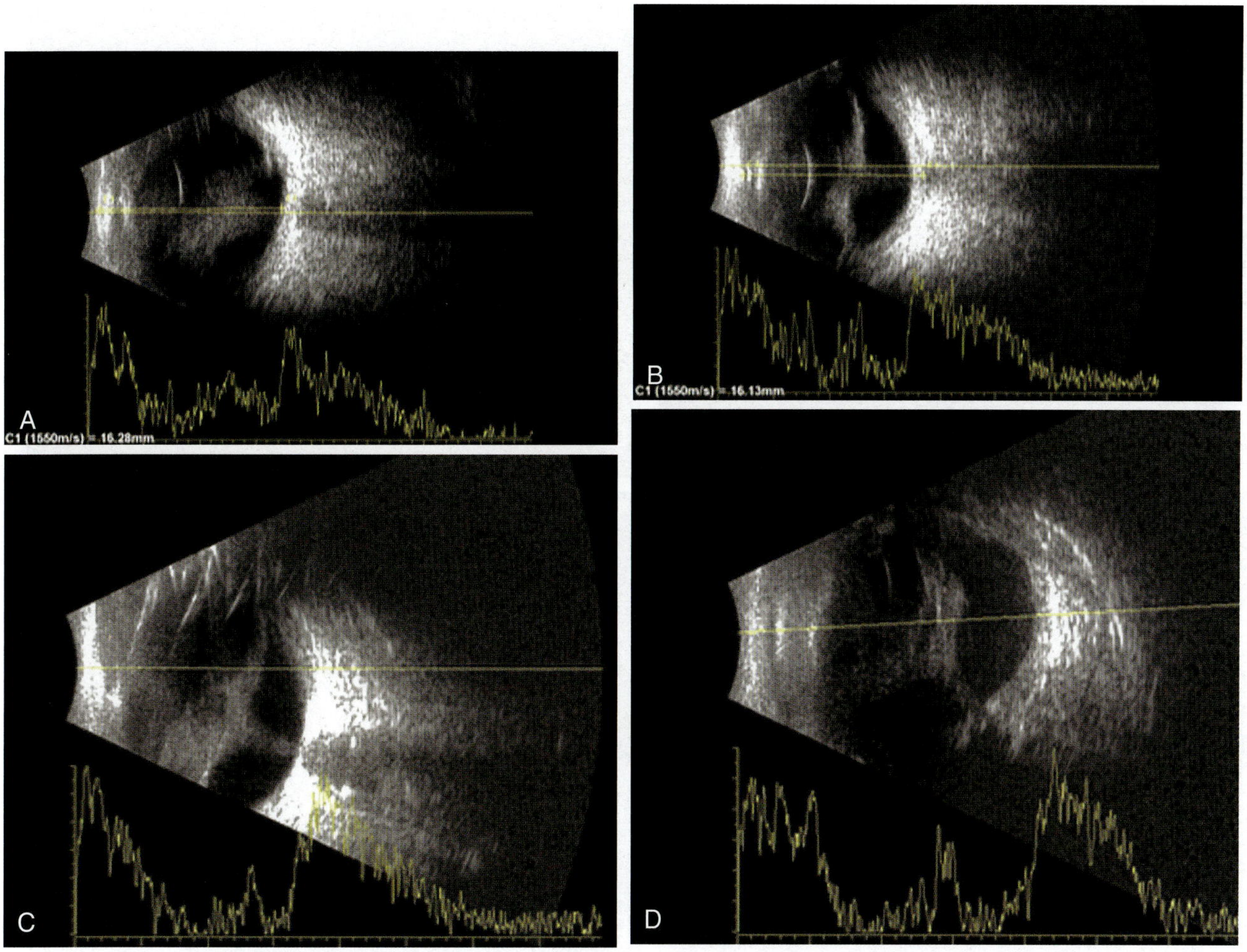

• **Fig. 12.3** A female infant was born at a gestational age of 25 weeks, with a birth weight of 725 g. The patient did not have an ophthalmological examination until the adjusted age of 1 year, when presented with retinal detachment. **(A–B)** A B-scan ultrasonographic exam was performed, showing small axial length in both eyes (**A**. AL OD: 16.28 mm; B. AL OS: 16.13 mm), and bilateral total closed funnel configuration retinal detachment **(C–D)**.

The use of ultrasonography in the management of ROP can be advantageous for premature neonates with poor pupillary dilation and hazy media, particularly in countries with a limited number of trained pediatric ophthalmologists and limited Retcam availability.

Ocular Toxocariasis

Toxocariasis is a zoonosis caused by the larvae of *Toxocara canis*, and, less frequently, *Toxocara cati*. There are two main syndromes caused by the larvae migrans: the visceral larva migrans, affecting major organs as liver and lungs, and the ocular larva migrans (OLV), a rare condition with challenging diagnosis.[6]

Clinical manifestations include diffuse endophthalmitis, and posterior pole and peripheral granuloma, which may have the following ultrasonographic findings:

- Granuloma: In B-scan ultrasonography, granuloma appears as a posterior pole or peripheral hyperechoic solid mass, with a regular surface in most cases. It presents a homogeneous internal reflectivity with vitreous membranes or bands adhered to the surface, that can extend from the mass to the posterior pole[7] and can be associated with retinal traction or detachment of folds. Calcifications might be observed, especially when ocular atrophy is present,[8] often erroneously leading to the suspicion of ocular retinoblastoma in children.
- Endophthalmitis: This clinical presentation occurs when the larva hatches from the cyst and dies, leading to an intense inflammatory process. Thus the ultrasonography findings are similar to endophthalmitis of any other etiology.
- Peripheral granulomas in UBM imaging and in peripheraly and anteriorly posited B-scans manifest as hyperechoic solid masses with rough borders.[9] The granulomas are encapsulated by a tissue, although they have a clear boundary with adjacent tissue, such as the ciliary body. Thick vitreous strands can be found on the surface of the granulomas or the adjacent eye wall. The other end extends to the vitreous or to the lens (Fig. 12.5). Detachment of

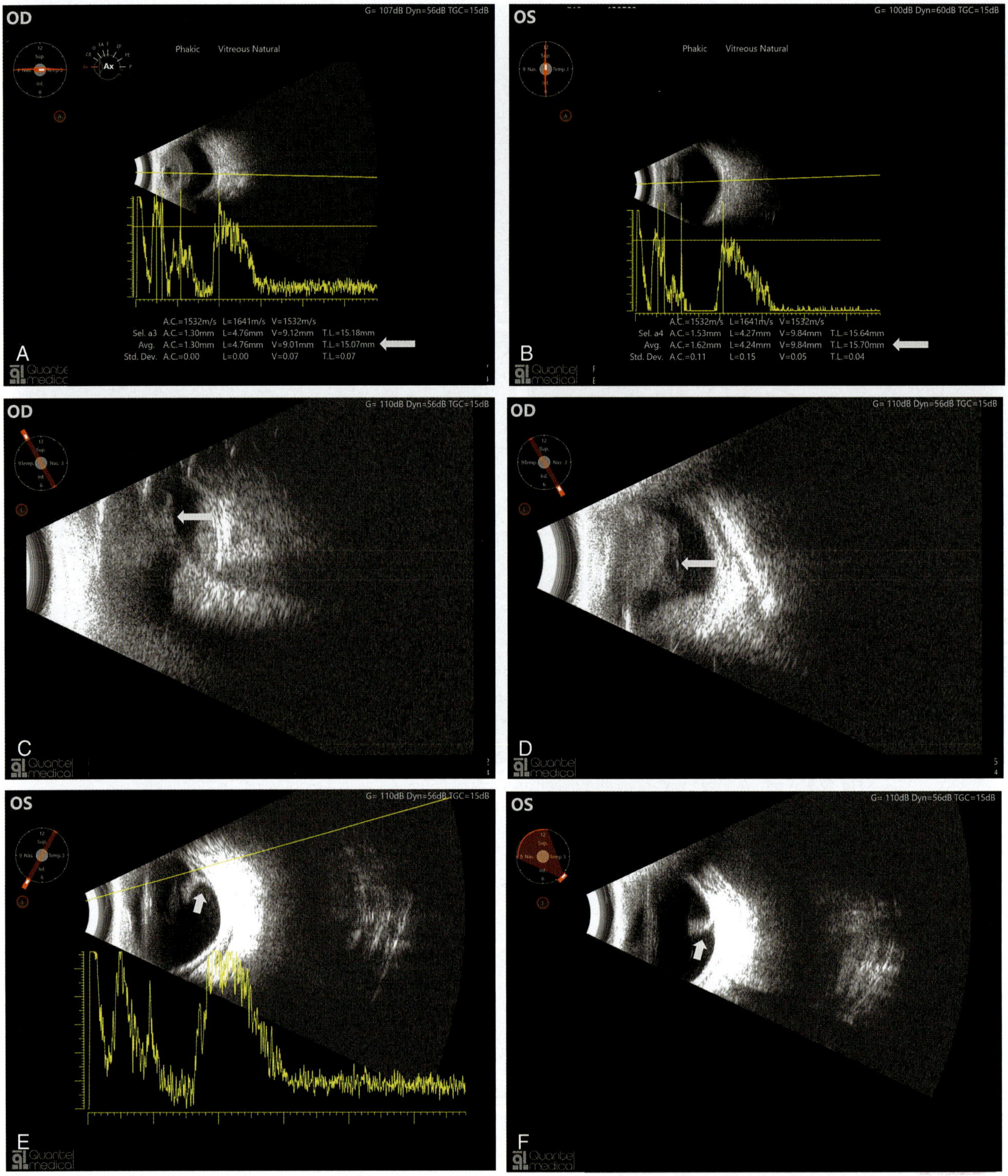

• **Fig. 12.4** B-scan ultrasonography of adjusted age of 28-day-old female infant. Her preterm birth was 4 months ago at 25 weeks gestational age and she had 926 g birth weight. Retinopathy of prematurity with retinal detachment was diagnosed in the right eye. A pediatric retina specialist evaluation demonstrated a retinal fold in the left eye. **(A–B)** B-scan ultrasound shows symmetric axial length in both eyes (**A**. Arrows show AL OD: 15.07 mm; **B**. AL OS: 15.70 mm), which were smaller than the normal reference for the age of 30 days old (normal reference for a 30-day-old infant, AL = 17.3–20.1 mm). **(C–D)** In the right eye, total retinal detachment (*arrows*), vitreoretinal proliferation, and dense subretinal content that moves according to head and eye position is observed. **(E-F)** In the left eye, longitudinal and transverse B-scan ultrasonograpgy of the superonasal meridian demonstrates a ridge and a localized tend-like retinal detachment.

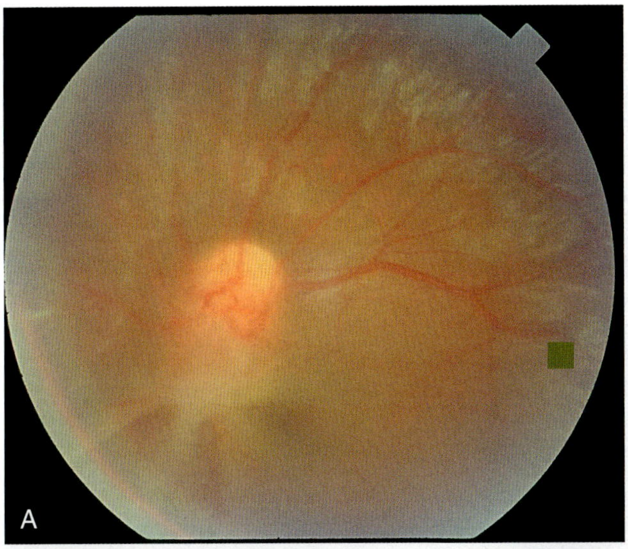

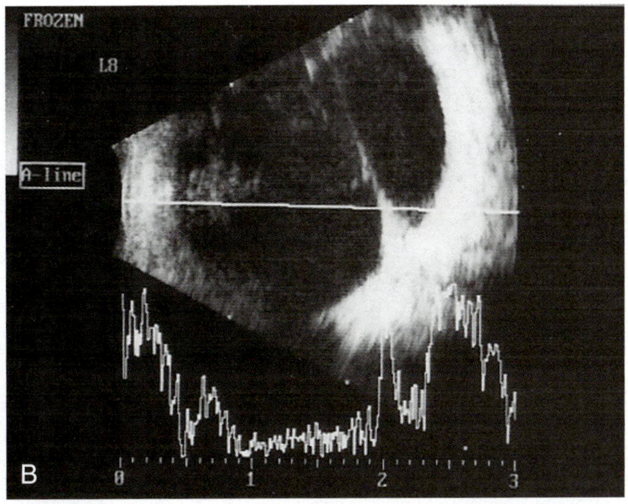

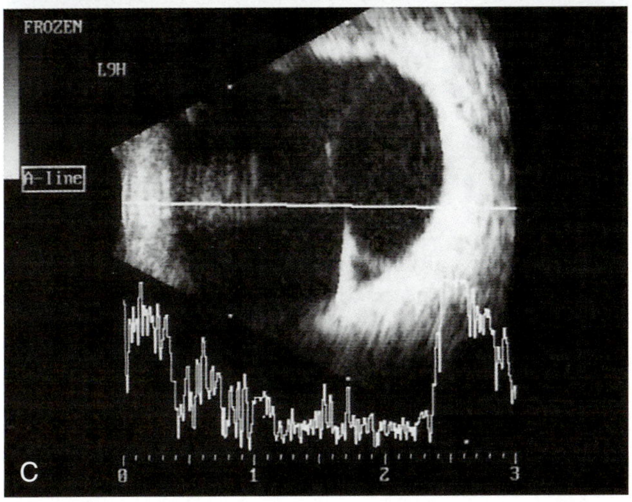

• **Fig. 12.5** A 6-year-old male patient presented with low visual acuity in the left eye. **(A)** Fundus examination and photography showed a unilateral white mass in the posterior pole (posterior pole granuloma) with an adherent vitreous membrane and moderate vitreous opacity. **(B)** B-scan ultrasound demonstrated a chorioretinal thickening in the posterior pole (posterior granuloma) with a vitreous membrane and retina traction **(C)**. Diagnosis: ocular toxocariasis.

the ciliary body or choroid usually occurs over the granulomas, whereas peripheral tractional retinal detachment can also be observed around the granulomas or the attachment points of vitreous strands.[9]

Ocular Toxoplasmosis

Ocular toxoplasmosis is caused by congential or acquired-*Toxoplasma gondii* infection. The disease most often presents as a focal necrotizing retinitis. It is associated with vitritis and often anterior uveitis. Active lesions accompanied by a severe vitreous inflammatory reaction have the classic "headlight in the fog" appearance. Less commonly, it may present as a papillitis. In cases of intense vitritis, epiretinal membranes and vitreoretinal traction adjacent to the lesion may occur.[10]

Ultrasonographic examination can identify vitreoretinal tractions due to the tight adherence of the vitreous on the retinochoroiditis site (Fig. 12.6), which can lead to tractional and rhegmatogenous retinal detachment, choroidal detachment, vitreous opacity, and papillary elevation.

In active lesions of toxoplasmic retinochoroiditis, B-scan ultrasonography demonstrates localized chorioretinal thickening and adjacent punctiform echoes in the vitreous, which is typical of vitreitis.

Congenital toxoplasmosis can show active lesions with localized thickening and vitreous strands, usually in the macular area.

Congenital Cataract

Cataracts may be unilateral or bilateral and can vary widely in size, morphology, and degree of opacification from a small white dot on the anterior capsule to total opacification of the lens. Consequently, the effect on vision, course of treatment, and prognosis may also be widely variable. It is the leading cause of leukocoria in children.[11]

The causes of infantile cataracts may be associated with systemic syndromes, intrauterine infections, genetic abnormalities, trauma, or could be idiopathic. They may be associated with other ocular pathologies like microphthalmia or aniridia.

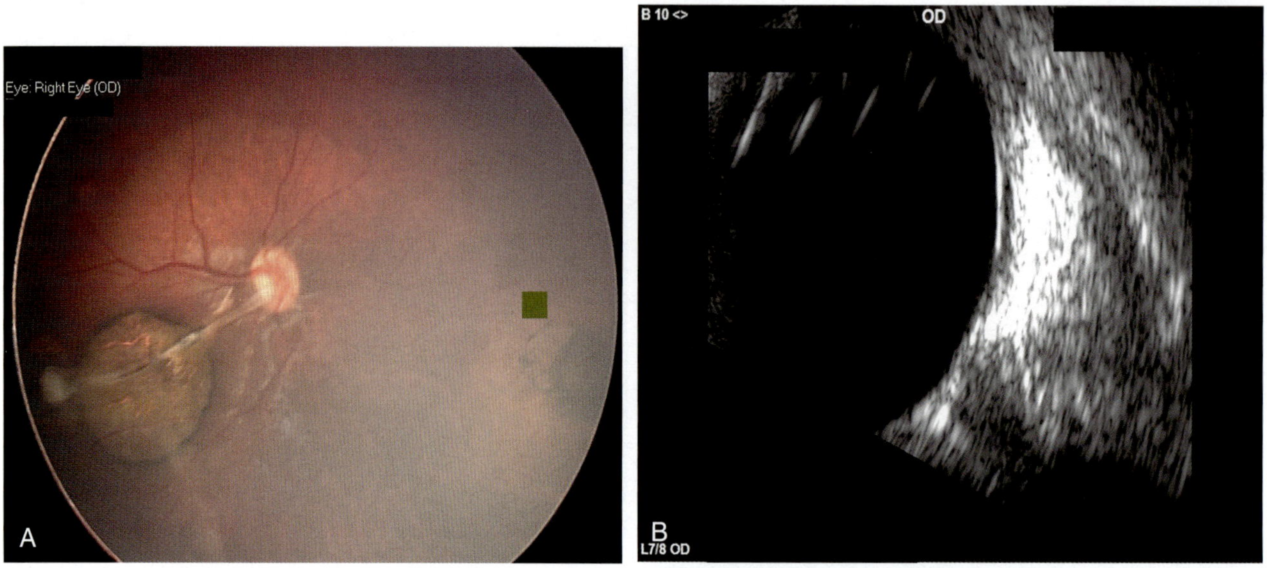

• **Fig. 12.6** A 5-week-old male infant presented with an abnormal red reflex test in the right eye. The family history was positive for toxoplasmosis infection during pregnancy. **(A)** Fundus examination and photography (RetCam) under anesthesia revealed a unilateral chorioretinal scar at the macular area in an inactive phase. **(B)** B-scan ultrasound demonstrated a vitreous strand from the optic disc to the lesion site inferotemporally at the macular area. Since the lesion was inactive, there was no chorioretinal thickening or inflammatory process.

B-scan ultrasound examination is essential to exclude other possible pathologies of the eye, which can be associated with congenital cataracts, such as persistent fetal vasculature and retinal detachment. The posterior pole is usually normal in a case of congenital cataract, and hyperreflectivity of the lens can be seen (Fig. 12.7).

Primary Congenital Glaucoma

Primary congenital glaucoma (PCG) results from elevated intraocular pressure (IOP) secondary to genetic abnormalities in the trabecular meshwork and anterior chamber angle. The elevated IOP causes rapid expansion of the infant's eye, resulting in buphthalmos, corneal enlargement, and Haab striae, which are breaks in the Descemet membrane that can lead to corneal edema and opacification.[12] The main symptoms are photophobia, epiphora, and blepharospasm. Other signs include deep anterior chamber, axial myopia, astigmatism, optic disc cupping, and anisometropia (present in unilateral PCG).

B-scan ultrasonography is helpful as the corneal opacification can jeopardize the visualization of the eye fundus. A-scan ultrasonography is useful to assess the ocular axial length, which is typically elongated,[13] and sometimes associated with posterior staphyloma and lens thinning. It is recommended to repeat the axial length measurement after 3–4 months to assess if the growth rate is greater than average. The average eye growth can be found in articles used as references.[13]

It is possible to detect disc cupping by B-scan ultrasonographic examination (Fig. 12.8),[14] although an identifiable optic disc cupping can be found in other conditions, such as an augmented physiological cupping. Thus, an identifiable cupping doesn't necessarily correspondend to a glaucomatous changes.

Persistent Fetal Vasculature

Persistent Fetal Vasculature (PFV), also known as Persistent Hyperplastic Primary Vitreous (PHPV), is a failure of the regression of fetal vessels within the eye. It is an important cause of infantile leukocoria and can result in several intraocular changes after infancy as the PFV can cause a retinal traction as the eye grows. Complications include glaucoma, cataracts, intraocular hemorrhages, retinal detachments, and/or phthisis that will further affect the child's vision/cosmesis of the eye.

PFV can affect both anterior and posterior segments of the eye. Isolated anterior PFV is unusual and it tends to have a better visual prognosis than the posterior subtype.[15] The anterior subtype has been defined as the presence of a retrolental opacity, elongated ciliary process, or cataract, but can also include a membranous transformation of the anterior vitreous face causing traction on the peripheral retina, a shallow anterior chamber, poor pupil dilation, and microphthalmos.[16] The posterior subtype presents a prominent stalk of tissue inserted over the optic disc but not extending to the anterior segment. The mixed subtype includes findings of the anterior and posterior subtypes combined, defined by a stalk of tissue extending from the optic nerve to the retrolental area causing an elevation of the vitreous membrane from the optic nerve, retinal folds or detachment, and varying degrees of optic nerve and retinal dysplasia.[17]

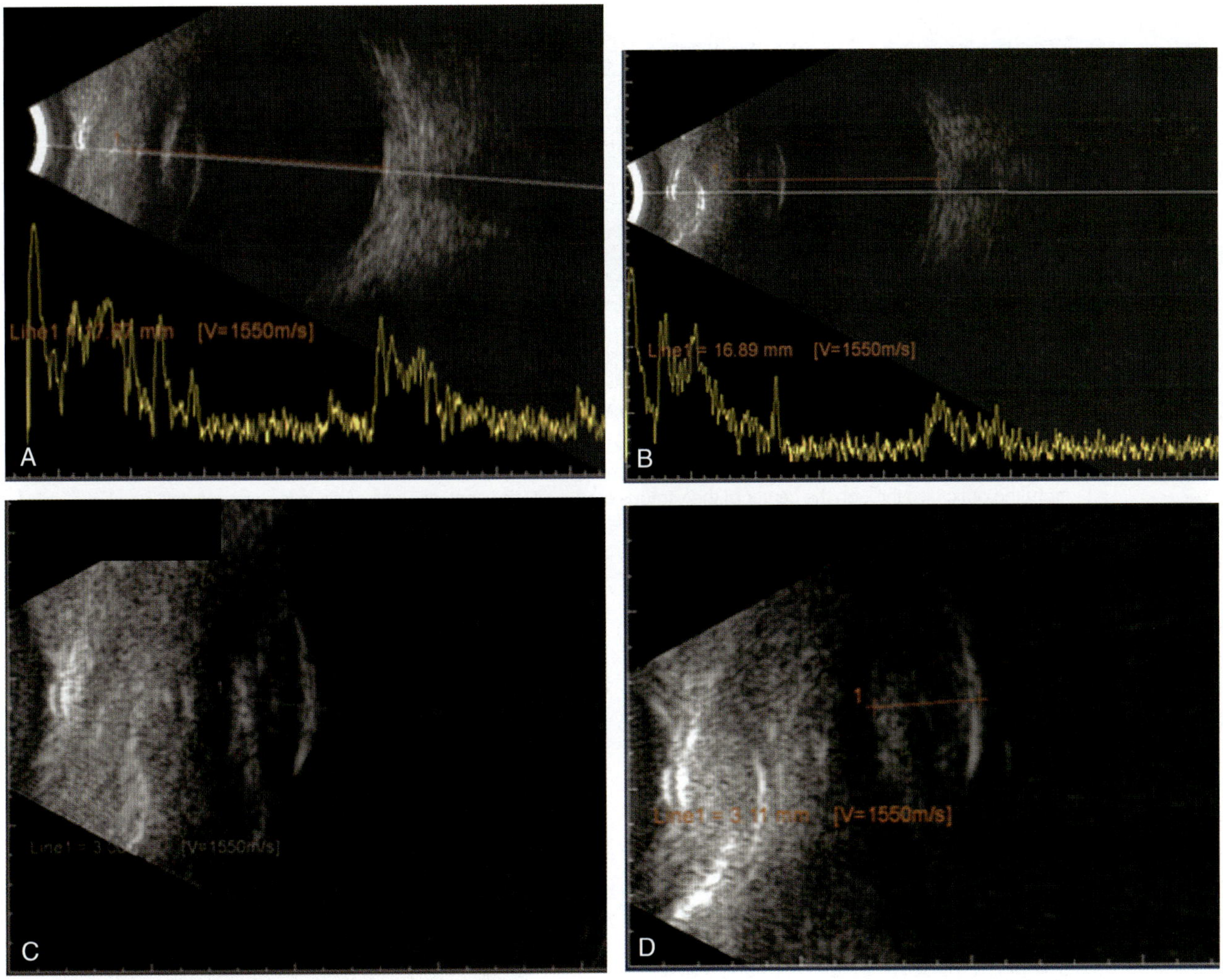

• **Fig. 12.7** A 3-month-old infant presented with bilateral leukocoria due to a congenital cataract. In both eyes, axial length was within normal limits **(A)** Axial length in the right eye: 17.07 mm; **(B)** Axial length in the left eye: 16.89 mm. **(C–D)** Hyperreflectivity of the lens was observed in both eyes. **C**. Lens thickness in OD: 3.00 mm; **D**. Lens thickness in OS: 3.11 mm. There were no obvious posterior abnormalities.

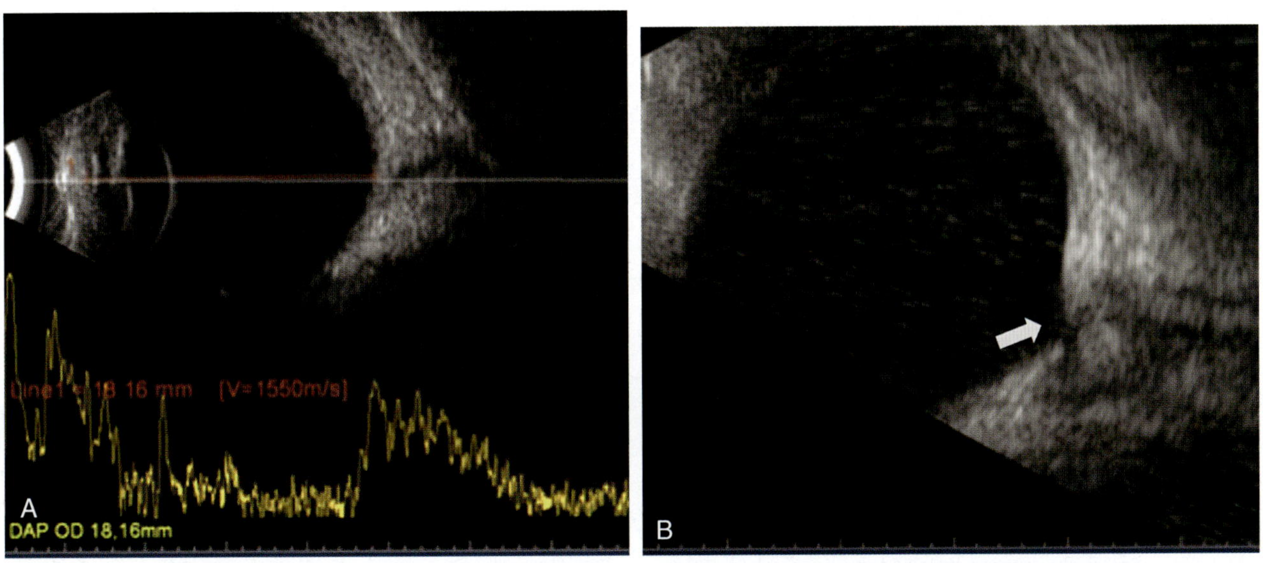

• **Fig. 12.8** A 1-month-old presented with unilateral leukocoria in the right eye. A B-scan ultrasound was taken. **(A)** Axial length was within normal limits (AL = 18.16 mm). (**B**) Optic disc cupping was evident (*arrow*), characterized by a large and deep interruption of the continuity of the ocular wall at the optic disc.

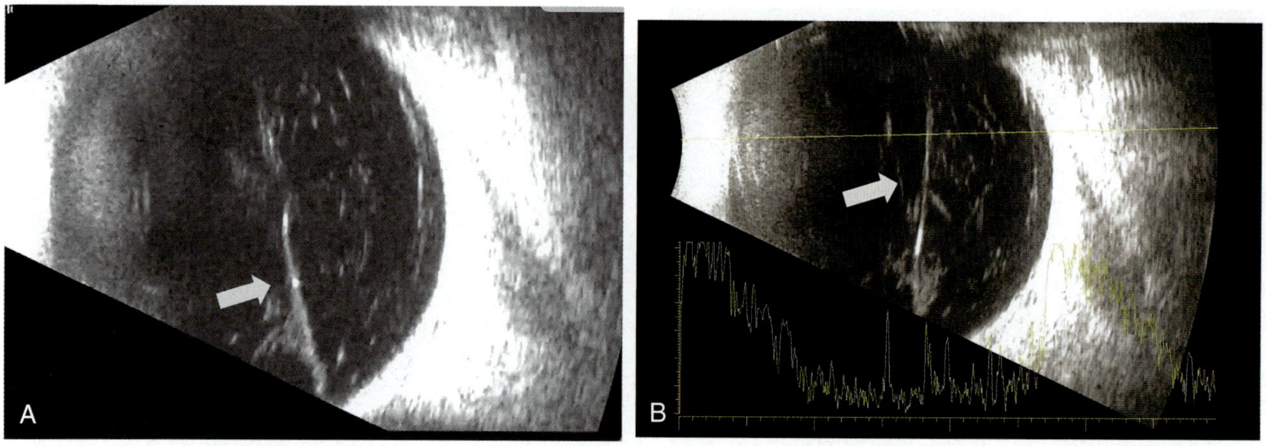

• **Fig. 12.9** B-scan ultrasonography of a 9-month-old male infant presenting with leukocoria in the right eye. **(A–B)** B-scan ultrasonography demonstrates a rectolental membrane or hyaloidal stalk extending from the optic disc through the center of the vitreous cavity until the posterior lens capsule (or a retrolental membrane). In this case, the stalk is thick close to the optic disc insertion and thin at the anterior portion.

PFV is diagnosed by direct visualization of any component of the persistent fetal vasculature on a fundus examination. In patients with poor view of the fundus, B-scan ultrasonography can be employed. Additionally, color Doppler ultrasonography can be quite useful to detect vasculature associated with PFV.

Typical ultrasonographic features of PFV include decreased anteroposterior diameter of the eye (small eyes), although differences can be subtle or even nonexistent in cases of buphthalmos associated with glaucoma. The crystalline lens is often thin and may present irregularities of the posterior capsule that can be related to retrolental membranes. The mixed subtype presents a vitreous band corresponding to the persistent hyaloid vessel extending from the posterior capsule lens to the optic disc (Fig. 12.9 and Video 12.1). The band can be thin and difficult to identify in some cases. In other cases, a color Doppler exam can identify patent blood vessels within this band.

Ultrasonography can be helpful in identifying some of the possible complications as retinal detachment, which is usually tractional in the peripapillary region but can be total in advanced cases.

Familial Exudative Vitreoretinopathy

Familial exudative vitreoretinopathy (FEVR) and ROP can have very similar clinical presentations, being the single most important difference in prematurity. Both present abnormal development of retinal vessels that can lead to blindness due to severe vitreoretinopathy. While ROP is related to prematurity, FEVR is associated with a genetic mutation, so it is a lifelong disease that requires close monitoring. Understanding the type of mutation is important to predict the disease prognosis, as it occurs in an X-linked, autosomal recessive or dominant inheritance pattern.

The disease is characterized by abnormal retinal vascular development that leads to progressive vitreoretinal features.[18] FEVR's clinical presentation includes retinal capillary dropout, vessel dragging, retinal folds, exudation, hemorrhage, neovascularization, vitreoretinal interface changes, and retinal detachment, which can be serous, tractional, and/or combined. Retinal detachments develops mainly during the first three decades of life due to poor vascularization in the peripheral retina.[19]

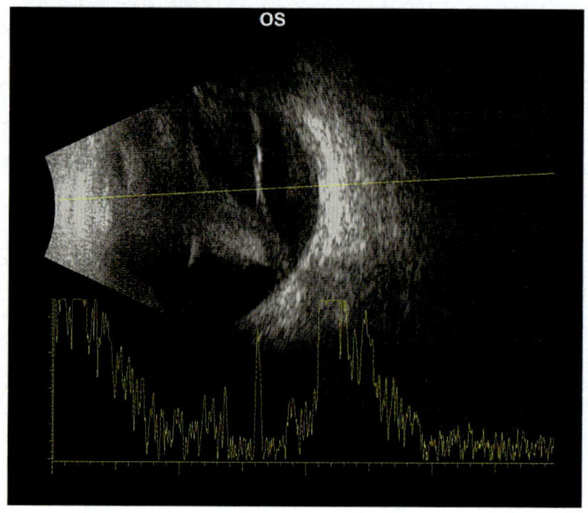

• **Fig. 12.10** A 4-month-old male infant with no history of prematurity presented with leukocoria in both eyes. B-scan demonstrates a normal axial length and total retinal detachment. Diagnostic hypothesis: familial exudative vitreoretinopathy (FEVR).

When presenting in the neonatal period, it can masquerade other pediatric retinal disorders like retinopathy of prematurity (ROP), Coat's disease, and persistent fetal vasculature (PFV).[20] Ultrasound is an important tool in the differential diagnosis, especially in more advanced cases of FEVR as genetic testing is not always available.

In earlier stages of FEVR other ancillary exams, such as fluorescein angiography, can be more helpful in detecting avascular peripheral areas and subtle vascular changes that can be easily overlooked by a routine fundus examination. Ultrasound is most commonly used in more advanced stages of the disease that involve retinal detachment and vitreous hemorrhage.

There is not much literature regarding typical ultrasonographic findings in FEVR but it includes serous and/or tractional retinal detachment and vitreous hemorrhage (Fig. 12.10).

References

1. Villegas VM, Hess DJ, Wildner A, Gold AS, Murray TG. Retinoblastoma. *Curr Opin Ophthalmol.* 2013;24(6):581–588.
2. Jones JH, Kroll AJ, Lou PL, Ryan EA. Coats' disease. *Int Ophthalmol Clin.* 2001 Fall;41(4):189–198.
3. Atta HR, Watson NJ. Echographic diagnosis of advanced Coats' disease. *Eye (Lond).* 1992;6(Pt 1):80–85.
4. Chiang MF, Quinn GE, Fielder AR, et al. International classification of retinopathy of prematurity, third edition. *Ophthalmology.* 2021;128(10):e51–e68.
5. Lee KF, Abdul Rahim A, Raja Azmi MN, et al. Ultrasonographic findings in eyes with retinopathy of prematurity in Malaysia. *Med J Malaysia.* 2013;68(1):39–43.
6. Despommier D. Toxocariasis: clinical aspects, epidemiology, medical ecology, and molecular aspects. *Clin Microbiol Rev.* 2003;16(2):265–272.
7. Wan WL, Cano MR, Pince KJ, Green RL. Echographic characteristics of ocular toxocariasis. *Ophthalmology.* 1991;98(1):2832.
8. Morais FB, Maciel AL, Arantes TE, Muccioli C, Allemann N. Ultrasonographic findings in ocular toxocariasis (Portuguese). *Arq Bras Oftalmol.* 2012;75(1):43–47.
9. Chen Q, Gu J, Jiang R, Zhou M, Chang Q. Role of ultrasound biomicroscopy in diagnosis of ocular toxocariasis. *Br J Ophthalmol.* 2018;102(5):642–646.
10. Park YH, Nam HW. Clinical features and treatment of ocular toxoplasmosis. *Korean J Parasitol.* 2013;51(4):393–399.
11. Haider S, Qureshi W, Ali A. Leukocoria in children. *J Pediatr Ophthalmol Strabismus.* 2008;45(3):179–180.
12. Weinreb RN, Grajewski AL, Papadopoulos M, Grigg J, Freedman SF. *Childhood Glaucoma: The 9th Consensus Report of the World Glaucoma Association.* Kugler Publications; 2013.
13. Sampaolesi R, Caruso R. Ocular echometry in the diagnosis of congenital glaucoma. *Arch Ophthalmol.* 1982;100(4):574–577.
14. Beatty S, Good PA, McLaughlin J, Tsaloumas M, O'Neill EC. Evaluation of optic disc cupping using high-resolution ocular ultrasound. *Eye (Lond).* 1998;12(Pt 1):54–60.
15. Yusuf IH, Patel CK, Salmon JF. Unilateral persistent hyperplastic primary vitreous: intensive management approach with excellent outcome beyond visual maturation. *BMJ Case Rep.* 2015;2015:bcr2014206525.
16. Nelson LB. *Pediatric Ophthalmology: Color Atlas and Synopsis of Clinical Ophthalmology.* 1st ed. Lippincott Williams & Wilkins; 2011.
17. Hunt A, Rowe N, Lam A, Martin F. Outcomes in persistent hyperplastic primary vitreous. *Br J Ophthalmol.* 2005;89:859–863.
18. Wood EH, Drenser KA, Capone A. Diagnosis and management of familial exudative vitreoretinopathy: a lifelong, progressive, and often asymmetric disease. *JAMA Ophthalmol.* 2019;137(9):1059–1060.
19. Mukai S, Mukai E, Puliafito CA. Familial exudative vitreoretinopathy. In: Berson EL, D'Amico DJ, Schepens CL, eds. *Principles and Practice of Ophthalmology.* Saunders; 1994:813–817.
20. Sızmaz S, Yonekawa Y, T Trese M. Familial exudative vitreoretinopathy. *Turk J Ophthalmol.* 2015;45:164–168.

13 Axial Eye Length Measurement

BERNADETE AYRES AND NORMA ALLEMANN

Axial eye length is one of the determinant factors for calculating intraocular lens (IOL) power when performing cataract surgery. Accurate axial eye length measurement is crucial for achieving the best postoperative refractive outcome. In fact, an error of 1.0 mm in the axial eye length measurement can result in a 3.75 D error in the power of the implanted lens, with greater magnitude in short eyes.

Using the e-norms methodology, Shammas et al.[1] established the average ocular biometric parameters in the cataract patient population. They found that axial eye length ranged from 22.50 mm to 24.50 mm (mean = 23.50 mm), with medium-long eyes between 24.51 mm and 24.99 mm and long eyes measuring 25.00 mm and longer; the medium-short eyes ranged from 22.01 mm to 22.49 mm, with the short eyes measuring 22.00 mm and shorter. Normal values for anterior chamber depth ranged from 2.50 mm to 3.50 mm (mean = 3.00 mm). Normal values for lens thickness ranged from 4.40 mm to 5.44 mm (mean = 4.92 mm).

The axial eye length can be measured by A-scan ultrasound or optical biometry. Ultrasound measures the axial length from the anterior surface of the corneal apex to the internal limiting membrane (ILM), whereas optical biometry measures the axial length from the anterior surface of the cornea to the photoreceptor layer (0.25 mm deeper than ILM). In theory, optical biometry reads longer than ultrasonic axial length. Optical biometry measures along the visual axis and has the advantage of being a noncontact method, user-friendly, and slightly more accurate than ultrasound biometry[2]; however, optical biometry can fail in acquiring measurements in eyes with dense cataracts.

Optical Biometers

Different technologies have evolved over the time that do not utilize ultrasound to perform measurements: axial length, anterior chamber depth, and lens thickness. Optical biometers also determine keratometry and other parameters needed for intraocular lens calculations. Different instruments are available: IOLMaster (Zeiss), Lenstar 900 (Haag-Streit), Eyestar (Haag-Streit), Argos (Alcon), AL-Scan (Nidek), Pentacam AXL (Oculus), and OA-2000 (Tomey), among others.

IOLMaster (Carl Zeiss AG, Germany)

The technology is based on partial-coherence interferometry using an infrared light (780 µm) to measure axial eye length (Fig. 13.1). Furthermore, it measures the corneal curvature, the anterior chamber depth, and the corneal diameter. It calculates the optimum IOL power by using the acquired biometry data, employing several IOL power calculation formulas built into its computer software.

Lenstar LS 900 (Haag-Streit AG, Köniz, Switzerland)

The system is based on optical low-coherence reflectometry, using a diode light source (820 µm) to measure the axial eye length (Fig. 13.2). In addition, the system provides a measurement of the corneal curvature, anterior chamber depth, crystalline lens thickness, and retina thickness. Most of the standard IOL prediction formulas are built into the system software.

Ultrasound Biometry

A-scan biometry is recognized as a reliable and reproducible technique for axial eye length measurement. The frequency commonly used in A-scan biometers ranges between 8 MHz and 12 MHz. The probe displays a fixation light that helps the alignment of the sound to the visual axis.

Settings and Care

Measurement mode. Most instruments provide the option of either a manual or automatic measurement mode. For good practice, the examiner should be skilled in both methods.

Gain. The gain should be set at a medium level in the beginning of the exam and is adjusted if necessary, avoiding high-level and false spikes.

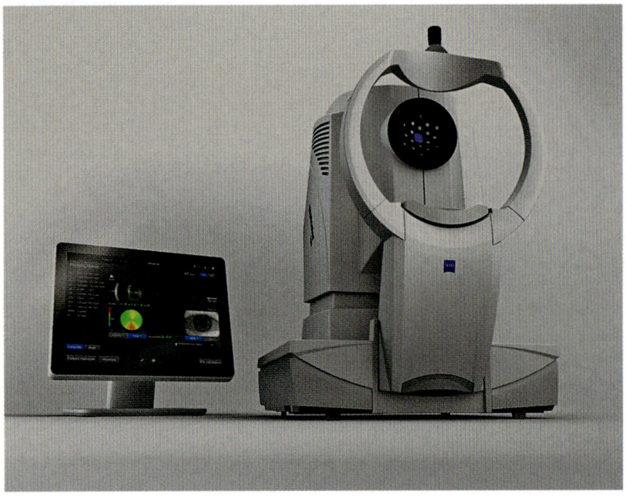

• **Fig. 13.1** Zeiss IOLMaster optical biometer.

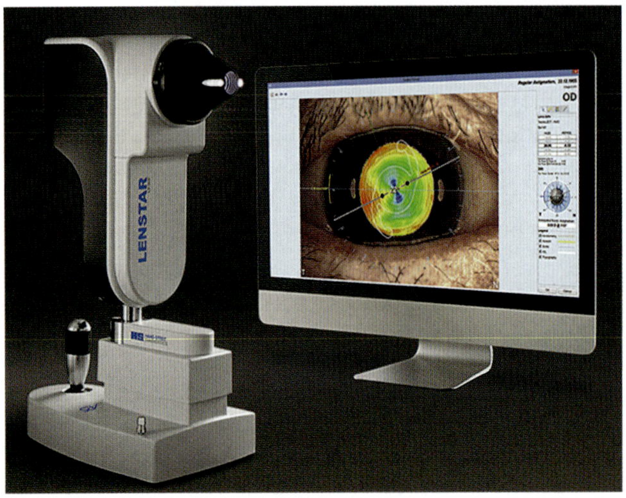

• **Fig. 13.2** Haag-Sreit Lenstar optical biometer.

Velocity settings. Accurate measurements of axial eye length require correct sound velocity settings. Biometers have phakic, pseudophakic, aphakic, dense cataract, and silicone-filled eye settings that can be selected based on the lens status of the patient.

Electronic gates. The electronic gates or calipers can have different presentations depending on the instruments. The biometers can provide between two and five gates. They can be a vertical superimposed line or a horizontal line. They should be placed on the ascendant segment or at the peak of the echo spike.

Transducer cleaning and disinfection. The probe must be cleaned and disinfected between each patient procedure. The sonographer must be aware of the various disinfection protocols with each associated transducer type. It recommends following manufacturer instructions, local law, and institutional infection control regulations.

Equipment calibration. The biometer calibration should be checked routinely according to the manufacturer's instructions.

TEACHING POINTS

Specification of a good ultrasound instrument for biometric exam

- A-scan and B-scan diagnosis capability.
- Immersion and contact modes.
- Automatic and manual capture mode.
- Eye type settings: phakic, dense cataract, silicone-filled, aphakic, and pseudophakic (PMMA, silicone, and acrylic).
- Automatic calculation of average and standard deviation of total length, anterior chamber depth, lens thickness, and vitreous length.
- A-scan biometry probe with patient's light fixation.

Exam

Before the ultrasound examination, the sonographer should inquire about previous ocular surgery, refractive errors, eye trauma, and systemic disease with ocular involvement. A patient with a history of retinal detachment repair with a scleral buckle has an eye longer axial length than the contralateral one. Taking a moment to explain the nature of the exam to the patient and expressing empathy can do wonders for your patient's comfort level. An external ocular exam can detect corneal anomalies, the density of the lens opacification, and the presence of a glaucoma filtering bleb.

Patient position. The examination should be performed preferentially with the patient supine, in primary gaze, looking up at the ceiling.

The sonographer is seated on the patient's right side, near the instrument screen and the patient's head, allowing the operator to simultaneously monitor the probe, the eye, and the image (Fig. 13.3).

Techniques. The axial eye length can be measured using either contact or immersion A-scan techniques (Fig. 13.4). In the contact technique, the probe is placed directly on the cornea. In the immersion technique, a scleral shell filled with fluid is placed over the cornea, and the probe is immersed in

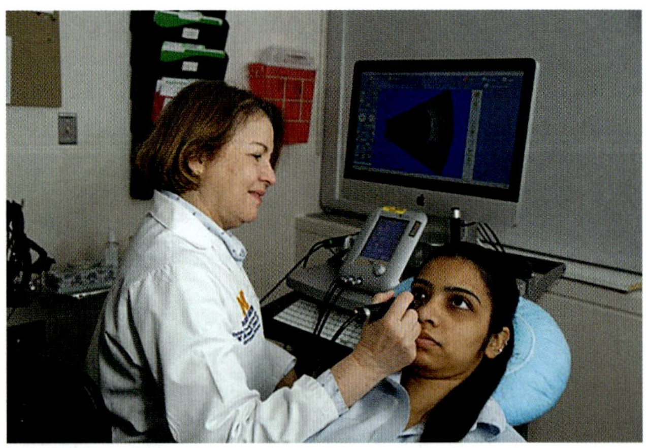

• **Fig. 13.3** Positioning the patient, equipment, and sonographer. The exam is best performed with the sonographer sitting and the patient supine. The sonographer is seated on the patient's right side near the instrument screen and the patient's head; therefore, the probe, the eye, and the image can be tracked simultaneously.

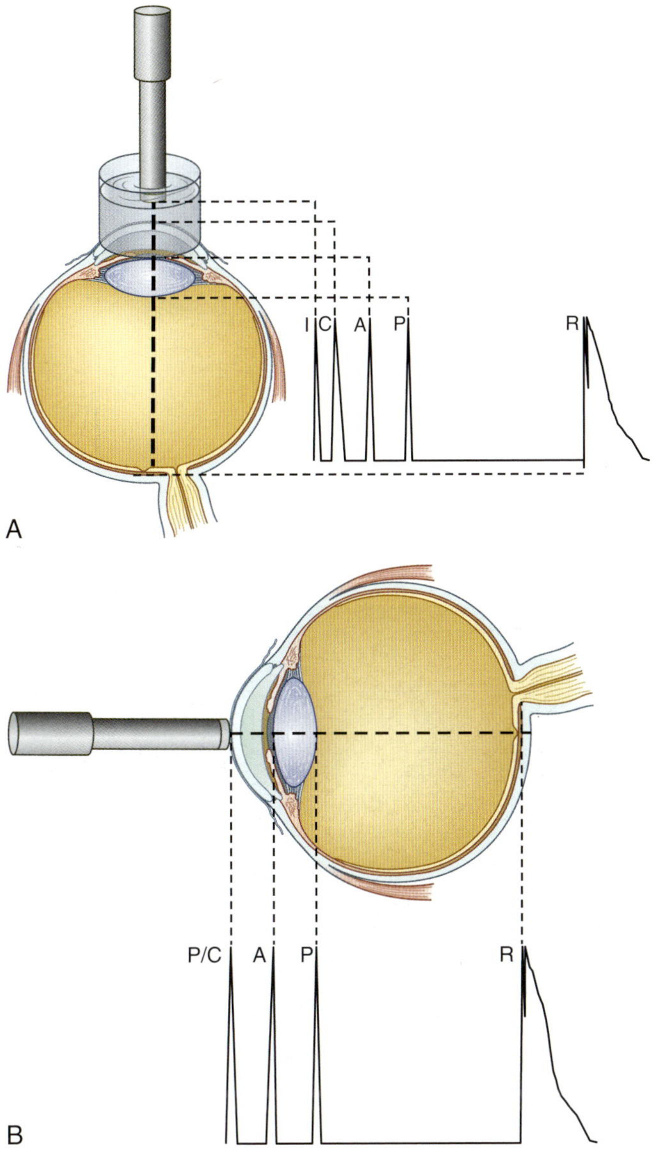

• **Fig. 13.4** Techniques for axial eye length measurement. **(A)** Immersion technique with the probe sunk in water bath avoiding a corneal contact. **(B)** Contact technique with the probe placed on the center of the cornea. I, *initial spike* of the tip of the probe; C, *cornea*; A, *anterior lens capsule*; P, *posterior lens capsule*; R, *retina*; P/C, *probe touching cornea*.

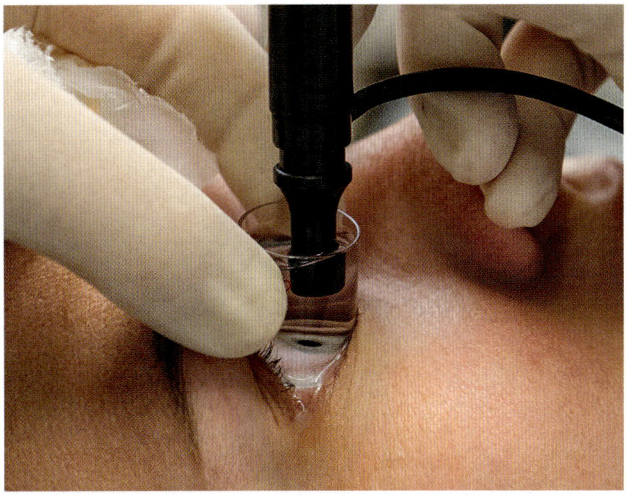

• **Fig. 13.5** Immersion A-scan technique. A scleral shell filled with fluid is placed on the corneoscleral limbus. The A-scan probe is immersed in the solution, keeping it approximately 5–10 mm from the cornea, aligned with the optical axis.

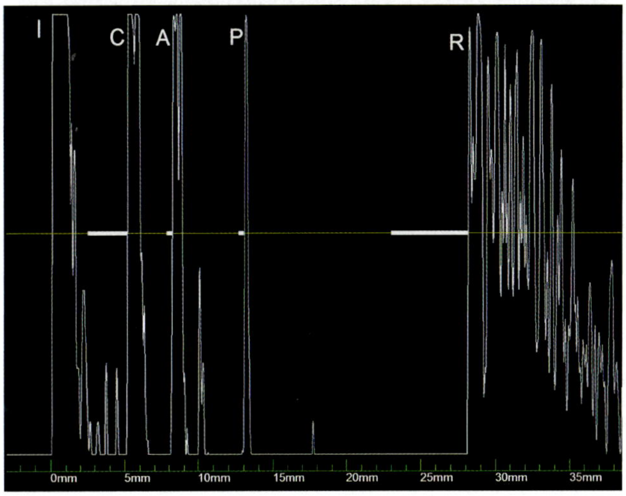

• **Fig. 13.6** Immersion A-scan of a phakic eye. I, *initial spike* of the probe tip; C, *cornea*; A, *anterior lens capsule*; P, *posterior lens capsule*; R, *retina*.

this fluid, keeping the tip of the probe away from the cornea. The measurements can be done in manual or automatic modes. The exam should always be taken bilaterally, except for a one-eyed patient.

Immersion technique. In this technique, the A-scan probe does not directly contact the cornea.

A drop of topical anesthesia is instilled in both eyes. A scleral shell is placed gently at the limbus, filling 2/3 full of saline solution carefully to avoid air bubbles. The patient is instructed to fixate in primary gaze. The shell must be held firmly in place to prevent fluid pouring. The ultrasound probe is immersed in the solution, keeping it approximately 5–10 mm from the cornea (Fig. 13.5 and Video 13.1). Monitoring the screen, the examiner directs the probe to the center of the cornea to align the sound beam precisely to the eye's optical axis. The gain is initially set at a medium-high level and then is turned down to improve the resolution and distinction of the spikes.

Using the immersion technique, in phakic eyes, the ultrasound displays five spikes. The first spike corresponds to the tip of the probe. The second spike, which has a double peak, corresponds to the cornea. The third and fourth spikes correspond to the anterior and posterior lens capsules, respectively. Finally, the fifth spike corresponds to the retina surface, followed by the scleral spike and a chain of orbital spikes (Fig. 13.6 and Video 13.2). The measurements need several repetitions to reach a confident average, excluding the extreme values and the lowest standard deviation.

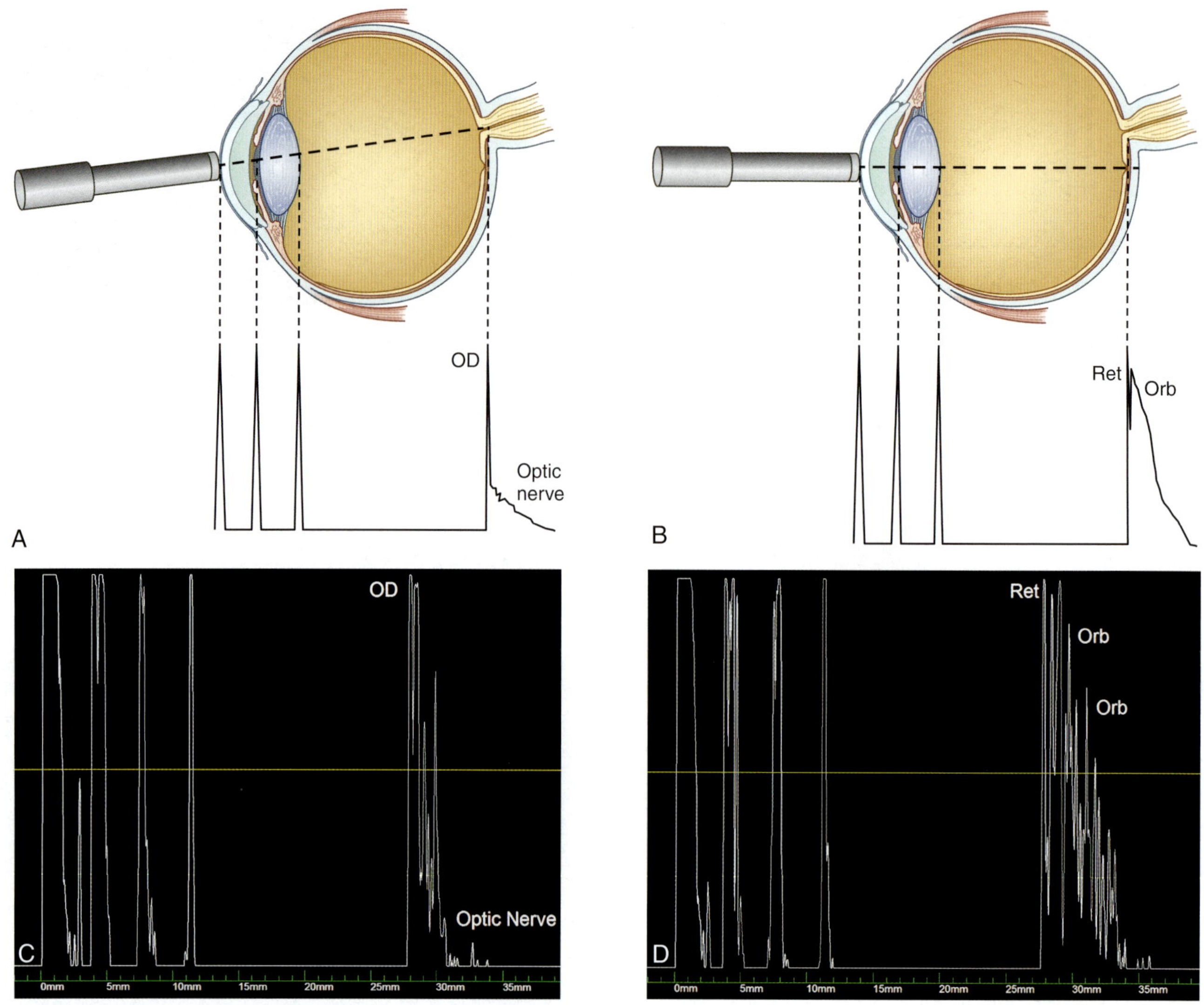

• **Fig. 13.7** Alignment of the sound beam to the visual axis. **(A)** Initially, the sound beam is aligned to the optic nerve, and the ultrasound shows low reflective spikes posterior to the sclera corresponding to the optic nerve. **(B)** The sound is slightly angled temporally toward the macula, and the ultrasound displays the orbital spikes (Orb) posterior to the retinoscleral layers (Ret). **(C)** The ultrasound shows incorrect sound beam alignment to the optic nerve. **(D)** The ultrasound shows correct sound beam alignment to the macula. OD, *optic disc*; Ret, *retina*; Orb, *orbit*.

When the ultrasound beam is correctly aligned with the center of the macula, all spikes will be steeply rising and of maximum height. Precise alignment to the macula is indicated by highly reflective orbital spikes. If the echogram shows low reflective spikes posterior to the sclera, it is most likely to be aligned to the optic nerve (Fig. 13.7A); in that event, the probe should be angled slightly temporally toward the macula (Fig. 13.7B and Video 13.3), therefore, the orbital spikes will be higher.

Using immersion technique for measurement of an aphakic eye, the ultrasound displays four spikes corresponding to the tip of the probe, the corneal spike, the iris or posterior lens capsule spike, and the retinal spike (Fig. 13.8).

Axial eye length measurement in pseudophakia (Fig. 13.9) is indicated for IOL exchange or comparison while doing biometry for the other eye. The ultrasound in pseudophakic eyes shows multiple artifact spikes posterior to the highly reflective IOL spike. The gain should be set down to distinguish the retinal spike from the reverberation

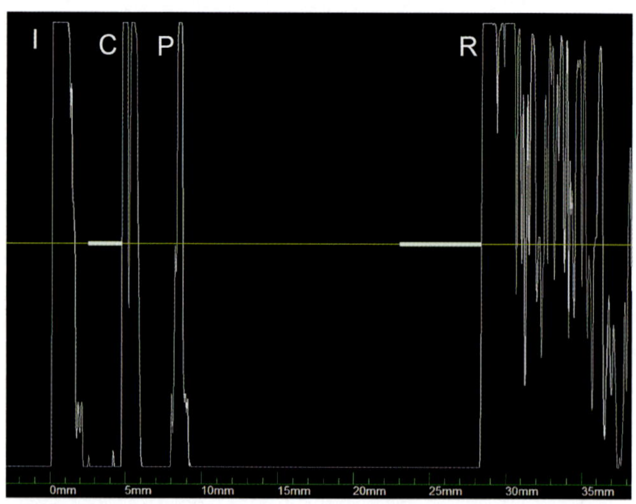

• **Fig. 13.8** Immersion A-scan of an aphakic eye. The spikes correspond to I, *initial spike* of the tip of the probe; C, *cornea*; P, *posterior lens capsule*; R, *retina*. The calipers are placed on the cornea and retina.

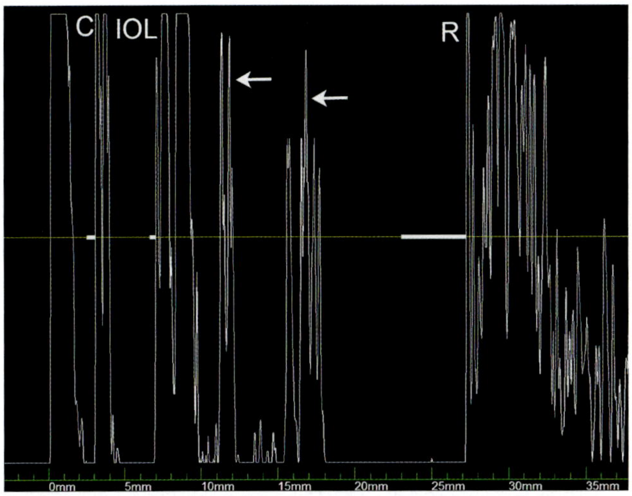

• **Fig. 13.9** Immersion A-scan of a pseudophakic eye. The intraocular lens implant (IOL) generates multiple reverberating spikes (*arrows*) with sound attenuation. C, *cornea*; R, *retina*.

TABLE 13.1 Correction Factors Added to Apparent Axial Length in Pseudophakia

IOL Type	Correction Factor
PMMA	+ 0.4 mm
Silicone	–0.8 mm
Acrylic	+ 0.2 mm
(IOL Thickness Unknown)	

artifact spikes in the vitreous cavity. Because the sound velocity of the different IOL materials differs, a proper correction factor must be added to the apparent axial length (Table 13.1). The A-scan measurement should be set the velocity to 1532 m/sec (aphakic velocity) and then applying a correction factor. For example, if at an ultrasound velocity of 1532 m/sec, a pseudophakic eye with an acrylic IOL, the apparent axial length measured 24.0 mm, the true axial length would be 24.0 + 0.2 = 24.2 mm. Modern instruments have the option for different types of IOLs velocities.

TEACHING POINTS

Ideal A-scan axial measurement

- Steeply rising high spikes form the cornea, anterior chamber, anterior and posterior lens capsule, and retina
- Maximally deep anterior chamber
- Maximal lens thickness
- Longest measurement at the macula
- Average the 5–10 most consistent results, giving the lowest standard deviation.

Types of immersion shells. Different shapes of immersion shells are available (Fig. 13.10), and the kind of shell to use is a matter of choice. Immersion biometry can be performed using an open cylinder shell (Hansen shell), an open conical shell (UBM immersion shell), or a fixed immersion shell (Prager Shell).

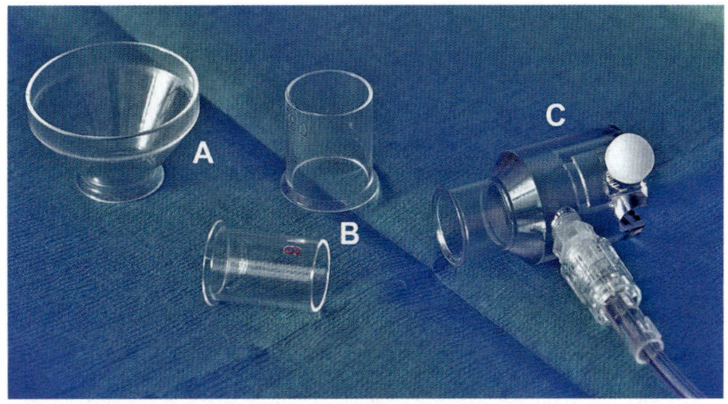

• **Fig. 13.10** Types of immersions shells. (A) UBM immersion shell, (B) Hansen shells, and (C) Prager shell.

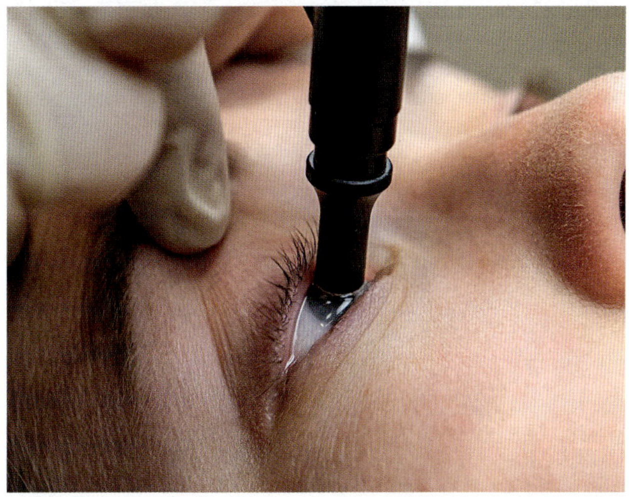

• **Fig. 13.11** Hand-held contact technique. The probe is placed gently on the center of the cornea, aligning the sound beam to the optical axis.

Contact Technique. In the contact technique, the probe is barely placed on the cornea's center, aligning the sound beam to the optical axis. The patient can be examined in a supine or upright position. The probe can be held directly by the examiner's hand, known as the hand-held method (Fig. 13.11); alternatively, the probe can be mounted in a Goldmann applanation unit, known as the applanation method. Care should be taken to avoid corneal compression and corneal abrasion. A maneuver of on-and-off touch on the cornea surface should be done to determine the minimal pressure to obtain high-quality echo spikes.

Using the contact technique, in a phakic eye, the ultrasound displays four spikes. The initial spike corresponds to the probe's tip on the cornea. The second and third spikes correspond to the anterior and posterior lens capsules. The fourth spike corresponds to the retina surface, followed by the scleral spike and a chain of orbital spikes (Fig. 13.12 and Video 13.4). In aphakic eye, the ultrasound displays spikes corresponding to the tip of the probe on the cornea, the iris or posterior lens capsule spike, and the retinal spike (Fig. 13.13). In pseudophakic eyes, the ultrasound shows an initial spike corresponding to the probe on the cornea,

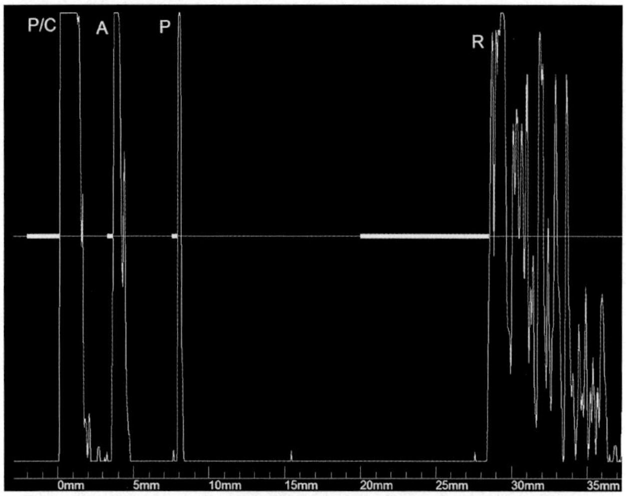

• **Fig. 13.12** Contact A-scan of a normal phakic eye. The calipers are positioned at the initial spike corresponding to the probe over the cornea (P/C), anterior lens capsule (A), posterior lens capsule (P), and retina (R).

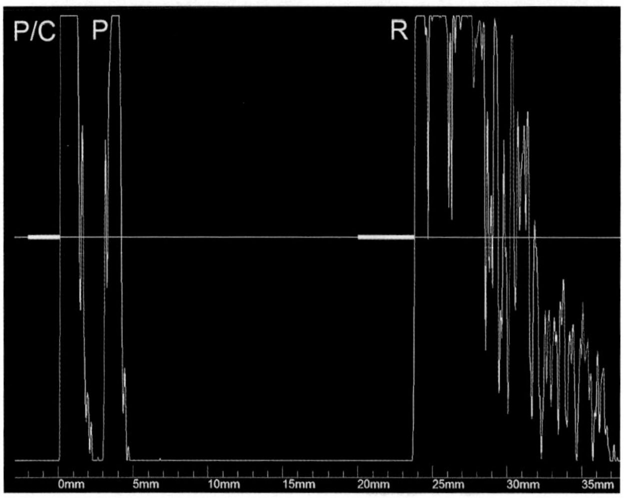

• **Fig. 13.13** Contact A-scan of an aphakic eye. The echogram displays three spikes corresponding to the probe on the cornea (P/C), posterior lens capsule (P), and retina (R).

a second high reflective spike from the IOL, followed by a chain of multiple spikes (Fig. 13.14).

Different IOL materials originate different appearances of the ultrasound; a polymethyl methacrylate (PMMA) IOL displays a long chain of multiple highly reflective spikes (Fig. 13.15), whereas a silicone implant displays a short chain of multiple spikes (Fig. 13.16).

B-mode biometry. A B-scan with a guided A-vector biometry is a reliable option for measuring axial eye length, especially in patients with asymmetric staphyloma or retinal detachment.[3]

The patient is positioned supine, and the instrument is set at a medium gain. After topical ocular anesthesia, a B-scan probe with a generous amount of coupling gel is gently approximated to the cornea using a horizontal axial approach (Fig. 13.17A). A UBM immersion shell can be

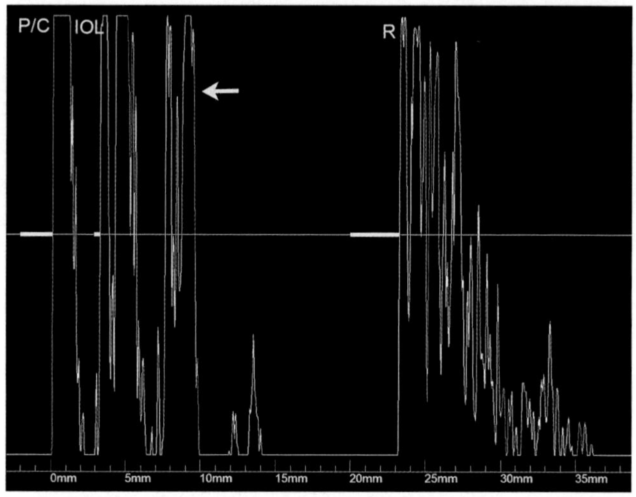

• **Fig. 13.14** Contact A-scan of a pseudophakic eye. The echogram shows an initial spike corresponding to a probe on the cornea (P/C), a second high reflective spike from the intraocular lens implant (IOL), followed by a chain of multiple spikes (*arrow*).

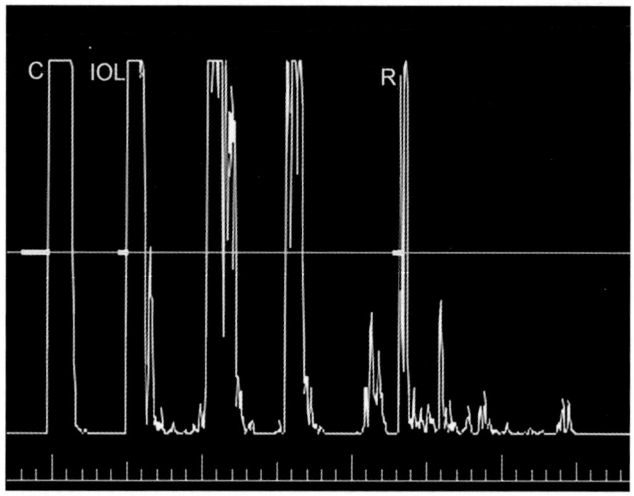

• **Fig. 13.15** Contact A-scan of a pseudophakic eye with PMMA intraocular lens implant. The PMMA IOL displays a long chain of multiple highly reflective spikes. C, *cornea*; IOL, *intraocular lens implant*; R, *retina*.

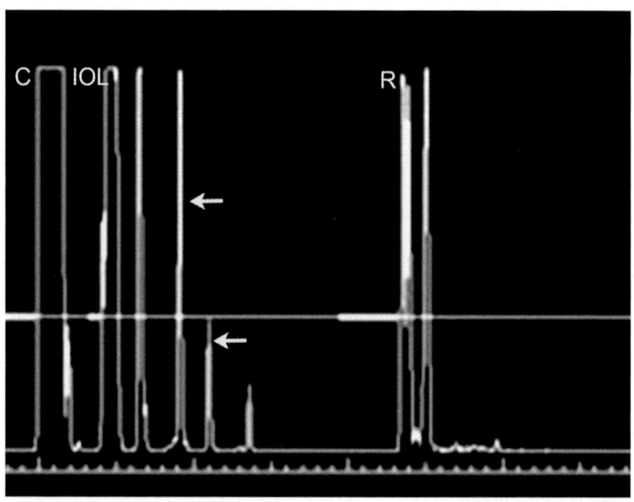

• **Fig. 13.16** Contact A-scan axial length of a pseudophakic eye with silicone IOL. The silicone IOL displays a short chain of multiple highly reflective spikes (*arrows*). C, *cornea*; IOL, *intraocular lens implant*; R, *retina*.

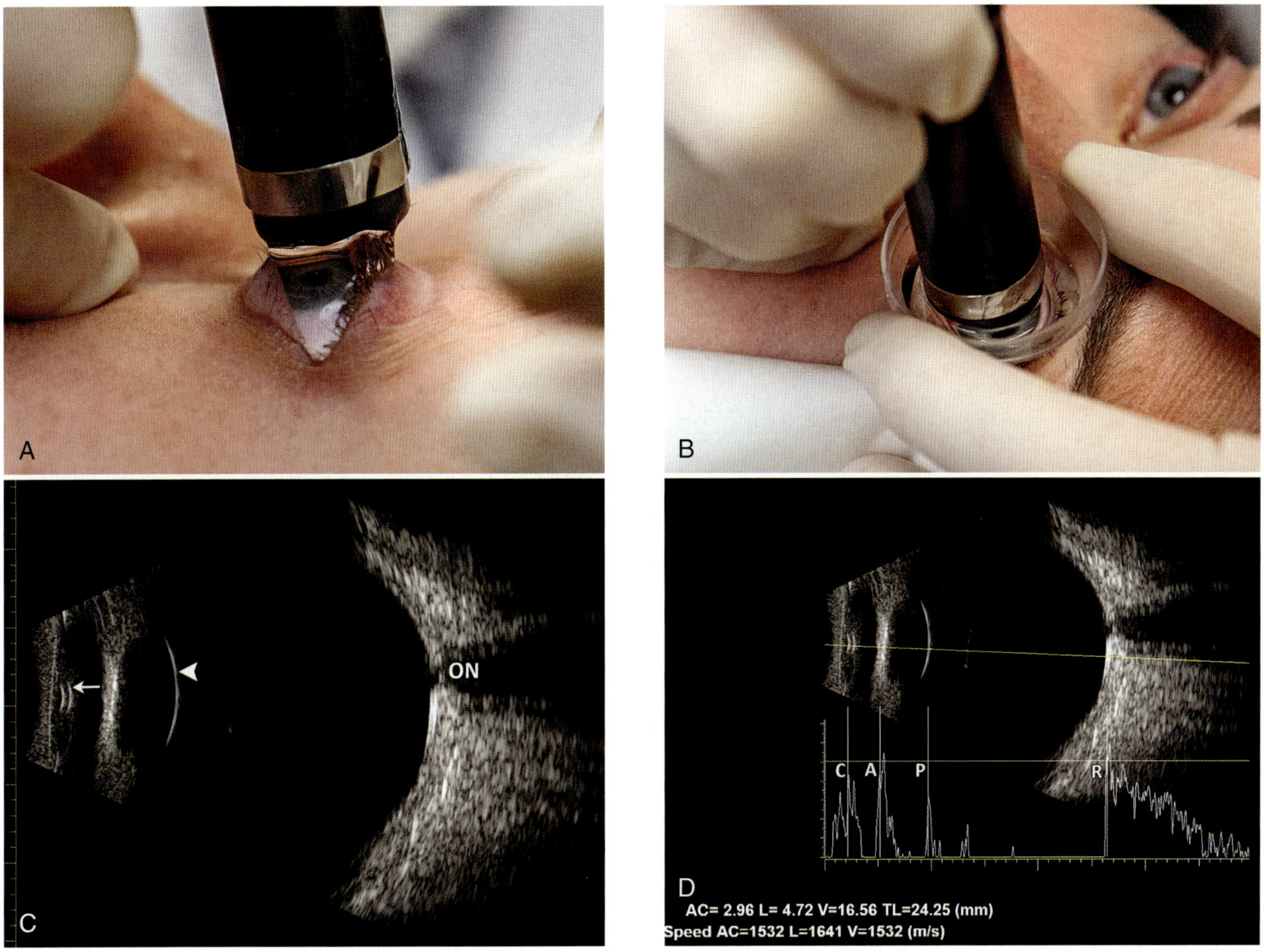

• **Fig. 13.17** B-mode biometry technique for axial eye length measurement. **(A)** A B-scan probe with a generous amount of gel is placed over the cornea in horizontal axial view. **(B)** B-scan biometry technique using a UBM immersion shell. **(C)** B-scan mode biometry of a phakic eye. Horizontal axial B-scan displays the corneal double arc lines (*arrow*), the posterior lens capsule (*arrowhead*), and the optic nerve (*ON*). **(D)** Horizontal axial B-scan with a superimposed vector A-scan aimed at the macula area with the calipers positioned at the cornea (*C*), anterior lens capsule (*A*), posterior lens capsule (P), and retina (*R*) using the correspondent sound velocities. The axial eye length measured 24.25 mm.

an alternative to the thick-layer gel method (Fig. 13.17B). The goal is to center the corneal double arc lines, the posterior lens capsule, and the optic nerve (Fig. 13.17C and Video 13.5). With this alignment, the vector A-scan is superimposed from the center of the cornea to the center of the macula, approximately 4.5 mm below the center of the optic nerve. In phakic eyes, the calipers are positioned at the vertex of the cornea, anterior and posterior lens capsule, and macula (Fig. 13.17D). Five high-quality measurements should be obtained.

TEACHING POINTS

Mitigating errors in biometry

Corneal compression
- Immersion technique must be the first-choice method.
- Minimize the corneal compression using the on-and-off maneuver when using the contact technique.

Incorrect velocity setting
- Select the correct sound velocity according to the eye type (phakic, aphakic, and pseudophakic/IOL type).

High gain setting
- The gain should be set at the lowest level at which a good reading is obtained.

Misalignment of the sound beam
- Look for highly reflective orbital spikes.

Measure both eyes and compare the symmetry between the eyes.
- If a difference of 0.3 mm or greater is found, a B-scan screening should rule out posterior segment anomalies.

Special Circumstances

Posterior staphyloma. The prevalence of posterior staphyloma increases from 1.4% in eyes with an axial length of 26.5–27.4 mm to 71.4% in eyes measuring 33.5–36.6 mm, and macular involvement is very common.[4] Optical

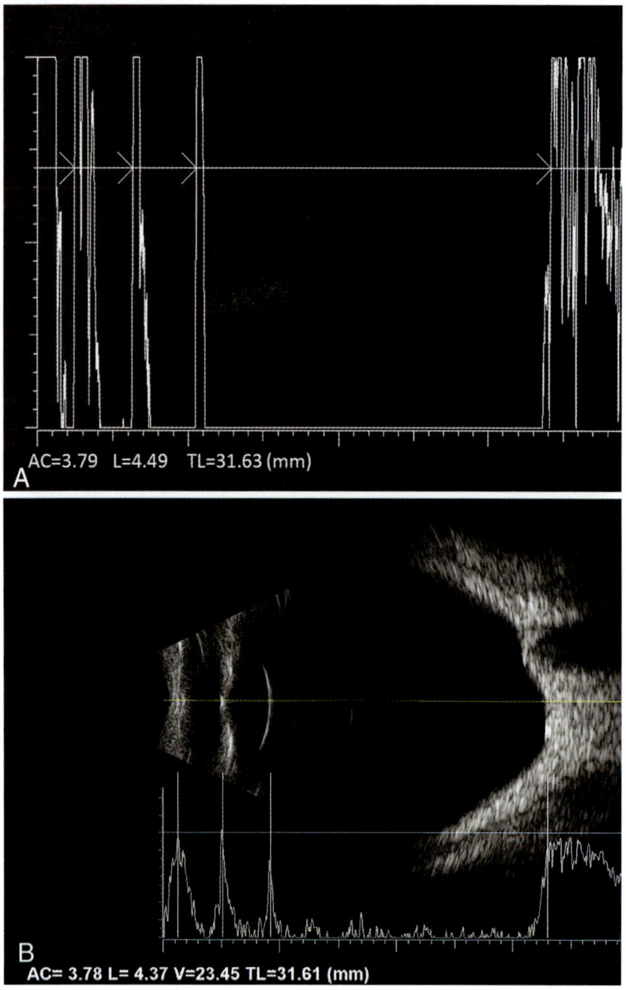

• **Fig. 13.18** Posterior staphyloma. **(A)** Immersion A-scan for axial measurement of a long eye with posterior staphyloma. **(B)** B-mode biometry shows the location of the peripapillary staphyloma and confirms the results.

biometry is expected to produce more precise axial length measurements for myopic eyes with posterior staphyloma because it uses macular fixation. A-scan measurement in eyes with posterior staphyloma can be challenging in displaying a steeply rising, maximum height retinal spike. B-scan biometry can be used to complement the immersion A-scan measurement (Fig. 13.18 and Video 13.6) for a commo decision on the final axial length value.

Ultrasound biometry in silicone oil-filled eyes. Because the speed of sound in silicone oil (987 m/s) is slower than in vitreous (1532 m/s), the apparent axial eye length is longer than the true one. Several techniques have been proposed to estimate the axial length in eyes filled with silicone oil, as follows:

1. Optical biometry is the preferential method to measure silicone oil-filled eyes.
2. Contact A-scan measurement with the patient sitting upright using a converted sound velocity of 987 m/s.
3. Intraoperative biometry with A-scan. After completely removing the silicone oil, the infusion cannula is kept in place to maintain the globe configuration. The axial length is measured using a sterilized A-scan probe.

Dislocated intraocular lens implant. Dislocation of IOL can result in an early or late complication of cataract surgery, prior vitreoretinal surgery, trauma, or zonular weakness. The dislocated IOL can be lying on the macula in the supine position, causing erroneous axial length measurement. Having the patient positioned upright will shift the IOL inferiorly, allowing correct measurement to the macula (Fig. 13.19). The velocity is set at aphakic.

Ectopia lentis (dislocated crystalline lens). Ectopia lentis is defined as a crystalline lens displacement, either partially or completely, due to zonular abnormalities. It can be a result of trauma, hereditary ocular disease, or part of systemic diseases like Marfan syndrome and homocystinuria. Using aphakic velocity, the patient must be examined in upright, moving the lens to the inferior quadrant (Fig. 13.20).

TEACHING POINTS

Immediately after the preoperative biometry assessment

- Check that the biometry results include the person's name, date of birth, and hospital number
- Check the biometry results with the patient's refractive status
- Use electronic data transfer to upload the biometry results to an electronic health record
- Do not transcribe the results by hand.

Keratometry

Keratometric measurement plays an essential role in determining IOL power in cataract surgery. Accurate refractive outcomes after cataract surgery require precise measurements of keratometric values. It should be noted that each 1.0 diopter error in K-reading will result in an IOL-power error of 1.3–1.7 diopter, depending on the IOL position.[5] Currently, the corneal power can be measured by manual keratometer, automated keratometer, corneal topography, built-in optical biometer keratometer, and topography or Scheimpflug topography (Pentacam and similar).

Normal values of corneal radius range from 42.50 to 44.82 diopters with a mean of 43.66 diopters.[1] Myopic eyes tend to have steeper cornea, as opposed to flatter corneas in hyperopic eyes. The measurements need to be taken from both eyes for comparison. The symmetry of the corneal radius between eyes is usually within one diopter. Extreme values below 40 diopters or above 46 diopters should be reviewed.

Keratometric measurements should always be performed before axial length measurement. Contact lens wear may affect the keratometry measurements. If the patient wears a contact lens, a contact lens hiatus of two weeks is recommended for a rigid contact lens and one week for a flexible contact lens before obtaining the final keratometry readings.[6]

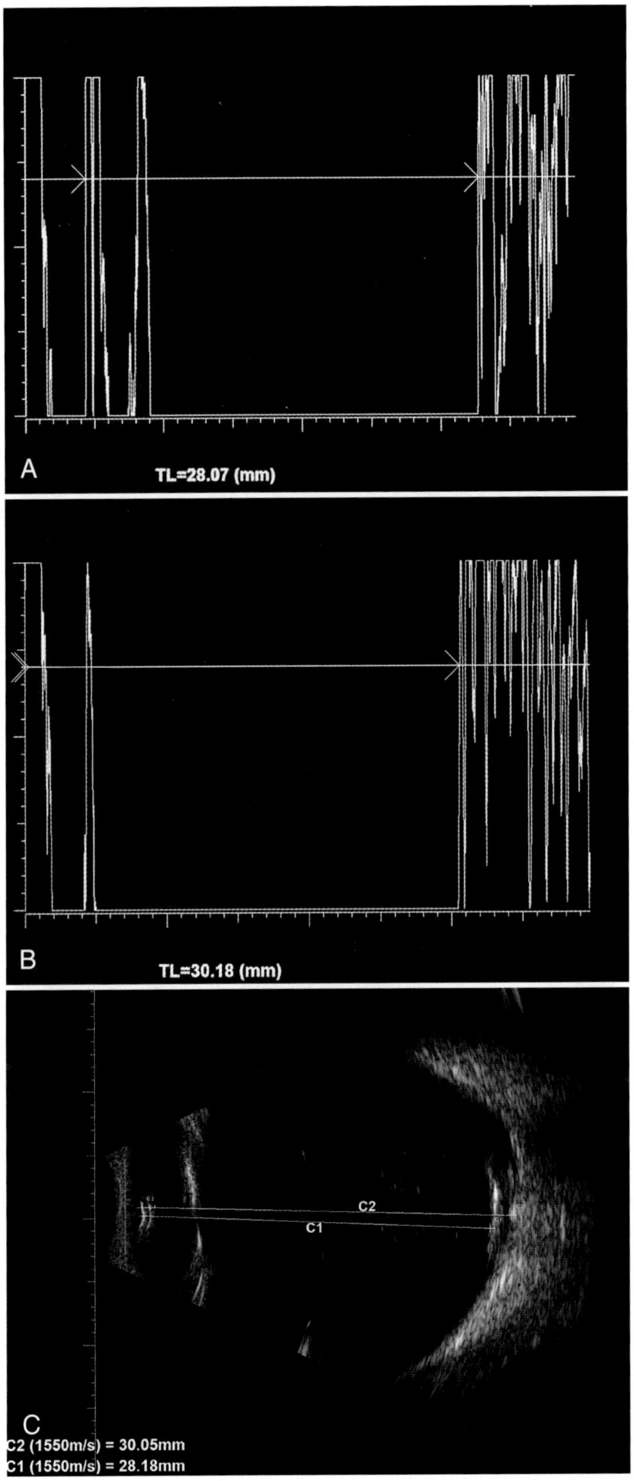

• **Fig. 13.19** **(A)** Immersion A-scan of a patient with dislocated IOL lying on the macula, examined in supine position; axial length measured to the IOL surface = 28.07 mm. **(B)** Immersion A-scan in the upright position, dislocating the IOL from the macula resulting in axial length = 30.18 mm. **(C)** Horizontal axial B-scan with dislocated IOL lying on the macula when the patient is supine; the axial measures shorter at the IOL surface (C1 = 28.1 mm) than at the retinal plane (C2 = 30.0 mm).

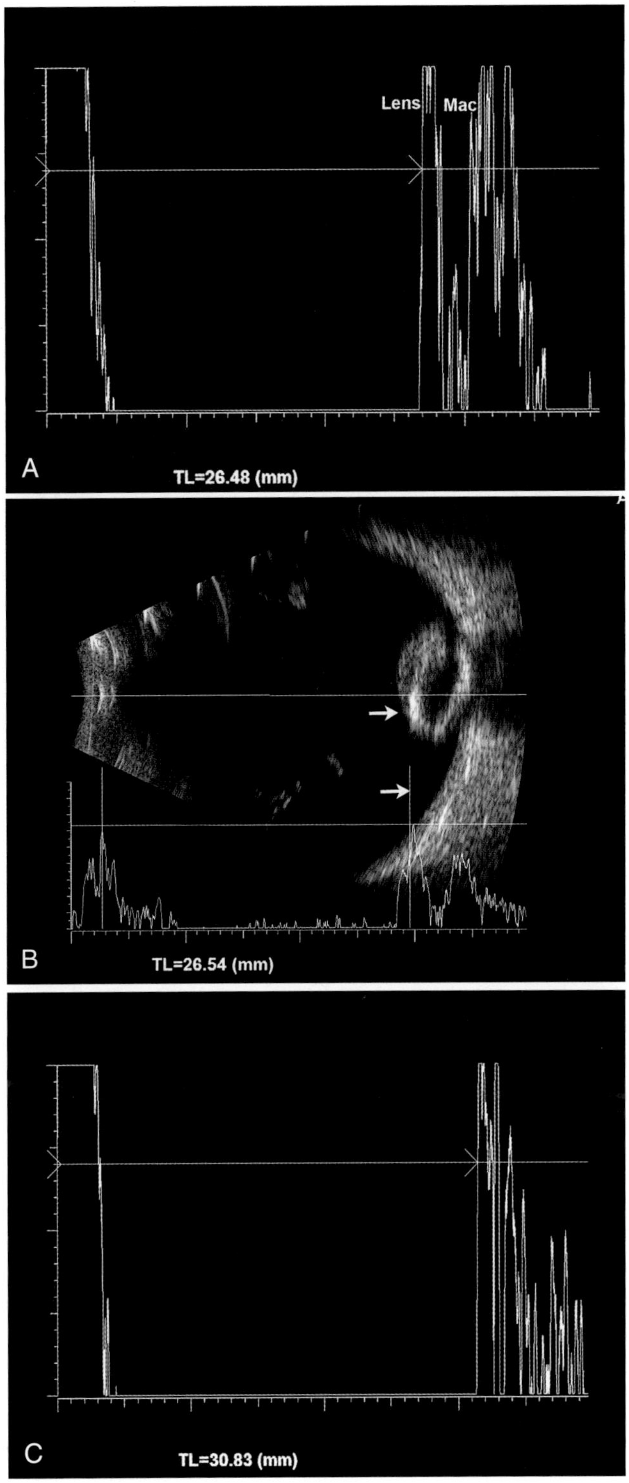

• **Fig. 13.20** **(A)** Immersion A-scan of a patient with a dislocated crystalline lens (arrows), examined in the supine position, measured to the lens seated on macula resulting in axial length = 26.48 mm. **(B)** B-mode biometry measured to the dislocated crystalline over the macula; axial length = 26.54 mm. **(C)** Immersion A-scan in the upright position, dislocating the crystalline from the macula resulting in axial length = 30.83 mm.

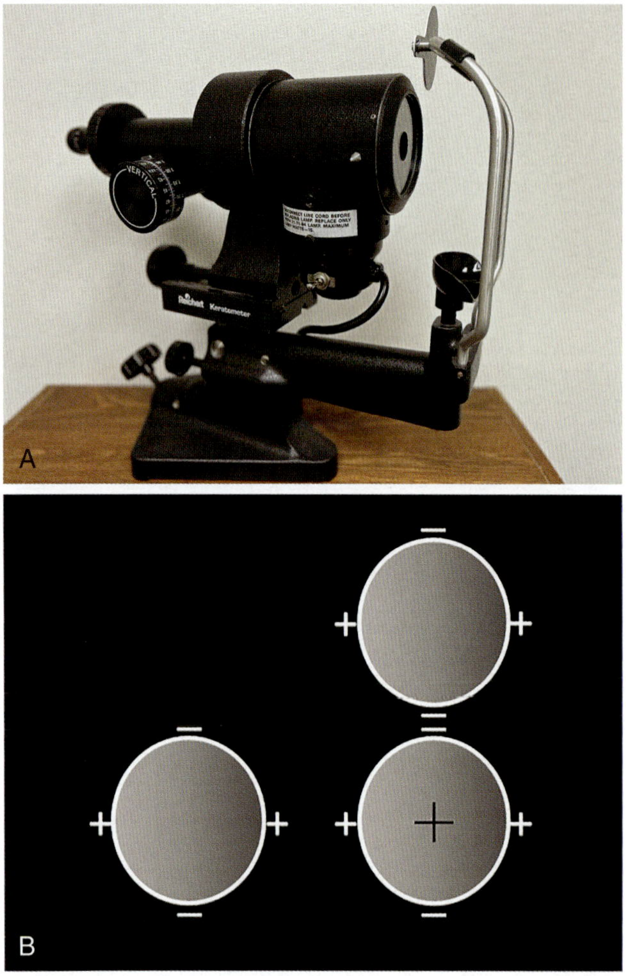

• **Fig. 13.21** **(A)** Manual keratometer. **(B)** The appearance of projected mires.

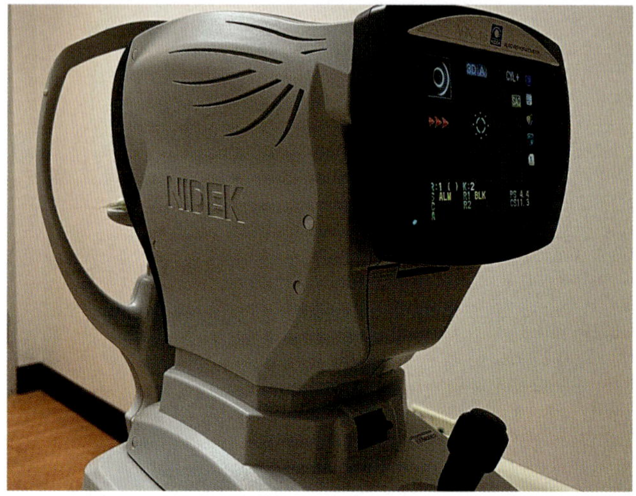

• **Fig. 13.22** Auto refractometer and auto keratometer instrument.

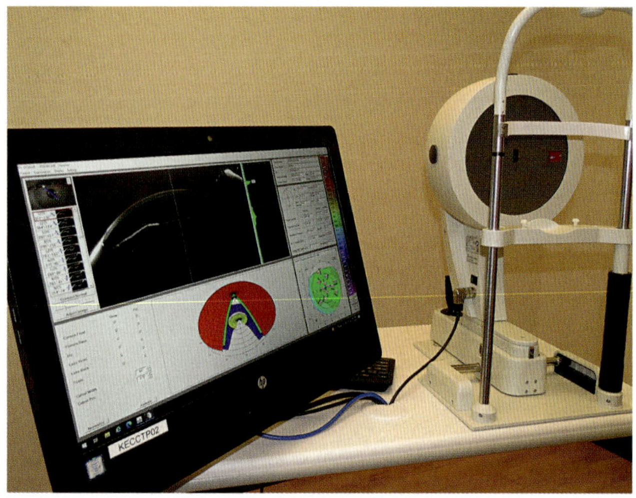

• **Fig. 13.23** Pentacam Scheimpflug device displaying a corneal tomographic map.

Manual Keratometry

Manual keratometry measures the anterior corneal curvature based on the power of a reflecting surface (Fig. 13.21). The instrument gives two anterior corneal curvature values (maximum and minimum) 90 degrees apart. The keratometer only measures a small cornea region at the 3–4 mm central zone and assumes a corneal index of refraction of 1.3375.

Automated Keratometry

Automated keratometers (Fig. 13.22) estimate corneal power by reading 4–6 points of the central corneal zone. This central zone varies from 2.25 mm to 4.00 mm, depending on the keratometer used. This device uses the corneal index of refraction of 1.3375. Often, the keratometry function is incorporated into autorefractors.

Lenstar Keratometry

For keratometry, Lenstar uses 32 measurement points placed on two concentric rings of 16 points, each at 1.65 mm and 2.3 mm.

IOLMaster Keratometry

The IOLMaster measures the curvature based on the relative position of six spots on the corneal in a hexagonal pattern with a diameter of about 2.5 mm. The newest version of the IOLMaster measures the anterior and posterior corneal surface to calculate total keratometry.

Pentacam Scheimpflug Camera Imaging

The Pentacam Scheimpflug device (Fig. 13.23) evaluates the anterior and posterior corneal surface and measures a simulated keratometry value. The unit also measures the posterior corneal radius, anterior corneal radius, and central corneal thickness. The computer software uses the correct indices of refraction to calculate the total corneal power. This measurement of the total corneal power is called the true-net corneal power and is different from the corneal vertex power measured by manual, automated, or simulated keratometry.[7] Pentacam Scheimpflug device is useful in various corneal conditions, including refractive surgery, phakic IOL implantation, and keratoconus diagnosis.

Intraocular Lens Power Calculation Formulas

Intraocular lens formulas have evolved through several generations, from theoretical formulas to regression analysis and more advanced mathematical models incorporating optical, linear regression, and artificial intelligence.

The intraocular lens power calculation formulas are based on the axial length, corneal refractive power, A-constant derived for each lens type and manufacturer, and postoperative anterior chamber depth (ACD).

The prediction of refractive outcomes has improved with optical biometry and modern formulas, and recently, surgeons have been able to achieve a postoperative spherical equivalent of 1.0 diopter in 90% of patients.[8] Currently, SRK/T, Barrett Universal II, and Hill-radial basis function (RBF) are very popular formulas among surgeons and have been proven accurate in predicting excellent refractive outcomes.

The SRK/T is a third-generation formula that combines a theoretical mathematical model with empirical regression to optimize the ACD. The SRK/T formula has good performance in a wide range of axial lengths, including long eyes.[9]

The Barrett Universal II formula is based on a theoretical model eye and retains the positive correlation of axial length and keratometry to ACD. It has excellent performance over a wide range of biometry values. Overall, the Barrett Universal II formula has the lowest prediction error in postoperative refractive outcomes.[10]

The Hill-radial basis function (RBF) calculator is a new method of IOL calculation that uses artificial intelligence and regression analysis of an extensive database of actual postsurgical refractive outcomes to predict the IOL power. The formula demonstrates good performance, including high myopic eyes.

To improve the postoperative ACD, Li et al.[11] proposed a machine learning method for postoperative ACD prediction based on postoperative optical biometry that can be incorporated into a variety of existing IOL power formulas to improve their accuracy in refraction prediction.

Intraocular Lens Power Calculation in Eyes With Previous Corneal Refractive Surgery

Accurate selection of IOL power is challenging in eyes that have undergone corneal refractive surgery such as excimer laser photorefractive keratectomy (PRK), laser-assisted in situ keratomileusis (LASIK), or radial keratotomy (RK).

Three categories of methods exist based on whether and how they use historical data acquired before the corneal refractive surgery:

1. When preoperative keratometry and/or refractive change are available. This method has been shown to provide excellent results when combined with the Double-K SRK/T formula and the Barrett true-K formula.
2. Clinical history method. Uses a combination of historical data and current corneal power values.
3. When preoperative keratometry and refractive change are not available, the formulas fall into two categories:
    a. Formulas that use anterior corneal power: Haigis-Land Barrett true-K no-history.
    b. Formulas based on measurement of both anterior and posterior corneal surfaces available in anterior segment OCT-based IOL calculation, total keratometry from the IOLMaster 700, and Pentacam Scheimpflug.[12,13]

The American Society of Cataract and Refractive Surgery (ASCRS) post-refractive IOL calculator is a web-based tool that assists physicians in selecting the appropriate IOL in patients with a history of prior refractive surgery. The ASCRS calculator incorporates many commonly used methods. Link: iolcalc.ascrs.org.

TEACHING POINTS

Safety checklist of A-scan axial measurement

Room
- Supine position relaxes the patient.
- Instrument should be calibrated.
- Probes and scleral shells should be cleaned and sanitized.

Patient
- Check the patient's past ocular history.
- Patient refraction before cataract, if available.
- Explain the nature of the procedure.
- Make sure that the patient's cornea is clear of ointments or fluids.

A-scan measurement
- Prioritize the immersion technique
- Select the appropriate sound velocity for the eye type (phakic, aphakic, or pseudophakic)
- Bilateral measurement, otherwise impossible (phthisical or enucleated eye)
- Check for gold-standard quality of the spikes and calipers' correct position
- OD/OS AL difference > 0.3mm, perform diagnostic B-scan

References

1. Shammas HJ, Jabre JF. Validating e-norms methodology in ophthalmic biometry. *BMJ Open Ophthalmol.* 2020;5:e000500.
2. Bhatt AB, Schefler AC, Feuer WJ, Yoo SH, Murray TG. Comparison of predictions made by the intraocular lens master and ultrasound biometry. *Arch Ophthalmol.* 2008;126(7):929–933.
3. Yang QH, Chen B, Peng GH, Li ZH, Huang YF. Accuracy of axial length measurements from immersion B-scan ultrasonography in highly myopic eyes. *Int J Ophthalmol.* 2014;18(7):441–445.

4. Curtin BJ, Karlin DB. Axial length measurements and fundus changes of the myopic eye. *Am J Ophthalmol.* 1971;71(1 Part 1):42–53.
5. Lin JT. Error Analysis of IOL Power Calculations. *Mastering the Technique s of IOL Power Calculations.* 2nd ed. New Delhi: Jaypee; 2008.
6. Meyer JJ, Kim MJ, Kim T. Effects of contact lens wear on biometry measurements for intraocular lens calculations. *Eye Contact Lens.* 2018;44(Suppl 1):S255–S258.
7. Shammas HJ, Hoffer KJ, Shammas MC. Scheimpflug photography keratometry readings for routine intraocular lens power calculation. *J Cataract Refract Surg.* 2009;35:330–334.
8. Sheard R. Optimising biometry for best outcomes in cataract surgery. *Eye (Lond).* 2014;2:118–125.
9. Aristodemou P, Knox Cartwright NE, Sparrow JM, Johnston RL. Intraocular lens formula constant optimization and partial coherence interferometry biometry: refractive outcomes in 8108 eyes after cataract surgery. *J Cataract Refract Surg.* 2011;37:50–56.
10. Melles RB, Holladay JT, Chang WJ. Accuracy of intraocular lens calculation formulas. *Ophthalmology.* 2018;125:169–178.
11. Li T, Stein J, Nallasamy N. AI-powered effective lens position prediction improves the accuracy of existing lens formulas. *Br J Ophthalmol.* 2021. https://doi.org/10.1136/bjophthalmol-2020-318321.
12. Savini G, Hoffer KJ. Intraocular lens power calculation in eyes with previous corneal refractive surgery. *Eye Vis (Lond).* 2018;5:18.
13. Wang L, Koch DD. Intraocular lens power calculations in eyes with previous corneal refractive surgery: review and expert opinion. *Ophthalmology.* 2021;128:e121–e131.

14 Ocular Trauma

NORMA ALLEMANN, GABRIELA ASSUMPÇÃO BRITO PEREIRA PELLEGRINI, AND ROSANA CRISTINA SCIENCIA DA SILVA PIZARRO

Ocular trauma can vary greatly in intensity and degree of involvement of ocular structures and adnexa. Therefore, early evaluation by a specialized professional is recommended, aiming for the correct diagnosis and for staging the severity of the condition, enabling guidance to carry out appropriate treatment.

Besides the differences in regional occupations and exposures,[1] ocular trauma remains an important cause of blindness all over the world, particularly in young and male patients.[2,3] Studies estimate that approximately 6–7%[1] of the admitted trauma patients have ocular manifestation, representing 10–15% of all eye disorders. Ocular trauma may be isolated or associated with head trauma and other complaints and it must be considered in order to prioritize the patient's necessities.

The three categories of ocular trauma, initially well documented by Coleman and colleagues in 1973,[4] were contusion and concussion injuries, perforating or laceration wounds, and foreign body injury. The ocular trauma is commonly classified into open and close trauma based on the mechanism of the trauma.[5]

In closed ocular trauma, the globe wall maintains its integrity. Differently, in the open globe trauma, the globe integrity was lost with corneoscleral rupture and can be classified into penetrating (entry wound) or perforating (entry and exit wound). In open globe injuries, special care with intraocular foreign body must be taken.[6]

The first Ocular Trauma Classification Group was created in 1997 to unify the language used in open-globe ocular trauma, leading to the development to a score of risk, the Ocular Score Table (OTS).[7] OTS is valued to standardize definitions of ocular trauma and to guide professionals to graduate severity and priority, estimating prognosis and favoring treatments. A higher OTS score is usually associated with a better prognosis. However, OTS is now over 20 years old, and recent studies suggest that a better final visual acuity can be acquired considering all the advances in technique and instrumentals in pars plana vitrectomy surgery.[8] In the pediatric population, a similar table can be used (POTS), considering the difficulty of obtaining the true initial visual acuity in young children.[9]

Imaging modalities in ocular trauma are useful for diagnosis and for documentation as legal practice, based on the gravity and poor prognosis that can impact in permanent vision loss.[10] Ultrasound biomicroscopy (UBM) and B-scan ultrasound are useful diagnostic modalities that can be used earlier as complementary examination commonly when the eye presents anterior and/or posterior media opacities, and difficulty to perform the complete ocular exam.[6] Even in clear media, UBM and B-scan can provide complementary information about the presence, location, size and nature of a foreign body, identifying angle recession, lens opacities, evaluate the extension of choroidal detachment, scleral laceration, and demonstrate orbital findings such as muscle rupture and localized hematoma and inflammatory signs of the eye wall.

It is well known that ocular ultrasound is a noninvasive, simple, and effective diagnostic method that can be used in bedside examination.[11] Particularly in ocular trauma, it is critical to assess and ensure the integrity of the globe before the ocular ultrasound. In cases of open globe injury, scleral laceration, or exposure of intraocular contents, B-scan ultrasound and UBM need to be postponed until postoperative evolution.[12] Eyelid edema, hematoma, or laceration may prevent an adequate eye opening. Pain is a common symptom in traumatic ocular injuries, and the exam must be executed with minimal contact and/or pressure to the globe. X-ray and orbital computed tomography imaging can be done complementary to the ocular exam and ultrasound. Magnetic resonance imaging must be avoided when metallic intra- or periocular foreign body is suspected.[13] Ocular trauma is usually unilateral, and it is always useful to examine the fellow eye for a comparative evaluation.

Knowledge about the mechanism of trauma and past ocular history, when possible, is always useful to refine the B-scan and UBM findings. Ocular trauma can lead to disorders of the anterior and/or posterior segments, and it is important to follow a standardized exam protocol to obtain as much information as possible from the exams.

For didactic purposes, the most common trauma findings will be divided into anterior and posterior segments.

Anterior Segment Findings in Ocular Trauma

Eyelid, cornea, anterior sclera, and conjunctiva can usually be evaluated in ocular examination. Often, the lesions are evident and can be diagnosed even without ophthalmic equipment. Visual acuity, eye movement, and pupillary reflex should be evaluated. Information about past ocular history and the trauma mechanism should be obtained. The trauma mechanism should be known to assess the possibility of experiencing an injury with an intraocular foreign body and its possible composition.[14]

UBM uses a high-frequency probe, which allows evaluation of the cornea, anterior chamber, angle, ciliary processes, lens, and zonular ligaments, even in cases with corneal opacities or hemorrhagic and/or inflammatory material in the anterior chamber.[15]

When UBM is not available or not suitable due to the eye injury, B-scan ultrasound using immersion or pseudoimmersion techniques (Clearscan) can provide information about the anterior segment.

Common findings in anterior segment traumatic lesions are listed in Table 14.1.

Hyphema usually does not allow a complete ocular exam. The echogenicity and distribution of the echoes in the anterior chamber can give information about its duration; if recent, the blood is usually fluid, mobile, and appears as low-reflectivity punctiform echoes. In longstanding hyphema, UBM may demonstrate clots as organized punctiform echoes with medium/high reflectivity and less mobility.

UBM is useful for localizing and measuring an anterior intraocular foreign body or even demonstrating a possible ocular penetration route. In ocular traumoa, anterior and/or posterior lens capsule might be ruptured, and lens material can be found in the anterior chamber and/or posterior chamber. B-scan ultrasound, particularly associated with pseudoimmersion or immersion technique, must be performed when there is posterior capsule rupture, lens or intraocular dislocation, or an intraocular foreign body[14] (Fig. 14.1 and Video 14.1).

TABLE 14.1 Most Frequent Anterior Segment Findings in Ocular Trauma

Cyclodialysis
Hyphema
Iridodialysis
Angle recession
Zonular ligaments dehiscence
Scleral rupture
Anterior corneoscleral laceration
Anterior and/or posterior lens capsule rupture
Lens opacity
Intraocular lens dislocation
Subconjunctival and/or subtenon's hemorrhage
Conjunctival laceration
Intraocular foreign body

Posterior Segment Findings in Ocular Trauma

Vitreous opacities, cataract formation with or without capsule rupture, lens dislocation to the posterior segment (Fig. 14.2 and Videos 14.2–14.4), and anterior chamber hemorrhage are frequently presented in ocular trauma not allowing detailed observation of the posterior segment.[16] Anterior chamber findings can guide the examiner about posterior segment injuries, such as corneal or scleral lacerations, for example.

B-scan ultrasonography can be performed in earlier phases of almost every case, contributing for a correct diagnosis and providing guidance for the treatment. Pain, edema, dense intraocular hemorrhage, and disorganization may mistake the correct diagnosis. In these cases, serial evaluation is usually valuable.

Vitreous may become more dense and organized in trauma. Vitreoschisis and posterior vitreous detachment may occur suddenly, leading to vitreous hemorrhage, retinal tears, and retinal detachment.[4] Choroidal detachment may be present and sometimes associated with ciliary body detachment, causing hypotony. Vitreous debris, clots, and impregnation of the posterior hyaloid are challenging findings to distinguish from retinal detachment. Gain reduction, observation of the membranes movements and after movements, and zooming in image details become important steps in a dynamic exam and must be tried to allow adequate evaluation.

In areas of posterior globe rupture, the vitreous usually becomes dense and incarcerated, as observed in Fig. 14.3 and Videos 14.5 and 14.6. This finding is important to be documented and further evaluated in a careful exam.

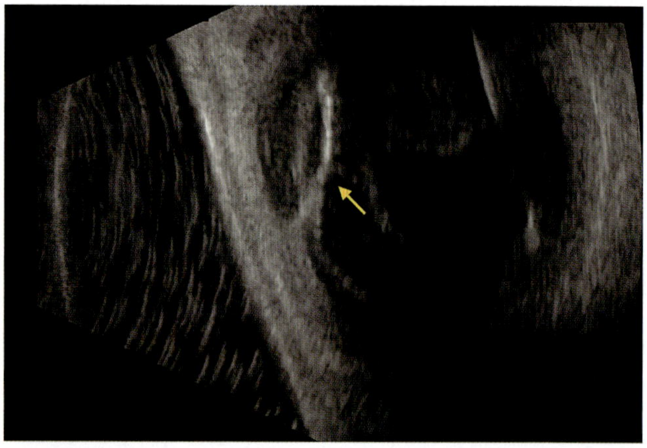

• **Fig. 14.1** Axial B-scan with pseudoimmersion. A localized irregularity of the posterior lens capsule suggested a rupture (*yellow arrow*). Internal high reflectivity of the lens and a reduced volume were compatible with traumatic cataract.

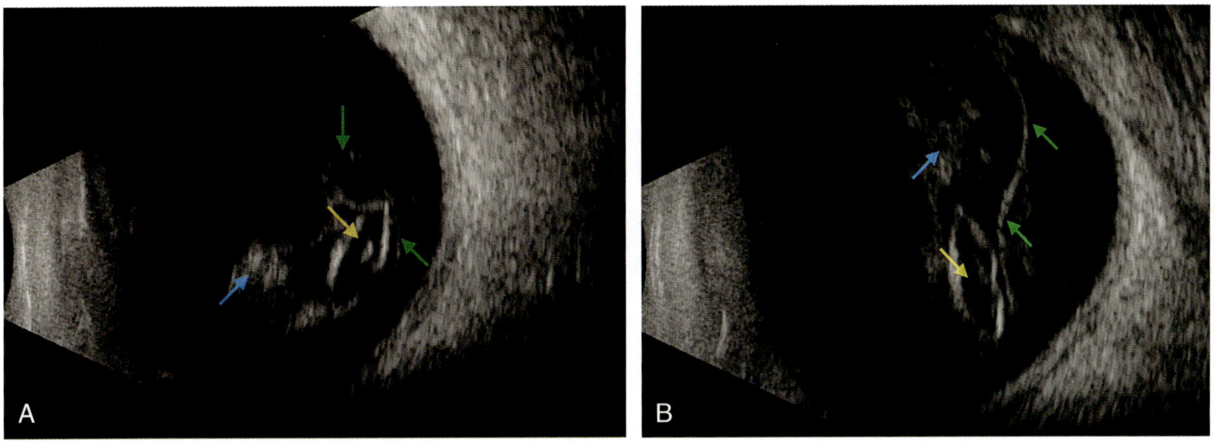

• **Fig. 14.2** Traumatic lens dislocation to the vitreous cavity. Transverse **(A)** and Longitudinal **(B)** B-scan showing a highly reflective lens (*yellow arrow*) positioned anterior to the detached posterior hyaloid (*green arrows*), surrounded by a dense cluster of echoes (*blue arrow*).

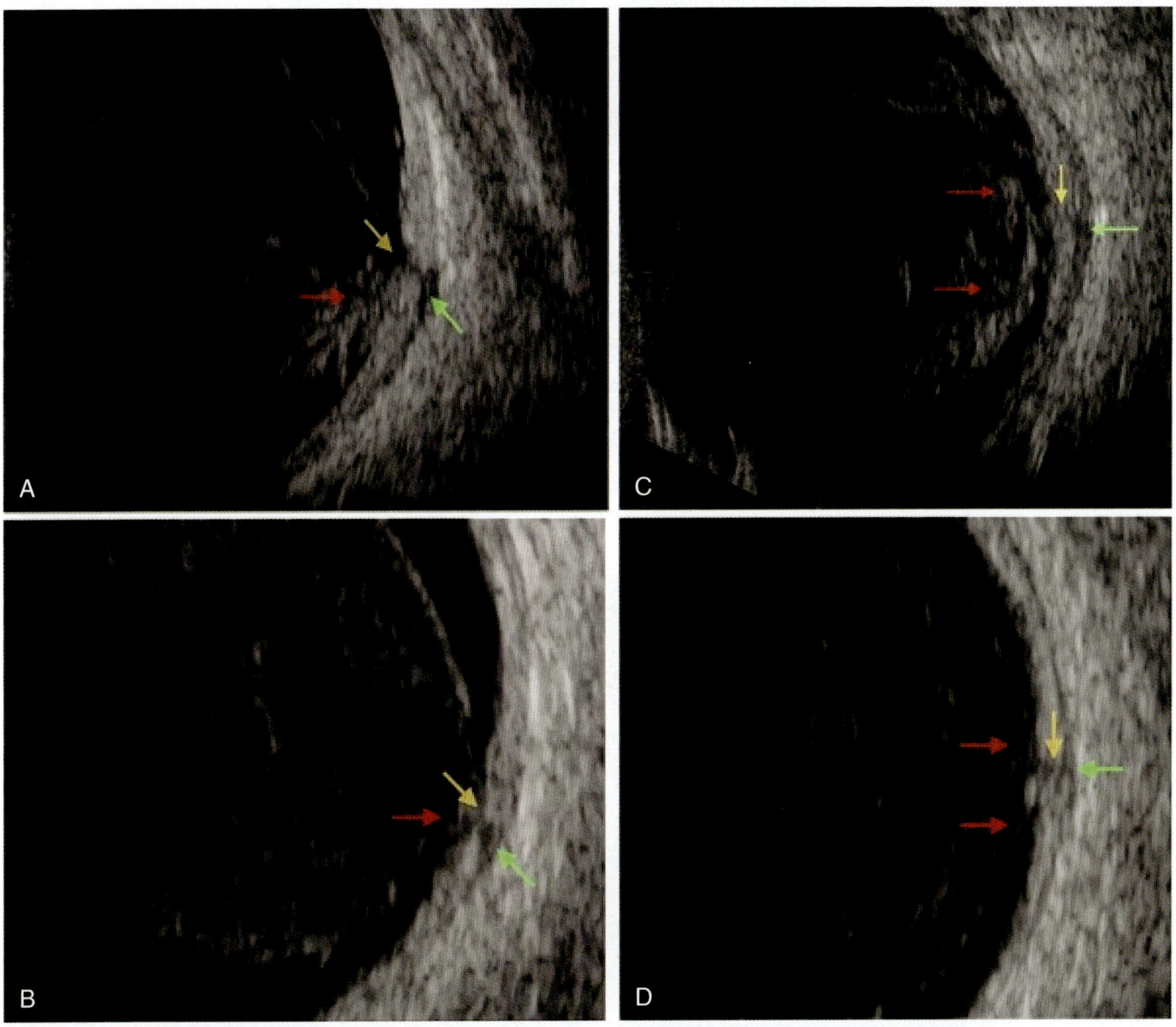

• **Fig. 14.3** Ocular wall rupture in **(A)** (longitudinal scan) and **(C)** (transversal scan) in the first exam and **(B)** (longitudinal scan) and **(D)** (transversal scan) 1 month later, evaluating the same area. B-scans show a slightly hypoechogenic band corresponding to interruption of scleral continuity (*yellow arrow*) with a localized posterior hematoma (*green arrow*) and vitreous adherence/incarceration (*red arrow*).

An area of hyporeflectivity in the subtenon's space and/or orbital fat adjacent to the presumed site of posterior scleral rupture might be present, representing a localized haematoma and this finding sometimes can guide the examiner about the scleral lesion.

When a foreign body is suspected, gain must be lowered and careful dynamic evaluation must be taken to distinguish a dense organized vitreous from a possible foreign body. Dislocated lens material and a dislocated intraocular lens mimic a foreign body. Metallic and acrylic foreign bodies are usually hyperreflective and present with sound artifacts, such as attenuation and reverberation, respectively[17] (Figs. 14.4–14.6 and Videos 14.7–14.9).

Organic foreign bodies are usually hyporreflective, and may present change their properties throughout serial exams due to decomposition.[17] It is important to measure the IOFB dimensions, determine its shape and characteristics, and its topography/location.

In traumatic lesions with IOFB, there is a high risk of endophthalmitis.[18] When metallic IOFB are involved, an early diagnosis may prevent siderosis.[19] Anterior and/or posterior vitrectomy are usually performed in these cases and a reliable ultrasound exam may allow surgical planning and adequate instrumentation, therefore contributing to a better outcome.

Common findings in posterior segment traumatic lesions are listed in Table 14.2.

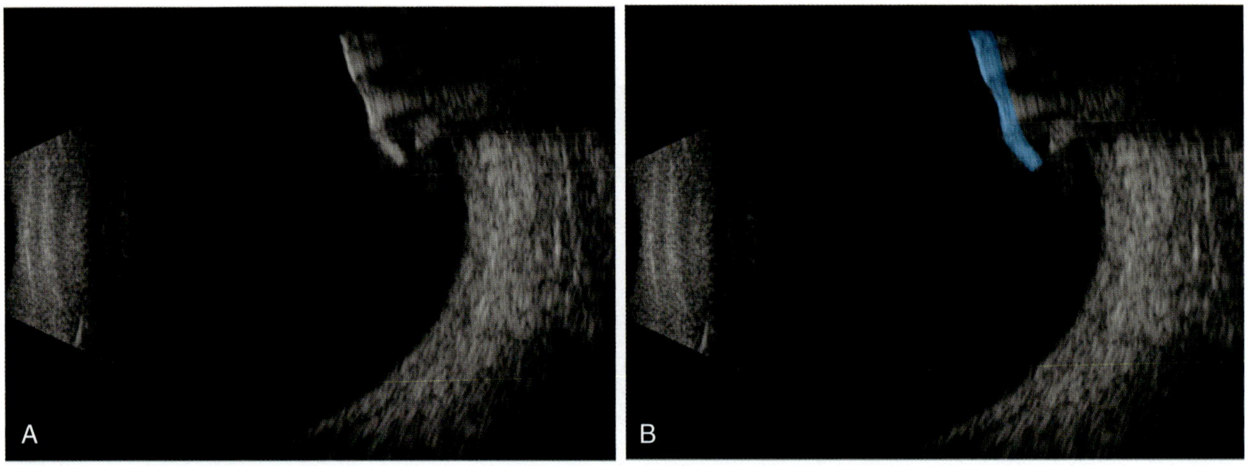

• **Fig. 14.4** Intraocular foreign body topograhy. **(A)** Longitudinal temporal B-scan shows a bright linear and continuous interface close to the posterior eye wall, determining acoustic reverberation and posterior shadowing, suggesting a metallic composition of the IOFB (in *blue* in **B**).

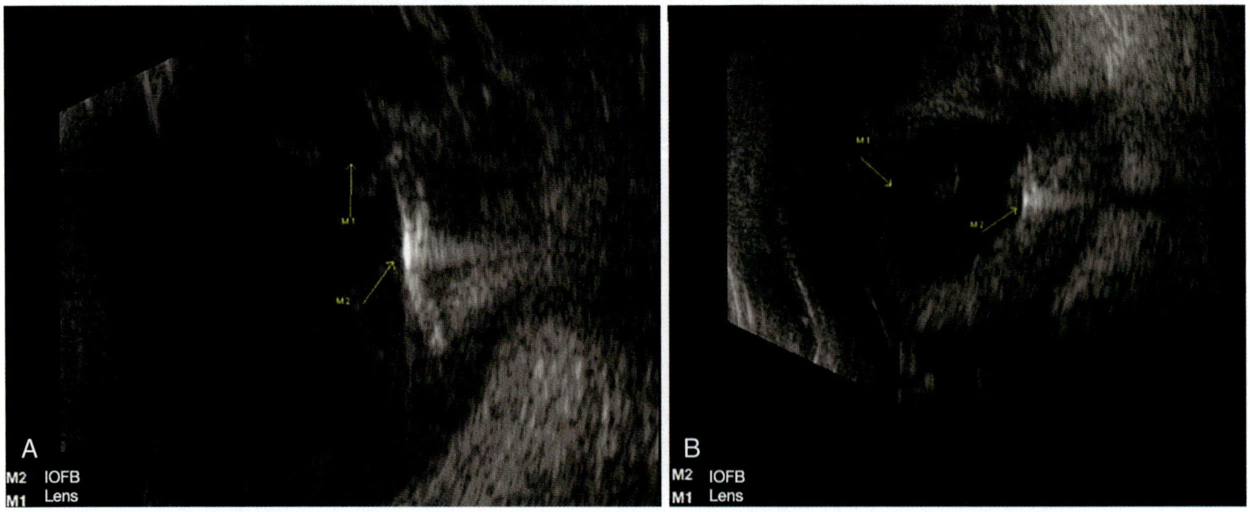

• **Fig. 14.5** IOFB anatomical relation to the lens. Longitudinal peripheral **(A)** and transverse **(B)** B-scans. Images show the proximity of the IOFB with the lens, which presented internal hyper reflectivity, compatible with traumatic cataract.

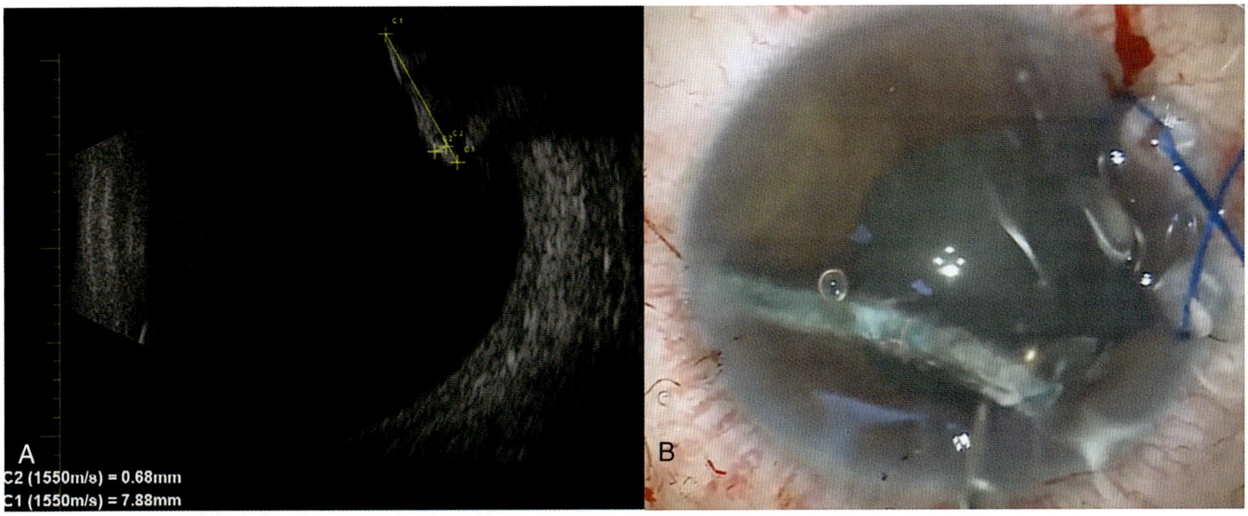

• **Fig. 14.6** IOFB measurement: B-scan and after removal. **(A)** Longitudinal B-scan measurement of the IOFB was approximately 7.88 mm in length and 0.68 mm in thickness. **(B)** After removal, the real IOFB measurement was close to 9 mm.

TABLE 14.2 Most Frequent Posterior Segment Findings in Ocular Trauma

Vitreous debris
Vitreous hemorrhage
Vitreous detachment
Subhyaloid hemorrhage
Subretinal hemorrhage
Retinal detachment
Choroidal thickening
Macular thickening
Scleral rupture
Pathological vitreous adhesions
Orbital hematoma or abscess
Choroidal detachment
Optic nerve avulsion
Intraocular foreign body

References

1. He CH, Poulsen DM, Parsikia A, Mbekeani JN. Characteristics of ocular trauma in the United States. *Arq Bras Oftalmol.* 2022;85(3):240–248. https://doi.org/10.5935/0004-2749.20220035.
2. Coelho J, Ferreira A, Kuhn F, Meireles A. Globe ruptures: outcomes and prognostic analysis of severe ocular trauma. *Ophthalmologica.* 2022;245(4):376–384.
3. Cruvinel IDL, Ghanem VC, Nascimento MA, Torigoe M, Kara-José N. Prognostic factors in open globe injuries. *Ophthalmologica.* 2003;217(6):431–435. https://doi.org/10.1159/000073075.
4. Coleman DJ, Jack RL, Franzen LA. Ultrasonography in ocular trauma. *Am J Ophthalmol.* 1973;75(2):279–288. https://doi.org/10.1016/0002-9394(73)91024-6.
5. Shah MA, Shah SM, Applewar A, Patel C, Shah S, Patel U. Ocular Trauma Score: a useful predictor of visual outcome at six weeks in patients with traumatic cataract. *Ophthalmology.* 2012;119(7):1336–1341. https://doi.org/10.1016/j.ophtha.2012.01.020.
6. Agarwal HC, Sood NN, Dayal Y. Ultrasonography in perforating ocular injuries. *Indian J Ophthalmol.* 1984;32(5):285–288.
7. Scott R. The Ocular Trauma Score. *Community Eye Health.* 2015;28(91):44–45.
8. Perez EA, Ramirez DA, Peterson JD, et al. The Ocular Trauma Score underestimates visual recovery for the most severe open-globe injuries. *Ophthalmol Retina.* 2023;7(7):612–619. https://doi.org/10.1016/j.oret.2023.01.021.
9. Acar U, Tok OY, Acar DE, Burcu A, Ornek F. A new ocular trauma score in pediatric penetrating eye injuries. *Eye (Lond).* 2011;25(3):370–374. https://doi.org/10.1038/eye.2010.211.
10. Vaghmare S, Rahul R, Prajna NV, Radhakrishnan N. Analysis on the completeness of case records of patients with penetrating ocular trauma following a multimodal intervention. *Indian J Ophthalmol.* 2022;70(8):2962–2965. https://doi.org/10.4103/ijo.IJO_223_22.
11. Kilker BA, Holst JM, Hoffmann B. Bedside ocular ultrasound in the emergency department. *Eur J Emerg Med.* 2014;21(4):246–253. https://doi.org/10.1097/MEJ.0000000000000070.
12. Blanch RJ, Bishop J, Javidi H, Murray PI. Effect of time to primary repair on final visual outcome after open globe injury. *Br J Ophthalmol.* 2019;103(10):1491–1494. https://doi.org/10.1136/bjophthalmol-2017-311559.
13. Williams S, Char DH, Dillon WP, Lincoff N, Moseley M. Ferrous intraocular foreign bodies and magnetic resonance imaging. *Am J Ophthalmol.* 1988;105(4):398–401. https://doi.org/10.1016/0002-9394(88)90305-4.
14. Moura MF, Hayashi I, Rocha DM, Allemann N. Evaluation of anterior segment foreign bodies with ultrasound biomicroscopy. *Arq Bras Oftalmol.* 2012;75(2):122–125. https://doi.org/10.1590/s0004-27492012000200010.
15. Ozdal MP, Mansour M, Deschenes J. Ultrasound biomicroscopic evaluation of the traumatized eyes. *Eye (Lond).* 2003;17(4):467–472. https://doi.org/10.1038/sj.eye.6700382.

16. Dastevska-Djosevska E. Ultrasonography in ocular trauma. *Pril (Makedon Akad Nauk Umet Odd Med Nauki)*. 2013;34(2):105–113.
17. Costa MA, Garcia PN, Barroso LF, Ferreira MA, Okuda EA, Allemann N. Composition of intraocular foreign bodies: experimental study of ultrasonographic presentation. *Arq Bras Oftalmol.* 2013;76(1):13–17. https://doi.org/10.1590/s0004-27492013000100005.
18. Sabaci G, Bayer A, Mutlu FM, Karagül S, Yildirim E. Endophthalmitis after deadly-weapon-related open-globe injuries: risk factors, value of prophylactic antibiotics, and visual outcomes. *Am J Ophthalmol.* 2002;133(1):62–69. https://doi.org/10.1016/s0002-9394(01)01320-4.
19. Acharya I, Raut AA. *Siderosis Bulbi*. StatPearls Publishing; 2023. https://www.ncbi.nlm.nih.gov/books/NBK567781.

15

Color Doppler in Ophthalmology

NORMA ALLEMANN AND MARIA HELENA MANDELLO RAMOS

Color Doppler is a noninvasive imaging method, applied to medicine since the 1980s, which combines real-time B-mode ultrasound with the Doppler technique, thus allowing the simultaneous analysis of the characteristics of anatomical structures and blood vessels encoded by colors.[1,2]

The first study to demonstrate the use of Doppler in the investigation of orbital vessels was published by Erickson in 1989. Between 1989 and 1991, Guthoff and Lieb published several other studies demonstrating the applicability of Doppler in the evaluation of ocular pathologies.[3–5]

Currently, Doppler is an important method of diagnostic investigation and monitoring of various ocular diseases.

Anatomy of the Orbital Vessels

The ophthalmic artery can originate from the internal carotid, meningeal, or anterior communicating arteries and is responsible for ocular perfusion. The ophthalmic artery penetrates the orbit through the optic canal and is located in fero-temporally to the optic nerve. It gives off branches including the central retinal artery, medial posterior short ciliary artery, and lateral posterior short ciliary artery.[4]

The central retinal artery is located in the inferior optic nerve and presents a simultaneous course with the central retinal vein within the optic nerve.

The posterior short ciliary arteries are located lateral to the optic nerve and supply the sclera, choroid, ciliary body, and iris.

The superior ophthalmic vein passes through the apex of the orbit to reach the cavernous sinus through the superior orbital fissure and is responsible for the most significant part of the venous drainage of the orbit.[5,6]

Technique

For the exam to be performed, the patient is positioned in a supine position. A large volume of gel is placed on the eyelids, followed by the linear transducer (3–12, 5–12, or 7–15 MHz). Compression of the probe on the eye can change the values of the resistance index and maximum systolic velocity of the retrobulbar vessels. Care is taken not to apply excessive pressure to the eye, avoiding artifacts.[4–8]

Color coding allows you to distinguish the direction of the flow in relation to the transducer; the flow approaching the transducer is shown in red, and the flow moving away from the transducer is shown in blue.[4,5]

The real-time ultrasound image works as an anatomical guide, orienting the location of the orbital vessels, intraocular and/or retrobulbar lesions to be studied.

A horizontal scan through the eyeball and orbit at the level of the optic nerve allows visualization of the central retinal artery/vein complex, which can be detected in the "acoustic shadow" that corresponds to the optic nerve (Fig. 15.1 and Video 15.1). The spectral analysis of this complex reveals an arterial component (pulsatile and positive, above the horizontal line) and a venous component (laminar, negative, below the horizontal line) (Fig. 15.2).

The posterior short ciliary arteries are visible lateral to the optic nerve. Its resistance index, under normal conditions, is always lower than that of the central retinal artery (Fig. 15.3).

To examine the ophthalmic artery, the probe should be oriented superiorly and nasally to the optic nerve. It presents an anterograde direction from the carotid siphon towards the eyeball and is coded in a red pattern. It presents a spectral profile similar to that of the internal carotid, with a maximum systolic peak, a dicrotic notch and, a smooth slope of the diastolic flow (Fig. 15.4 and Video 15.2).[9–11]

The superior ophthalmic vein presents a pattern that can change depending on breathing, the cardiac cycle and the gradient between the veins of the nose and the cavernous sinus. It normally presents a low and continuous speed (Figs. 15.5 and 15.6 and Video 15.3).

Blood flow (peak systolic velocity) and resistance indices are quantitative parameters used to evaluate orbital arteries (Table 15.1) and veins (Table 15.2).[7–10] In color Doppler imaging, spectral analysis allows qualitative evaluation of the blood flow.

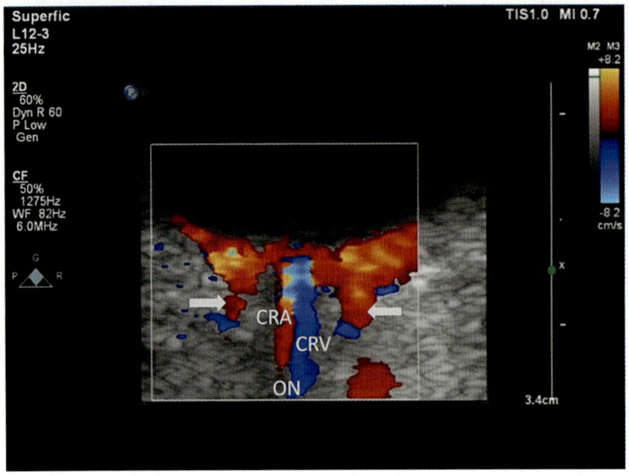

• **Fig. 15.1** Normal arterial anatomy. Axial horizontal scan through the globe shows the central retinal artery (CRA) and accompanying central retinal vein (CRV) within the anterior portion of the optic nerve shadow (ON). On both sides of the optic nerve the short posterior ciliary arteries can be identified (*arrows*).

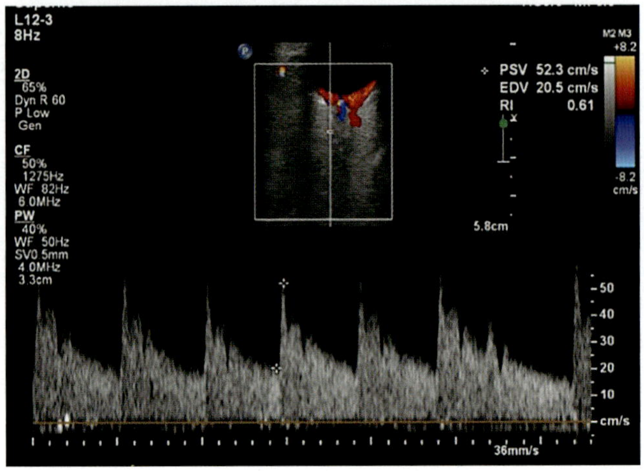

• **Fig. 15.4** Spectral analysis of the ophthalmic artery shows a steep maximum systolic peak, often a dicrotic notch, and low diastolic flow velocity.

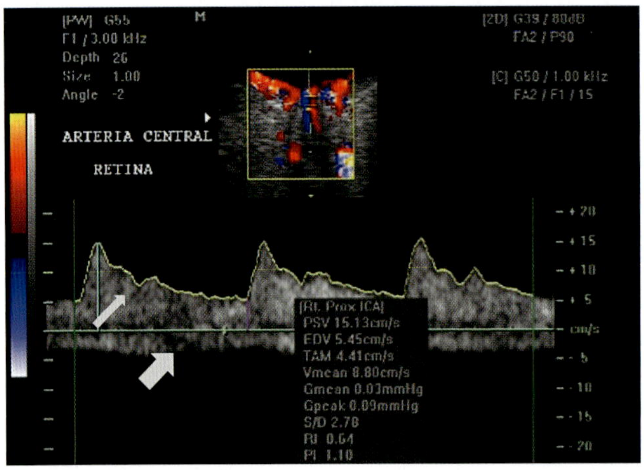

• **Fig. 15.2** In the spectral analysis, the CRA presents a positive, pulsatile flow above the horizontal line (*thin arrow*), and the CRV presents a laminar flow below the horizontal line (*arrow*).

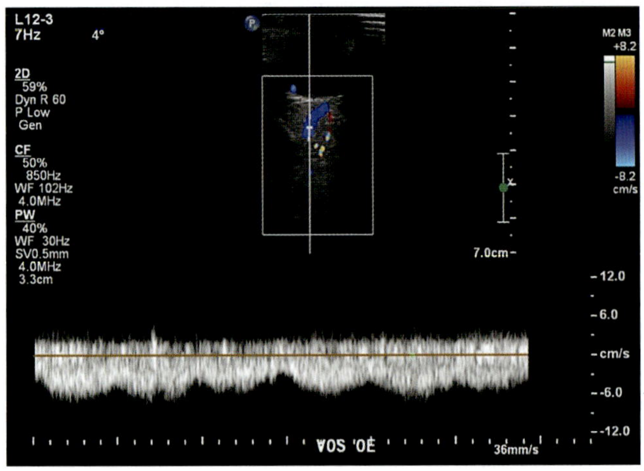

• **Fig. 15.5** Color Doppler of the superior ophthalmic vein demonstrates the characteristic continuous, non-pulsatile venous flow.

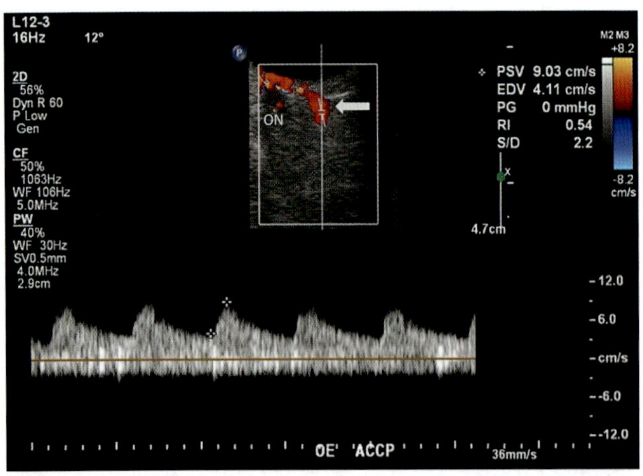

• **Fig. 15.3** Posterior short ciliary artery. Using color Doppler, the posterior ciliary artery (*arrow*) can be seen lateral to the optic nerve (ON) and presents, under normal conditions, a resistance index lower than that of the central retinal artery.

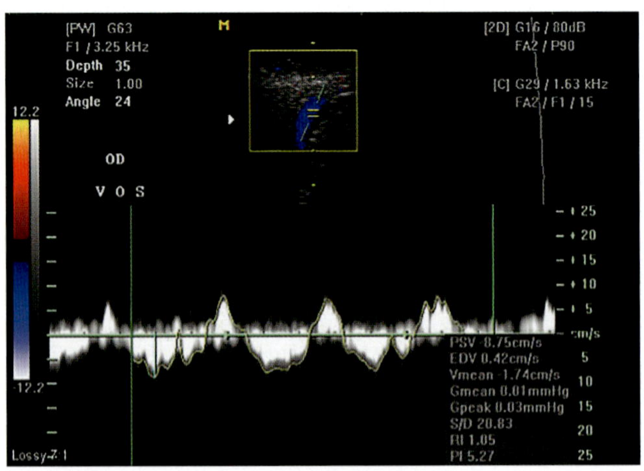

• **Fig. 15.6** Alternate flow within the superior ophthalmic vein – normal variant, color and pulsed Doppler.

TABLE 15.1 Blood Flow and Resistance Indices in Orbital Arteries in Normal Subjects

Doppler Index	Kaiser et al.[7]	Fukukita et al.[8]	Berges et al.[9]
PSV OA	38.9 ± 0.5	35.8 ± 8.4	45.0 ± 10.0
RI OA	0.75 ± 0.006	0.776 ± 0.035	0.75 ± 0.05
PSV CRA	11.1 ± 0.1	11.3 ± 3.1	15.0 ± 3.0
RI CRA	0.70 ± 0.005	0.627 ± 0.038	0.62 ± 0,05
VSM ACCP	11.27 ± 0,1	10.2 ± 2.8	12.0 ± 3.0
IR ACCP	0.68 ± 0.005	0.614 ± 0.06	0,53 ± 0.08

CRA, central retinal artery; *OA*, ophthalmic artery; *PCA*, posterior ciliary arteries; *PSV (cm/s)*, Peak systolic velocity; *RI*, resistance index.

TABLE 15.2 Blood Flow Velocities in Orbital Veins in Normal Subjects[10]

	Maximum Velocity	Minimum Velocity
CRV	6.7 ± 2.4	2.7 ± 0.7
SOV	10.2 ± 3.8	4.3 ± 2.4

CRV, Central retinal vein; *SOV*, superior ophthalmic vein. Blood flow velocities in cm/s.

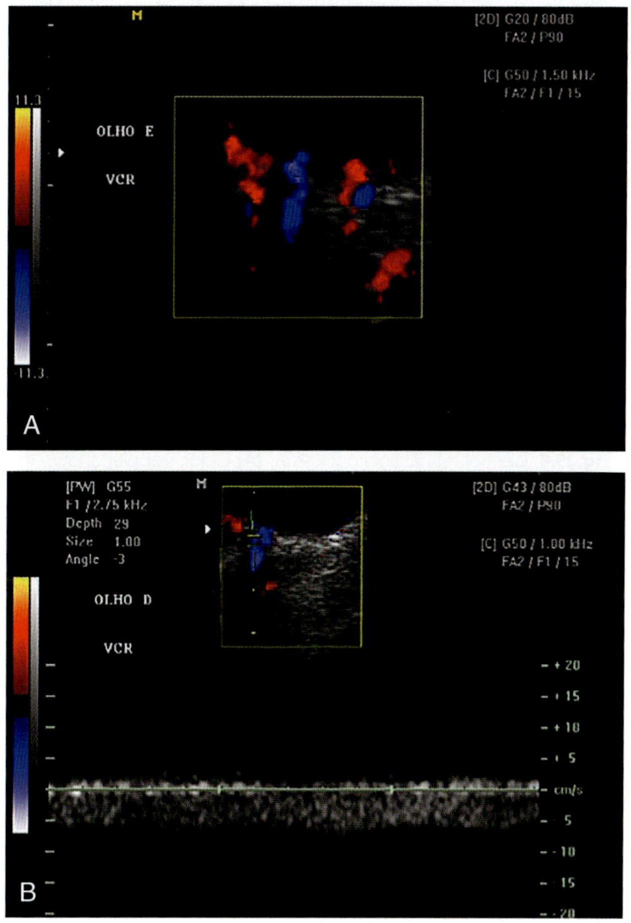

• **Fig. 15.7** Retinal artery occlusion. **(A)** Color Doppler shows the absence of arterial color Doppler signals within the optic nerve. **(B)** No arterial waveform is shown on spectral analysis.

Indications

Central Retinal Artery Occlusion

Central retinal artery occlusion is a blockage of blood flow throught the central retinal artery secondary to embolus, thrombosis, or vasculitis. The clinical picture usually presents with sudden loss of vision. Embolic occlusion of central retinal occlusion is a risk factor for stroke and mortality from cardiovascular disease.

Depending on the time of evolution, the color Doppler imaging may show an absence of flow in the central retinal artery or a reduction in the maximum systolic velocity and an increase in the resistance index with or without identification of the embolus (condensate of highly echogenic echoes close to the surface of the optical disc). There may also be a concomitant change in flow in the central retinal vein[11] (Fig. 15.7).

Central Retinal Vein Occlusion

The clinical picture of central retinal vein occlusion (CRVO) presents with a moderate to severe decrease in visual acuity. The main risk factors are high blood pressure, age, hyperlipidemia, glaucoma, diabetes, and increased blood viscosity. It can progress to neovascularization of the retina and iris, leading to neovascular glaucoma.

On color Doppler, an absence or reduction in venous flow velocity is observed, which may or may not be associated with a reduction in maximum systolic velocity and an increase in the resistance index of the central retinal artery, as shown in Fig. 15.8.[12,13]

Optic Disc Drusen

Optic disc drusen (ODD) is more common in Caucasians. It is usually bilateral, and patients are usually asymtomatic. However, it can increase in size and cause visual field defects

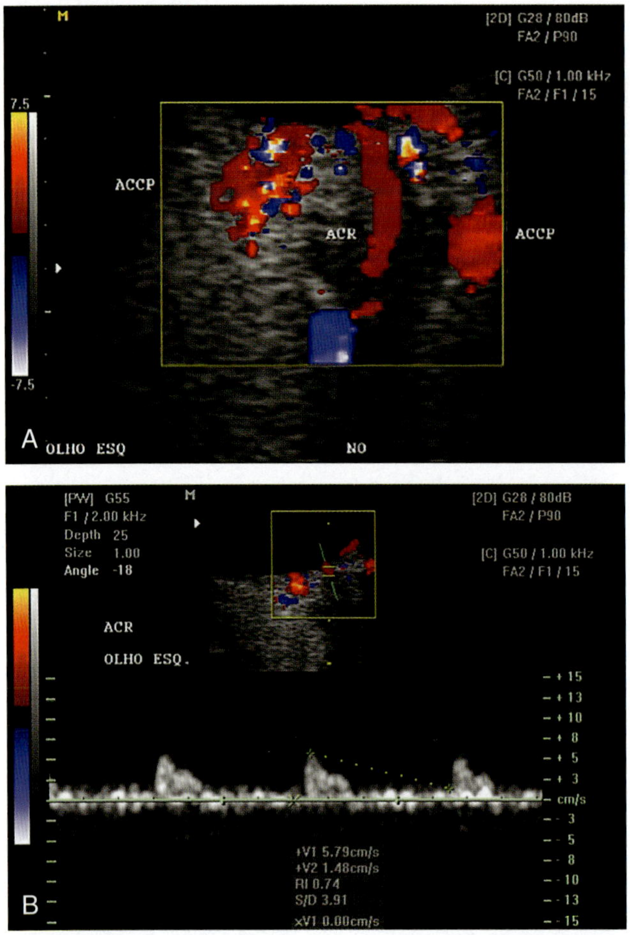

• **Fig. 15.8** Central retinal vein occlusion. **(A)** Color Doppler shows the absence of venous color Doppler signals within the optic nerve. **(B)** In the spectral analysis, an absence of flow in the central retinal vein and a reduction in maximum systolic velocity with an increase in the resistance index of the central retinal artery are observed.

and changes in the blood flow of the central retinal artery,[14] as shown in Fig. 15.9.

Glaucoma

Intraocular pressure and changes in the hemodynamics of the retrobulbar vessels are risk factors for the progression of glaucoma. The study of the vascularization of the retrobulbar vessels may show a reduction in maximum systolic velocity and an increase in the resistance index of the central retinal and posterior short ciliary arteries. Hemodynamic parameters improve with adequate control of the intraocular pressure,[7–8] as shown in Fig. 15.10.

Epidermoid Cyst

Benign tumor that originates from the incarceration of the embryonic ectoderm at the site of fetal cleft closure.

Superficial epidermoid cysts usually present in childhood as an encapsulated nodule often located in the temporal region. They are painless, firm in consistency, and slow growing (Fig. 15.11).

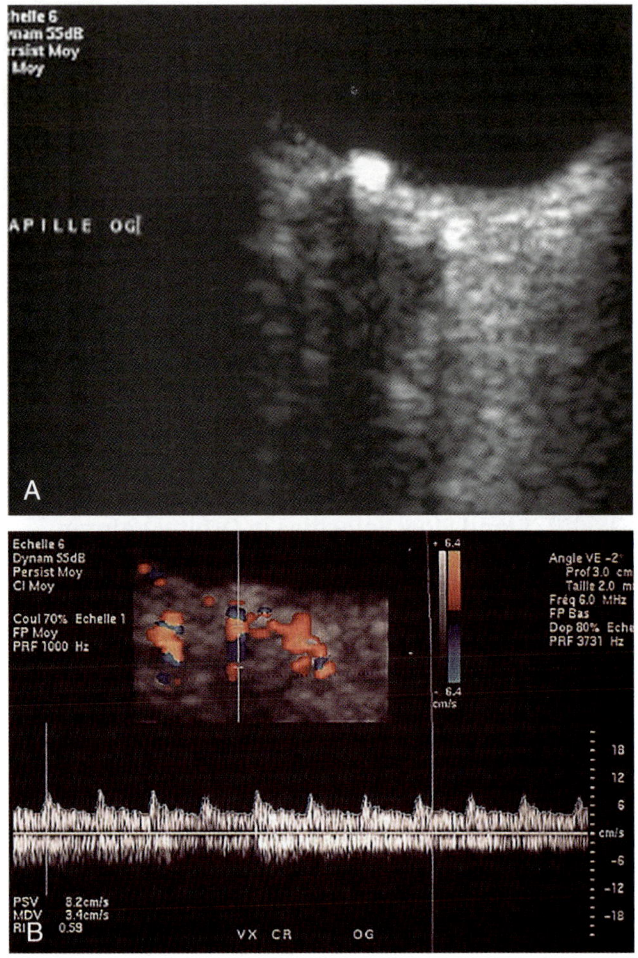

• **Fig. 15.9** Optic disc drusen. **(A)** Large optic disc drusen, visible as a highly reflective structure with posterior shadowing at the optic nerve. **(B)** Color Doppler imaging: blood flow spectrum in the central retinal artery in a patient with optic disc drusen, presenting decreased peak-systolic velocity.

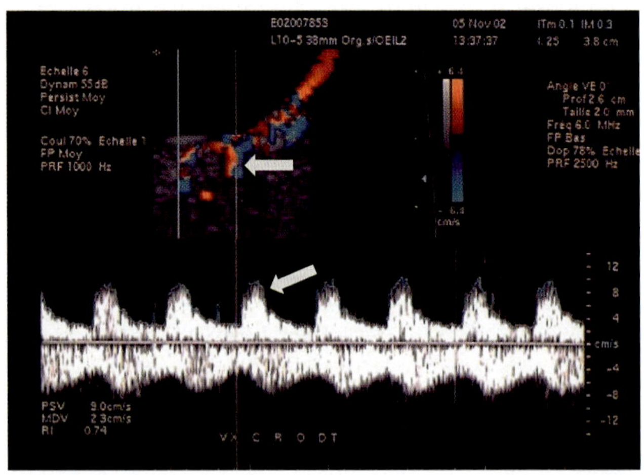

• **Fig. 15.10** Glaucoma. In a patient with glaucoma, an increase in the resistance index (IR: 74) in the central retinal artery (*arrows*) is observed.

Persistent Fetal Vasculature

Persistent fetal vasculature (PVF) is a congenital developmental anomaly of the eye, resulting from failure of regression of the hyaloid vascular system and primary vitreous.

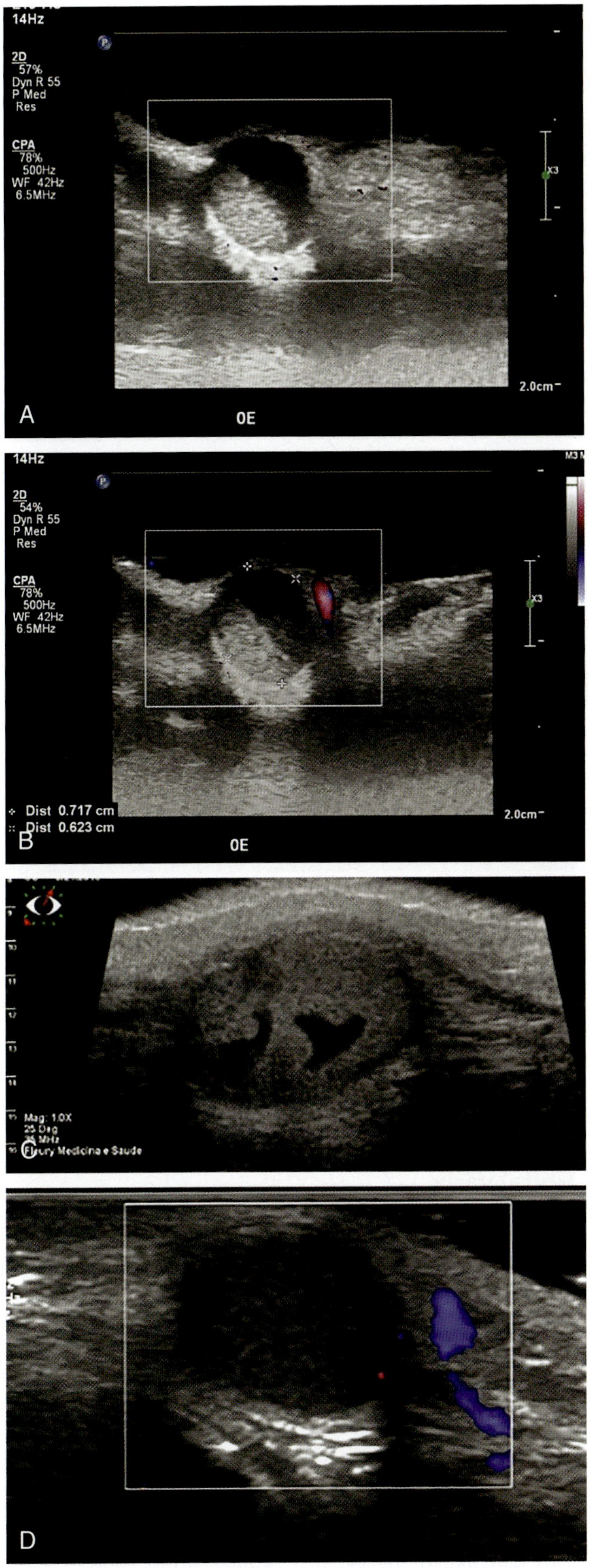

• **Fig. 15.11** Epidermoid cyst. **(A–B)** Color Doppler: Well-defined lesion with a thin wall, predominantly low internal echogenicity and no internal vascularization. **(C)** UBM, 50 MHz, pseudoimmersion technique shows a well-defined oval shaped lesion. **(D)** Color Doppler does not detect internal blood flow.

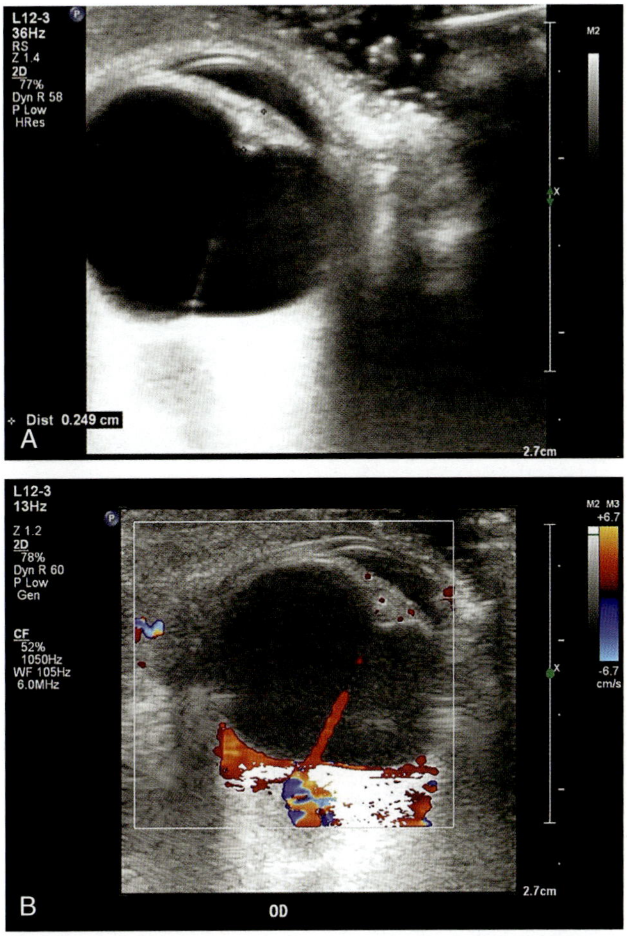

• **Fig. 15.12** **(A)** B-scan ultrasound demonstrates a linear interface with medium-to-high echogenicity inserted in optic disc and extending to the topography of the posterior lens capsule. **(B)** Color Doppler detects blood flow confirming the presence of a patent hyaloid artery.

PFV is classified into three presentations: anterior form (retrolental fibrovascular membrane, elongation of the ciliary processes, cataract, and microphthalmia), posterior form (linear interface in the prepapillary region, tractional retinal detachment, hypoplasia of the optic nerve, or macula), and mixed form (anterior and posterior findings).

Ultrasound may reveal an eye with an anteroposterior diameter below the normal limits for the age group, increased echogenicity of the lens (cataract), presence of a hyperechoic retrolental membrane, membranous echo that extends from the papilla to the vitreous or even the posterior region of the lens, and tractional retinal detachment. When evaluating these structures using color Doppler, it is possible to assess the presence or absence of persistent vascularization in the retrolental membrane and in the hyaloid artery[15–18] (Fig. 15.12).

Carotid Cavernous Fistula

Carotid cavernous fistula is an anomalous communication between the carotid arterial system and the cavernous sinus, characterized by the flow of arterial blood from

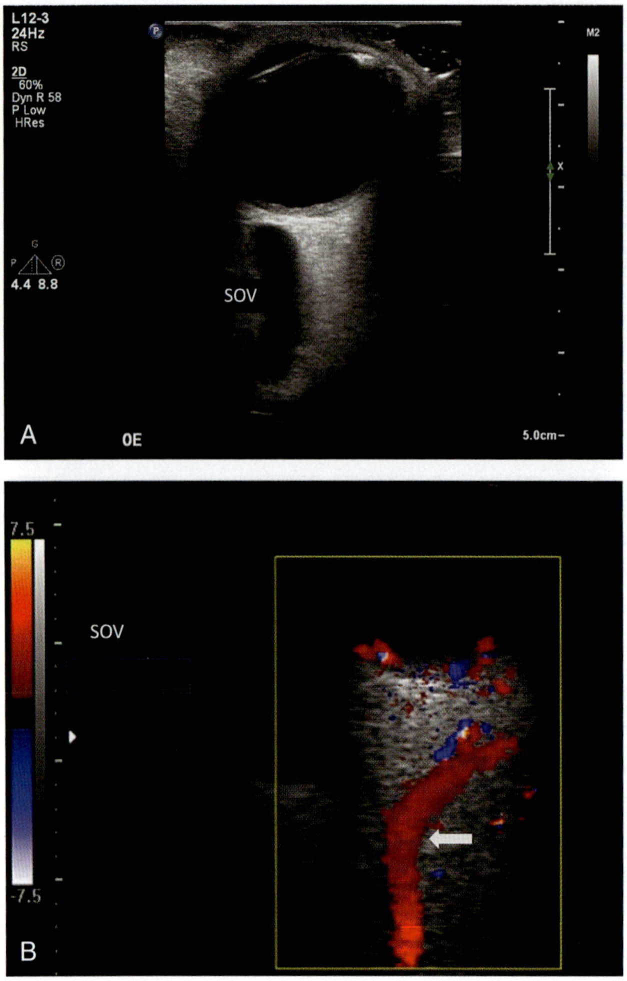

• **Fig. 15.13** Carotid cavernous fistula. **(A)** B-mode ultrasound: Enlarged caliper of the superior ophthalmic vein (SOV). **(B)** Color Doppler flow reveals an enlarged superior ophthalmic vein, color-coded in red (*arrow*), which indicates the presence of reversed flow.

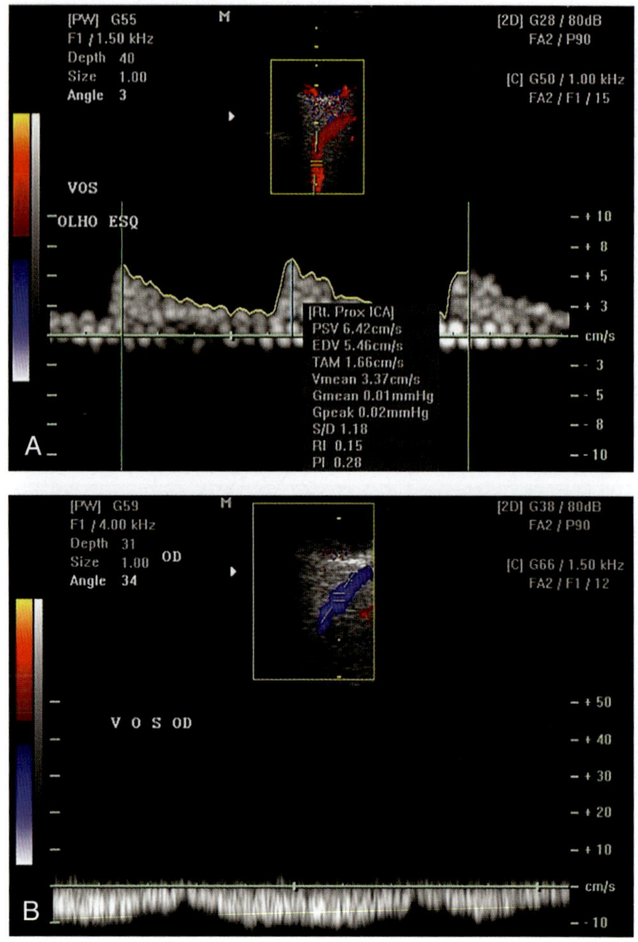

• **Fig. 15.14** Carotid cavernous fistula. **(A)** Left eye. Color Doppler spectral trace showed evidence of arterialization of the superior ophthalmic vein. Spectral analysis shows a very low resistance index (RI = 0.15). **(B)** Right eye. Color Doppler showed a normal-size superior ophthalmic vein with anterograde flow.

a high-pressure system of the internal or external carotid artery to the low-pressure venous system of the cavernous sinus.

Anatomically, they can be divided into two types: direct carotid cavernous fistula (direct communication between the internal carotid artery and cavernous sinus) and indirect carotid cavernous fistula or indirect communications or dural arteriovenous malformations of the cavernous sinus (indirect communications, through the meningeal branches, originating from the internal or external carotid or both and the cavernous sinus).

In most cases, direct carotid cavernous fistulas present a high output and important ocular manifestations such as pulsatile proptosis, congestion of the episcleral veins, diplopia, and reduction in eye movements due to paresis of the cranial nerves III, IV, and VI, reduced visual acuity, conjunctival chemosis, papillary edema, increased intraocular pressure, flow reversal with arterialization of the ophthalmic vein.[19–20]

By performing color Doppler, one can observe a dilated superior ophthalmic vein, color-coded in red. In the spectral analysis, the flow appears positive, arterialized and with a low resistance index (less than 0.60). (Figs. 15.13 and 15.14 and Video 15.4).

Orbital Varix

Clinically, orbital varix is manifested by the presence of intermittent, non-pulsatile proptosis, which increases with physical exertion like Valsalva maneuver.

Using color Doppler imaging, an increase in the diameter of the superior ophthalmic vein can be seen during the Valsalva maneuver with a change in the direction of blood flow.[21]

Superior Ophthalmic Vein Thrombosis

Superior ophthalmic vein thrombosis is rare. Risk factors for superior ophthalmic vein thrombosis include the Virchow's triad: damage to the vascular endothelium, venous stasis (decreased blood flow), and changes in blood constitution (hypercoagulability).

The etiology is divided into aseptic and infectious causes. Orbital cellulitis, sinusitis, and cavernous sinus thrombosis

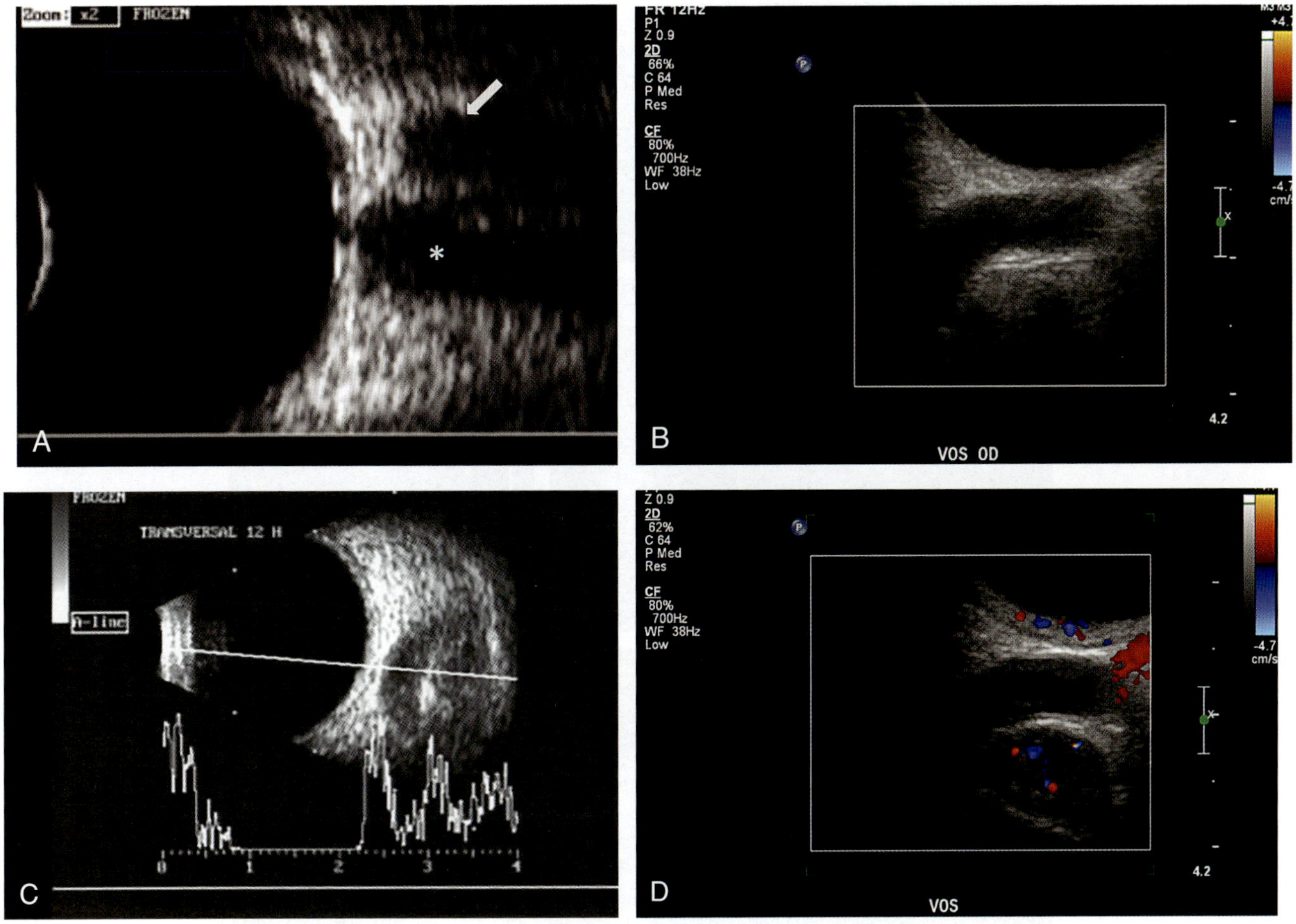

• **Fig. 15.15** Superior ophthalmic vein thrombosis. **(A)** B-scan ultrasound axial scan, demonstrates an enlarged superior ophthalmic vein (*arrow*) located superiorly to the optic nerve (*). **(B)** Color Doppler demonstrates enlarged SOV and no internal blood flow. **(C–D)** One month later. **(C)** B-scan demonstrates enlargement of the SOV with heterogeneous internal reflectivity. **(D)** A mild blood flow can be detected in the SOV, possibly the beginning of revascularization.

are the primary infectious causes. Aseptic causes include orbital vascular malformation (dural arteriovenous fistula, carotid-cavernous fistula), systemic and autoimmune conditions (systemic lupus, thyroid disease, ulcerative colitis), trauma, hematological changes (antiphospholipid syndrome, orbital inflammatory diseases), hormonal therapy (tamoxifen, oral contraceptive. The associated signs and symptoms are pain, proptosis, ptosis, chemosis, ophthalmoplegia, and reduced visual acuity.[22–24]

When suprior ophthalmic vein thrombosis developed, an enlarged superior ophthalmic vein with no blood flow is observed at the early stages, and, during follow-up, mild blood flow can be detected, indicating revascularization of the thrombosed vein (Fig. 15.15).

Ocular Ischemic Syndrome

Ocular ischemic syndrome can occur with amaurosis fugax and scotoma and is secondary to stenosis or occlusion of the ipsilateral internal carotid artery. Using color Doppler, a decrease in maximum systolic velocity and an increase in the resistance index of the posterior short ciliary and central retinal arteries can be observed, as well as the presence or absence of inversion of blood flow in the ophthalmic artery.[10]

Vascular Anomalies

Vascular anomalies can be divided into two large groups: vascular tumors and vascular malformations.[25–27]

Vascular Malformations

Vascular malformations are anomalies resulting from the abnormal development of progressively enlarged vessels. They are composed of an atypical architecture of isolated or combination vascular structures of veins, lymphatic vessels, or arteries.

These malformations can be divided into high-flow and low-flow vascular malformations based on their hemodynamic properties. Low-flow vascular malformations include venous, lymphatic, capillary, and venolymphatic malformations (Fig. 15.16). Those with high flow include arteriovenous malformations and fistulas. There are mixed vascular malformations that can make up different vascular groups and can have high or low flow.[26]

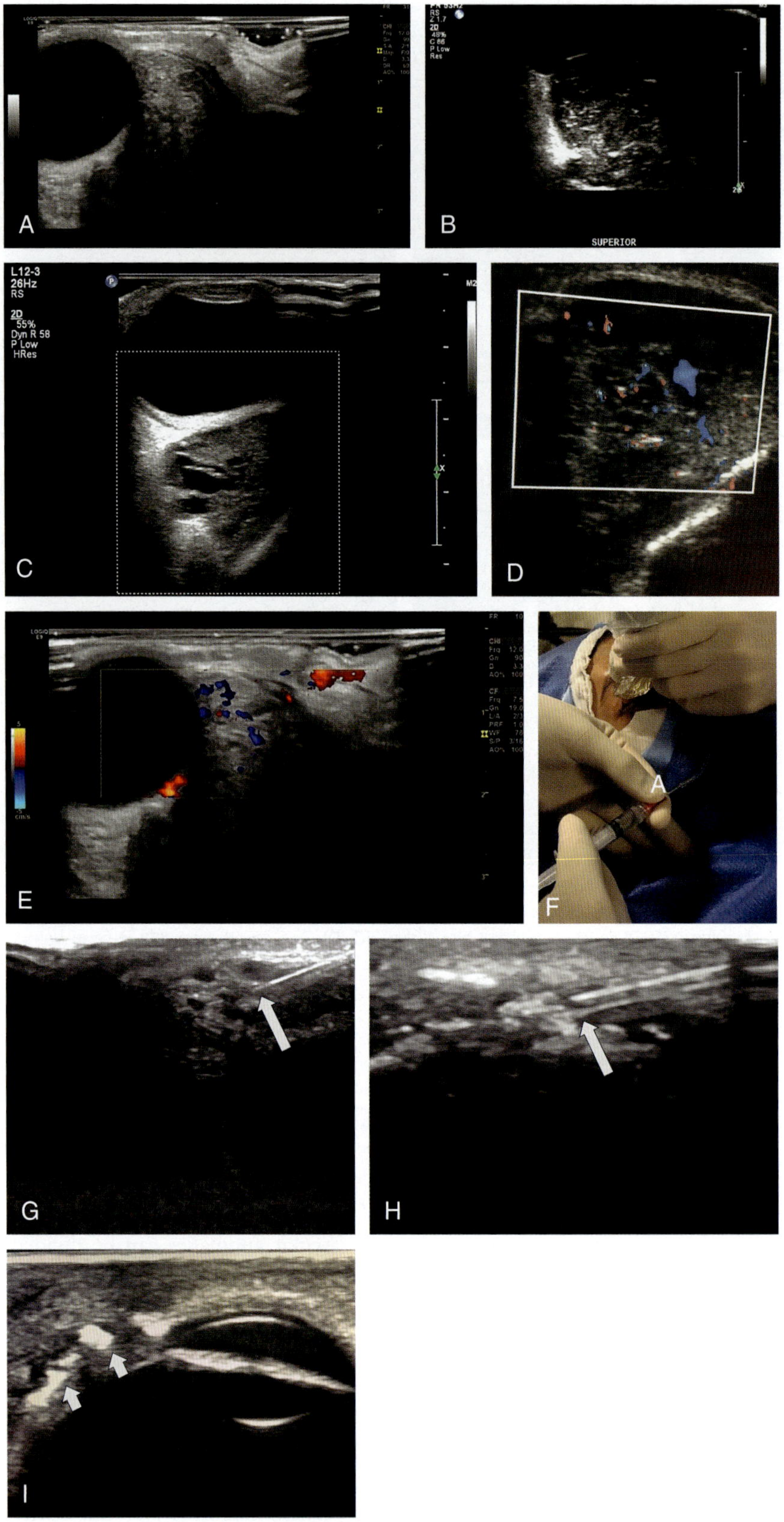

• **Fig. 15.16** Venolymphatic malformation of the orbit. **(A–C)** B-scan ultrasound demonstrates poorly limited lesion with heterogeneous internal echogenicity, composed of septa and cystic spaces with the presence of venous lakes. **(D–E)** Color Doppler demonstrates venous lakes and highlights the presence of blood flow in the cyst wall. **(F)** Injection in place in the operating room under anesthesia. **(G)** During treatment, ultrasonography monitors the topography of the cystic spaces in order to adequately locate the injection of the sclerosing agent. **(H)** The tip of the needle can be seen in the B-scan images (arrows). **(I)** After application, the sclerosing agent appears as a hyperreflective collection in the injection area (*short arrows*).

Venolymphatic Malformation

Venolymphatic malformations are rare and typically appear early in life. These lesions have a venous and lymphatic component and may grow rapidly secondary to infection or hemorrhage.

Currently, treatment options may include observation, oral treatment (sirolimus or sildenafil), surgery, and sclerotherapy.

The sclerotherapy technique consists of an ultrasound-guided aspiration of the cystic content, followed by the injection of the sclerosing agent (Fig. 15.16). The mechanism of action is based on the inflammatory reaction provoked, with consequent occlusion and fibrosis of cysts and lymphatic channels.[26]

Periocular or Orbital Hemangioma

Periocular or orbital hemangiomas are among the most common soft-tissue tumors in infants.

These lesions normally demontrate three phases of growth, plateau phase and then spontaneous involution or secondary to the use of corticosteroids or beta-blockers.

The clinical history associated with color Doppler ultrasound and MRI findings that demonstrate a hyper-vascularized tumor lesion with low-resistance vessels defines the diagnosis in most cases. Appearance is usually a local swelling with a purple coloration[27] (Fig. 15.17).

Arteriovenous Malformations

Arteriovenous malformations are high-flow lesions and are characterized by the presence of multiple arteriovenous shunts. On examination, these lesions present with local pulsatility and thrill on palpation.

Arteriovenous malformations can be differentiated from hemangioma by the absence of a soft-tissue mass.

Examination using color Doppler allows the identification of increased blood flow in arteries and veins related to malformation and the presence of arteriovenous shunts without the interposition of cellular stroma[26] (Fig. 15.18).

Intraocular Lesions

Retinoblastoma

Retinoblastoma is the most common ocular tumor in childhood. Leukocoria, a white pupillary reflex, is the most common presenting sign.

On B-scan ultrasonography, retinoblastoma usually appears as a solid lesion, irregular in shape, with heterogeneous echogenicity, areas suggestive of calcification, and the presence of internal blood flow[18] (Fig. 15.19). It may be associated with retinal detachment and vitreous cellularity.

Choroidal Hemangioma

Choroidal hemangioma is a benign vascular tumor that presents in a circumscribed or diffuse form; the latter is often associated with Sturge–Weber Syndrome.

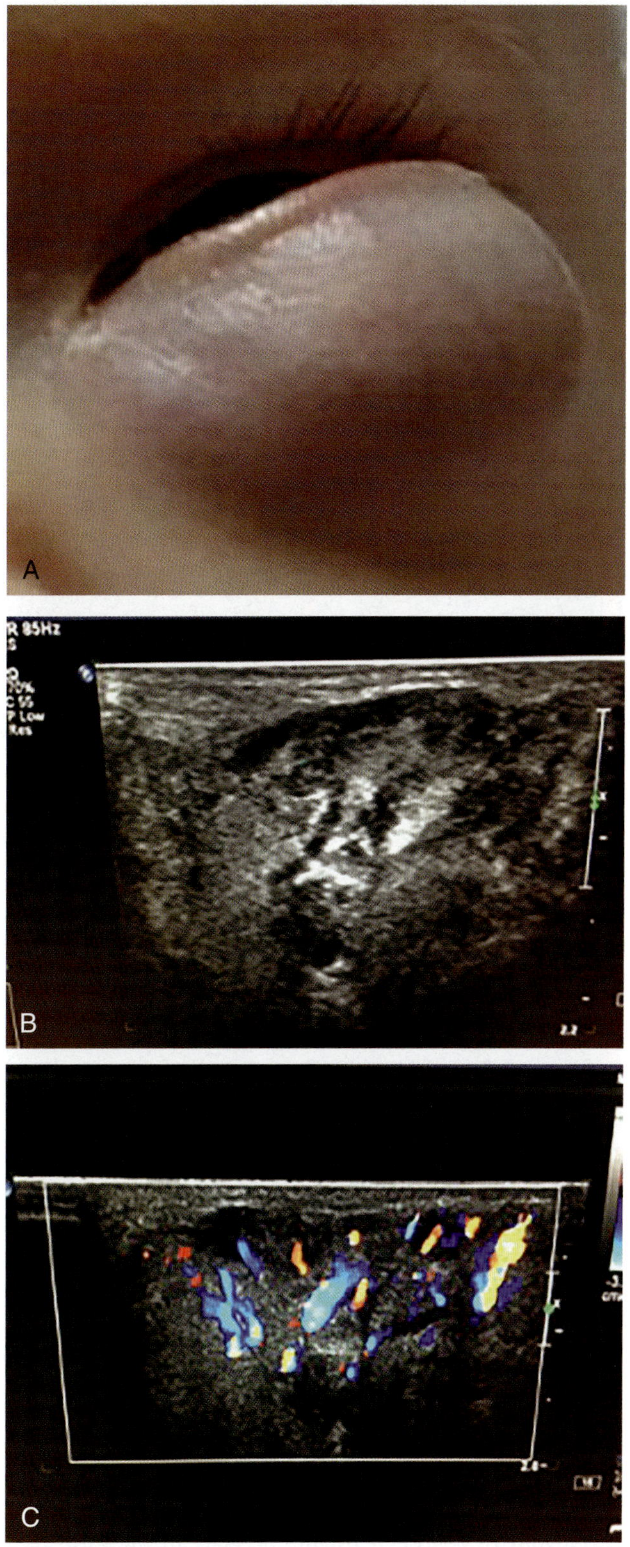

• **Fig. 15.17 (A)** Clinical appearance of a capillary hemangioma of the lower eyelid presenting a purple color. **(B–C)** B-scan and color Doppler sonographies show the tumor that involves the lower eyelid with vascular elements (hyperreflective at B-scan) with high vessel density and signs of arteriovenous shunting.

Circumscribed tumors manifest insidiously, with diagnosis commonly made after the appearance of secondary symptoms in the fourth decade of life. The most frequent location is posterior to the equator, or in the macula or

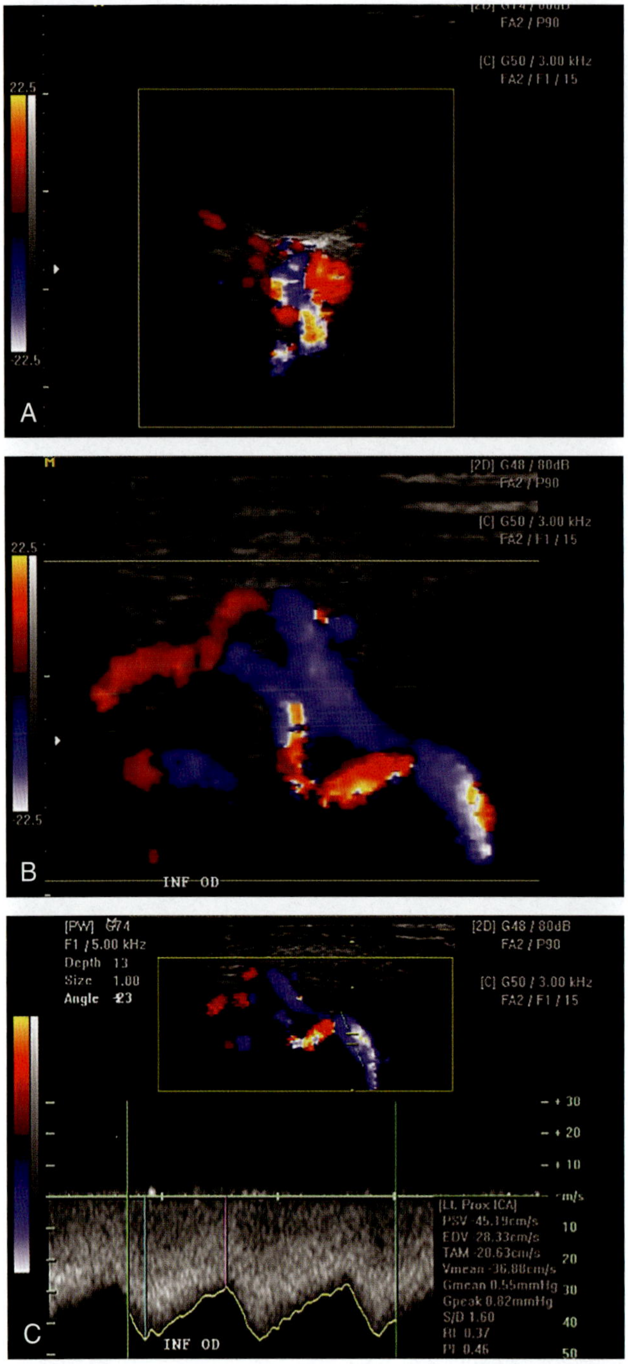

• **Fig. 15.18** Arteriovenous malformation and color Doppler exam. **(A)** Demonstrates the orbital topography of the malformation. **(B)** Detail of arteriovenous shunting. **(C)** Spectral analysis shows high-velocity blood flow.

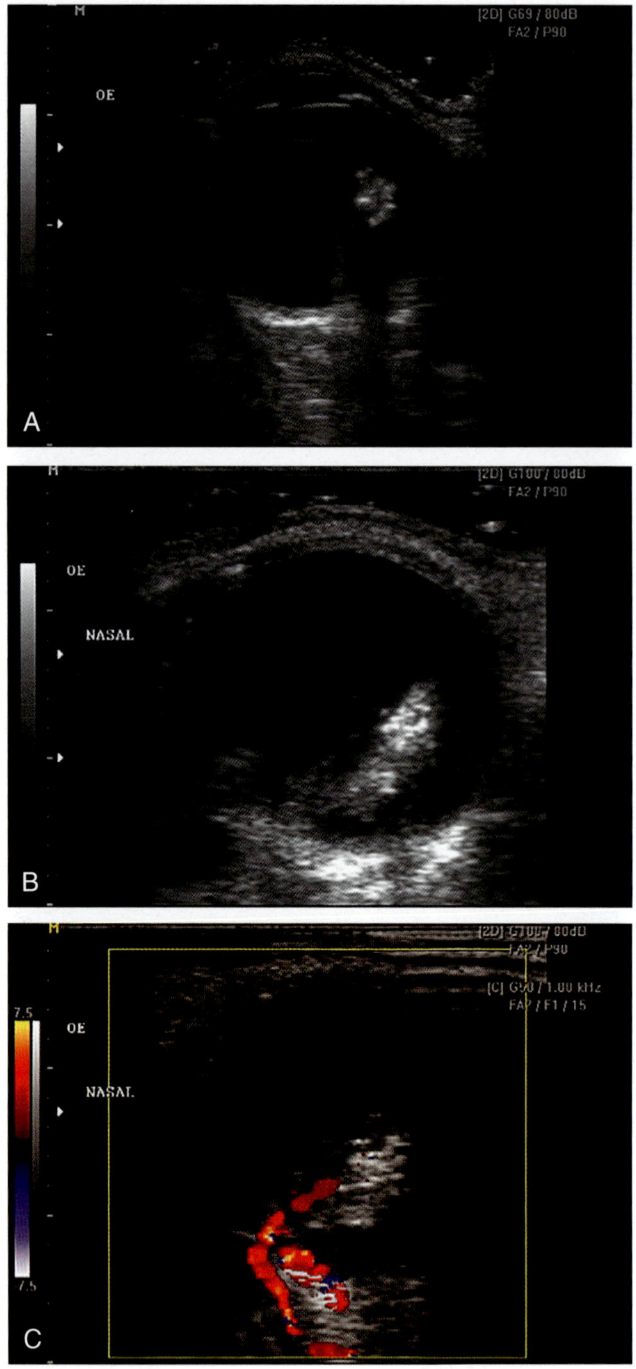

• **Fig. 15.19** Retinoblastoma. **(A–B)** B-scan ultrasonography demonstrates an irregular shaped solid intraocular lesion with areas of calcification. **(C)** Color Doppler confirms arterial blood flow to the tumor. Shadowing artifacts are seen in the area with high level of calcification.

juxtapapillary region. It usually presents in the form of a dome-shaped, orange-colored choroidal mass. Associated exudative retinal detachment or vitreous hemorrhage can be observed, resulting in decreased visual acuity and central visual field defect, as well as metamorphopsia.[27–29]

On B-scan ultrasonograhy, the tumor appears as a sessile or dome-shaped choroidal lesion with high internal reflectivity. On color Doppler imaging, diffuse vascularization of the tumor is observed[18,28–29] (Fig. 15.20 and Video 15.5).

Uveal Melanoma

Uveal melanoma can develop in the ciliary body or choroid. It also can involve both structures simultaneously (ciliochoroidal melanoma).

Choroidal melanoma is the most common primary intraocular tumor in adults. Ocular symptoms depend on the location and size of the tumor. If the tumor is close to the macula, the patient usually presents with visual complaints such as

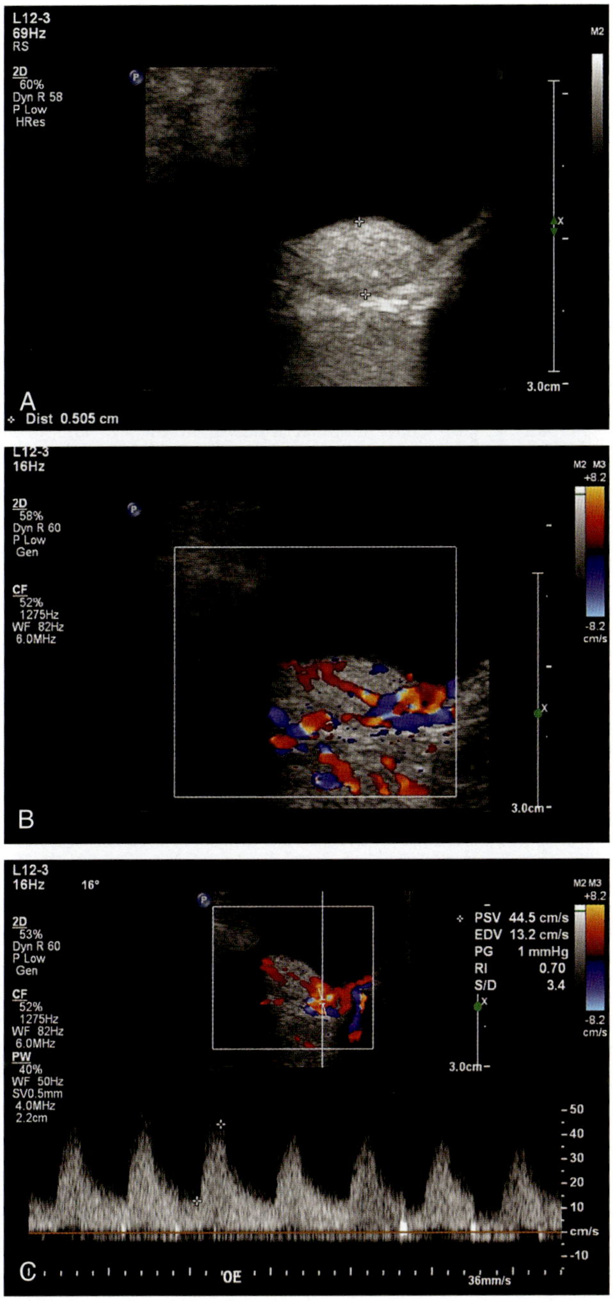

• **Fig. 15.20** Choroidal hemangioma. **(A)** B-scan demonstrates a dome-shaped solid lesion with high internal echogenicity. Measured height: 5.05 mm. **(B)** Color Doppler shows marked internal hypervascularity. **(C)** Spectral analysis shows a peak systolic velocity of 44.5 cm/s and a resistance index of 0.70.

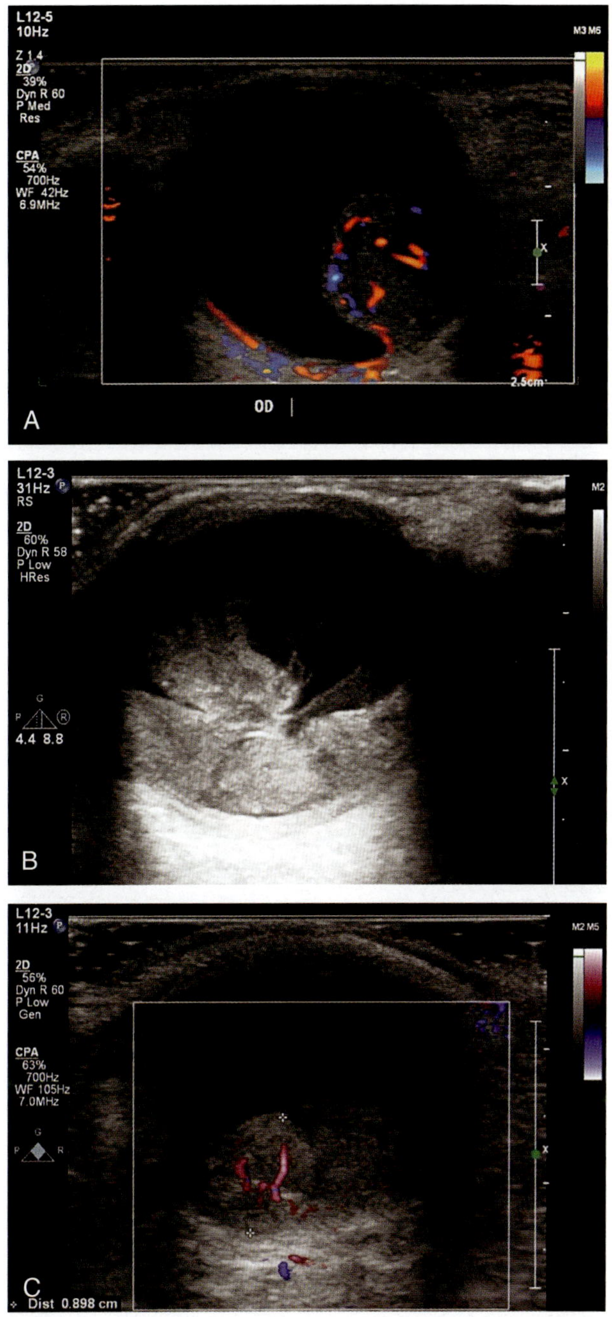

• **Fig. 15.21** Choroidal melanoma. **(A)** Color Doppler shows superficial and deep arteries inside the dome-shaped lesion. **(B–C)** Malignant uveal melanoma and vitreous, subhyaloid, and subretinal hemorrhage. **(B)** B-scan shows hemorrhagic material hindering the limits of a choroidal lesion. **(C)** Color Doppler shows the internal blood flow of the tumor.

decreased visual acuity, but if it is at the periphery, it can grow to large size until the patient notices visual changes.

Color Doppler imaging is useful both in the assessment of internal vascularization and in the follow-up of patients undergoing brachytherapy. In response to treatment through brachytherapy, an increase in internal echogenicity, a reduction in vascularization, and an increase in the resistance index of intra-tumoral arteries are observed.[10,30]

Ultrasonographic and color Doppler features of choroidal melanoma include dome- or mushroom-shaped solid choroidal lesion with medium to low internal reflectivity. Internal reflectivity is greater at the apex of the lesion, which progressively attenuates with the formation of the Kappa angle, and the presence of internal vascularization[18,30] (Fig. 15.21 and Video 15.6).

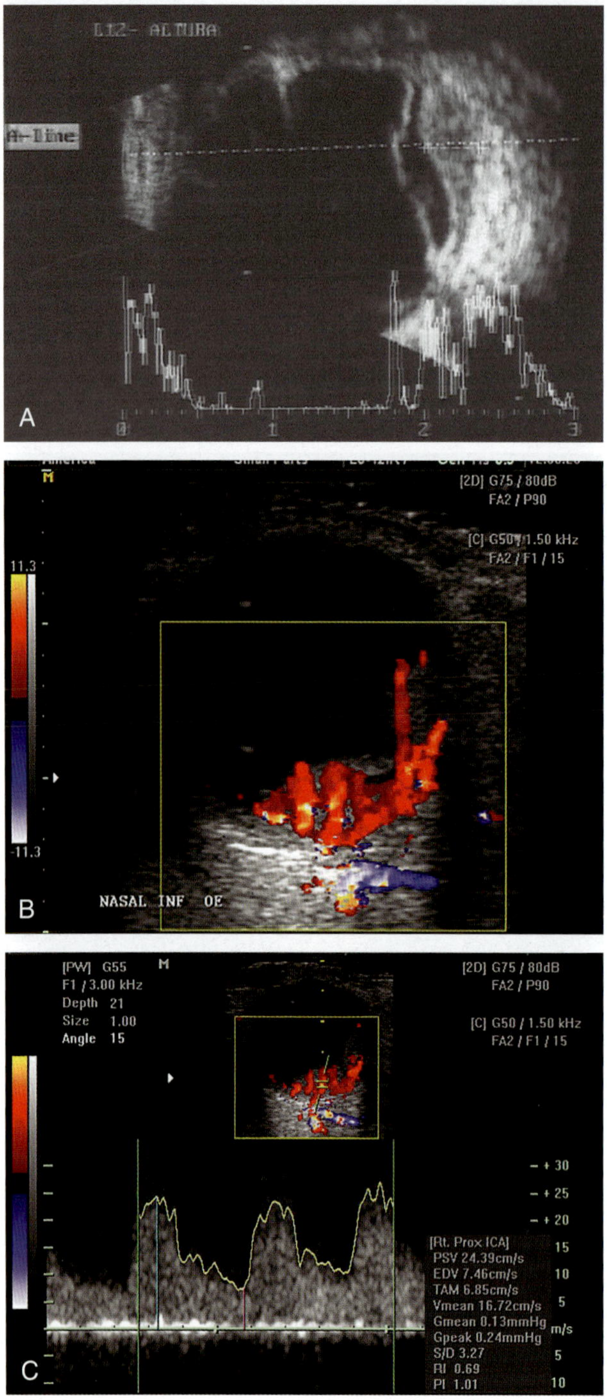

• **Fig. 15.22** Metastatic choroidal lesion. **(A–B)** Irregularly shaped choroidal lesion, medium-to-high internal reflectivity, demonstrating internal vascularity on color Doppler. **(C)** Spectral analysis shows that intralesional arteries present moderate peak systolic velocity and low resistance index.

Metastasis

Metastatic tumor to the uvea is the most common intraocular malignancy and can present as a single or multifocal, convex or placoid mass. Its main location is in the posterior pole and is often associated retinal detachment,[18,31] as can be seen in Fig. 15.22.

References

1. Erickson SJ, Mewissen MW, Foley WD, et al. Stenosis of the internal carotid artery: assessment using color dopplerimaging compared with angiography. *Am J Roentgenol.* 1989;152:1299–1305.
2. Duck F, Starritt H, Aindow JD, Perkins MA, Hawkins AJ. The output of pulse-echo ultrasound equipment: a survey of powers, pressures and intensities. *Br J Rad.* 1985;58:989–1001.
3. Guthoff RF, Berger RW, Winker P, Helmke K, Chumbley LC. Doppler ultrasonography of the ophthalmic and central retinal vessels. *Arch Ophthamol.* 1991;109:532–536.
4. Lieb WE, Cohen SM, Merton DA, Shields JA, Mitchell DG, Goldberg BB. Color Doppler imaging of the eye and orbit: technique and normal vascular anatomy. *Arch Ophthalmol.* 1991;109:527–531.
5. Erickson SJ, Hendrix LE, Massaro BM, et al. Color Doppler flow imaging of the normal and abnormal orbit. *Radiology.* 1989;173:511–516.
6. Hayreh SS. Arteries of the orbit in the human Being. *Br J Surg.* 1963;50:938–953.
7. Kaiser HJ, Schoetzay A, Stümpfig D, Flammer J. Blood-flow velocities of the extraocular vessels in patients with high-tension and normal-tension primary open-angle glaucoma. *Am J Ophthalmol.* 1997;123:320–327.
8. Fukukita M, Ido M, Osawa S, et al. Retrobulbar hemodynamic effects of nipradilol in normal and normal-tension glaucoma eyes. *J Ophthalmol.* 2011;2011:652904. doi:10.1155/2011/652904.
9. Koskas P, Bergès O, Lecler A. Écho-Doppler. *Bergès Oet cols. Échographiede l'oeil et de l'orbite.* Sauramps Medical; 2022:43–48.
10. Tranquart F, Bergès O, Koskas P, et al. Color Doppler imaging of orbital vessels: personal experience and literature review. *J Clin Ultrasound.* 2003;31d:258–273.
11. Williamson TH, Baxter GM, Dutton GN. Color Doppler velocimetry of the optic nerve head in arterial occlusion. *Ophthalmology.* 1993;100:312–317.
12. Baxter GM, Williamson TH. Color Doppler flow imaging in central retinal vein occlusion: a new diagnostic technique? *Radiology.* 1993;187:847–850.
13. Keyser BJ, Flaharty PM, Sergott RC. Color Doppler imaging of arterial blood flow in central retinal vein occlusion. *Ophthalmol.* 1994;101:1357–1361.
14. Palmer E, Gale J, Crowstond JG, Wellsa AP. Optic nerve head drusen: an update. *Neuroophthalmology.* 2018;42:1–15.
15. Shastry BS. Persistent hyperplastic primary vitreous: congenital malformation of the eye. *Clin Exp Ophthalmol.* 2009;37(9):884–890.
16. Reese AB. Persistent hyperplastic primary vitreous (PHPV). *Am J Ophthalmol.* 1955;40:317.
17. Goldberg MF. Persistent fetal vasculature (PFV): an integrated interpretation of signs and symptoms associated with persistent hyperplastic primary vitreous (PHPV). *Am J Ophthalmol.* 1997;124:587–626.
18. Yang W, Hu S, Wang J, Wang L, Zheng B. Color Doppler imaging diagnosis of intra-ocular tumor. *Chin Med J (Engl).* 1997;110(9):664–666.
19. Phelps CD, Thompson HS, Ossoinig KC. The diagnosis and prognosis of atypical carotid-cavernous fistula (red-eyed shunt syndrome). *Am J Ophthalmol.* 1982;93(4):423–436.
20. Miller NR. Diagnosis and management of dural carotid-cavernous sinus fistulas. *Neurosurg Focus.* 2007;23(5):E13.

21. Lieb WE, Merton DA, Shields JA, Cohen SM, Mitchell BBG. Color Doppler imaging in the demonstration of an orbital varix. *Br J Ophthalmol.* 1990;74:305–308.
22. van der Poel NA, de Witt KD, van den Berg R, de Win MM, Mourits MP. Impact of superior ophthalmic vein thrombosis: a case series and literature review. *Orbit.* 2019;38(3):226–232.
23. Sotoudeh H, Shafaat O, Aboueldahab N, Vaphiades M, Sotoudeh E, Bernstock J. Superior ophthalmic vein thrombosis: what radiologist and clinician must know? *Eur J Radiol Open.* 2019;6:258–264.
24. Khurram R, Naidu V, Butt MF, Durnford L, Joffe M. Superior ophthalmic vein thrombosis secondary to COVID-19: an index case. *Radiol Case Rep.* 2021;16(5):1138–1143.
25. Yarmand F, Seyyedmajidi M, Shirzad A, Foroughi R, Bakhshian A. Lymphangiohemangioma of buccal mucosa: report of a rare case. *J Oral Maxillofac Surg Med Pathol.* 2015;21:282–285.
26. Wassef M, Blei F, Adams D, et al. Vascular anomalies classification: recommendations from the International Society for the Study of Vascular Anomalies. *Pediatrics.* 2015;136:e203–e214.
27. Chiller KG, Passaro D, Frieden IJ. Hemangiomas of infancy: clinical characteristics, morphologic subtypes, and their relationship to race, ethnicity, and sex. *Arch Dermatol.* 2002;138(12):1567–1576.
28. Singh AD, Kaiser PK, Sears JE. Choroidal hemangioma. *Ophthalmol Clin North Am.* 2005;18(1):151–161.
29. Frossard JC, Covre EP, Conci LS, Alves DLS, Harchbart KK, Saraiva FP. Choroidal hemangioma and the challenge of differential diagnosis. *Rev Bras Oftalmol.* 2020;79(4):273–275.
30. Shields CL, Manalac J, Das C, Ferguson K, Shields JA. Choroidal melanoma: clinical features, classification, and top 10 pseudomelanomas. *Curr Opin Ophthalmol.* 2014;25(3):177–185.
31. Shields CL, Shields JA, Gross NE, Schwartz GP, Lally SE. Survey of 520 eyes with uveal metastases. *Ophthalmol.* 1997;104(8):1265–1276.

16

Guideline to Develop Ultrasound Reports

LILIANE ANDRADE ALMEIDA KANECADAN AND NORMA ALLEMANN

Introduction

With the advancement of technology, ocular ultrasound equipment has shown significant improvements in image quality. Training of examiners, standardization of the examination technique, and the increase in availability are factors that contribute to the increasing indication of ultrasound examination in the ophthalmological practice. As important as the good performance of the exam is the quality report carried out by the sonographer, which requires a good knowledge of the anatomy of the eye and orbit, as well as the wide variety of diseases that affect this region.

The high level of diagnostic accuracy of experienced sonographers (90–99%) has been demonstrated in numerous studies across the different subspecialties of medicine.[1] For this reason, there is a great expectation that the sonographer not only performs the ultrasound examination but also provides the diagnostic interpretation and prepares a good report of the examination performed.[1] The purpose of this chapter is to provide a detailed overview of practices in reporting ophthalmic ultrasound examinations.

Report Structure

There is a consensus in the literature on what the structure of an ultrasound report should be.[2,3] In general, an ultrasound report includes the following sections:

(1) Title
(2) Patient identification
(3) Requesting physician
(4) Equipment on which the examination was performed and the type of transducer (10, 35, or 50 MHz)
(5) Indications: history and clinical information
(6) Technique used, for example, direct eye contact, transpalpebral contact, immersion, pseudo-immersion
(7) Findings
  (7.1) Eye globe
    a) Anteroposterior diameter or axial length
    b) Crystalline lens
    c) Internal space or Intraocular Cavity: Retina, Vitreous and Choroid
    d) Ocular wall
    e) Optic disc
  (7.2) Retrobulbar Space
    a) Optic nerve
    b) Extrinsic muscles
    c) Retrobulbar fat
(8) Conclusion
(9) Name of the examining physician
(10) Inclusion of reference standards in footnotes (when necessary)

Title. The title must clearly identify the type of examination and the eye that was examined, for example, ocular ultrasound of the right or left eye or both eyes.

Patient identification. It is important that the report contains correct identification, such as the patient's full name, date of birth, and one of the following items: address, medical insurance, and medical record number of the clinic where the exam is being carried out. The date and time of the exam are also relevant data to be included in the report. By inserting the correct information, the sonographer ensures that the report can reach the patient and the requesting doctor in electronic and/or printed form.

Requesting physician. The name of the doctor to whom the report will be addressed.

Equipment. The instrument on which the examination was performed and the type of transducer. The specifications of the equipment must be included, such as brand and type and which transducer was used to carry out the eye examination.

Indication

History and clinical information. Patient history and clinical information can be obtained from different sources:

a) the requesting doctor
b) other medical records
c) the patient to the sonographer during the examination
d) clinical observation carried out by the sonographer

Many patients have complex histories, including multiple comorbidities, serial investigations (laboratory and imaging), interventions, complex conditions, or extensive use of medications, but it is not practical to include all information in the report.[4] In these cases, the sonographer must select the most relevant information to assist in the ultrasound examination.

In cases of previous changes in the orbit or lacrimal sac, clinical examination of the area can be performed, for instance, in superficial masses, evaluate anatomical location, shape, compressibility, fluctuation, smooth or irregular edges, associated with skin changes and phlogistic signs.

Technique used. The report should contain information about the technique used for assessment: direct ocular contact or transpalpebral contact; if immersion or pseudo-immersion techniques were used to evaluate the anterior segment of the eye or the eyelids; transocular, periocular, or paraocular evaluation; or orbital lesions.

Findings. In the report, the findings must present a logical sequence, in the order in which the examination was carried out or in the order of clinical priority[1] and preferably described herein.[5] In this chapter, we will describe the evaluation of the posterior segment of the eye.

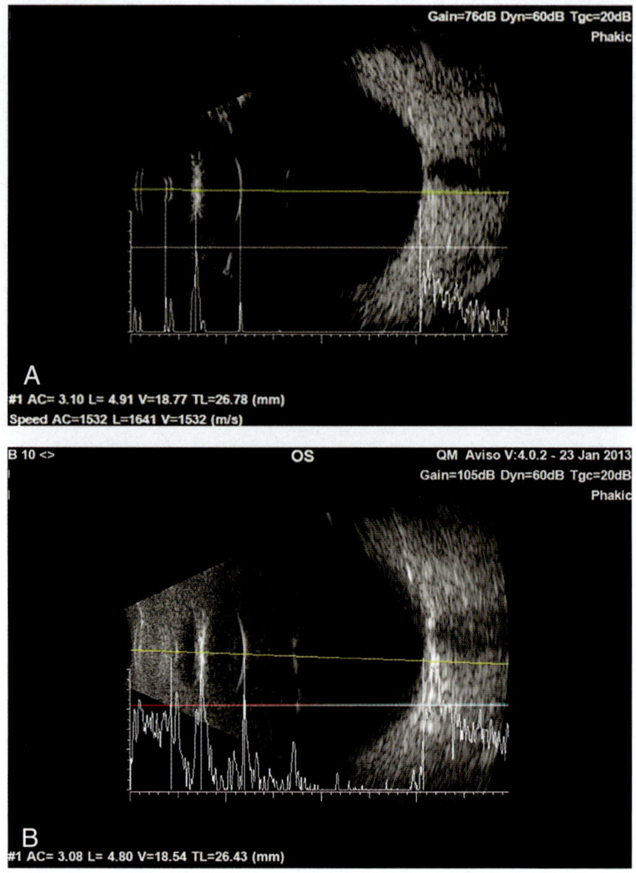

• **Fig. 16.1** Axial length measurement. **(A)** Immersion technique, coupling media allows visualization of the two linear peaks correspondent to anterior and posterior echoes of the cornea, at the left side of the image. **(B)** Contact technique, sound beam surpasses the eyelid barrier and disposes the images for the lens and vitreous cavity.

Posterior segment

1. Ocular Globe
   a) Anteroposterior diameter or axial length (Fig. 16.1)
      i) Evaluate symmetry, considering asymmetrical differences in diameter above 1 mm
      ii) Approximated axial length
      iii) Comparison with normality according to age group
         - for children, Table 16.1 can be used as a reference to axial length growth[6]

   b) Crystalline Lens (Fig. 16.2)
      i) Normal
         - high reflectivity echoes that correspond to interfaces capsular, in normal topography (phakia).

      ii) Cataract
         - globose crystalline, with high internal reflectivity
         - unstructured echoes (crystalline lens in reabsorption)

      iii) Aphakia
         - absence of interfaces corresponding to the lens

      iv) Subluxation or dislocation
         - interfaces corresponding to the lens are found to be displaced

      v) Pseudophakia
         - high reflectivity interfaces, corresponding to the intraocular lens implant, which can be topical or displaced

   c) Vitreous Cavity (Fig. 16.3)
      i) Anechoic or absence of acoustic interfaces in the vitreous cavity
      ii) Posterior vitreous detachment
         - membranous echo of low/medium/high/heterogeneous reflectivity, mobile, inserted in a papillary area or in the wall (partial detachment) or without adhesion to the wall (total detachment)
         - impregnated hyaloid: homogeneously or with areas of impregnation

      iii) Vitreoschisis
         - membranous echoes, parallel to each other, with the same mobility, corresponding to the delamination of the vitreous cortex

      iv) Hemorrhagic and/or inflammatory and/or infectious vitreous/subhyaloid/subretinal process
         - pointlike echoes of low or medium reflectivity, mobile
         - with organization: membranous and punctate echoes forming "echo condensates" in the vitreous cavity, with heterogeneous reflectivity, mobile or slightly mobile

      v) Synchysis scintillans
         - dense pointlike echoes of high reflectivity, mobile, which remain visible with decreasing equipment gain, dispersed in the vitreous cavity during the movement of the eyeball and which are deposited when the eye is at rest

      vi) Asteroid hyalosis

TABLE 16.1 Correlation Between Axial Length and Age in Normal Eye[6]

Age	Axial Length (mm)	95% Confidence Interval of the Forecast Line (mm)	
1 month	18.7	18.2 a 19.1	17.3 a 20.1
2 months	19.4	19.0 a 19.7	18.0 a 20.7
3 months	19.8	19.4 a 20.1	18.4 a 21.1
4 months	20.0	19.8 a 20.3	18.7 a 21.4
5 months	20.3	20.0 a 20.5	18.9 a 21.6
6 months	20.4	20.2 a 20.7	19.1 a 21.8
7 months	20.6	20.3 a 20.8	19.3 a 21.9
8 months	20.7	20.5 a 20.9	19.4 a 22.0
9 months	20.8	20.6 a 21.1	19.5 a 22.2
10 months	20.9	20.7 a 21.2	19.6 a 22.3
11 months	21.0	20.8 a 21.3	19.7 a 22.4
12 months = 1 year	21.1	20.9 a 21.3	19.8 a 22.4
18 months = 1.5 year	21.5	21.3 a 21.8	20.2 a 22.8
24 months = 2 years	21.8	21.5 a 22.1	20.5 a 23.1
30 months = 2.5 years	22.0	21.7 a 22.3	20.7 a 23.3
36 months = 3 years	22.2	21.9 a 22.5	20.8 a 23.5
42 months = 3.5 years	22.3	22.0 a 22.7	21.0 a 23.7
48 months = 4 years	22.5	22.1 a 22.8	21.1 a 23.8
54 months = 4.5 years	22.6	22.2 a 22.9	21.2 a 23.9
60 months = 5 years	22.7	22.3 a 23.1	21.3 a 24.0
66 months = 5.5 years	22.8	22.4 a 23.2	21.4 a 24.1
72 months = 6 years	22.9	22.5 a 23.3	21.5 a 24.2
78 months = 6.5 years	22.9	22.5 a 23.3	21.6 a 24.3
84 months = 7 years	23.0	22.6 a 23.4	21.6 a 24.4

From: Sampaolesi R, Zarate J, Sampaolesi JR. The Glaucomas: Volume 1 - Pediatric Glaucomas. Springer Science & Business Media, Nov 2008.

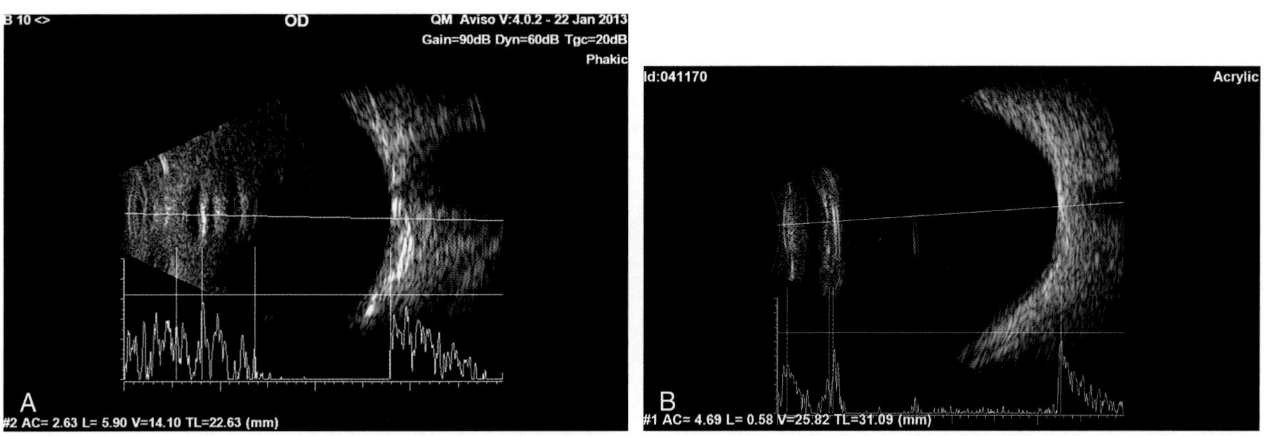

• **Fig. 16.2** Ultrasound evaluation of the lens status. **(A)** Hyperreflective crystalline lens, phakic eye. **(B)** Pseudophakic eye, linear highly reflective interface corresponds to the intraocular lens implant.

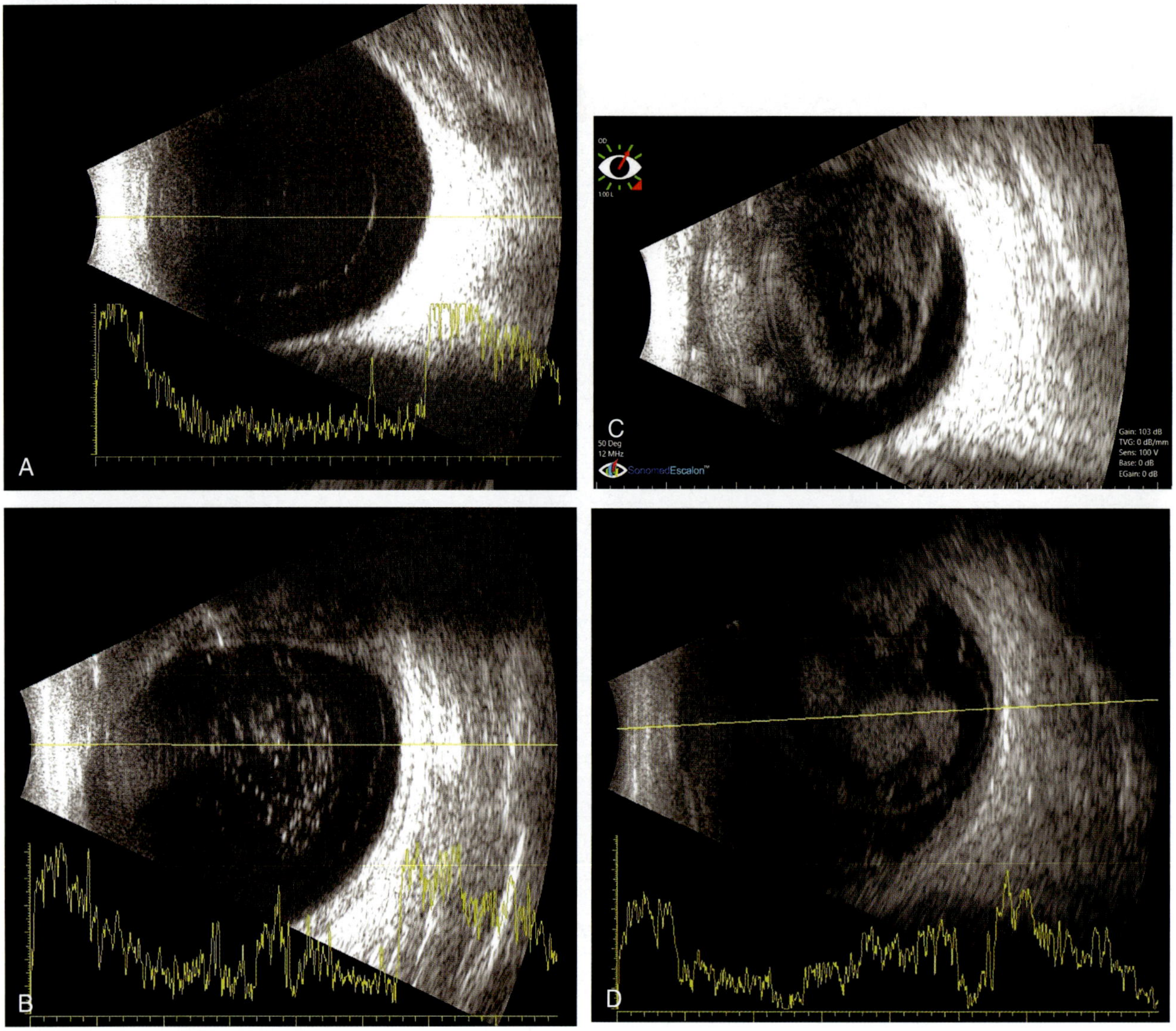

• **Fig. 16.3** Ultrasound evaluation of the vitreous. **(A)** Linear and continuous vitreous interface detached from the ocular wall: posterior vitreous detachment. **(B)** Linear structure correspondending to the posterior hyaloid, and observation of round-shaped and highly reflective particles in the vitreous, characteristic of asteroid hyalosis. **(C)** Posterior vitreous detachment and dense punctiform and membranous vitreousinterfaces in vitreous hemorrhage. **(D)** Endophthalmitis: observe the linear structure detached from the ocular wall (posterior hyaloid detachment), dense vitreous condensates and debris, and sub-hyaloid debris.

- dense pointlike echoes of high reflectivity, mobile, which remain visible with the reduction of equipment gain, dispersed in the vitreous cavity, which mobilize as a block and have a band of anechoic vitreous posterior to these echoes

vii) Silicone oil (Fig. 16.4)
- image compatible with the presence of a vitreous substitute substance, totally or partially filling the vitreous cavity, which causes acoustic artifact of artificial lengthening of the echogram, straightening of the wall, and posterior shadowing and which remains or is mobilized with the change in the patient's position

viii) Emulsified silicone oil
- fragments of dense and dispersed linear echoes in the vitreous cavity

ix) Gas or air in the vitreous cavity
- intravitreal element or element filling the vitreous cavity, which causes acoustic shadowing artifacts and prevents the evaluation of posterior structures, which remains or moves with the patient's change in position

x) Perfluorocarbon
- one or multiple elements causing acoustic reverberation artifact located in the anterior segment or vitreous cavity or in the wall or subretinal space

xi) Retinal detachment (Fig. 16.5)
- membranous echo of high reflectivity, little mobile (low amplitude or "guitar string" movements) or fixed, e.g., inserted in the papillary area and extending anteriorly to the equator

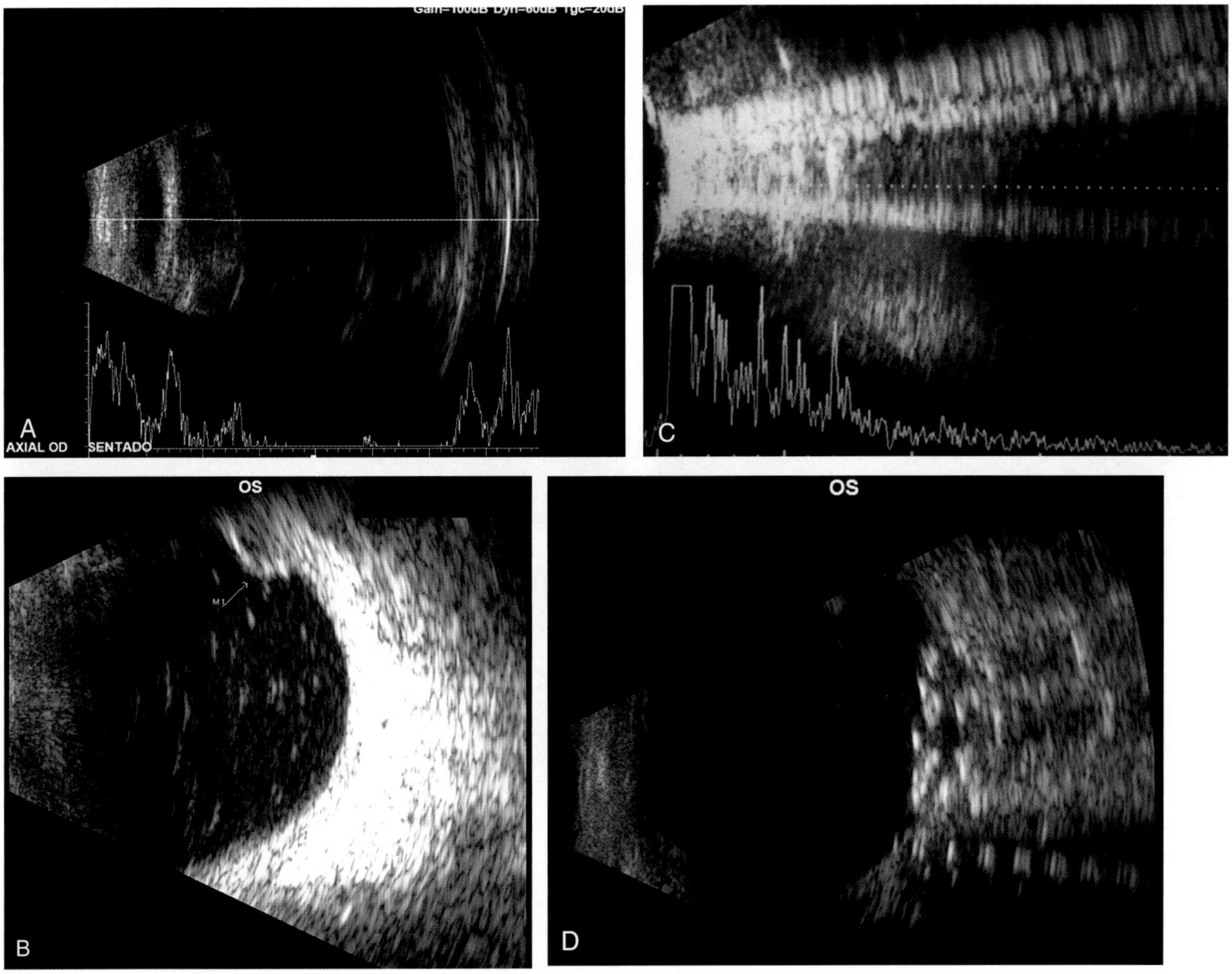

• **Fig. 16.4** Vitreoretinal surgery postoperative conditions. **(A)** Vitreous cavity filled with silicone oil and artifacts related to a different sound speed (slower): rectification of the posterior ocular wall, attenuation of posterior structure, artificial elongation of the echogram. **(B)** After silicone oil removal, some round particles can be seen in the cavity, but no artifacts hinder the evaluation of the retina. Peripheral vitreous remnants can be evidenced. **(C)** Gaseous element placed in the anterior chamber determines artifacts (comet tails) hindering the evaluation of the posterior segment. **(D)** Heavy vitreous substitute adherent to the posterior wall determines reverberation artifacts.

- rupture: linear echo of high reflectivity, with or without mobility, discontinuous from the wall
- tractional: the hyaloid adheres and causes punctate traction or in a segment of high-reflectivity, fixed membranous echo, compatible with "tent" or "tabletop" tractional retinal detachment

xii) Retinal detachment with cyst
- rounded structure with thin walls, juxtaposed to the detached retina

xiii) Choroidal detachment (Fig. 16.6)
- membranous echo of high reflectivity, without mobility, with a flat shape (parallel to the wall) or dome-shaped, with a double peak of high reflectivity in mode A

d) Ocular wall

i) Calcification
- high reflectivity element, which remains visible when the equipment gain decreases and which causes acoustic artifacts from subsequent shadowing

ii) Staphyloma (Fig. 16.7)
- focal increase in wall concavity or localized increase in wall curvature

iii) Glaucoma drainage device
- high reflectivity interface arranged parallel to the external ocular wall, with acoustic shading of its edges and underlying (measuring ????...... mm) and overlying (measuring ...????... mm) anechoic spaces, compatible with drainage implant with adjacent filtration ampullae

iv) Circumferential scleral introflexion
- high-reflectivity or low-reflectivity scleral element, which causes 360-degree wall introflexion and acoustic artifact from posterior shadowing

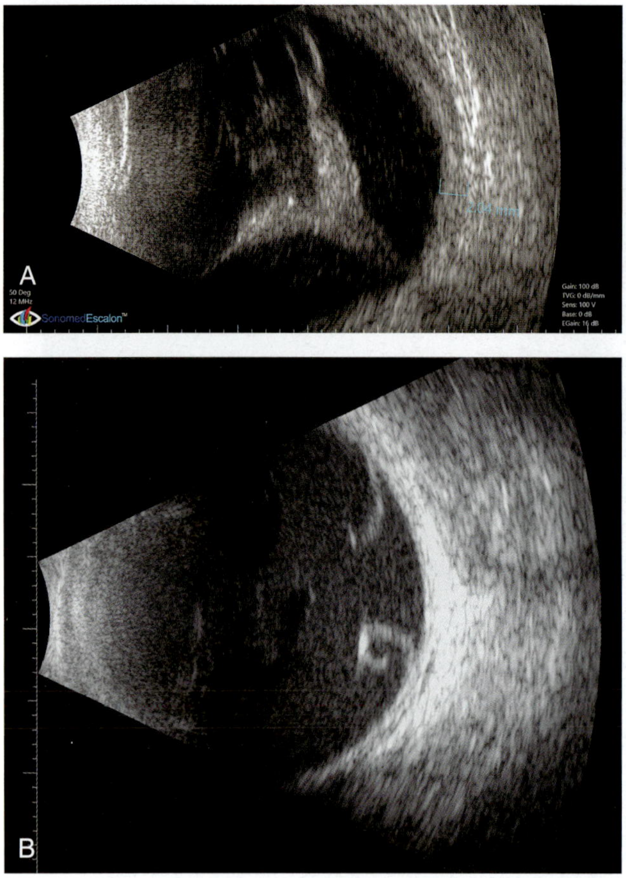

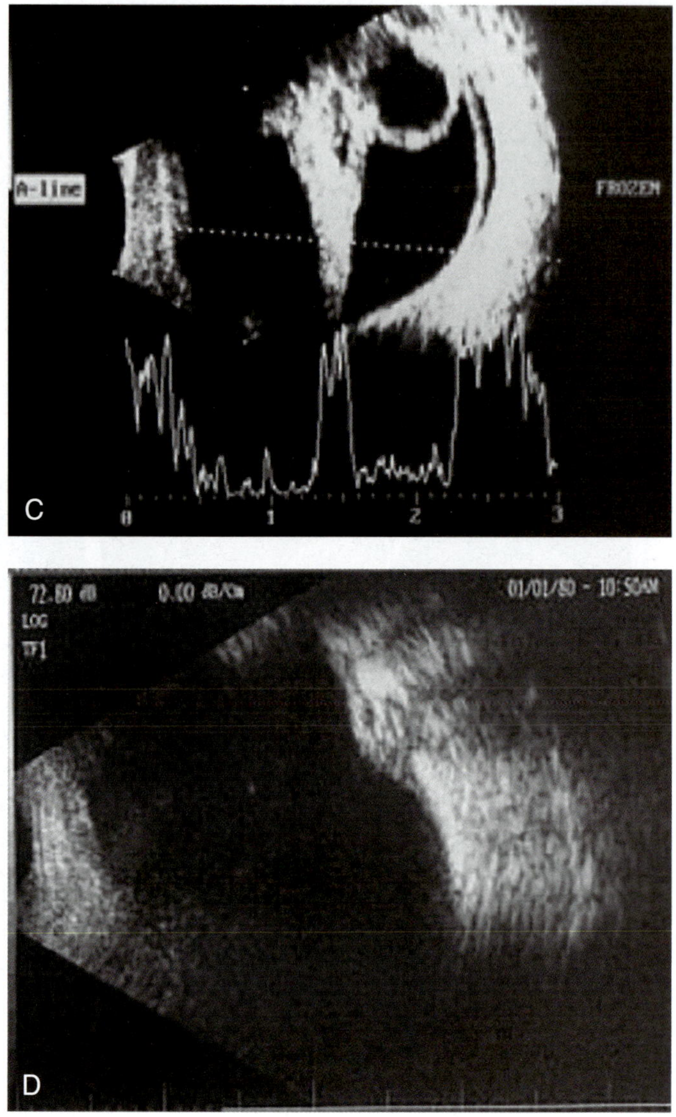

• **Fig. 16.5** Evaluation of the retina. **(A)** Retinal detachment in V-shape, observation of thickening of the retina and the ocular wall, subretinal debris. **(B)** Transverse peripheral scan at the retinal tear site. Observe the elevated retinal flaps with bending edges. **(C)** Total retinal detachment, V-shape with dense proliferative vitreoretinopathy and a peripheral loop. Sometimes, a choroidal detachment can be observed in chronic cases of retinal detachment. **(D)** After retinopexy, the peripheral scleral indentation can be noticed.

v) Diffuse scleritis
- Tenon's edema: low echogenicity interface, parallel to the thickened scleral wall, corresponding to edema of the Tenon's layer
- "T" sign: low echogenicity interface parallel to the wall, showing in the axial section in continuity with the optic nerve

vi) Solid lesions
- description: - topographic (location, extension, and shape)
- quantitative (reflectivity and internal structure)
- kinetics (internal vascularization)

2. Retrobulbar Space (Fig. 16.8)
   a) Optic nerve
      i) Description of the equipment gain and whether the approach is axial, longitudinal, or transverse
      ii) Describe the diameter, internal reflectivity, and structure characteristics (Table 16.2).
      iii) Comparison with the nerve of the contralateral eye[7,8]
   b) Extraocular muscles
      i) Description of equipment gain and whether the approach is longitudinal (evaluate tendon) or transverse (evaluate diameter)
      ii) Describe the diameter and internal reflectivity
      iii) Comparison with the contralateral muscles and with normal values (Table 16.3)[9]
   c) Retrobulbar fat
      i) Description of the equipment gain and whether the approach is transocular, or paraocular
      ii) Description of the reflectivity and density of the tissue [7]
      iii) In the presence of solid or cystic lesions, describe limits, topographic (location, extension, and shape), quantitative (reflectivity and internal structure), and kinetic (assess presence of liquid level) characteristics.

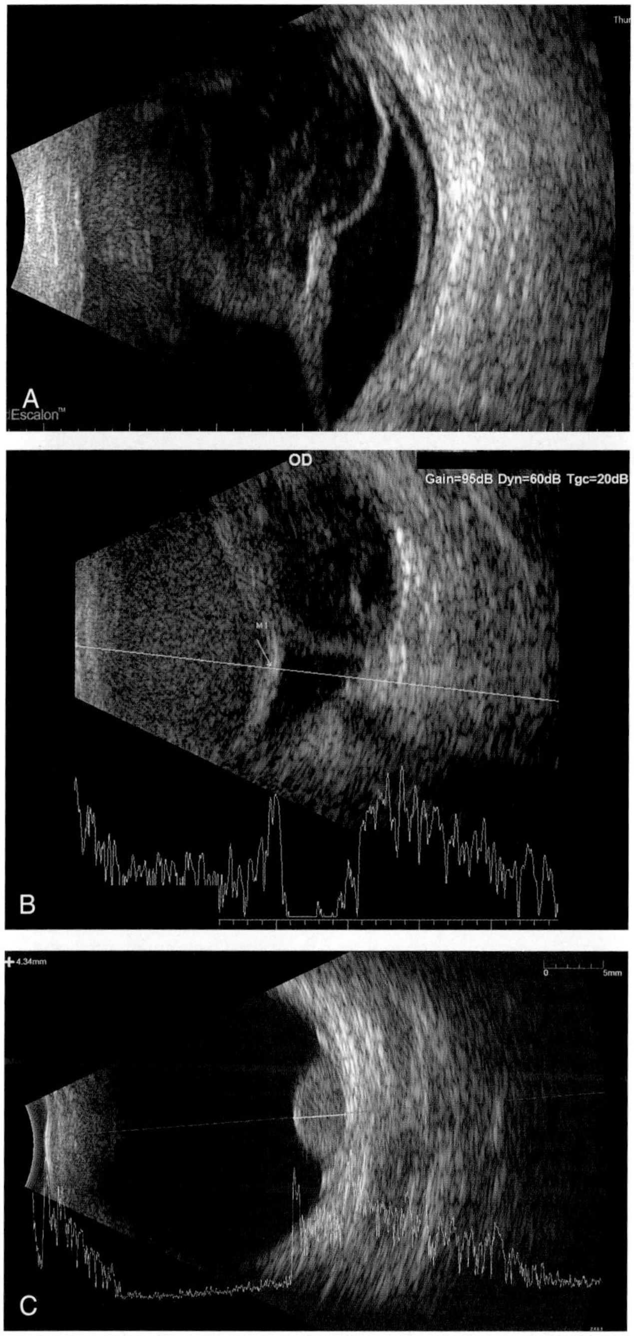

• **Fig. 16.6** Evaluation of the choroid. **(A)** A case of total retinal detachment presents shallow serous choroidal detachment. **(B)** Hemorrhagic choroidal detachment (punctiform interfaces) and choroids from each side of the globe touch at the center of the vitreous cavity (kissing choroidal). **(C)** Choroidal dome-shaped tumor characteristic of choroidal melanoma.

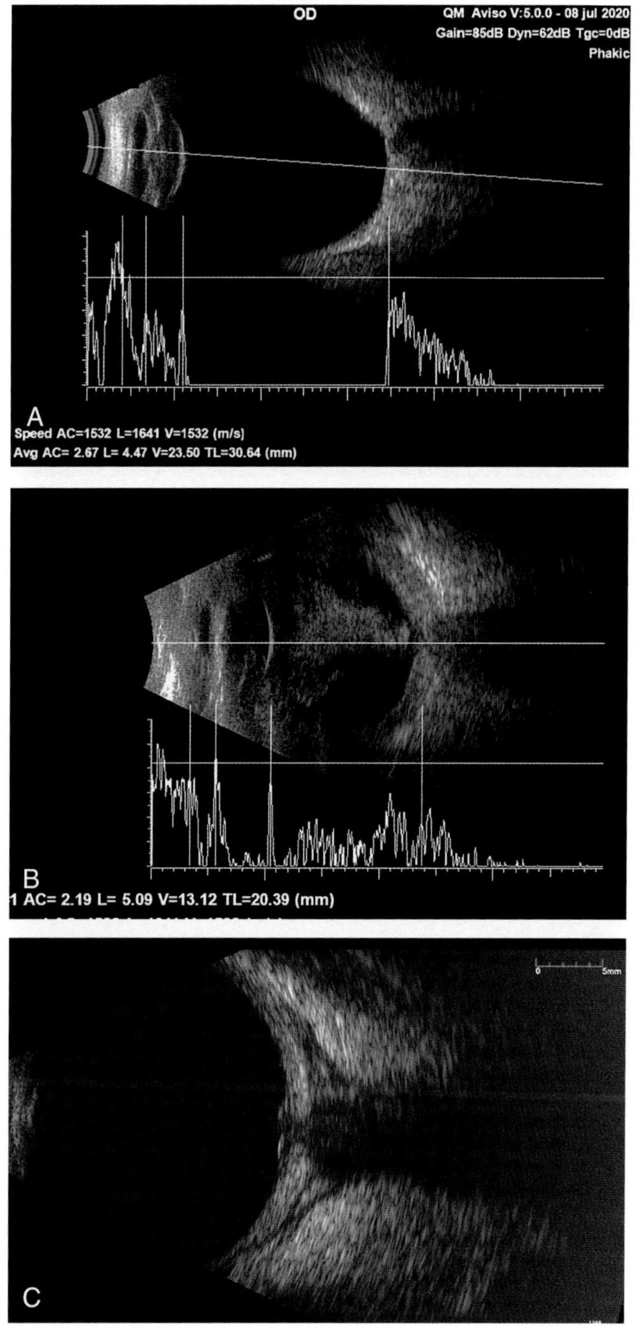

• **Fig 16.7** Evaluation of the sclera and the ocular wall. **(A)** High myopia, observing an elongated axial length, and excessive curvature. **(B)** High hyperopia, observing small axial length and ocular wall thickening. **(C)** Scleritis, noting fluid accumulation in the posterior episcleral space and around the optic nerve.

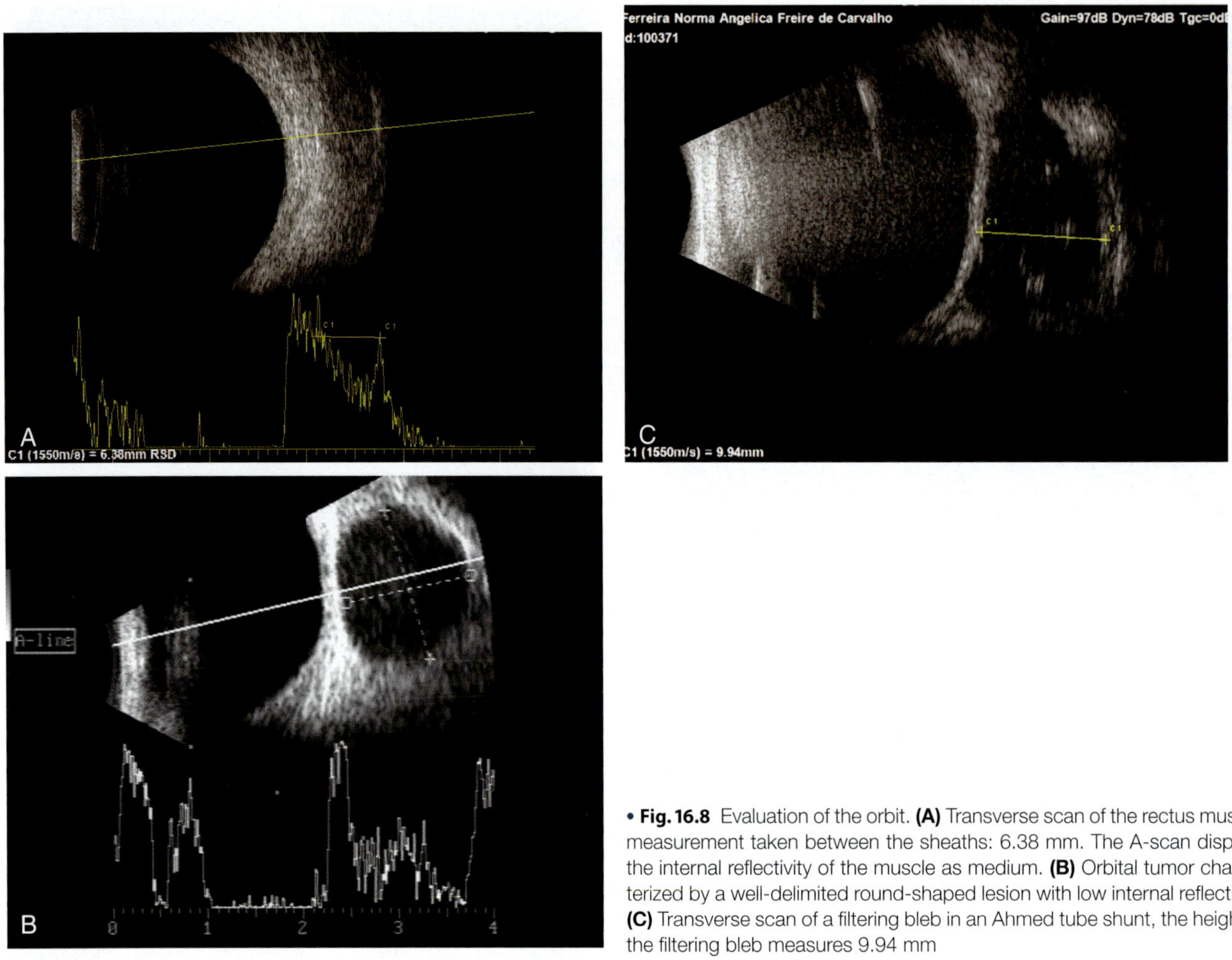

• **Fig. 16.8** Evaluation of the orbit. **(A)** Transverse scan of the rectus muscle, measurement taken between the sheaths: 6.38 mm. The A-scan displays the internal reflectivity of the muscle as medium. **(B)** Orbital tumor characterized by a well-delimited round-shaped lesion with low internal reflectivity. **(C)** Transverse scan of a filtering bleb in an Ahmed tube shunt, the height of the filtering bleb measures 9.94 mm

TABLE 16.2 Normal Reference Values for Optic Nerve Diameter Measured 3 mm From the Scleral Limit of the Optic Disc

Dura - dura mater	4.0 a 5.3 mm
Arachnoid – arachnoid	3.2 a 4.0 mm
Pia - pia mater	2.8 a 3.4 mm

Comparison With Previous Sonographic Exam

When reviewing current ultrasound features with previous exam, the presence or absence of changes should be clearly stated. In serial exams, the sonographer must assess for changes in appearance, shape, and dimensions in structures or lesions over time as well as measure the size of structures and lesion to quantify any change, especially in cases

TABLE 16.3 Indicates the Limits of 95% Confidence for Rectus Muscle Diameter, as the Difference of the Diameter of Correspondent Contralateral Muscles

Muscle	Normal Values (mm)	Difference Between Contralateral Muscles (mm)
Medial rectus	2.3–4.7	0.5
Lateral rectus	2.2–3.8	0.4
Superior rectus/levator complex	3.9–6.8	0.8
Inferior rectus	1.6–3.6	0.4
Sum of all muscles	11.9–6.9	1.2

of tumor surveillance. In addition, measuring the axial eye length is essential to monitor congenital glaucoma or globe atrophy progression.

Conclusions or Impressions

In the conclusions, clear and summarized information must be introduced from that cited in the body of the report. It should be avoided to give new information that is not found in the description of the ultrasound findings. The conclusion should be brief and aim to answer the clinical question.[1]

References

1. Necas M. The clinical ultrasound report: guideline for sonographers. *AJUM*. 2018;21(1):9–23.
2. Society and College of Radiographers and British Medical Ultrasound Society. Guidelines for Professional Ultrasound Practice. 2021. 190p. https://www.bmus.org/static/uploads/resources/2021_SoR_and_BMUS_guidelines_v1.0_.pdf.
3. Michael R. Hobson's choice: The new ACR Practice Guideline for Communication. *Appl Radiol.* 2012;19–20. doi: 10.37549/AR1878.
4. Hall FM. Language of the radiology report. *Am J Roentgenol.* 2000;175(5):1239–1242.
5. Byrne SF, Green LG. *Ultrasound of the Eye and Orbit.* 2nd ed. Mosby; 2010.
6. Byrne SF, Gendron EK, Glaser JS, Feuer W, Atta H. Diameter of normal extraocular recti muscles with echography. *Am J Ophthalmol.* 1991;112(6):706–713.
7. Cennamo G, Rosa N, La Rana A, Pastena B. Standardized A-scan echography and the normal optic nerve. Experience with the new Mini A equipment. *Acta Ophthalmol Suppl (1985).* 1992;204:87–89.
8. Edwards H, Smith J, Weston M. What makes a good ultrasound report? *Ultrasound.* 2014;22:57–60.
9. Sampaolesi R, Zarate J, Sampaolesi JR. *The Glaucomas: Volume 1 - Pediatric Glaucomas.* Springer Science & Business Media; 2008.

Index

Note: Page numbers followed by "*f*" indicate figures, "*t*" indicate tables, and "*b*" indicate boxes.